RIT - WALLACE LIBRARY
CIRCULATING LIBRARY BOOKS

OVERDUE FINES AND FEES FOR ALL BORROWERS

- Recalled = $1/ day overdue (no grace period)
- Billed = $10.00/ item when returned 4 or more weeks overdue
- Lost Items = replacement cost+$10 fee
- All materials must be returned or renewed by the duedate.

ANNALS OF
THE NEW YORK ACADEMY
OF SCIENCES

Volume 1050

EDITORIAL STAFF

Director, Publishing and New Media
SARAH GREENE

Managing Editor
JUSTINE CULLINAN

Associate Editor
STEFAN MALMOLI

The New York Academy of Sciences
2 East 63rd Street
New York, New York 10021

AUTOIMMUNITY

CONCEPTS AND DIAGNOSIS
AT THE CUTTING EDGE

ANNALS OF THE NEW YORK ACADEMY OF SCIENCES
Volume 1050

AUTOIMMUNITY

CONCEPTS AND DIAGNOSIS
AT THE CUTTING EDGE

Edited by M. Eric Gershwin and Yehuda Shoenfeld

The New York Academy of Sciences
New York, New York
2005

Library of Congress Cataloging-in-Publication Data

International Congress on Autoimmunity (4th: 2004: Budapest, Hungary)
    Autoimmunity: concepts and diagnosis at the cutting edge / edited by M. Eric Gershwin and Yehuda Shoenfeld.
        p.; cm. — (Annals of the New York Academy of Sciences; v. 1050)
    Includes bibliographical references and index.
    ISBN 1-57331-516-8 (cloth: alk. paper) — ISBN 1-57331-517-6 (pbk.: alk. paper)
    1. Autoimmunity—Congresses. 2. Autoimmune diseases—Congresses.
    [DNLM: 1. Autoimmunity—Congresses. 2. Autoimmune Diseases—diagnosis—Congresses.
QW 545 I61a 2005] I. Gershwin, M. Eric, 1946– II. Shoenfeld, Yehuda. III. Title. IV. Series.
    Q11.N5 vol. 1050
    [QR188.3]
    616.97′8—dc22

                                                                    2005012032

GYAT / PCP
Printed in the United States of America
ISBN 1-57331-516-8 (cloth)
ISBN 1-57331-517-6 (paper)
ISSN 0077-8923

ANNALS OF THE NEW YORK ACADEMY OF SCIENCES
Volume 1050
June 2005

AUTOIMMUNITY

CONCEPTS AND DIAGNOSIS AT THE CUTTING EDGE

Editors
M. ERIC GERSHWIN AND YEHUDA SHOENFELD

This volume comprises part of the proceedings of the **Fourth International Congress on Autoimmunity**, which was supported by the American Autoimmune Related Diseases Association (AARDA) and the Associazione Patologie Autoimmuni Internazionale (APAI), and held November 3–7, 2004, in Budapest, Hungary.

CONTENTS

Part II. Diagnostic Considerations of Autoimmunity

Part III. Infection and Autoimmunity

Foreword

On November 3–7, 2004, in Budapest, Hungary, at the Fourth International Congress on Autoimmunity, more than 1000 scientists from 50 countries met and discussed the state of the art/science in autoimmunity. It was a fitting occasion not only because incredible and exciting new discoveries were discussed, but also there were awards given for careers in excellence to Professors Donato Alarcon-Segovia, Ian Mackay, and Noel Rose.

In fact, the very first textbook on autoimmune diseases was written by Professor Mackay and his mentor, Professor Macfarlane Burnet, in 1963. In the preface to that textbook, only approximately 40 years ago, it was written that "one of the greatest developments in medicine during recent years has been the growing recognition of the importance of processes in which the immune mechanisms of the body are, as it were, turned against the body's own components." More importantly, the authors wrote: "This topic is in many ways in a prescientific phase. Many clinical scientists are skeptical of the reality of autoimmune processes...." We doubt that there are many people that remain skeptical and, in fact, it is estimated that nearly 1 in 31 Americans suffers from an autoimmune disease. There are also suggestions that the incidences of autoimmune diseases are increasing, although such increments may be more due to increased diagnosis and recognition. It is, however, crystal clear that the immune system plays a critical role not only in specific autoimmune pathology, but also as contributors to the pathology mediated by inflammation in many other diseases. The first real description of an autoimmune disease was that of hemolytic anemia, in which it was noted that antibody can lyse red blood cells, an observation in 1904 by Donath and Landsteiner. The use of adjuvants for an experimental induction of autoimmunity was noted in 1943, but it was really the demonstration of the rheumatoid factor in 1941, the Coombs' test in 1945, and the mother of all serologic tests, the LE cell prep in 1948, that augured the modern phase of autoimmunity and immunopathology. The number of recognized autoimmune diseases continues to increase—perhaps the best example being the phospholipid antibody syndrome, initially described in 1983. An enormous explosion in data has resulted from our knowledge of the major histocompatibility complex, the production of monoclonal antibodies, and the subsequent identification of distinct cell phenotypes and the resultant demonstration of an enormous battery of accessory and secondary molecules and messengers, including complement, cytokines, chemokines, and a host of cognate receptors. The list can go on and on.

The purpose of this volume is to include a cross section of the work presented at the Fourth International Congress on Autoimmunity. [Note that a companion volume of the *Annals* (Volume 1051) contains a further compendium of additional papers.] It does not include each and every paper presented. A number of papers that do not appear in this issue have appeared in *Autoimmunity Reviews* and in *Clinical and Developmental Immunology*. However, the work presented herein is considerably more broad and covers three main areas: general principles of autoimmunity; new

Ann. N.Y. Acad. Sci. 1050: ix–x (2005). © 2005 New York Academy of Sciences.
doi: 10.1196/annals.1313.130

discoveries in the diagnosis of autoimmunity; and infection and autoimmunity. The authors have been advised to be imaginative and to be as illustrative as possible so that their papers can be not only user-friendly, but also to have the potential for use as a teaching resource. We prefer that the papers be new and perhaps controversial, rather than just simply a review of the existing literature. The Fourth International Congress on Autoimmunity developed on the heels of three previous congresses and its success will lead to the Fifth International Congress in two years. Autoimmunity is certainly not the doubtful science that some had suggested at the time of Professor Mackay's 1963 textbook, and we note that Confucius was believed to have said that the light is always darkest on the other side of the lantern. The future is the brightest side of all and we all look forward to the improvements that will lead to better health for our patients.

—M. Eric Gershwin
—Yehuda Shoenfeld

Posttranslational Modifications of Self-Antigens

HESTER A. DOYLE AND MARK J. MAMULA

Section of Rheumatology, Department of Internal Medicine, Yale University School of Medicine, New Haven, Connecticut 06520, USA

ABSTRACT: Although the immune system has developed mechanisms to distinguish "self" from "non-self," the presence of autoimmune diseases demonstrates that these mechanisms can be bypassed. The posttranslational modification of self-antigens is one way in which "new" antigens are created for which immune tolerance does not exist. We review some of the posttranslationally modified self-antigens associated with autoimmune diseases, how they arise, and how they break immune tolerance.

KEYWORDS: posttranslational modifications; autoimmunity; T cells; antibody; antigen processing; MHC class II

INTRODUCTION

When one thinks of posttranslational modifications, events such as phosphorylation and glycosylation come to mind. These posttranslational modifications, as well as others, are frequently required for the proper functioning of numerous biological molecules; without them, processes such as cell signaling and DNA replication would not occur. However, modifications occur within proteins that are not to the benefit of the host organism. Such is the case with regard to the posttranslational modifications of self-proteins to which the immune system has not developed tolerance. These modifications can be the result of the addition of molecules to a protein, such as a phosphate molecule or a sugar moiety (TABLE 1). They also can be the result of a conversion of an amino acid to a distinct structure, as in the deimination of arginine to citrulline or the deamidation of aspartic acid/asparagine to isoaspartic acid (TABLE 1).

All 20 primary amino acids are capable of undergoing some type of posttranslational modification. However, certain factors determine whether those modifications will take place. First, the location of the amino acid within the protein sequence affects both the type and frequency of modifications that may arise. Flanking residues can influence the conformation of the protein, potentially altering whether an enzyme has access to a certain amino acid or is exposed to a certain environment. The cellular location of the modifying enzyme, if required, will determine whether the modifica-

Address for correspondence: Hester A. Doyle, Ph.D., Section of Rheumatology, Yale University School of Medicine, P.O. Box 208031, New Haven, CT 06520–8031. Voice: 203-737-6052; fax: 203-785-7053.

hester.doyle@yale.edu

Ann. N.Y. Acad. Sci. 1050: 1–9 (2005). © 2005 New York Academy of Sciences.
doi: 10.1196/annals.1313.001

TABLE 1. Common posttranslational modifications

Modification	Amino acids altered
Additions	
Acetylation	Lysine, serine
Glycosylation	Asparagine, serine
Hydroxylation	Proline, lysine
Methylation	Arginine, histidine, lysine
Phosphorylation	Serine, threonine, tyrosine
Conversions	
Deamidation/Isoaspartylation	Aspartic acid, asparagine
Citrullination/Deimination	Arginine

tion occurs at all. Finally, previous modifications or proteolytic cleavages within a protein influence subsequent amino acid modifications within the same protein.[1]

AUTOIMMUNE RESPONSES TO MODIFIED SELF-ANTIGENS

The immune system has evolved the ability to discriminate between self and non-self. Lymphocytes that react strongly to self-antigens in the thymus and bone marrow are deleted. Although a wide variety of peripheral self-antigens are expressed in the thymus, the posttranslational modification of any self-antigen in the periphery may not be represented in the thymus.[2] Thus, a "new" self-antigen arises for which there is no immune tolerance. TABLE 2 lists some of the autoimmune diseases in which modified self-antigens are known to influence autoimmune responses or tissue pathology.

Of the organ-specific autoimmune diseases, rheumatoid arthritis and multiple sclerosis have been noted to have several self-antigens that undergo posttranslational modifications.[3–6] Citrullination (the enzymatic deimination of arginine to citrulline) received much attention after it was discovered that rheumatoid arthritis patients have autoantibodies specific for citrullinated fillagrin (an epidermal protein) but not to the noncitrullinated form.[7] Although fillagrin is not found in the synovium, autoantibodies against other citrullinated proteins (such as fibrin and vimentin) have been detected in the synovium of rheumatoid arthritis patients, suggesting that these autoantibodies contribute to disease pathogenesis.[3] In addition to citrulline, type II collagen undergoes several posttranslational modifications, namely hydroxylation of proline and lysine and glycosylation of hydroxylyines.[4,8] In murine collagen-induced arthritis (a model for rheumatoid arthritis), T-cell hybridomas derived from mice immunized with type II collagen recognize type II collagen (256–270). Post-translational modifications, especially glycosylation of a single lysine residue at position 264, gave rise to 5 different T-cell determinants.[4] Interestingly, the degree to which collagen is hydroxylated or glycosylated influences the incidence and severity of disease.[8] Mice immunized with type II collagen produced in a yeast expression system (hydroxylated prolines, unhydroxylated lysines, and no glycosyla-

TABLE 2. Autoimmune diseases and their associated posttranslational modifications

Disease	Modifications	Antigens modified
Multiple sclerosis/EAE	Phosphorylation	αB-crystallin
	Citrullination	MBP
	Acetylation	MBP
Collagen-induced arthritis	Glycosylation	Type II collagen
	Hydroxylation	
Rheumatoid arthritis	Citrullination	Fillagrin
		Fibrin
		Vimentin
SLE	Phosphorylation	Multiple
	Deamidation	snRNP D, H2B
	Mannose modification	Multiple
	Methylation	Sm D1, D3

tion) or a baculovirus expression system (hydroxylated prolines, underhydroxylated lysines, underglycosylated) failed to induce arthritis to the same degree, or with the same incidence, as tissue-derived type II collagen.

Citrulline-modified residues also have been detected in myelin basic protein (MBP), a common autoantigen in multiple sclerosis. One isoform of MBP, designated MBP-C8, has 6 of the 19 arginyl residues citrullinated and is increased in the brain tissue of multiple sclerosis patients.[9] T-cell lines specific for citrullinated MBP-C8 are able to induce experimental allergic encephalomyelitis (EAE) (the murine model of multiple sclerosis) when injected into rats.[5] In humans, CD4[+] T-cell lines from both multiple sclerosis patients and healthy control subjects recognized MBP-C8.[10] However, multiple sclerosis patients had either more T-cell lines that responded to MBP-C8, T cells that responded with greater sensitivity to MBP-C8, or both compared with healthy control subjects.[11] In EAE, reactivity is directed toward the myelin basic protein (MBP Ac1–11) that requires acetyl modifications at its N-terminus. Encephalogenic T-cell clones of MBP Ac1–11 induce EAE, although the nonacetylated form fails to stimulate T cells or to induce disease.[6]

Systemic autoimmune diseases, such as systemic lupus erythematosus (SLE), also have immune responses directed toward posttranslationally modified self-antigens. For example, the spontaneous conversion of an asparagine residue or an aspartic acid residue to an isoaspartyl residue renders cytochrome c and snRNP D peptides immunogenic in murine models of SLE autoimmunity.[12] Mice develop T-cell responses to the isoaspartic acid peptides but not the native aspartic acid peptides. However, mice also develop autoantibodies that recognize both the isoaspartic peptides and the native aspartic acid peptides. These autoantibodies can diversify to recognize other antigens such as dsDNA. In addition, isoaspartic acid residues have been found in histone H2B, a common autoantigen in spontaneous and drug-induced lupus.[13] Finally, patients with SLE have been shown to have autoantibodies that react to the C-terminus of snRNP, which contains symmetrical dimethyl arginines[14] as well as phosphorylated serine/arginine-rich residues of the SR protein (a family of pre-mRNA splicing factors). Interestingly, some autoantibodies were directed at dephosphorylated SR proteins that normally would exist in a phosphorylated state.[15]

Several interesting points can be gleaned about the immune response to posttranslationally modified self-antigens. In general, T-cell responses to these modified antigens tend to be specific for the modified form of self-antigen and do not recognize the unmodified form, as is the case with citrullinated MBP, isoaspartic cyt c, and snRNP D. Further evidence of T-cell specificity for modified antigens comes from a recent study in which TCR contact residues of guinea pig MBP (72–85) were either glycosylated or citrullinated. T cells specific for the wild-type peptide did not recognize the modified MBP (72–85) peptides. Conversely, T cells specific for the modified peptides did not recognize the wild-type MBP (72–85).[16] This study also suggests that T-cell recognition with regard to glycosylated amino acids was dependent on both the sugar residue and the amino acid side chain.

In contrast to T-cell responses, B-cell responses to posttranslationally modified self-antigens tend to be more diverse in that antibodies recognize not only the modified but also the native self-antigen. For example, the antibody response in mice immunized with isoaspartic snRNP D peptides is directed at both the isoaspartic and native (aspartic) forms of snRNP D.[12] Furthermore, sera from these mice also react to other lupus autoantigens after breaking immune tolerance to the modified self-antigen.[12] This reaction suggests that the posttranslational modification of a particular self-antigen promotes epitope spreading, a phenomenon known to occur in virtually all autoimmune diseases, including diabetes,[17] lupus,[18] and multiple sclerosis.[19]

HOW POSTTRANSLATIONAL EVENTS OCCUR

Posttranslational modifications occur during many normal cellular events, such as aging. Isoaspartic acid formation occurs spontaneously under physiological conditions and increases as proteins age. Isoaspartic acids are known to accumulate in proteins with relatively long half-lives, perhaps as a marker for protein degradation.[20] αB-Crystallin, a major lens protein with a long half-life, is another protein that accumulates isoaspartic residues and undergoes phosphorylation with age.[21,22] Cell proliferation, as occurs with mitogen stimulation, can even increase the amount of isoaspartic residues within T and B cells.[12]

Cellular stress, such as infection, trauma, or apoptosis, also induces many posttranslational modifications. For example, proteins in apoptotic cells can undergo phosphorylation,[23] ubiquination,[24] transglutamination,[25] citrullination,[26] and oxidation.[27] Intracellular proteins are phosphorylated as a result of caspase activation and subsequent cleavage of intracellular kinases. Although the structural integrity of the cell is maintained during apoptosis, studies have shown that certain phosphorylated proteins clinically associated with SLE are found on the surface of cells within apoptotic blebs.[28] SLE patient sera immunoprecipitates phosphorylated proteins from apoptotic cells.[29] Antiphospholipid antibodies, associated with antiphospholipid syndrome and SLE, also recognize apoptotic cells.[30,31] Oxidized low-density lipoproteins have been found on apoptotic cells, and mice immunized with apoptotic cells develop high titers of autoantibodies to various oxidized epitopes, whereas mice immunized with viable or necrotic cells do not.[32] These data indicate that the posttranslationally modified self-antigens found on apoptotic cells are "new" antigens capable of eliciting an immune response.

MECHANISMS BEHIND THE BREAKDOWN OF TOLERANCE TO MODIFIED SELF-ANTIGENS

The most obvious way in which posttranslational modifications could break immune tolerance is that the modified self-antigen is not represented in the thymus, and therefore reactive T cells escape tolerance and migrate into the periphery. However, a second mechanism may be that antigen processing of proteins and peptides containing posttranslational modifications is different than for the unmodified counterparts. In support of this second mechanism, citrullinated MBP is digested at a greater rate by cathepsin D—an aspartic protease involved in major histocompatibility complex (MHC) class II antigen processing—than MBP lacking citrulline residues.[33] The β-peptide linkage connecting an isoaspartic acid residue and its C-terminus neighbor are not recognized by most proteases and peptidases.[34] These observations suggest that the modified amino acid alters which epitopes are or are not generated during antigen processing. This concept is further supported by recent studies of the protease asparagine endopeptidase (AEP). Individuals with multiple sclerosis expressing HLA-DR2 have T cells that recognize the dominant epitope MBP (84–102). The asparagine at position 94 of MPB (84–102) is cleaved on its C-terminus by AEP. Using IL-2 production by a T-cell hybridoma specific for MBP (85–99) (the minimal immunogenic epitope) as a readout, high AEP activity resulted in decreased IL-2 production because of a decrease in the amount of MBP (85–99) generated from the full-length protein. Conversely, when AEP activity was low, the amount of MBP (85–99) generated increased, and T-cell stimulation was enhanced. These investigators suggested that because AEP is expressed in the thymus, MBP (85–99) is destroyed in the thymus, and thus autoreactive T cells escaped into the periphery.[35] Furthermore, an interesting speculation to this process is that asparagine residues are susceptible to deamidation, which results in the formation of aspartic acid or isoaspartic acid within the protein. Currently it is unclear whether AEP would be able to cleave after asparagine residues if they were posttranslationally modified. If AEP could not cleave an isoaspartic acid residue, then presumably antigens such as MBP (82–104) would be generated, especially in the periphery. FIGURE 1 illustrates how an alteration in the ability of a posttranslationally modified self-antigen to be enzymatically processed properly could result in a new epitope being generated for which no immune tolerance exists.

After antigen processing takes place, the next potential step affected by posttranslational modifications is the binding of the epitope to MHC class II molecules. There appears to be no clear-cut answer as to how posttranslational modifications affect MHC binding. Depending on the type of posttranslational modification, the affinity of the modified peptide for a MHC molecule can vary. Competition assays using MHC class II molecules demonstrated that different posttranslational modifications of MBP (72–85) resulted in either a low, an intermediate, or a similar affinity for MHC compared with the wild-type peptide.[16] We have demonstrated that isoaspartic acid residues in cytochrome c or snRNP D peptides bind MHC class II just as well as the unmodified peptides.[12] In another study, phosphorylation of αB-crystallin at

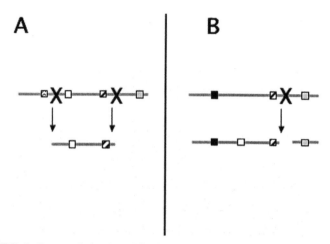

FIGURE 1. Posttranslational modification of self-antigens can alter antigen processing. In the native form of a self-protein, there are specific cleavage sites (represented by ✕) for proteases that form distinct peptides **(A)**. When an amino acid within this self-protein is posttranslationally modified (represented by ■), proteases may not be able to cleave after these modified amino acids, resulting in a new peptide for which no tolerance exists **(B)**. This is one way in which posttranslationally modified self-proteins become immunogenic.

Ser 45 did not prevent binding to murine MHC class II molecules. In fact, computer-assisted modeling suggested that the phosphate group pointed out of the MHC-peptide binding cleft where it was likely to have direct contact with the TCR.[22] In contrast to these studies, citrullinated peptides of vimentin, a rheumatoid arthritis autoantigen, have a greater affinity for HLA-DRB1*0401 than the unmodified peptide does.[36] Because the conversion of arginine to citrulline results in the loss of positive charges, the alteration of the net charge of the molecule could alter MHC binding. All of these examples illustrate that individual modifications in the context of a particular self-antigen may have varying effects on MHC class II binding.

FUTURE IMPACT OF POSTTRANSLATIONALLY MODIFIED SELF-ANTIGENS ON AUTOIMMUNE DISEASE

In the postgenomic age, the impact of posttranslationally modified self-antigens on autoimmune responses and autoimmunity is beginning to be appreciated. Although the relevance of each modification in the context of a particular self-antigen will have to be determined, there is evidence that modified self-antigens play an important role in not only disease pathogenesis but also diagnostics. The presence of autoantibodies against citrullinated fillagrin has been exploited to develop more sensitive assays for rheumatoid arthritis. These autoantibodies are highly diagnostic for rheumatoid arthritis and can be detected early in disease.[37] Second-generation cyclic citrullinated fillagrin-derived peptides (CCP2) have improved the sensitivity (80%) as well as the specificity (98%) of citrullinated peptides as a diagnostic marker for rheumatoid arthritis.[38]

Immunotherapy for autoimmune diseases is another area in which posttranslationally modified self-antigens may be useful. N-Palmitoylated proteolipid protein (PLP) peptides (a palmitic acid side chain attached to the N terminus via the amide group) completely suppress or reduce acute and chronic relapsing EAE in SJL mice.[39] This suppression is in contrast to the S-palmitoylated PLP peptides (a palmitic acid side chain attached via a thioester linkage) that are immunogenic.[40] A phosphorylated synthetic peptide of the 70K snRNP protein when administered to the lupus-prone mouse strain MRL/lpr decreased certain disease symptoms such as proteinuria and anti-DNA antibodies while prolonging the survival of the mice.[41] These studies suggest that modified antigens potentially act as antagonists and may offer some benefit as therapeutic agents.

CONCLUSIONS

The posttranslational modification of self-antigens in autoimmune diseases represents one way in which immune tolerance is bypassed and may even represent an initiating factor for disease. Autoimmune responses to modified self-antigens will have to be evaluated on an individual basis to determine if and how they contribute to disease pathogenesis. As is the case with several modified self-antigens, autoimmune responses may prove useful not only in determining pathogenesis but also in diagnosing and even treating autoimmune diseases.

REFERENCES

1. WOLD, F. 1981. *In vivo* chemical modification of proteins (post-translational modification). Annu. Rev. Biochem. **50:** 783–814.
2. DERBINSKI, J. *et al.* 2001. Promiscuous gene expression in medullary thymic epithelial cells mirrors the peripheral self. Nat. Immunol. **2:** 1032–1039.
3. MASSON-BESSIERE, C. *et al.* 2001. The major synovial targets of the rheumatoid arthritis-specific antifilaggrin autoantibodies are deiminated forms of the α- and β- chains of fibrin. J. Immunol. **166:** 4177–4184.
4. CORTHAY, A. *et al.* 1998. Epitope glycosylation plays a critical role for T cell recognition of type II collagen in collagen-induced arthritis. Eur. J. Immunol. **28:** 2580–2590.
5. CAO, L., D. SUN & J.N. WHITAKER. 1998. Citrullinated myelin basic protein induces experimental autoimmune encephalomyelitis in Lewis rats through a diverse T cell repertoire. J. Neuroimmunol. **88:** 21–29.
6. ZAMVIL, S.S. *et al.* 1986. T-cell epitope of the autoantigen myelin basic protein that induces encephalomyelitis. Nature **324:** 258–260.
7. GIRBAL-NEUHAUSER, E. *et al.* 1999. The epitopes targeted by the rheumatoid arthritis-associated antifilaggrin autoantibodies are posttranslationally generated on various sites of (pro)filaggrin by deimination of arginine residues. J. Immunol. **162:** 585–594.
8. MYERS, L.K. *et al.* 2004. Relevance of posttranslational modifications for the arthritogenicity of type II collagen. J. Immunol. **172:** 2970–2975.
9. MOSCARELLA, M.A. *et al.* 1994. Myelin in multiple sclerosis is developmentally immature. J. Clin. Invest. **94:** 146–154.
10. MARTIN, R. *et al.* 1994. Citrulline-containing myelin basic protein is recognized by T-cell lines derived from multiple sclerosis patients and healthy individuals. Neurology **44:** 123–129.
11. TRANQUIL, L.R. *et al.* 2000. Enhanced T cell responsiveness to citrulline-containing myelin basic protein in multiple sclerosis patients. Mult. Scler. **6:** 220–225.
12. MAMULA, M.J. *et al.* 1999. Isoaspartyl post-translational modification triggers autoimmune responses to self-proteins. J. Biol. Chem. **274:** 22321–22327.

13. YOUNG, A.L. *et al.* 2001. Structural integrity of histone H2B *in vivo* requires the activity of protein L-isoaspartate O-methyltransferase, a putitive protein repair enzyme. J. Biol. Chem. **276:** 37161–37165.

14. BRAHMS, H. *et al.* 2000. The C-terminal RG dipeptide repeats of the spliceosomal Sm proteins D1 and D3 contain symmetrical dimethylarginines, which form a major B-cell epitope for anti-Sm autoantibodies. J. Biol. Chem. **275:** 17122–17129.

15. NEUGEBAUER, K.M. *et al.* 2000. SR proteins are autoantigens in patients with systemic lupus erythematosus: importance of phosphoepitopes. Arthritis Rheum. **43:** 1768–1778.

16. HAAN, E.C. *et al.* 2005. Limited plasticity in T cell recognition of modified T cell receptor contact residues in MHC class II bound peptides. Mol. Immunol. **42:** 355–364.

17. OTT, P.A. *et al.* 2004. T cells recognize multiple GAD65 and proinsulin epitopes in human type 1 diabetes, suggesting determinant spreading. J. Clin. Immunol. **24:** 327–339.

18. MONNEAUX, F. & S. MULLER. 2002. Epitope spreading in systemic lupus erythematosus: identification of triggering peptide sequences. Arthritis Rheum. **46:** 1430–1438.

19. LEHMANN, P.V. *et al.* 1992. Spreading of T cell autoimmunity to cryptic determinants of an autoantigen. Nature (Lond.) **358:** 155–157.

20. TARCSA, E. *et al.* 2000. Ca^{2+}-free calmodulin and calmodulin damaged by *in vitro* aging are selectively degraded by 26 S proteasome without ubiquitination. J. Biol. Chem. **275:** 20295–20301.

21. TAKEMOTO, L.J. 1995. Degradation of aspartyl and asparaginyl residues of lens proteins *in vivo*. *In* Deamidation and Isoaspartate Formation in Peptides and Proteins. D.W. Aswad, Ed.: 157–165. CRC Press. Boca Raton, FL.

22. VAN STIPDONK, M.J.B. *et al.* 1998. T cells discriminate between differentially phosphorylated forms of B-crystallin, a major central nervous system myelin antigen. Int. Immunol. **10:** 943–950.

23. RATHMELL, J.C. & C.B. THOMPSON. 1999. The central effectors of cell death in the immune system. Annu. Rev. Immunol. **17:** 781–828.

24. HERSHKO, A. & A. CIECHANOVER. 1998. The ubiquitin system. Annu. Rev. Biochem. **67:** 425–479.

25. PIACENTINI, M. & V. COLIZZI. 1999. Tissue transglutaminase: apoptosis versus auto-immunity. Immunol. Today **20:** 130–134.

26. ASAGA, H., M. YAMADA & T. SENSHU. 1998. Selective deimination of vimentin in calcium ionophore-induced apoptosis of mouse peritoneal macrophages. Biochem. Biophys. Res. Commun. **243:** 641–646.

27. KADL, A. *et al.* 2004. Apoptotic cells as sources for biologically active oxidized phospholipids. Antioxid. Redox. Signal. **6:** 311–20.

28. CASCIOLA-ROSEN, L.A., G. ANHALT & A. ROSEN. 1994. Autoantigens targeted in systemic lupus erythematosus are clustered in two populations of surface structures on apoptotic keratinocytes. J. Exp. Med. **179:** 1317–1330.

29. UTZ, P.J. *et al.* 1997. Proteins phosphorylated during stress-induced apoptosis are common targets for autoantibody production in patients with systemic lupus erythematosus. J. Exp. Med. **185:** 843–854.

30. PRICE, B.E. *et al.* 1996. Anti-phospholipid autoantibodies bind to apoptotic, but not viable, thymocytes in a beta 2-mglycoprotein I-dependent manner. J. Immunol. **157:** 2201–2208.

31. LEVINE, J.S. *et al.* 1999. Apoptotic cells as immunogen and antigen in the antiphospholipid syndrome. Exp. Mol. Pathol. **66:** 82–98.

32. CHANG, M. *et al.* 2004. Apoptotic cells with oxidation-specific epitopes are immunogenic and proinflammatory. J. Exp. Med. **200:** 1359–1370.

33. PRITZKER, L.B. *et al.* 2000. Deimination of myelin basic protein. 1. Effect of deimination of arginyl residues of myelin basic protein on its structure and susceptibility to digestion by cathepsin D. Biochemistry **39:** 5374–5381.

34. JOHNSON, B.A. & D.W. ASWAD. 1990. Fragmentation of isoaspartyl peptides and proteins by carboxypeptidase Y: release of isoaspartyl dipeptides as a result of internal and external cleavage. Biochemistry **29:** 4373–4380.

35. MANOURY, B. *et al.* 2002. Destructive processing by asparagine endopeptidase limits presentation of a dominant T cell epitope in MBP. Nat. Immunol. **3:** 169–174.

36. HILL, J.A. *et al.* 2003. Cutting edge: the conversion of arginine to citrulline allows for a high-affinity peptide interaction with the rheumatoid arthritis-associated HLA-DRB1*0401 MHC class II molecule. J. Immunol. **171:** 538–541.
37. NIJENHUIS, S. *et al.* 2004. Autoantibodies to citrullinated proteins in rheumatoid arthritis: clinical performance and biochemical aspects of an RA-specific marker. Clin. Chim. Acta **350:** 17–34.
38. ZENDMAN, A.J., E.R. VOSSENAAR & W.J. VAN VENROOIJ. 2004. Autoantibodies to citrullinated (poly)peptides: a key diagnostic and prognostic marker for rheumatoid arthritis. Autoimmunity **37:** 295–299.
39. LOUIS, J.S. *et al.* 2001. Tolerance induction by acylated peptides: suppression of EAE in the mouse with palmitoylated PLP peptides. J. Neuroimmunol. **115:** 79–90.
40. GREER, J.M. *et al.* 2001. Thiopalmitoylation of myelin proteolipid protein epitopes enhances immunogenicity and encephalitogenicity. J. Immunol. **166:** 6907–6913.
41. MONNEAUX, F. *et al.* 2003. T cell recognition and therapeutic effect of a phosphorylated synthetic peptide of the 70K snRNP protein administered in MR/lpr mice. Eur. J. Immunol. **33:** 287–296.

Expression and Reexpression of Recombination Activating Genes

Relevance to the Development of Autoimmune States

SOPHIE HILLION, CAROLINE ROCHAS, PIERRE YOUINOU, AND CHRISTOPHE JAMIN

Laboratory of Immunology, Brest University, Medical School, Brest, France

ABSTRACT: Like all antibodies, autoreactive antibodies are generated in developing B cells in the bone marrow by variable (V), diversity (D), and joining (J) recombination under the regulation of recombination activating gene (RAG) 1 and RAG2 proteins. Deletion, anergy, and receptor edition prevent the emergence of autoreactive B cells. In the periphery, somatic hypermutation during the course of germinal center responses can lead to the emergence of autoreactive and low-affinity antibody-producing B cells. Deletion and receptor revision regulate autoreactive and inappropriate B cells. Defects in central or peripheral tolerance mechanisms associated with RAG expression could contribute to the appearance of autoreactive B cells. We demonstrate the presence of RAG+ B cells in CD5-expressing cells outside germinal centers. Our data suggest that receptor revision in the periphery also may occur in unusual sites when B cells are induced to express CD5. This revision may correspond to a novel regulation checkpoint in which impaired control of RAG expression could generate autoreactive B cells and lead to autoimmune states.

KEYWORDS: RAG; B cells; autoimmunity

RECEPTOR EDITING IN TOLERANCE ACQUISITION

During B-cell genesis, recombination of variable (V), diversity (D), and joining (J) immunoglobulin (Ig) genes ensures repertoire diversity, that is, the development of efficient responses to a universe of potential pathogens. Recombination activating gene (RAG) 1 and RAG2 proteins are involved in the Ig gene rearrangement. They bind to and cleave DNA at recombination signal sequences (RSS) that flank Ig gene segments.[1] Two waves of high RAG expression can thus be observed in developing B cells. The first initiates the recombination of Ig heavy (H) chain genes, and the second appears for the assembly of Ig light (L) chain genes (FIG. 1). Because Ig genes are randomly selected, autoreactive antibodies may be produced in the bone

Address for correspondence: Professor Pierre Youinou, Laboratory of Immunology, Brest University Medical School Hospital, BP824, F29609 Brest, France. Voice: +(33)-2-98-22-33-84; fax: +(33)-2-98-22-38-47.

youinou@univ-brest.fr

Ann. N.Y. Acad. Sci. 1050: 10–18 (2005). © 2005 New York Academy of Sciences.
doi: 10.1196/annals.1313.002

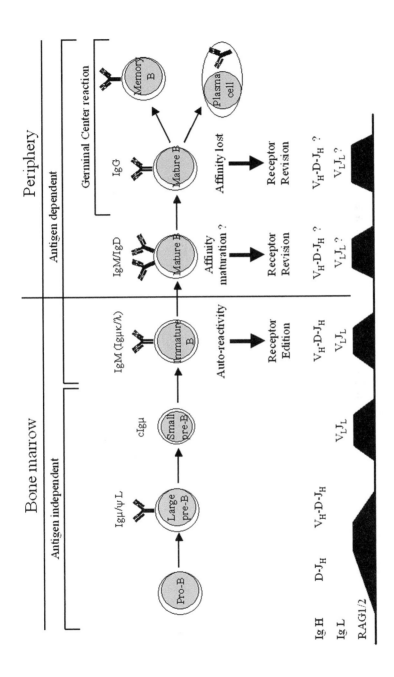

FIGURE 1. Schematic representation of B cell development. Stages of B-cell development, status of the immunoglobulin heavy (IgH) and light (IgL) chain gene rearrangements, and intensity of RAG1 and RAG2 expression are shown. Receptor edition in the bone marrow and receptor revision in the periphery are indicated.

marrow. Three mechanisms that regulate autoreactivity when cells are stimulated with antigens have been documented. Thus, deletion through apoptosis,[2] tolerance through anergy,[3] and receptor editing[4] prevent the emergence of self-reactive antibodies (Abs). Only 10 to 20% of immature B cells in the bone marrow reach the periphery, and 3% contribute to the mature B-cell pool,[5] indicating the importance of these mechanisms in restricting the development of autoreactive cells. Further, one-fourth of all Abs in the human immature B cell compartment produced self-reactive Abs.[6] This observation highlights that defects in 1 or several of these process of tolerance mechanisms could contribute to the development of autoimmunity.

As shown in FIGURE 1, a third wave of RAG expression can appear in developing cells when an autoreactive B-cell receptor (BCR) emerges. This relates mainly to the editing of Ig L chain genes in B cells that escape deletion. Using autoAb (H + L) transgenic (Tg) mice, it was demonstrated that escaped cells in normal mice always bear the Tg H chain but in association with an endogenous L chain after Ig L gene edition, resulting in the loss of self-reactivity.[7] Although 47% of λ^+ cells have evidence for κ rearrangement in normal mice,[8] almost all λ^+ cells carry previous genes rearranged in humans.[9] Overall, 25% of the normal repertoire result from secondary rearrangements, suggesting that receptor editing plays an important role in the formulation of the normal Ab repertoire. Furthermore, gene editing of autoAb–producing B cells also may involve the H chain.[10] This has been reported to be caused by the presence of cryptic RSS embedded in the coding region of the V_H genes.[11,12] Because 5–12% of the human Ab repertoire is produced by V_H replacement, receptor editing of the V_H chain may be an essential event. It is pertinent to reflect on the processes that trigger deletion, anergization, or receptor edition of autoreactive B cells in the bone marrow. Again, Tg mouse models have helped to clarify this crucial point, suggesting that the choice of tolerance mechanisms in B cells depends on BCR affinity for autoantigens. Thus, a high degree of BCR cross-linking promotes deletion by apoptosis, whereas a low degree of cross-linking triggers anergy. Noteworthy in this respect is that an intermediate level of BCR cross-linking triggers persistent expression of RAG that could induce receptor editing. Indeed, because of low BCR levels, self-reactive B cells might sustain RAG1 and RAG2 expression until they produce a non–self-reactive receptor. Cells that fail to undergo successful editing would die by apoptosis.

RECEPTOR EDITING IN THE DEVELOPMENT OF AUTOIMMUNITY

Receptor editing appears to be a powerful mechanism for inducing and maintaining tolerance. Consequently, defects in Ig gene edition or aberrant RAG protein expression could have a profound impact on the development of an autoimmune repertoire. It has thus been shown that, in some circumstances, defects in receptor editing permit the emergence of autoreactivity. This was especially evident in systemic lupus erythematosus (SLE), where some reexpression of second L chain without editing the first V region favored the development of autoreactive B cells.[13] Further, an increased frequency of abnormal D-D junction with secondary rearrangement of Ig H chain genes in lupus-prone MRL mouse has been observed.[14] These aberrant recombinations might thus contribute to the appearance of autoimmunity.

RECEPTOR REVISION DURING POSITIVE SELECTION

Maturation of B cells is associated with decreased RAG expression together with an increase in the level of BCR expression. This leads us to suggest that B cells with a non–self-reactive BCR will turn off their V(D)J recombination. Therefore, secondary RAG expression was initially thought to be restricted to the bone marrow and to immature B cells. However, RAG proteins have been detected in *in vitro* activated mature B cells.[15] Further, RAG expression also was observed in mature germinal center B cells.[16] Although some investigators thought this was caused by the migration of immature transitional type 2 B cells to the spleen,[17] others have demonstrated the presence of mature RAG+ cells in human tonsil tissues.[18] In line with these observations, several reports provide compelling evidence that a peripheral V(D)J recombination may occur at the level of centrocyte development, after somatic hypermutation.[19] Thus, a fourth wave of RAG expression could be identified in germinal centers that contributes to receptor revision (FIG. 1). This secondary peripheral Ig gene recombination would result in the generation of high-affinity Abs for efficient immune responses.[20] Although high-affinity BCR is positively selected, thus ending B-cell differentiation, low-affinity and self-reactive BCR are eliminated by apoptosis. We suggest that intermediate signals could maintain or induce RAG1 and RAG2 expression to obtain higher BCR affinity.

RECEPTOR REVISION AND AUTOIMMUNE DISEASES

It is intriguing to note that a high frequency of RAG+ B cells was observed in the peripheral repertoire in autoimmune individuals. This was the case in patients with SLE in which single-cell RT-PCR analysis revealed that 8% of peripheral blood B cells expressed RAG1 and RAG2 mRNA. This finding was in contrast to less than 3% of B lymphocytes in healthy control subjects,[21] indicating a 3-fold increase in the frequency of RAG1- and RAG2-expressing B cells in SLE patients. These activated B cells may participate in abnormal immune regulation associated with SLE. Although RAG mRNA was hardly detectable in B cells from the peripheral blood of patients with rheumatoid arthritis (RA) as determined by RT-PCR, higher levels of RAG1 and RAG2 mRNA expression were found in B cells from RA synovial tissues.[22] RAG-mediated Ig L chain rearrangement associated with RSS DNA breaks was thus evidenced in one-third of RA synovia. This finding suggests that receptor revision of L chain genes may contribute to the local production of autoAbs in ectopic germinal centers. Replacement of the V_H gene also has been demonstrated in RA synovial B cells, where almost 8% of the clones with V_HDJ_H variants were apparently generated by receptor revision.[23] The presence of RAG-expressing cells and the identification of RSS DNA breaks also suggest that these secondary rearrangements could occur in ectopic germinal centers in RA synovial tissues. This may contribute to the generation of autoreactive B cells, which may play a role in the immunopathogenesis of RA. Ectopic intrathyroidal secondary lymphoid follicles also were described in autoimmune thyroid diseases.[24] Germinal center–like structures and the occurrence of high levels of RAG1 and RAG2 mRNA expression strongly suggest that receptor revision takes place in intrathyroidal lymphoid follicles and may contribute to the generation of high-affinity autoAbs to thyroid antigens. Overall, these data indicate that chronic stimulation of the immune system in autoimmune diseases may reveal receptor revision. Because RAG expression is switched off by high BCR levels[19] but maintained by low BCR signals, one can speculate that in the case of autoreactive BCR, autoantigens could induce a receptor downregulation from the cell surface. Consequently, this could disrupt signals from the cell surface that are required to repress RAG expression.[25] Aberrant receptor revision favors the maintenance or the appearance of autoreactive B cells, which is associated with defect in apoptosis (i.e., defect in selection against autoreactivity).

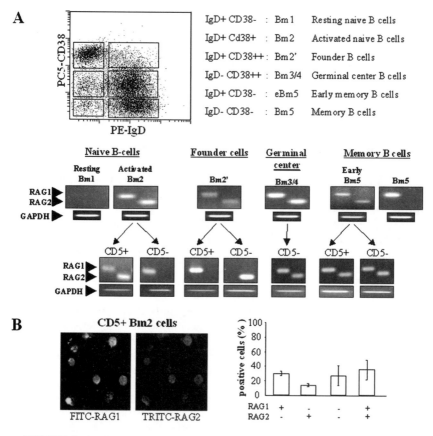

FIGURE 2. RAG1 and RAG2 expression in human mature B-cell subsets. (**A**) Tonsillar B-cell subsets, identified by the surface expression of CD19, CD38, IgD, and CD5, were sorted by flow cytometry and specific RAG1, RAG2, and GAPDH mRNA amplified by RT-PCR. (**B**) Purified CD5+ Bm2 cells were stained with anti-RAG1 and anti-RAG2 antibodies revealed with appropriate secondary agents for the detection of RAG1 and RAG2 proteins. The frequencies of single RAG1 or RAG2 positive cells as well as those of RAG1 and RAG2 double-negative or double-positive cells were determined (mean ± SD of 3 experiments).

RECEPTOR REVISION OUTSIDE GERMINAL CENTERS

There is compelling evidence that the process of somatic hypermutation is not restricted to germinal centers[26] and that peripheral RAG$^+$ B cells may be identified outside germinal centers.[27] This suggests that Abs can be generated outside the conventional sites and, consequently, that autoAbs could be produced there. It is possible to hypothesize that low BCR signals could influence RAG expression outside germinal centers. Specifically, it is established that CD5$^+$ B cells are confined to the mantle zone of germinal centers,[28] that the CD5 molecule has a negative influence on BCR signals thus raising receptor threshold,[29] and that CD5$^+$ B cells may produce autoAbs.[30,31] The CD5 molecule may thus contribute to the triggering of receptor revision, which could ultimately lead to the production of autoAbs in some circumstances. This view signifies the possibility of finding RAG expression in activated CD5$^+$ B cells outside germinal centers. To test this possibility, we sorted human mature B cell subpopulations based on IgD and CD38 expression[32] and examined RAG1 and RAG2 mRNA expression. These studies revealed RAG$^+$ B cells outside germinal centers (FIG. 2A). When the subpopulations were further separated according to CD5 expression, we observed that activated naïve CD5$^+$ B cells (Bm2 cells) expressed both RAG1 and RAG2 mRNA outside germinal centers. Immunofluorescence staining confirmed the coexpression of RAG1 and RAG2 proteins in approximately 25% of CD5$^+$ Bm2 cells (FIG. 2B).

We then carried out *in vitro* experiments to confirm the association between the presence of CD5 and RAG upregulation. CD5$^-$ Bm2 cells were sorted and stimulated with anti-IgM Abs on CD40L-transfected fibroblasts (FIG. 3). These results revealed the induction of CD5 on the cell surface concomitantly with the appearance of RAG1 and RAG2 mRNA. Remarkably, when the cells were further separated based on CD5 expression, only CD5$^+$ B cells displayed both RAG proteins (FIG. 3). These data indicate that activated naïve CD5$^+$ B cells revise their BCR before they enter germinal centers.

CD5$^+$ B lymphocytes are known to be involved in the production of polyreactive and autoAbs in autoimmune diseases.[33] Our observations suggest that these cells are antigen driven and activated. In this setting and depending on BCR affinity, CD5 could be induced on the surface of B cells, thus raising the BCR threshold. Consequently, the diminished BCR signals would contribute to the upregulation of RAG and the revision of the BCR before entrance of the cells into germinal centers. Acquisition of a revised BCR with higher affinity would then promote initiation of the germinal center reaction with the loss of CD5 expression.[34] This would represent a fifth wave of RAG expression (FIG. 1).

In this respect, the emergence of autoreactive B cells in autoimmune diseases could be ascribed to a faulty control of CD5 expression or to a defective regulation of receptor revision. Similar to the other tolerance checkpoints for receptor edition and intragerminal center receptor revision, a lack in apoptosis associated with an impaired control of RAG expression would favor the opportunity to generate autoAb-secreting B cells before the cells enter germinal centers.

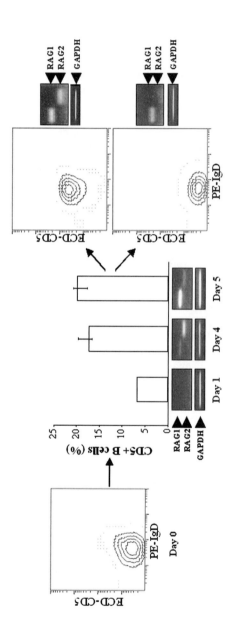

FIGURE 3. *In vitro* induction of CD5, RAG1, and RAG2 in Bm2 cells. Bm1 and Bm2 cells negative for CD5 were sorted and cultured on CD40L-transfected fibroblasts with 1 µg/mL anti-IgM antibodies. Frequency of CD5⁺ cells was evaluated by flow cytometry and RAG1, RAG2, and GAPDH mRNA amplified by RT-PCR. Cells turned positive for CD5 and cells still negative were separated, and expression of mRNA was analyzed as above.

ACKNOWLEDGMENTS

This work was supported by a grant from the Ministère de l'Enseignement Supérieur et de la Recherche. The editorial assistance of Professor Rizgar A. Mageed is greatly appreciated. Thanks are also due to Simone Forest and Cindy Séné for secretarial assistance.

REFERENCES

1. GELLERT, M. 2002. V(D)J recombination: RAG proteins, repair factors, and regulation. Annu. Rev. Biochem. **71:** 101–132.
2. NEMAZEE, D. & K. BUERKI. 1989. Clonal deletion of autoreactive B lymphocytes in bone marrow chimeras. Proc. Natl. Acad. Sci. USA **86:** 8039–8043.
3. GOODNOW, C.C., J. CROSBIE, S. ADELSTEIN, *et al.* 1988. Altered immunoglobulin expression and functional silencing of self-reactive B lymphocytes in transgenic mice. Nature **334:** 676–682.
4. GAY, D., T. SAUNDERS, S. CAMPER, *et al.* 1993. Receptor editing: an approach by autoreactive B cells to escape tolerance. J. Exp. Med. **177:** 999–1008.
5. HAO, Z. & K. RAJEWSKY. 2001. Homeostasis of peripheral B cells in the absence of B cell influx from the bone marrow. J. Exp. Med. **194:** 1151–1164.
6. WARDEMANN, H., S. YURASOV, A. SCHAEFER, *et al.* 2003. Predominant autoantibody production by early human B cell precursors. Science **301:** 1374–1377.
7. RADIC, M.Z., J. ERIKSON, S. LITWIN, *et al.* 1993. B lymphocytes may escape tolerance by revising their antigen receptors. J. Exp. Med. **177:** 1165–1173.
8. RETTER, M.W. & D. NEMAZEE. 1998. Receptor editing occurs frequently during normal B cell development. J. Exp. Med. **188:** 1231–1238.
9. BRAUNINGER, A., T. GOOSSENS, K. RAJEWSKY, *et al.* 2001. Regulation of immunoglobulin light chain gene rearrangements during early B cell development in the human. Eur. J. Immunol. **31:** 3631–3637.
10. WILSON, P.C., K. WILSON, Y.J. LIU, *et al.* 2000. Receptor revision of immunoglobulin heavy chain variable region genes in normal human B lymphocytes. J. Exp. Med. **191:** 1881–1894.
11. RADIC, M.Z. & M. ZOUALI. 1996. Receptor editing, immune diversification, and self-tolerance. Immunity **5:** 505–511.
12. ZHANG, Z., M. ZEMLIN, Y.H. WANG, *et al.* 2003. Contribution of Vh gene replacement to the primary B cell repertoire. Immunity **19:** 21–31.
13. LI, Y., H. LI, & M. WEIGERT. 2002. Autoreactive B cells in the marginal zone that express dual receptors. J. Exp. Med. **195:** 181–188.
14. KLONOWSKI, K.D. & M. MONESTIER. 2000. Heavy chain revision in MRL mice: a potential mechanism for the development of autoreactive B cell precursors. J. Immunol. **165:** 4487–4493.
15. HIKIDA, M., M. MORI, T. TAKAI, *et al.* 1996. Reexpression of RAG-1 and RAG-2 genes in activated mature mouse B cells. Science **274:** 2092–2094.
16. HAN, S., B. ZHENG, D.G. SCHATZ, *et al.* 1996. Neoteny in lymphocytes: Rag1 and Rag2 expression in germinal center B cells. Science **274:** 2094–2097.
17. GARTNER, F., F.W. ALT, R.J. MONROE, *et al.* 2000. Antigen-independent appearance of recombination activating gene (RAG)-positive bone marrow B cells in the spleens of immunized mice. J. Exp. Med. **192:** 1745–1754.
18. GIRSCHICK, H.J., A.C. GRAMMER, T. NANKI, *et al.* 2001. RAG1 and RAG2 expression by B cell subsets from human tonsil and peripheral blood. J. Immunol. **166:** 377–386.
19. MEFFRE, E., F. PAPAVASILIOU, P. COHEN, *et al.* 1998. Antigen receptor engagement turns off the V(D)J recombination machinery in human tonsil B cells. J. Exp. Med. **188:** 765–772.
20. MAGARI, M., T. SAWATARI, Y. KAWANO, *et al.* 2002. Contribution of light chain rearrangement in peripheral B cells to the generation of high-affinity antibodies. Eur. J. Immunol. **32:** 957–966.

21. GIRSCHICK, H.J., A.C. GRAMMER, T. NANKI, *et al.* 2002. Expression of recombination activating genes 1 and 2 in peripheral B cells of patients with systemic lupus erythematosus. Arthritis Rheum. **46:** 1255–1263.
22. ZHANG, Z., X. WU, B.H. LIMBAUGH, *et al.* 2001. Expression of recombination-activating genes and terminal deoxynucleotidyl transferase and secondary rearrangement of immunoglobulin kappa light chains in rheumatoid arthritis synovial tissue. Arthritis Rheum. **44:** 2275–2284.
23. ITOH, K., E. MEFFRE, E. ALBESIANO, *et al.* 2000. Immunoglobulin heavy chain variable region gene replacement as a mechanism for receptor revision in rheumatoid arthritis synovial tissue B lymphocytes. J. Exp. Med. **192:** 1151–1164.
24. ARMENGOL, M.P., M. JUAN, A. LUCAS-MARTIN, *et al.* 2001. Thyroid autoimmune disease: demonstration of thyroid antigen-specific B cells and recombination-activating gene expression in chemokine-containing active intrathyroidal germinal centers. Am. J. Pathol. **159:** 861–873.
25. JANKOVIC, M., R. CASELLAS, N. YANNOUTSOS, *et al.* 2004. RAGs and regulation of autoantibodies. Annu. Rev. Immunol. **22:** 485–501.
26. WILLIAM, J., C. EULER, S. CHRISTENSEN, *et al.* 2002. Evolution of autoantibody responses via somatic hypermutation outside of germinal centers. Science **297:** 2066–2070.
27. MERU, N., A. JUNG, I. BAUMANN, *et al.* 2002. Expression of the recombination-activating genes in extrafollicular lymphocytes but no apparent reinduction in germinal center reactions in human tonsils. Blood **99:** 531–537.
28. DONO, M., V.L. BURGIO, C. TACCHETTI, *et al.* 1996. Subepithelial B cells in the human palatine tonsil. I. Morphologic, cytochemical and phenotypic characterization. Eur. J. Immunol. **26:** 2035–2042.
29. BIKAH, G., J. CAREY, J.R. CIALLELLA, *et al.* 1996. CD5-mediated negative regulation of antigen receptor-induced growth signals in B-1 B cells. Science **274:** 1906–1909.
30. CASALI, P., S.E. BURASTERO, M. NAKAMURA, *et al.* 1987. Human lymphocytes making rheumatoid factor and antibody to ssDNA belong to Leu-1$^+$ B-cell subset. Science **236:** 77–81.
31. HARDY, R.R., K. HAYAKAWA, M. SHIMIZU, *et al.* 1987. Rheumatoid factor secretion from human Leu-1$^+$ B cells. Science **236:** 81–83.
32. LIU, Y.J. & C. ARPIN. 1997. Germinal center development. Immunol. Rev. **156:** 111–126.
33. YOUINOU, P. & P.M. LYDYARD. 2001. CD5$^+$ B cells in nonorgan-specific autoimmune diseases: a fresh look. Lupus **10:** 523–525
34. YOUINOU, P., C. JAMIN & P.M. LYDYARD. 1999. CD5 expression in human B-cell populations. Immunol. Today **20:** 312–316.

B Lymphocytes Are Required for Development and Treatment of Autoimmune Diseases

PIERRE YOUINOU, CHRISTOPHE JAMIN, JACQUES-OLIVIER PERS, CHRISTIAN BERTHOU, ALAIN SARAUX, AND YVES RENAUDINEAU

Brest University Medical School, Brest, France

ABSTRACT: Recent studies have revealed that B cells serve extraordinarily diverse functions within the immune system in addition to antibody production. These functions contribute to autoimmunity. They initiate the development of lymphoid architecture and regulate dendritic and T-cell function through cytokine production. Receptor editing is also essential to prevent autoimmunity. Both abnormalities in the distribution of B-cell subsets and the benefits of ablative B-cell therapy of autoimmune states confirm their importance. Results from transgenic models have demonstrated that the sensitivity of B cells to antigen receptor cross-linking correlates to autoimmunity, with particular reference to negative signaling by CD5 and CD22. These mechanisms maintain tolerance by recruiting *src*-homology 2 domain-containing protein tyrosine phosphatase-1. These findings open new prospects for immunotherapy of autoimmune diseases.

KEYWORDS: B lymphocyte; autoimmune disease; dendritic cell; T lymphocyte; B-cell antigen receptor; CD5

Major advances recently have revived and refined our understanding of autoreactive B cells.[1] Humoral abnormalities, most notably in systemic lupus erythematosus (SLE), have even been explained by intrinsic B-cell hyperactivity.[2] New works have indeed incorporated B lymphocytes in the afferent arm of the immune response rather than confined them in the efferent phase. For example, according to Klinman and Steinberg,[3] connective tissue diseases (CTD) clearly arise from polyclonal B-cell activation.

In this respect, it is not surprising that characteristics suggestive of the breakdown of normal antibody (Ab) regulation have been identified in the relatives of patients[4–6] with SLE, rheumatoid arthritis (RA), or primary Sjögren's syndrome (pSS) that might predispose the family members to full-blown diseases similar to that of their probands. The finding of enhanced immunoglobulin (Ig) production in response to mitogens is consistent with this propensity for IgG production in the peripheral blood of relatives.

Address for correspondence: Professor Pierre Youinou, Laboratory of Immunology, Brest University Medical School Hospital, BP824, F29609 Brest Cedex, France. Voice: +33-298-22-33-84; fax: +33-298-22-38-47.

youinou@univ-brest.fr

Ann. N.Y. Acad. Sci. 1050: 19–33 (2005). © 2005 New York Academy of Sciences.
doi: 10.1196/annals.1313.003

Concomitantly, additional complexity was defined in the B-cell compartment. It follows that models based on a single B-lymphocyte population could not be sustained anymore; thus, new subpopulations of B cells need to be delineated. The earliest concept that B cells are exclusively committed to the production of Ig also has been reconsidered. Owing to latest breakthroughs in their functions, it has become apparent that they accomplish various tasks other than the production of autoAb. Any of these may be faulty, and any of the resulting inadequacies may be involved in the autoimmune process. Consequently, B-cell tolerance and tolerance breakdown warrant being reanalyzed in light of the previously mentioned recent insights. Survival and selection of B lymphocytes are determined by antigens (Ag) and, therefore, B-cell Ag receptor (BCR) specificity, but the signal transduction is finely tuned by a dozen coreceptors and thereby adjusted by numerous protein tyrosine kinases (PTK) and protein tyrosine phosphatases (PTP).

In practice, we have witnessed that numerous initially promising therapies for CTD have proved disappointing over the past 20 years. Novel approaches, such as targeting B-cell subsets or autoAb,[7] have since been derived from awareness of B-cell involvement in humans and compelling studies in mice. A number of groups have subsequently embarked on trials using B-cell ablative therapy to treat autoimmune diseases. Not only do these treatments remove autoAb efficiently, but the patients feel remarkably improved. Hence, it is beyond any doubt that preliminary results represent one of the keys to understanding how the process is initiated and completed. Encouraging results have been obtained so far.

SUBPOPULATIONS OF B LYMPHOCYTES

Classification According to the Expression of CD5

CD5 was first described as a T-cell marker, then discovered on malignant human B cells, and finally shown to characterize some B-lymphocytes in human tonsils and peripheral blood.[8] Increased levels of circulating CD5[+] B cells have been reported by Youinou et al.[9,10] and others[11,12] in RA and pSS. This fluctuating expression of CD5 correlates with disease activity in various autoimmune conditions. For example, it is of note that those pSS patients with monoclonal Ig had higher levels of CD5[+] B cells than the remainder,[9] as could be predicted from the frequent occurrence of lymphoma in this disorder.

CD5[+] B lymphocytes are associated with the production of low-affinity autoAb[13] and a propensity for malignant transformation,[14] giving rise to lymphomas, most notably chronic lymphocytic leukemia. To come full circle, leukemic cells can be induced to release autoAb by phorbol ester.[15] Intriguingly, the proportion of B cells that express CD5 is relatively constant in a given individual,[16] so that their enhancement is a feature of selected RA families rather than a peculiarity of the RA patients themselves compared with their own healthy relatives.[5]

Some controversy still exists about their lineage origins, although a great deal of effort has been put into trying to understand the significance of CD5[+] cells. The activation view implies that the CD5[+] B cells can be generated from CD5[−] B cells,[17] whereas the lineage paradigm posits the existence of separate progenitors for CD5[+] and CD5[−] B cells.[18] A new nomenclature[19] distinguishes B1 from B2 lymphocytes.

The former population encompasses CD5[+] B cells, and the latter population encompasses the conventional B cells. However, it is unclear whether B1 lymphocytes constitute a naïve population of cells. Therefore, we have proposed[8] that different reasons may exist for B cells to harbor CD5, depending on the consequences of ligation of this receptor on their surface. In this respect, the B1 population has been subdivided into B1a and B1b subpopulations.[20] The B1b "sister population" lacks surface CD5 but shares the other attributes of B1a cells, such as natural Ab production and the low density of the high molecular weight isoform of the common leukocyte antigen CD45. In addition to a feedback mechanism,[21] the distribution of B cells into B1 and B2, as well as B1a and B1b, is regulated, at least in the mouse, by the major histocompatibility class 2 haplotype[22] and the level of interleukin (IL)-10.[23]

B Lymphocyte Ontogenesis

B cells originate in the liver during fetal life and in the bone-marrow (BM) after birth[24] where they pass through a sequence of clear-cut intermediate stages. The sizable diversity of the BCR repertoire proceeds from the ordered rearrangement of the gene segments variable (V), diversity (D), and joining (J) of the Ig heavy chain locus and those of the gene segments V and J of its light chain locus.

Pre-B cells are referred to as immature B lymphocytes. They migrate to the periphery. Such an escape depends on the signal delivered by the Ag, but it is uncertain whether this applies to all immature B lymphocytes or whether the signal is restricted to a fraction of those cells. After BCR-mediated maturation, they are pushed into leaving the primary lymphoid tissues to settle down in the secondary lymphoid organs (SLO). This view implies a massive death of B cells that has never been observed in the BM. Hence, it remains possible that a handful of immature B cells leaves this central organ and carries on maturing, as recirculating B lymphocytes.

Maturation of B Cells in the Germinal Centers

Those cells that have just reached the SLO turn into transitional B lymphocytes type 1, type 2, and type 3,[25] at least in the mouse, and, step by step, achieve immune maturation. Only mature B lymphocytes gain entry into the lymphoid follicles to launch a new germinal center (GC). Subsequent noncirculating B cells consist of marginal zone B cells[26] and follicular B cells.[27,28] Note that within the marginal zone, subsets differentiate into early Ab-forming cells, whereas, in response to a T-dependent Ag, others give rise to GCs with hypermutation. Furthermore, they proliferate within exocrine glands of certain mouse models of pSS[29] and spur on lymphomas in some patients with pSS.[30] Marginal zone lymphocytes would thus be key in the development of autoimmune settings. Access to lymphoid follicles depends on specific chemokines, but maintenance signals also are delivered from the BCR. The importance of the ongoing lymphoid follicles competition is supported by the presence of ectopic GCs at sites of inflammation in pSS,[31] RA,[32] and Hashimoto's thyroiditis,[33] as well as by the demonstration that the autoAg-induced engagement of the BCR occurs locally, be it IgG in the rheumatoid synovium,[34] double-stranded (ds) DNA in kidneys from SLE,[35] or RNP particles in exocrine tissues from pSS.[36] Even more important, autoAb can develop outside GCs via somatic hypermutations of Ig genes, which recently was established in the MRL *lpr/lpr* mouse model of

TABLE 1. Mature B (Bm) lymphocyte subsets within germinal centers

Subpopulation	IgD	CD38	CD23	CD27
Bm1 (naïve)	+	−	−	−
Bm2 (activated)	+	+	+	−
Bm2′ (germinal center founder)	+	++	+	−
Bm3 (centroblast)	−	++	−	−
Bm4 (centrocyte)	−	++	−	−
Early Bm5 (antibody or memory)	−	+	−	−
Bm5 (antibody-secreting cell)	−	−	−	+

SLE.[37] Some B lymphocytes undergo apoptosis, whereas others resist programmed cell death. The capacity of T lymphocytes to promote B-cell proliferation would proceed from the insertion of the CD40 ligand into its receptor.[38]

Surface markers have been unraveled by further analysis of B cells in the GC.[39] In particular, IgD and CD38 have been useful in characterizing 7 developmental stages. Mature B (Bm) cell subpopulations differ with respect to the expression of these 2 markers (TABLE 1). Naïve IgD$^+$ CD38$^-$ Bm1, once activated as IgD$^+$ CD38$^+$ Bm2, differentiate into GC founder IgD$^+$ CD38^{++} Bm2′, IgD$^-$ CD38^{++} Bm3, and Bm4, ending up as early IgD$^-$ CD38$^+$, Bm5 and ultimately IgD$^-$ CD38$^-$ Bm5 cells. These include memory B cells that express CD27 and plasma cells (PC) that do not. There appear to be two types of long-lived memory B cells; one is resting in specialized microanatomical niches of SLO, such as the mantle zone of the spleen, and another is activated in the BM. This long-lived PC pool can intervene in natural immunity.[40] Throughout the sequence from Bm1 to Bm5, a fraction of each B-cell subset leaks into the peripheral blood. Their distribution is skewed in autoimmune patients so that characteristic signatures of B-cell subset abnormalities have been identified. According to Bohnhorst et al.[41] and our unpublished results, there appears to be increased levels of GC founder cells in pSS. This is also the case for pre-GC and PC precursors in juvenile SLE.[42] In contrast, the number of memory B cells is reduced in pSS.[41,43] It is possible that preferential accumulation of CD27$^+$ memory B cells in the inflamed parotid glands[44] entails their reduction in the peripheral blood. Active SLE is, by contrast, characterized by an increase in circulating PC that is normalized by immunosuppressive therapy.[45] Such significant abnormalities in B cell subpopulations occur in RA patients[41,43] (also our unpublished results). However, CD20$^+$ CD38$^-$ B lymphocytes with defective proliferative responsiveness may be found[46] in RA synovial fluid. B-cell subset disturbances are thus specific for each disease.

VARIOUS FUNCTIONS OF B CELLS

B cells are central to the development of autoimmunity. Evidence comes from the combinations of autoAbs that characterize various conditions, the finding that polyclonal B-cell activation is the earliest and most common abnormality of lupus mice, and the finding that B lymphocytes spontaneously produce Ig, of which they switch

TABLE 2. B lymphocytes produce autoantibodies

- Complete absence of T-cell infiltrates in MRL *lpr/lpr* mice homologous for the deletion *JH/JH*.

- The IgM MRL/MpJ-*Fas^lpr* mice have a transgene encoding surface immunoglobulins, but not permitting its secretion. They develop nephritis characterized by cellular infiltration.

NOTE: From references 84–86.

TABLE 3. Function of B cells in addition to antibody production

- Shaping of the splenic architecture: dendritic cells and T lymphocytes

- Antigen presentation (in particular, CD5-expressing and rheumatoid factor–making B cells)

- Production of cytokines to trigger polarization of naïve T lymphocytes into T helper 1 (Th1) or Th2

the isotype in the absence of T-cell help. Reininger *et al.* elegantly established that long-term *in vitro* proliferating fetal liver pre-B cell lines derived from autoimmune-prone mice differentiate in SCID mice, up to the production of high levels of auto-Ab.[47] The authors pursued this issue by showing that murine pre-B cells lead to a marked hyperglobulinemia in their mice.[48]

The involvement of autoAb remains, nonetheless, debated. Though a flurry of results suggest that B lymphocytes do not purely and simply act as precursors of auto-Ab-secreting cells, efforts to identify how they contribute to autoimmunity have gathered provocative conclusions. These findings have indeed become more and more difficult to combine into only one model. For example, MRL *lpr/lpr* mice (TABLE 2) that lack B lymphocytes (i.e., mice homologous for the deletion *JH/JH*) are preserved of nephritis,[49] and those that have B cells with membrane but not secreted Ig (i.e., IgM MRL/MpJ-*Fas^lpr* mice) develop nephritis.[50] Thus, an essential role for B cells in nephritis may not be through autoAb. How can we reconcile such statements with previous observations that SLE is associated with circulating anti-ds DNA–enriched immune complexes, induced by passively transferred polyclonal or monoclonal autoAb and caused by immune complex deposition? In fact, B lymphocytes are now endowed with other functions (TABLE 3). Likewise, in nonobese diabetic mice,[51] these lymphocytes are required, even though the autoimmune process itself is elicited by activated T cells.

Influence of B Lymphocytes on Cells in Their Vicinity

There is recent evidence that tumor necrosis factor (TNF)-α, lymphotoxin (LT)-α, and LT-β permit organization of the spleen. Indeed, LT-α, LT-β, TNF-α receptor-I, and TNF-α KO mice show abnormal splenic architecture, as well as those in which LT-α or LT-β genes are disrupted. Although it is still not exactly apparent why defects create such derangements, the lack of dendritic cells (DC) appears most intriguing in TNF- or LT-KO mice.[52] Interrelationships were initially predicted from

SCID mice devoid of mature B lymphocytes and DC.[53] Converging proofs have since been furnished by experiments in which B cells induced DC, thanks to the expression of membrane LT-α.[54]

Owing to the impulse of T-cell differentiation on autoimmune susceptibility, pathways of T lymphocytes into T helper (Th) 1 and Th2 have been the focus of feverish research. It has been advocated that OX40 receptor/OX40 ligand juncture from DC coordinates the cytokine-mediated differentiation of both Th1 and Th2 cell help for B cells. However, Ag-specific interaction of B and T lymphocytes, along with the engagement of OX40 receptor on activated T cells by OX40 ligand on stimulated B cells, induces IL-4 production, restrains interferon (IFN)-γ synthesis, and favors the differentiation of Th2 and PC under the influence of this very IL-4 that has just been released.[55] B cells are also necessary for the induction of the T-cell contact sensitivity in certain murine models. All in all, B lymphocytes influence the formation of follicular DC and superintend T-cell migration. In such a Th1/Th2 frame, TNF-α released by T-cell–activated macrophages might be protective[56] in SLE.

B Lymphocytes as Ag-Presenting Cells

In addition, B cells act[57] as Ag-presenting cells (APC): any Ag-specific B lymphocyte can indeed take up, internalize, process, and return peptides from the nominal Ag to a neighboring T cell or to another B cell. This process would improve T-cell immunity and magnify the ultimate Ab response. B1a cells are particularly suitable to the membrane expression of multispecific auto Ab and thus most appropriate to stretch out self-components to B-1, B-2, or T lymphocytes. The fact that splenic B-1a cells behave as potent APCs explains that they induce 2-fold greater levels of IFN-γ release than B-2 cells in the NZBM2410 mouse.[58] Other experiments[59] have temptingly suggested that B cells binding IgG containing immune complex Ab via membrane rheumatoid factor present their Ag very rapidly. It is possible that, in the bulk of natural autoAb, physiological rheumatoid factor comes from the B1 population. This raises the issue of their effect as inflammatory mediators, all the more because T-cell activation could be B cell-dependent in RA.[60] Synovial tissues that are infiltrated by T cells, macrophages, and DC but that lack B cells do not activate adoptively transferred T-cell clones, leaving the possibility of a critical function for B cells in T-cell activation. In fact, Ag presentation involves B lymphocyte synapses, which extracts intact Ag from APC and contributes to the generation of peptide-MHC for T lymphocyte synapse formation in a sort of relay race.[61] This subtle organization renders B cells, especially those with specificity for ds DNA and rheumatoid factor, critical APCs in the presentation of nuclear Ag.

Polarized Cytokine Production by B Cells

Cytokines are involved in disease activity, namely IL-6, which stimulates the final stages of B-lymphocyte maturation and is abundantly produced in SLE.[62] Given the constitutive expression of IL-6 receptors and their part in the excessive cell function in SLE, T-cell help could be dispensable in dysregulation of B cells. Another candidate is IL-10,[63] as indicated by 6 experiments: (1) B-1a cells are the main source of B cell-derived IL-10;[64] (2) continuous treatment of normal mice with anti-IL-10 Ab depletes B-1 but not B-2 cells;[65] (3) antisense oligodeoxynucleotides specific for IL-

10 mRNA inhibit the growth of murine leukemic B-1 cells *in vitro*;[66] (4) IL-10 is elevated in the serum of patients with SLE;[67] (5) antiagonist is beneficial in the management of refractory SLE;[68] and (6) we have, ourselves,[23] sorted B-1a, B-1b, and B-2 lymphocytes from normal and IL-10-KO mice and identified IL-10 mRNA.

The cliché of two T-cell families, Th1 and Th2, has been acknowledged. These effector cells produce distinct spectra of cytokines compatible with the kind of response required to particular Ag: Th1 cells secrete IFN-γ and IL-2, whereas Th2 cells produce IL-4, IL-5, and IL-6.[69] The latter set of cytokines favors activation of B lymphocytes. In addition, Th1 cytokines enhance further production of Th1 cells, while inhibiting Th2 cells, and the other way round. B cells produce cytokines, such as IL-10, IL-6, and TNF-α, albeit at low levels, but they also acquire the ability to express IL-2, IFN-γ, IL-4, and IL-12 when stimulated with Ag in the presence of Th1 cells.

An exciting issue emerges that naïve B cells differentiate into B cells with different cytokine profiles, after stimulation with Ag and Th1 or Th2. The resulting polarized B cells are B effectors (Be) 1 and Be2, respectively.[70] In return, they impart functional capacities to the T lymphocytes. Be1 cells, by virtue of IFN-γ and Ag presentation to T cells, promote Th1, whereas IL-4 from Be2 cells encourages Th2. The fact that Th1/Th2 and Be1/Be2 cells cross-regulate the differentiation of naïve B and T lymphocyte supports the concept of a sequence of amplifying mechanism. If out of control, such B cells lead to autoimmunity. The precise origin of the Be1 and Be2 cells remains to be defined, but the positive feedback amplification occurs at sites of inflammation because assessment of circulating Be1 and Be2 in SLE[71] has not seen differences between patients and normal subjects.

B-CELL TOLERANCE AND TOLERANCE BREAKDOWN

The B-Cell Ag Receptor

The Ag Binds to the BCR: The encounter of the Ag with its BCR sets up an essential checkpoint for tolerance to the self. Recent work has brought new insights into the stoichiometry of these components, that is, a binding subunit, the membrane Ig, and a signaling subunit with Ig-α (CD79a) and Ig-β (CD79b) proteins. These Ig-like ectodomains are both necessary, and their intracytoplasmic tails carry immuno-receptor tyrosine-based activation motifs (ITAM), which constitute as many docking sites for PTK and the subsequent transduction of the signal. High-affinity interactions between autoAg and membrane-bound Ig lead to apoptosis of immature B cells.[72] The ensuing affinity maturation for exoAg takes place in the GC: centroblasts undergo hypermutations, and, as the sequence goes on, centrocytes emerge, either with low-affinity cells that endure apoptosis or with high-affinity cells that change into Ab forming cells.

The Transduction Machinery: Cross-linking of the BCR switches on a number of PTK, including *syk* and *Lyn* and *btk*, which are *src*-family members. Downstream, the phosphatidylinositol-3 kinase and serine/threonine kinase Akt transduction pathway can promote cell survival by activating protein kinases C (PKC) and implicating the three families of mitogen-activated kinases (MAP): p38, the C-*Jun* NH$_2$-terminal kinase families (which are both pro-apoptotic), and the extracellular-regulated kinase family (which is antiapoptotic). Once activated, phospholipase C generates diacylglycerol and inositol-1,4,5-triphosphate from membrane phosphatidylinositol-4,5-biphosphate. These messengers are required for activation of PKC and release of Ca^{2+}, respectively. MAP kinases are then activated by PKC, which has just been tyrosine phosphorylated, and intracellular Ca^{2+}, which has just been mobilized. Either or both may be defective, and either offers novel avenues for therapy of autoimmune diseases.

Implications with Respect to Tolerance: There is compelling evidence that recruitment of mature short-lived B cells into the recirculating pool of lymphocytes is dependent on BCR engagement by such autoAg.[73] Additional mechanisms of self-tolerance in the periphery silence mature B cells that have dodged central tolerance. Interestingly, by downregulating Ig surface expression, chronic lymphocytic leukemia B lymphocytes[74,75] keep inducing BCR-mediated survival signals, whereas the level required for apoptosis cannot be reached. Molecular aberrations also have been observed in autoimmune settings. These include signaling defects and abnormal apoptosis of autoreactive lymphocytes.[76] Clearly, autoAg are involved here because most of those targeted in SLE are clustered into apoptotic bodies,[77] and such an intracellular localization predisposes for autoAb production.[78] It may be safely stated that signaling is abnormal in SLE.

Coordinated and Intricate Mechanisms of Self-Tolerance

Regulation of Signaling Thresholds: Despite the complexity of the mechanisms involved in tolerance, they are not foolproof at all. During the course of an immune response, coreceptors lift and lower the BCR threshold by modulating the activation of molecules necessary to the transduction. This machinery is stimulated by CD19 and CD21 and dampened down by CD22,[79] CD72, and CD5. The latest receptor is physically[80] and functionally[81] associated with the BCR, and B cells that are equipped with the CD5 receptor express more of the CD5 ligand, CD72, than B cells that are not.[82] It is also interesting that ligation of CD5 triggers apoptosis in resting B cells, but not in resting T cells,[83] and extends the proliferative response of B1a cells activated with anti-IgM and IL-2.[84]

CD32, which is one of the high-affinity receptors for the Fc part of IgG, is involved in preventing the BCR response.[85] CD22 also is endowed with a potent role as a regulator, but we found its expression normal in B lymphocytes from SLE patients.[86] All these glycoproteins carry ITAM and immunoregulatory tyrosine-inhibiting motifs (ITIM), which recruit PTP to reverse the effects of PTK, namely SH2-containing protein tyrosine phosphatase (SHP)-1 for CD22, CD72, and CD5, and SH2-containing inositol polyphosphate 5-phosphatase (SHIP) for CD32. *Lyn* is required to phosphorylate CD22 and to link SHP-1 to the CD22/BCR complex. Mice in which *Lyn*, CD22, or SHP-1 has been disrupted have autoAb-releasing hyperactive B cells. A lupus-like disease develops in those lacking the ITIM-encoding gene, or *Lyn*, CD22, or SHP-1.[87]

Negative regulation is normally offset by commensurate coreceptors that amplify the signals. They include CD19 and various isoforms, RA, RB, RC, and RO of CD45.[88] Enhancing the density of CD19 expression renders B lymphocytes hyperresponsive to transmembrane signals and induces autoAb production. Modest increases may indeed shift the balance between tolerance and immunity to immunity.

Thus, patients with systemic sclerosis overexpress CD19 by as few as 20%.[89] These findings indicate that coreceptors are regulated through molecular interactions on the B-cell surface. Any defect is liable to promote autoimmunity.

Anergy in Self-Reactive B Cells: Constant tickling of BCR by self-Ag transmits tolerogenic signals by activation feedback processes that render the cell anergic. Again, tolerance is governed by BCR signaling thresholds. Hippen *et al.*[90] demonstrated in double-transgenic (Tg) mice that CD5 contributes to maintain tolerance in anergic B cells: those B lymphocytes of mice Tg for anti-hen egg lysozyme (HEL) Ab and membrane HEL Ag undergo apoptosis based on their robust activation. They rather become anergic if the mice are Tg for soluble HEL, but this tolerance is broken if this model for B-cell anergy is bred onto the CD5-KO background.

Secondary Changes in the BCR Specificity: The importance of self Ag in negative selection in the BM has been underlined recently. Therefore, a role in the positive selection of B cells is essential. By altering the specificity of their BCR in the BM, autoreactive B cells may initiate new Ig light chain rearrangements.[91] The system can get rid of self-reactive BCR generated by the recombination process, not only through classical deletion but also through continued recombination. Editing immature B cells transcribe recombinase-activating genes, RAG1 and RAG2, and synthesize the recombination signal sequence-specific endonucleases that activate V(D)J reorganizations.[92] The genes are then switched off by a feedback mechanism initiated by the BCR.

Nonetheless, Ag-receptor genes can be reactivated in response to Ag in mature B cells. This mechanism is supported by the description of secondary rearrangements in a number of systems: for example, RAG1 and RAG2 may be reexpressed in a subset of activated mature murine B-cell population within the GC of draining lymph nodes. If, once reexpressed, gene products are functional, an unfavorable surface Ig receptor gains an additional chance to be revised, and autoreactive B cells arising by hypermutations in the centroblast of GC gain an unexpected chance to escape deletion.[93] Alternatively, the interpretation has been asserted that new BCR assembly in cells that fail to bind Ag may contribute to repertoire diversification by improving the affinity. As a matter of fact, Ag receptor engagement does not turn off the V(D)J recombination machinery, for good, in human tonsil B cells.

Using cell sorting and three RT-PCR ligation-mediated PCR on one and a single B lymphocyte, we have very recently found[94] that activated mature CD5[+] human tonsil B lymphocytes express both *RAG* gene mRNA, assemble the proteins, and display the subsequent DNA cleavages. Double immunofluorescence staining enabled the detection of the corresponding two enzymes in one-third of CD5[+] Bm2 lymphocytes. To further elucidate the link between CD5 expression and *RAG* transcription, CD5-nonexpressing Bm1 and Bm2 lymphocytes were sorted and stimulated with anti-IgM and CD40 ligand to generate a CD5[+] B cell population anew and coexpress RAG1 and RAG2 again. One may speculate that control of CD5 expression or receptor revision before the cells enter the GC may be inadequate in CTD.

Tuning the Response of the BCR

The Lipid Raft Model: After its engagement, the BCR, along with proteins involved in signaling, partitions into microdomains of the cell membrane[95] that are enriched in ganglioside M1. These lipid rafts (LR) can be visualized by conjugated cholera toxin B that binds to ganglioside M1, although the BCR is seen by conjugated anti-IgM. Overlay of red and green stain is seen yellow in activated but not in resting B lymphocytes, indicating that the BCR have moved into these transduction micro-domains.

One mechanism by which CD19 and CD32 operate is to prolong their residency within the LR. CD19 defers the exclusion of the BCR from the LR,[96] and CD32 recruits SHIP.[97] This mechanism is strengthened by the report that LR composition is altered in SLE and by our finding that the BCR resides for a long time in the LR of pSS patients, when entry into the domains should be inhibited in tolerant B lymphocytes.

Cytokinetic Survival Factors: The fate of B cells is adjusted by survival factors. One of the most potent is the B-cell activating factor of the TNF family (BAFF), which protects B lymphocytes from apoptosis, increases their number, and promotes autoAb production. Furthermore, patients with SLE, RA, and pSS[29] harbor elevated levels of BAFF. They correlate with the titer of autoAb in pSS. It is interesting that the cytokine is produced at sites of inflammation, but it is not surprising that it is aberrantly expressed by B lymphocytes in chronic lymphocytic leukemia. Three cognate receptors have been uncovered for this growth factor: B-cell maturation Ag, transmembrane activator and Ca^{2+} modulator, and cyclophilin ligand receptor and the third BAFF receptor (BR3). BAFF is a positive regulator, provided it binds to BR3. Interestingly, its overexpression benefits exclusively self-reactive B cells and facilitates their migration into otherwise forbidden microenvironments, such as the synovial membrane in RA or the exocrine glands in pSS.[98] Another major advance has been that BAFF upregulates CD19, which is consistent with the fact that B cells carry more CD19 molecules in patients than in control subjects. After its release by B cells, the CD5 molecule behaves the same way.[99] It may interact with one of its ligands, such as CD72, compete for receptor occupancy, and deliver a costimulatory signal to resting B lymphocytes.

Genetic Regulation of CD5 Expression: We have recently identified[100] a novel regulatory motif upstream of the noncoding region of the *cd5* gene: this was termed E1B. Compared with the known exon 1, renamed E1A, it creates a new level of CD5 regulation, as established at the transcriptional and translational levels. The E1B-containing transcripts code for a truncated protein that is retained intracellularly. As a result, the amount of E1A-containing transcripts is downregulated, and the protein membrane expression is diminished. Translocation of SHP-1 (which reduces the BCR signal) and, thereby, activation of the cell, is prevented. Studies of transfected cells may hint to closer ties between the gene and the synthesis of the CD5 molecule. In this setting, the strength of the BCR-mediated signaling might lead to the expansion of autoreactive B lymphocytes.

One may assume that B lymphocyte depletion[7] from the pre-B to the mature B cell stages is relevant to the treatment of SLE, Wegener's granulomatosis, auto-immune thrombocytopenic purpura, myasthenia gravis, and dermatomyositis. We also have become aware that BAFF antagonists, monoclonal Ab, or BAFF decoys, ameliorate autoimmune states progression. Unfortunately, little clinical data are available. Based on the tight regulation of PTK and PTP, novel approaches aimed at modulating B lymphocyte function should be designed in the near future. Yet, much remains to be learned about the importance of B cells in the development of CTD.

REFERENCES

1. LIPSKY, P.E. 2001. Systemic lupus erythematosus: an autoimmune disease of B cell hyperactivity. Nat. Immunol. **2:** 764–766.
2. DAVIDSON, A. & B. DIAMOND. 2001. Autoimmune diseases. N. Engl. J. Med. **345:** 340–350.
3. KLINMAN, D.M. & A.D STEINBERG. 1987. Systemic autoimmune diseases arise from polyclonal B cell activation. J. Exp. Med. **165:** 1755–1760.
4. YOUINOU, P., G. SÉMANA, S. MULLER, *et al.* 1997. Interaction between HLA class II determinants and TCR elements promote the antibody production to extractable nuclear antigen-related peptides. Hum. Immunol. **52:** 12–21.
5. YOUINOU, P., P. LE GOFF, G. MERDRIGNAC, *et al.* 1990. The relation between CD5-B lymphocytes in rheumatoid arthritis patients and their relatives. Arthritis Rheum. **33:** 339–348.
6. REVEILLE, J.D., R.W. WILSON, T.T. PROVOST, *et al.* 1984. Primary Sjögren's syndrome and other autoimmune diseases in families. Prevalence and immunogenetic studies in six kindreds. Ann. Intern. Med. **101:** 748–756.
7. LOONEY, R.J. 2002. Treating human autoimmune disease by depleting B cells. Ann. Rheum. Dis. **61:** 863–866.
8. YOUINOU, P., C. JAMIN & P.M. LYDYARD. 1999. CD5 expression in human B-cell populations. Immunol. Today **20:** 312–316.
9. YOUINOU, P., L.E. MACKENZIE, J. JOUQUAN, *et al.* 1987. CD5-positive B cells in patients with rheumatoid arthritis: phorbol ester-mediated enhancement of detection. Ann. Rheum. Dis. **46:** 17–22.
10. YOUINOU, P., L.E. MACKENZIE, G. LE MASSON, *et al.* 1988. CD5-expressing B lymphocytes in the blood and salivary glands of patients with primary Sjögren's syndrome. J. Autoimmun. **1:** 185–194.
11. PLATER-ZYBERK, C., R.N. MAINI, K. LAM, *et al.* 1985. A rheumatoid arthritis B cell subset expresses a phenotype similar to that in chronic lymphocytic leukemia. Arthritis Rheum. **28:** 971–976.
12. DAUPHINÉE, M., Z. TOVAR & N. TALAL. 1988. B cells expressing CD5 are increased in Sjögren's syndrome. Arthritis Rheum. **31:** 642–647.
13. LYDYARD, P.M., L.E. MACKENZIE, P. YOUINOU, *et al.* 1992. Specificity and idiotype expression of IgM produced by CD5$^+$ and CD5$^-$ cord blood B cells. Ann. N.Y. Acad. Sci. **651:** 527–535.
14. YOUINOU, P., L.E. MACKENZIE, A. LAMOUR, *et al.* 1993. Human CD5-positive B cells in lymphoid malignancy and connective tissue disease. Eur. J. Clin. Invest. **23:** 139–150.
15. BRÖKER, B.M., A. KLAJMAN, P. YOUINOU, *et al.* 1988. Chronic lymphocytic leukemia cells secrete multispecific autoantibodies. J. Autoimmun. **1:** 469–481.
16. KIPPS, T.J., J.H. VAUGHAN. 1987. Genetic influence on the levels of circulating CD5$^+$ B lymphocytes. J. Immunol. **139:** 1060–1064.
17. WORTIS, H.H. & R. BERLAND. 2001. Cutting edge commentary: origins of B-1 cells. J. Immunol. **166:** 2163–2166.
18. HERZENBERG, L.A. 2000. B-1 cells: the lineage question revisited. Immunol. Rev. **175:** 9–19.
19. KANTOR, A. 1991. A new nomenclature for B cells. Immunol. Today **12:** 388–391.
20. KASSIAN, M.T., H. IKEMATSU & P. CASALI. 1992. Identification and analysis of a novel surface CD5-B lymphocyte subset producing natural antibodies. J. Immunol. **148:** 2690–2702.
21. LALOR, P.A., L.A. HERZENBERG, S. ADAMS, *et al.* 1989. Feedback regulation of murine Ly-1B cell development. Eur. J. Immunol. **19:** 507–513.
22. PERS, J.O., C. JAMIN, P.M. LYDYARD, *et al.* 2002. The *H2* haplotype regulates the distribution of B cells into B1a, B1b and B2 subsets. Immunogenetics **54:** 208–211.
23. PERS, J.O., C. JAMIN, P. YOUINOU, *et al.* 2003. Role of IL-10 in the distribution of B cell subsets in the mouse B1 cell population. Eur. Cytokine Netw. **14:** 178–185.
24. DEFRANCE, T., M. CASAMAYOR-PALLEJA & P.H. KRAMMER. 2002. The life and death of a B cell. Adv. Cancer Res. **86:** 195–225.

25. ALLMAN, D., R.C. LINDSLEY, W. DEMUTH, et al. 2001. Resolution of three nonprolifera-
    tive immature splenic B cell subsets reveals multiple selection points during peripheral
    B cell maturation. J. Immunol. **167:** 6834–6840.
26. MARTIN, F. & J.F. KEARNEY. 2002. Marginal-zone B cells. Nat. Rev. Immunol. **2:** 323–335.
27. LIU, Y.J. & C. ARPINC. 1997. Germinal center development. Immunol. Rev. **156:** 111–126.
28. MACLENNAN, I.C.M. 1994. Germinal centers. Annu. Rev. Immunol. **12:** 117–139.
29. GROOM, J., S.L. KALLED, A.H. CUTLER, et al. 2002. Association of BAFF/BLyS over-
    expression and altered B cell differentiation with Sjögren's syndrome. J. Clin. Invest.
    109: 59–68.
30. ROYER, B., D. CAZALS-HATEM, J. SIBILIA, et al. 1997. Lymphomas in patients with
    Sjögren's syndrome are marginal zone B cell neoplasms, arise in diverse extranodal
    and nodal sites, and are not associated with viruses. Blood **90:** 766–775.
31. SALOMONSSON, S., M.V. JONSSON, K. SKARSTEIN, et al. 2003. Cellular basis of ectopic
    germinal center formation and autoantibody production in the target organ of
    patients with Sjögren's syndrome. Arthritis Rheum. **48:** 3187–3201.
32. SCHRÖDER, A.E., A. GREINER, C. SEYFERT, et al. 1996. Differentiation of B cells in the
    nonlymphoid tissue of the synovial membrane of patients with rheumatoid arthritis.
    Proc. Natl. Acad. Sci. U.S.A. **93:** 221–225.
33. ARMENGOL, M.P., M. JUAN, A. LUCAS-MARTIN, et al. 2001. Demonstration of thyroid
    antigen-specific B cells and recombination-activating gene expression in chemokine-
    containing active intrathyroidal germinal centers. Am. J. Pathol. **159:** 861–873.
34. YOUINOU, P., W.J.W. MORROW, A.W. LETTIN, et al. 1984. Specificity of plasma cells in
    the rheumatoid synovium. I. Immunoglobulin class of antiglobulin-producing cells.
    Scand. J. Immunol. **20:** 307–315.
35. CASSESE, G., S. LINDENAU, B. DE BOER, et al. 2001. Inflamed kidney of NZB/w mice
    are a major site for the homeostasis of plasma cells. Eur. J. Immunol. **31:** 2726–2732.
36. TENGNER, P., A.K. HALSE, H.J. HAGA, et al. 1998. Detection of anti-Ro/SSA and anti-
    La/SSB autoantibody-producing cells in salivary glands from patients with Sjögren's
    syndrome. Arthritis Rheum. **41:** 2238–2248.
37. WILLIAM, J., C. EULER, S. CHRISTENSEN, et al. 2002. Evolution of autoantibody
    responses via somatic hypermutation outside the germinal centers. Science **297:**
    2066–2070.
38. GRAMMER, A.C. & P.E. LIPSKY. 2001. CD40-mediated regulation of immune responses
    by TRAF-dependent and TRAF-independent signaling mechanisms. Adv. Immunol.
    76: 61–178.
39. LIU, Y.J. & J. BANCHEREAU. 1996. The paths and molecular controls of peripheral B
    cells development. Immunologist **6:** 55–66.
40. GRAMMER, A.C. & P.E. LIPSKY. 2002. CD154-CD40 interactions mediate differentiation
    to plasma cells in healthy individuals and persons with systemic lupus erythematosus.
    Arthritis Rheum. **46:** 1417–1429.
41. BOHNHORST, J.Ø., M.B. BJØRGAN, J.E. THOEN, et al. 2001. Bm1-Bm5 classification of
    peripheral blood B cells reveals circulating germinal center founder cells in healthy
    individuals and disturbance in the B cell subpopulations in patients with primary
    Sjögren's syndrome. J. Immunol. **167:** 3610–3618.
42. ARCE, E., D.G. JACKSON, M.A. GILL, et al. 2001. Increased frequency of pre-germinal
    center B cells and plasma cell precursors in the blood of children with systemic lupus
    erythematosus. J. Immunol. **167:** 2361–2369.
43. POTTER, K.N., C.I. MOCKRIDGE, A. RAHMAN, et al. 2002. Disturbances in peripheral
    blood B cell subpopulations in autoimmune patients. Lupus **11:** 872–877.
44. HANSEN, A., M. ODENHAHL, K. LE REITER, et al. 2002. Diminished peripheral blood
    memory B celles and accumulation of memory B cells in the salivary glands of
    patients with Sjögren's syndrome. Arthritis Rheum. **46:** 12160–12171.
45. ODENDAHL, M., A. JACOBI, A. HANSEN, et al. 2000. Disturbed peripheral B lymphocyte
    homeostasis in systemic lupus erythematosus. J. Immunol. **165:** 5970–5979.
46. REPARON-SCHUIJT, C., W.E.J. VAN ESCH, C. VAN KOOTEN, et al. 2001. Presence of a
    population of CD20⁺ CD38⁻ lymphocytes with defective proliferative responsiveness
    in the synovial compartment of patients with rheumatoid arthritis. Arthritis Rheum.
    44: 2029–2037.

47. REININGER, L., T. RADASZKIEWICZ, M. KOSCO, *et al.* 1992. Development of autoimmune disease in SCID mice populated with long-term *in vitro* proliferating (NZB×NZW) F1 pre-B cells. J. Exp. Med. **176:** 1343–1353.
48. REININGER, L., T.H. WINKLER, C.P. KALBERER, *et al.* 1996. Intrinsic B cell defects in NZB and NZW mice contribute to systemic lupus erythematosus in (NZB×NZW) F1 mice. J. Exp. Med. **184:** 853–861.
49. CHAN, O.T.M., M.J. SCHLOMCHIK. 1998. A new role for B cells in systemic autoimmunity: B cells promote spontaneous T cell activation in MRL-*lpr/lpr* mice. J. Immunol. **160:** 51–59.
50. CHAN, O.T.M., L.G. HANNUM, A.M. HABERMAN, *et al.* 1999. A novel mouse with B cells but lacking serum antibody reveals an antibody-dependent role for B cells in murine lupus. J. Exp. Med. **189:** 1639–1648.
51. NOORCHASHM, H., N. NOORCHASHM, J. KERN, *et al.* 1997. B cells are required for the initiation of insulitis and sialitis in nonobese diabetic mice. Diabetes **46:** 491–496.
52. DE TOGNI, P., J. GOELLNER, N.H. RUDDLE, *et al.* 1994. Abnormal development of peripheral lymphoid organs in mice deficient in lymphotoxin. Science **264:** 703–707.
53. KAPASI, Z.F., G.F. BURTON, L.D. SHULTZ, *et al.* 1993. Induction of functional follicular dendritic cell development in severe combined immunodeficiency mice influence B and T cells. J. Immunol. **150:** 2648–2658.
54. GONZALEZ, M., F. MACKAY, J.L. BROWNING, *et al.* 1998. The sequential role of lymphotoxin and B cells in the development of splenic follicles. J. Exp. Med. **187:** 997–1007.
55. FLYNN, S., K.M. TOELLNER, C. RAYKUNDALIA, *et al.* 1998. CD4 T cell cytokine differentiation: the B cell activation molecule, OX40 ligand, instructs CD4 T cells to express interleukin-4 and upregulates expression of the chemokine receptor Bbr-1. J. Exp. Med. **188:** 297–304.
56. GOMEZ, D., P.A. CORREA, L.M. GOMEZ, *et al.* 2004. Th1/Th2 cytokines in patients with systemic lupus erythematosus: is tumor necrosis factor alpha protective? Semin. Arthritis Rheum. **33:** 404–413.
57. SCHULTZ, K.R., J.P. KLARNET, R.S. GIENI, *et al.* 1990. The role of B cells for *in vivo* T cell response to a Friend virus-induced leukemia. Science **249:** 921–923.
58. MOHAN, C., L. MOREL, P. YANG, *et al.* 1998. Accumulation of splenic B-1a cell with potent antigen-presenting capability in NZM2410 lupus-prone mice. Arthritis Rheum. **41:** 1652–1662.
59. ROOSNEK, E. & A. LANGEVECCHIA. 1991. Efficient and selective presentation of antigen-antibody complexes by rheumatoid factor B cells. J. Exp. Med. **173:** 487–489.
60. TAKEMURA, S., P.A. KLIMIUK, A. BRAUN, *et al.* 2001. T cell activation in rheumatoid synovium in B cell-dependent. J. Immunol. **167:** 4710–4718.
61. DUSTIN, M.L. & L.B. DUSTIN. 2001. The immunological relay race: B cells take antigen by synapse. Nat. Immunol. **2:** 480–482.
62. LINKER-ISRAELI, M., R.J. DEANS, D.J. WALLACE, *et al.* 1991. Elevated levels of endogenous IL-6 in systemic lupus erythematosus. A putative role in pathogenesis. J. Immunol. **147:** 117–123.
63. MOORE, K.W., R. DE WAAL MALEFYT, R.L. COFFMAN, *et al.* 2001. Interleukin-10 and the interleukin-10 receptor. Ann. Rev. Immunol. **19:** 683–765.
64. O'GARRA, A., R. CHANG, N. GO, *et al.* 1992. Ly-1 B (B-1) cells are the main source of B cell-derived interleukin 10. Eur. J. Immunol. **22:** 711–717.
65. ISHIDA, H., R. HASTINGS, J. KEARNEY, *et al.* 1992. Continuous interleukin-10 antibody administration depletes mice of Ly-1 B cells, but not conventional B cells. J. Exp. Med. **175:** 1213–1220.
66. PENG, B., N.H. MEHTA, H. FERNANDES, *et al.* 1995. Growth inhibition of malignant CD5$^+$ B (B-1) cells by antisense IL-10 oligonucleotide. Leuk. Res. **19:** 159–167.
67. LLORENTE, L., Y. RICHAUD-PATIN, R. FIOR, *et al.* 1994. *In vivo* production of interleukin-10 by non-T cells in rheumatoid arthritis, Sjögren's syndrome and systemic lupus erythematosus: a potential mechanism of B lymphocyte hyperactivity in autoimmunity. Arthritis Rheum. **37:** 1647–1655.
68. LLORENTE, L., Y. RICHAUD-PATIN, C. GARCIA-PADILLA, *et al.* 2003. Clinical and biological effects of anti-interleukine-10 monoclonal antibody administration in systemic lupus erythematosus. Arthritis Rheum. **43:** 1790–1800.

69. MOSMANN, T.R. & S. SAD. 1996. The expanding universe of T-cell subsets: Th1, Th2 and more. Immunol. Today **17:** 138–146.

70. HARRIS, D.P., L. HAYNES, P.C. SAYLES, *et al.* 2000. Reciprocal regulation of polarized cytokine production by effector B and T cells. Nat. Immunol. **1:** 475–482.

71. AMEL KASHIPAZ, M.R., M.L. HUGGINS, P. LANYON, *et al.* 2003. Assessment of Be1 and Be2 cells in systemic lupus erythematosus indicates elevated interleukin-10-producing CD5+ B cells. Lupus **12:** 356–363.

72. HEALY, J.I. & C.C. GOODNOW. 1998. Positive *versus* negative signaling by lymphocyte antigen receptors. Ann. Rev. Immunol. **16:** 645–6770

73. LAM, K.P., R. HÜHN & R. RAJEWSKY. 1997. *In vivo* ablation of surface immunoglobulin on mature B cells by inducible gene targeting results in rapid cell death. Cell **90:** 1073–1083.

74. RENAUDINEAU, Y., S. NÉDELLEC, C. BERTHOU, *et al.* 2005. Role of B cell antigen receptor associated molecules and lipid rafts in CD5-induced apoptosis of B CLL cells. Leukemia **19:** 223–229.

75. NÉDELLEC, S., Y. RENAUDINEAU, C. BERTHOU, *et al.* 2005. B cell response surface IgM cross-linking identifies different prognostic groups of B-chronic lymphocytic leukemia patients. J. Immunol. **174:** 3749–3756.

76. LIOSSIS, S.M.C., B. KOVACS, G. DENNIS, *et al.* 1996. B cells from patients with systemic lupus erythematosus display abnormal antigen receptor-mediated early transduction events. J. Clin. Invest. **98:** 2549–2557.

77. CASCIOLA-ROSEN, L.A., G. ANHALT & A. ROSEN. 1994. Autoantigens targeted in systemic lupus erythematosus are clustered in two populations of surface structures on apoptotic keratinocytes. J. Exp. Med. **179:** 1317–1330.

78. FERRY, H., M. JONES, D.J. VAUX, *et al.* 2003. The cellular location of self-antigen determines the positive and negative selection of autoreactive B cells. J. Exp. Med. **198:** 1415–1425.

79. NITSCHKE, L., R. CARSETTI, B. OCKER, *et al.* 1997. CD22 is a negative regulator of B cell receptor signaling. Curr. Biol. **7:** 133–143.

80. LANKESTER, A.C., G.M.W. VAN SCHIJNDEL, J.L. CORDELL, *et al.* 1994. CD5 is associated with the human B cell antigen receptor complex. Eur. J. Immunol. **24:** 812–816.

81. JAMIN, C., R. LE CORRE, J.O. PERS, *et al.* 1997. Modulation of CD72 by ligation of B cell receptor complex molecules on CD5+ B cells. Int. Immunol. **9:** 1001–1009.

82. JAMIN, C., A. LAMOUR, Y.L. PENNEC, *et al.* 1993. Expression of CD5 and CD72 on T and B cell subsets in rheumatoid arthritis and Sjögren's syndrome. Clin. Exp. Immunol. **92:** 245–250.

83. PERS, J.O., C. JAMIN, R. LE CORRE, *et al.* 1998. Ligation of CD5 on resting B cells, but not on resting T cells, results in apoptosis. Eur. J. Immunol. **28:** 4170–4176.

84. JAMIN, C., R. LE CORRE, P.M. LYDYARD, *et al.* 1996. Anti-CD5 extends the proliferative response of human CD5+ B cells activated with anti-IgM and interleukin-2. Eur. J. Immunol. **26:** 57–62.

85. GERGELY, J. & G. SÁRMAY. 1996. Fc RII-mediated regulation of human B cells. Scand. J. Immunol. **44:** 1–10.

86. HUCK, S., R. LE CORRE, P. YOUINOU, *et al.* 2001. Expression of B cell receptor-associated signaling molecules in human lupus. Autoimmunity **33:** 213–224.

87. BLASIOLI, J. & C.C. GOODNOW. 2002. Lyn/CD22/SHP-1 and their importance in autoimmunity. Curr. Dir. Autoimmun. **5:** 151–160.

88. HATHCOCK, K.S., H. HIRANO, S. MURAKAMI, *et al.* 1992. CD45 expression by B cells. Expression of different isoforms by subpopulations of activated B cells. J. Immunol. **149:** 2286–2294.

89. SATO, S., M. HASEGAWA, M. FUJIMOTO, *et al.* 2000. Quantitative genetic variation in CD19 expression correlates with autoimmunity. Immunology **165:** 6635–6643.

90. HIPPEN, K.L., L.E. TZE & T.W. BEHRENS. 2000. CD5 maintains tolerance in anergic B cells. J. Exp. Med. **191:** 883–889.

91. TIEGS, S.L., D.M. RUSSEL & D. NEMAZEE. 1993. Receptor editing in self-reactive bone marrow B cells. J. Exp. Med. **177:** 1009–1020.

92. OETTINGER, M.A., D.G. SCHATZ, C. GORKA, *et al.* 1990. RAG1 and RAG2, adjacent genes that synergistically activate V(D) recombination. Science **248:** 1517–1523.

93. HAN, S., B. ZHENG, D.G. SCHATZ, *et al.* 1996. Neoteny in lymphocytes: RAG1 and RAG2 expression in germinal center B cells. Science **274:** 2094–2097.
94. HILLION, S., P. YOUINOU & C. JAMIN. 2005. Expression of recombination activating genes in peripheral B cells outside germinal centers is regulated by CD5. J. Immunol. In press.
95. PIERCE, S.K. 2002. Lipid rafts and B cell activation. Nat. Rev. Immunol. **2:** 96–105.
96. CHERUKURI, A., P.C. CHENG, H.W. SOHN, *et al.* 2001. The CD19/CD21 complex functions to prolong B cell antigen receptor signaling from lipid rafts. Immunity **14:** 169–179.
97. AMAN, M.J., A.C. TOSELLO-TRAMPONT & K. RAVICHANDRAN. 2001. Fc RII B1/SHIP-mediated inhibitory signaling in B cells involves lipid rafts. J. Biol. Chem. **276:** 46371–2001.
98. THIEN, M., T.G. PHAN, S. GARDAM, *et al.* 2004. Excess BAFF rescues self-reactive B cells from peripheral deletion and allows them to enter forbidden follicular and marginal zone niches. Immunity **20:** 785–798.
99. JAMIN, C., G. MAGADUR, A. LAMOUR, *et al.* 1991. Cell-free CD5 in patients with rheumatic diseases. Immunol. Lett. **31:** 79–84.
100. RENAUDINEAU, Y., R.A. MAGEED & P. YOUINOU. 2005. An alternative exon 1 of human *cd5* gene regulates CD5 protein expression. Blood. In press.

BAFF Overexpression Is Associated with Autoantibody Production in Autoimmune Diseases

JACQUES-OLIVIER PERS,[a] CAPUCINE DARIDON,[a] VALÉRIE DEVAUCHELLE,[b] SANDRINE JOUSSE,[b] ALAIN SARAUX,[b] CHRISTOPHE JAMIN,[a] AND PIERRE YOUINOU[a]

[a]Department of Immunology and [b]Department of Rheumatology, Brest University Medical School, Brest, France

ABSTRACT: The B-cell activity factor (BAFF) acts as a positive regulator of B-cell function. To gain further insight into the understanding of B-cell hyperactivity in autoimmune diseases, the serum level of BAFF was determined in 43 systemic lupus erythematosus (SLE) patients, 58 primary Sjögren's syndrome (pSS) patients, 28 rheumatoid arthritis (RA) patients, and 68 normal control subjects using an in-house sandwich ELISA. A commercial kit was used to detect soluble CD23 (sCD23) reflecting B-cell activation. In-house assays for the detection of autoantibodies also were used. We found an increased level of BAFF in SLE, pSS, and RA sera compared with normal subjects (respectively, 10.6 ± 8.5, 15.8 ± 12.9, 9.7 ± 1.5 ng/mL vs. 4.6 ± 2.9 ng/mL, $P < .001$). sCD23 released on B-cell activation also was found to be elevated in SLE, pSS, and RA compared with normal sera. However, no correlation was found between the circulating BAFF and the level of sCD23. By contrast, we observed that high levels of BAFF were associated with the presence of autoantibodies (anti–double-stranded DNA antibodies in SLE, anti-SSA antibodies in pSS, and rheumatoid factors in RA). Our data suggest that BAFF is influential in driving antibody production rather than activation of the B lymphocytes in autoimmune diseases.

KEYWORDS: BAFF; autoantibodies; systemic lupus erythematosus; Sjögren's syndrome; rheumatoid arthritis

Polyclonal hyperglobulinemia is a common aspect in non-organ-specific autoimmune diseases, including rheumatoid arthritis (RA), systemic lupus erythematosus (SLE), and primary Sjögren's syndrome (pSS).[1] The profile of autoantibodies in any individual disease is relatively specific, indicating unique pathogenic features for each disease. Nevertheless, the global elevations in serum immunoglobulins (Igs) observed across patients with different connective diseases suggest that common factors contribute to this dysregulation. One of the most potent is the B-cell activity

Address for correspondence: Professor Pierre Youinou, Laboratory of Immunology, Brest University Medical School Hospital, BP824, F29609, Brest, France. Voice: +(33)-2-98-22-33-84; fax: +(33)-2-98-22-38-47.

youinou@univ-brest.fr

Ann. N.Y. Acad. Sci. 1050: 34–39 (2005). © 2005 New York Academy of Sciences.
doi: 10.1196/annals.1313.004

factor of the tumor necrosis factor (TNF) family (BAFF).[2,3] Indeed, BAFF is an effective costimulator of B-cell expansion and function. Recombinant soluble BAFF costimulates B cells *in vitro* to proliferate and secrete Ig,[2–4] and *in vivo* administration of recombinant BAFF to mice promotes B lymphocytosis and hypergammaglobulinemia.[2] Overproduction of BAFF in BAFF transgenic (Tg) mice leads B cells to proliferate, produce autoantibody, and ultimately develop kidney failure similar to that of SLE with respect to the symptoms. Moreover, aging BAFF Tg mice also present a pSS-like disease, demonstrating inflammation and destruction of salivary glands.[5]

In addition to the attendant polyclonal hypergammaglobulinemia, the Tg mice develop elevated titers of multiple autoantibodies, including antinuclear antibodies, anti–double-stranded DNA antibodies (anti-dsDNA), rheumatoid factors (RF), circulating immune complexes, and Ig deposits in kidneys.[6]

These observations raised the possibility that BAFF contributes to B-cell hyperactivity in human non-organ-specific autoimmune diseases. Indeed, elevated levels of BAFF were found in sera from patients with SLE,[7] RA,[8] and pSS.[5] We assessed BAFF levels in sera from patients with SLE, RA, and pSS and showed a correlation with autoantibody titer in these diseases.

SERUM LEVELS OF BAFF ARE INCREASED IN PATIENTS WITH CONNECTIVE TISSUE DISEASES

Using a sandwich enzyme-linked immunosorbent assay (ELISA), we measured the levels of BAFF in the sera of 44 patients with SLE, 28 patients with RA, 58 patients with pSS, and 68 control subjects. All the patients satisfied the diagnostic criteria for the respective disease.[9–11] Control subjects were healthy volunteer donors, sex- and age-matched to the patients. None had connective tissue diseases, RF, anti-nuclear Abs, or anti-Ro (SSA) or anti-La (SSB) Abs. The serum levels of BAFF in all the samples from patients with connective tissue diseases were found to be significantly higher than normal control subjects. Indeed, although the serum BAFF levels in normal control subjects were less than 5 ng/mL, the BAFF levels were higher than 2 standard deviations (SD) above the mean of the control subjects in 23 of 44 patients with SLE ($P < .001$) and in 35 of 58 patients with SS ($P < .001$) (FIG. 1). Of note, levels of BAFF were moderately elevated in sera from patients with RA (9.7 ± 1.4 ng/mL, $P < .05$, compared with normal subjects).

Such results are consistent with other findings.[7,8,12] Variability in serum BAFF levels should not be surprising, given the great heterogeneity among patients with connective tissue diseases. However, murine studies suggest that relatively modest elevations in serum BAFF may be associated with development of clinical disease.[6]

SOLUBLE CD23 DID NOT CORRELATE WITH ABNORMAL PRODUCTION OF BAFF IN CONNECTIVE TISSUE DISEASES

CD23 is a B-cell differentiation and early activation marker expressed on mature B cells that is lost after isotype switching. The soluble form of CD23 (sCD23) is produced by cleavage of the cell surface molecule and may be involved in the regulation

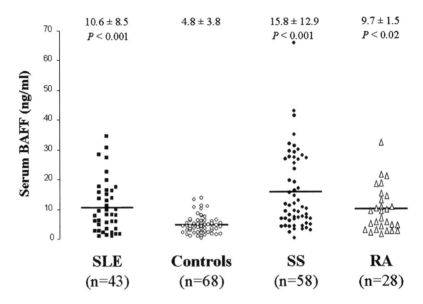

FIGURE 1. Individual serum B-cell activity factor (BAFF) levels in 44 systemic lupus erythematosus (SLE) patients, 58 Sjögren's syndrome (SS) patients, 28 rheumatoid arthritis (RA) patients, and 68 control subjects. Sera were assayed by ELISA based on the use of a monoclonal IgG1 anti-BAFF antibody (Ab) as a capture agent and several layers of poly-clonal Abs as revealing agents. To avoid confounding effects of rheumatoid factor activity, an irrelevant monoclonal IgG1 was required as a negative control. The absorbance values in the monoclonal IgG1 control wells were subtracted from the corresponding anti-BAFF Ab capture wells. The median serum BAFF concentrations (in ng/mL) of each group were as follows: normal, 4.8; SLE, 10.6; SS, 15.8; RA, 9.7.

of IgE production. Elevated levels of sCD23 were found in the sera of patients with enhanced B-cell activation and humoral immunity, including SLE, SS, and RA.[13]

To assess whether B-cell activity was associated with BAFF levels, we evaluated the levels of sCD23 with regard to the levels of BAFF. Although BAFF can function as a B-cell stimulator,[7] BAFF levels did not correlate to that of sCD23 (FIG. 2A). Furthermore, we did not observe any correlation between the sCD23 levels and the autoAbs titers.

INCREASED CIRCULATING BAFF IS ASSOCIATED WITH NON-ORGAN-SPECIFIC AUTOABS IN SLE

To determine whether increased levels of BAFF play a role in the production of autoAbs, the sera of SLE patients were divided into 2 groups according to their BAFF levels. The cutoff level for BAFF was set at 2 SD above the mean of the 68 normal sera, that is, 8.5 ng/mL (TABLE 1).

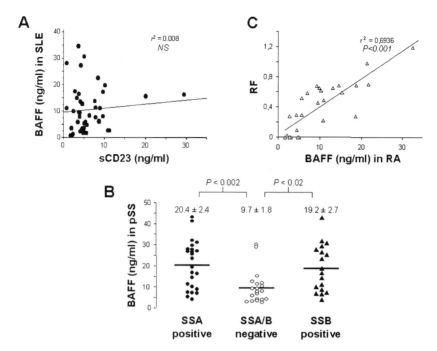

FIGURE 2. Correlation between serum levels of B-cell activity factor (BAFF) and soluble CD23 (sCD23) in systemic lupus erythematosus (SLE), anti-SSA or anti-SSB antibodies (Abs) in primary Sjögren's syndrome (pSS), and rheumatoid factor (RF) in rheumatoid arthritis (RA). **(A)** No correlation between sCD23 and serum level of BAFF was observed for the 44 patients with SLE. **(B)** Among the 58 patients with pSS, BAFF levels were higher in patients with anti-SSA and anti-SSB Abs. **(C)** Correlation between serum levels of BAFF and serum RF (IgM) was evaluated in RA. P values were determined by the Spearman correlation test.

TABLE 1. Antinuclear and related autoantibodies in 44 SLE sera and circulating levels of BAFF

	No. of positive (%)				
	dsDNA	Histone	Cardiolipin	SSA	SSB
Group I ($n = 23$)	13 (57)	11 (48)	11 (48)	2 (9)	2 (9)
Group II ($n = 21$)	5 (24)	4 (19)	4 (19)	1 (5)	1 (5)
Difference	$P < .03$	$P < .05$	$P < .05$	NS	NS

NOTE: The cutoff level for BAFF was set at 2 SD above the mean of 44 normal sera, that is, 8.5 ng/mL. Patients fell into 2 groups: those with elevated level (group I) and those with normal level (group II) of circulating BAFF.

The SLE patients with high levels of BAFF (group I) exhibited significantly higher levels of anti-dsDNA ($P < .03$), antihistone ($P < .05$), and anticardiolipin ($P < .05$) Abs compared with the SLE patients displaying low levels of BAFF (group II). The increased levels of BAFF associated with the production of anti-dsDNA Abs suggest that BAFF might be involved in the B-cell tolerance loss driven by dsDNA in SLE. BAFF might be a primary factor that acts directly on the B cells to drive the production of anti-dsDNA Abs in a T-cell–independent manner. Furthermore, BAFF level appears to be associated with antihistone and anticardiolipin Abs. Because deficiencies in apoptosis can lead to the development of lupus-like disease, BAFF also might play an anti-apoptotic role in B-cell tolerance loss. Indeed, blockades of BAFF function with soluble form of BAFF receptors decrease severely and prolong the survival in animal lupus model.[14]

INCREASED CIRCULATING BAFF IS ASSOCIATED WITH ANTI-SSA OR ANTI-SSB ABS IN PSS AND WITH RF IN RA

In pSS, BAFF levels were higher in patients with anti-SSA Abs ($P < .002$) or with anti-SSB Abs ($P < .02$) compared with patients without detectable levels of these autoAbs (FIG. 2B). In RA, serum RF titers (IgM) were correlated with serum BAFF levels (FIG. 2C) ($P < .0001$), but no association was observed between circulating BAFF and anti-CCP Abs.

Therefore, pro-survival BAFF signaling might counterbalance the pro-apoptotic signals induced by the B-cell receptor (BCR). Maturation occurs only when the survival signals outweigh the death signals. Overexpression of BAFF might disturb the balance. Hence, B cells might be able to survive to stronger death signals triggered by autoantigens. This would lead to the emergence of autoreactive B cells.

B cells from BAFF Tg mice express higher levels of Bcl-2 than those from wild-type mice and might develop autoimmune disorders similar to those of Bcl-2 Tg mice.[15] Consequently, the level of BAFF needs to be tightly regulated to maintain B-cell survival without triggering autoimmunity.

Moreover, excess BAFF level leads to the expansion of a subset of B cells named marginal zone (MZ) B cells,[5] which are able to activate naïve T cells. In addition, expansion of the MZ B-cell population correlates with certain autoimmune diseases. These cells have been detected in inflamed tissues in mice and humans.[16] The most important functional feature of the MZ B cells is their very early participation in immune responses. These properties occur because MZ B cells appear to have a lower stimulating threshold than recirculating immature B cells for activation, proliferation, and differentiation into Ab-secreting cells. Furthermore, MZ B cells are key players in T-independent immune responses. Consequently, further analysis of the BAFF captation effect on these cells obviously should be analyzed. Recently, BAFF was shown to stimulate T-cell activation, another aspect that may contribute to autoimmunity.[17]

New elements about BAFF biology indicate that this factor may be involved in connective tissue diseases, and antagonists of this cytokine are thus likely to provide attractive new treatments of rheumatic diseases.

REFERENCES

1. YOUINOU, P., W. MANGOLD, J. JOUQUAN *et al.* 1987. Organ specific autoantibodies in non-organ-specific autoimmune diseases with special reference to rheumatoid arthritis. Rheumatol. Int. **7:** 123–126.
2. MOORE, P.A., O. BELVEDERE, A. ORR *et al.* 1999. BLyS: member of the tumor necrosis factor family and B lymphocyte stimulator. Science **285:** 260–263.
3. SCHNEIDER, P., F. MACKAY, V. STEINER *et al.* 1999. BAFF, a novel ligand of the tumor necrosis factor family, stimulates B cell growth. J. Exp. Med. **189:** 1747–1756.
4. YAN, M., S.A. MARSTERS, I.S. GREWAL *et al.* 2000. Identification of a receptor for BLyS demonstrates a crucial role in humoral immunity. Nat. Immunol. **1:** 37–41.
5. GROOM, J., S.L. KALLED, A.H. CUTLER *et al.* 2002. Association of BAFF/BLyS overexpression and altered B cell differentiation with Sjögren's syndrome. J. Clin. Invest. **109:** 59–68.
6. MACKAY, F., S.A. WOODCOCK, P. LAWTON *et al.* 1999. Mice transgenic for BAFF develop lymphocytic disorders along with autoimmune manifestations. J. Exp. Med. **190:** 1697–1710.
7. ZHANG, J., V. ROSCHKE, K.P. BAKER *et al.* 2001. Cutting edge: a role for B lymphocyte stimulator in systemic lupus erythematosus. J. Immunol. **166:** 6–10.
8. CHEEMA, G.S., V. ROSCHKE, D.M. HILBERT *et al.* 2001. Elevated serum B lymphocyte stimulator levels in patients with systemic immune-based rheumatic diseases. Arthritis Rheum. **44:** 1313–1319.
9. TAN, E.M., A.S. COHEN, J.F. FRIES *et al.* 1982. The 1982 revised criteria for the classification of systemic lupus erythematosus. Arthritis Rheum. **25:** 1271–1277.
10. ARNETT, F.C., S.M. EDWORTHY, D.A. BLOCH *et al.* 1987. The American Rheumatism Association 1987 revised criteria for the classification of rheumatoid arthritis. Arthritis Rheum. **31:** 315–324.
11. VITALI, C., S. BOMBARDIERI, R. JOUSSON *et al.* 2002. Classification criteria for Sjögren's syndrome: a revised version of the European criteria proposed by the American-European consensus group. Ann. Rheum. Dis. **61:** 554–558.
12. MARIETTE, X., S. ROUX, J. ZHANG *et al.* 2003. The level of BLyS (BAFF) correlates with the titre of autoantibodies in human Sjögren's syndrome. Ann. Rheum. Dis. **62:** 168–171.
13. BANSAL, A., T. ROBERTS, E.M. HAY *et al.* 1992. Soluble CD23 levels are elevated in the serum of patients with primary Sjögren's syndrome and systemic lupus erythematosus. Clin. Exp. Immunol. **89:** 452–455.
14. GROSS, J.A., S. JOHNSTON, R. MUDRI *et al.* 2000. Taci and BCMA are receptors for a TNF homologue implicated in B-cell autoimmune disease. Nature **404:** 995–999.
15. STRASSER, A., S. WHITTINGHAM, D.L. VAUX *et al.* 1991. Enforced BCL2 expression in B-lymphoid cells prolongs antibody responses and elicits autoimmune disease. Proc. Natl. Acad. Sci. USA **88:** 8661–8665.
16. MACKAY, F., F. SIERRO, S.T. GREY *et al.* 2005. The BAFF/APRIL System: an important player in systemic rheumatic diseases. Curr. Dir. Autoimmun. **8:** 234–265.
17. NG, L.G., A.P. SUTHERLAND, R. NEWTON *et al.* 2004. B cell-activating factor belonging to the TNF family (BAFF)-R is the principal BAFF receptor facilitating BAFF costimulation of circulating T and B cells. J. Immunol. **173:** 807–817.

Histo-Blood Group Antigens as Allo- and Autoantigens

URS E. NYDEGGER,[a] HENDRIK TEVAEARAI,[a] PASCAL BERDAT,[a]
ROBERT RIEBEN,[b] THIERRY CARREL,[a] PAUL MOHACSI,[b]
AND WILLY A. FLEGEL[c]

[a]Clinic for Cardiovascular Surgery, University Hospital/Inselspital, Bern, Switzerland

[b]Swiss Cardiovascular Center, Bern, Switzerland

[c]Department of Transfusion Medicine, University Hospital, Ulm, Germany

ABSTRACT: The science of blood groups has made giant steps forward during the last decade. Blood-group typing of red blood cells (RBCs) is performed on more than 15 million samples per year in Europe, today much less often for forensic reasons than for clinical purposes such as transfusion and organ transplantation. Specific monoclonal antibodies are used with interpretation on the basis of RBC agglutination patterns, and mass genotyping may well be on its way to becoming a routine procedure. The discovery that most blood group systems, whose antigens are by definition found on RBCs, are also expressed in multiple other tissues has sparked the interest of transplantation medicine in immunohematology beyond the HLA system. The one and only "histo-blood group" (HBG) system that is routinely considered in transplantation medicine is ABO, because ABO antigen–incompatible donor/recipient constellations are preferably avoided. However, other HBG systems may also play a role, thus far underestimated. This paper is an up-to-date analysis of the importance of HBG systems in the alloimmunity of transplantation and autoimmune events, such as hemolytic anemia.

KEYWORDS: ABO; alloimmunity; antigen; autoimmune; disease; histo-blood group (HBG); immune complex; red blood cell (RBC)

INTRODUCTION

During most of the last century, blood groups were regarded as "peripheral" blood groups in the strict sense of the word. In fact, they were considered antigenic structures on the surface of circulating red blood cells (RBCs) only, where they were initially discovered, although several of them were later found on white blood cells and platelets as well. With the discovery in the mid-20th century of the human leukocyte antigen (HLA) system on human leukocytes, the strict separation of blood

Address for correspondence: Urs E. Nydegger, M.D., Clinic for Cardiovascular Surgery, Inselspital, CH-3010 Bern, Switzerland. Voice: +41-31-6322329; fax: +41-31-6322919; or Willy A. Flegel, M.D., Department of Transfusion Medicine, University Hospital Ulm, Helmholtzstrasse 10, D-89081 Ulm, Germany. Voice: +49-731-150600; fax: +49-731-150602.

urs.nydegger@insel.ch; waf@ucsd.edu

Ann. N.Y. Acad. Sci. 1050: 40–51 (2005). © 2005 New York Academy of Sciences.
doi: 10.1196/annals.1313.006

TABLE 1. Tissue distribution of selected blood group systems among the 29 recognized systems according to ISBT numerical and system name terminology

ISBT no.	System name	System symbol	Blood cells other than RBC or in soluble form	Solid tissues: histological localization
001	ABO	ABO	WBCs, T cells, etc., on many plasma proteins and in soluble form	Universally expressed on most epithellial and endothelial cells; aberrant expression often observed in malignant cells
002	MNS	MNS	None	None
003	P	P1		Endothelial cells, fibroblasts, smooth muscle cells of digestive tract and urogenital tissue, interstitial cells of human placenta, tumor cells
004	Rhesus	RH	None	None
005	Lutheran	LU	WBCs, T cells	Basal layer of epithelium and endothelium of blood vessels
006	Kell	KEL		Erythroid tissue and testis, brain, heart, skeletal muscle
008	Duffy	FY		Endothelial cells of capillary and post-capillary venules, epithelial cells of kidney collecting ducts, lung alveoli, and Purkinje cells of cerebellum
009	Kidd	JK		Renal medulla
010	Diego	DI		Bone tissue, inner ear (?)
014	Dombrock	DO		Erythroid cells in adult bone marrow or fetal liver, lymph nodes, testes, spleen, fetal heart
015	Colton	CO		Original example of the aquaporin (AQP) family of water channel proteins AQP1: proximal tubules of nephron capillaries, ciliary and lens epithelium, hepatic bile ducts, gall bladder
017	Chido/ Rogers	CH/RG	Plasma protein passively adsorbed onto blood cells	Synthesized primarily by liver monocytes/macrophages
020	Gerbich	GE	Erythroid tissue	Wide variety of tissues including fetal liver and renal endothelium
021	Cromer	CROM	WBCs, T cells soluble in plasma and urine	Apical surfaces of trophoblasts in placenta, endothelial and epithelial tissues
022	Knops	KN	B cells	Follicular dendritic cells

NOTE: The classification of blood group systems is defined by the ISBT Committee on Terminology of Red Blood Cell Antigens (http://www.iccbba.com/ppage107.htm).

cell antigens from tissue antigens began to stagger. The emerging organ transplantation medicine began to see HLA as alloantigens that need to be typed in donor and recipient tissues, because a perfect match of its highly polymorphic antigens would form the basis for prolonged graft survival. In the 1960s, the pioneers of organ transplantation, among them Thomas Starzl, recognized the *noli me tangere* of the ABO system. Indeed, it was thought (and it still may be so) that strict adherence to ABO identity/compatibility was mandatory lest hyperacute rejection result. However a few reports surprisingly described the absence of immediate or delayed problems after transplantation of ABO-incompatible organs.[1,2] Indeed, in some ABO-incompatible kidney transplantations, the graft was flushed with large volumes of preservative solution before being transplanted. It was believed that the most hidden RBCs remaining in the donor kidney glomeruli could thus be eliminated.[1]

The International Society of Blood Transfusion (ISBT) Committee on Terminology of Red Blood Cell Antigens recognized in its latest summary 29 different blood group systems of either carbohydrate or proteinaceous constitution[3] (TABLE 1). By definition, all display various degrees of allogeneic polymorphism (FIG. 1). Many systems are now recognized as having either physiologic (e.g., the protein expressed by the Kell system is an enzyme) or pathological (e.g., the Duffy protein is a receptor for *Plasmodium vivax*) functions.[4] Using oligonucleotide arrays we will very soon be able to genotype the majority of clinically relevant alleles of the ABO, Rhesus, Kell, Duffy, Kidd, MNS, Diego, Colton, and Dombrock systems on a single slide. A multicentric evaluation of this new technique is in progress (e.g., http://www.bloodgen.com).

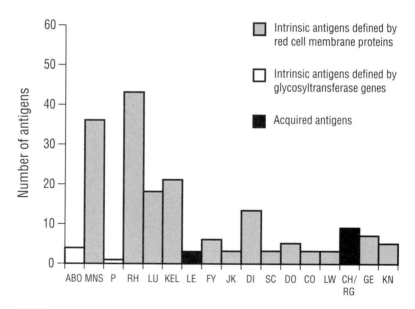

FIGURE 1. Twenty-three important blood group systems with their assigned antigens. Blood group systems are listed by their abbreviations on the abscissa (see also TABLE 1). The corresponding number of known alloantigens in a given blood group system reflecting its polymorphism is shown on the ordinate.

TABLE 2. Links for histo-blood group information on the Internet

URL	Comment
http://www.bioc.aecom.yu.edu/bgmut/index.htm	Olga Blumenfeld's excellent work on blood groups is an ideal introduction to the field.
http://www.iccbba.com/ppage107.htm	Classification of blood group systems and antigens according to the International Society of Blood Transfusion (ISBT) Committee on Terminology of Red Blood Cell Antigens.
http://jove.prohosting.com/~scarfex/blood/groups.html	The Web site of the immunohematologists' exchange group explains blood groups for the public audience.
http://www.uni-ulm.de/~wflegel/RH/	The Rhesus Site details research-grade immunohematologic and genetic results in the field of the RH blood group.
http://www.immune-complex.ch	This is the Web site to explore the consequences of immune complex formation in organ rejection.
http://www.ncbi.nlm.nih.gov/entrez/	Online Mendelian Inheritance in Man (OMIM) via PubMed: select the OMIM option in "search" and fill in the topic (e.g., "ABO system") at the "for" prompt.

Such typing has the advantage of being independent of analytical antibodies with their variable properties, that is, affinity, titer, and agglutinating capacity. The polymorphic forms that occur with a high incidence in all populations worldwide are products of a restricted number of different alleles of common genes displaying variable incidences (from less than 0.1% to as much as 99%); rare alleles are often associated with defined geographic and/or ethnic distributions. Several Web sites provide the investigator with details on the biological and medical aspects of the different blood group systems (TABLE 2). The data are based on identification of blood group phenotypes using analytical antibodies with known specificity and, thus, in most cases, focus on DNA variations that occur within or affect the extracellular regions of the expressed protein, or that affect sugars. So far, all information indicates that each serological phenotype (common or rare) corresponds to a particular mutation(s) or DNA alteration. Hence, each serological phenotype can be attributed to one or more distinct alleles of the underlying blood group gene.

By definition, blood group genes are expressed in erythroid tissues. Their products are membrane-associated proteins or sugars. In the case of proteins, they themselves represent the antigens. In the case of glycosyltransferases these enzymes synthesize membrane-associated sugars that represent the antigenic epitopes. In a few cases the gene product is adsorbed to the RBC surface from plasma (e.g., Lewis and Chido-Rodgers antigens).

The prime reason for this review is that recent findings show a wider distribution of blood group antigens in human and animal organs, although blood group antigens remain largely confined to erythroid tissues. Blood group antigens with a wider organ distribution are often found on nonerythroid blood cells, on membrane surfaces of solid organ tissues as well in soluble form in various body fluids (TABLE 2). Here, we refrain from discussing their role in transfusion medicine because this topic has been covered extensively in the transfusion literature. We set out to analyze the importance of blood groups in autoimmunity and tissue transplantation.

EXPRESSION OF HISTO-BLOOD GROUPS IN TISSUE

Ever since the discovery of the ABO system by Landsteiner in 1900, researchers have aimed at defining the biochemical properties of the A, B, AB, and O(H) antigens. The first attempts to isolate these antigens from RBCs were not successful because the antigens are insoluble in water and elutions yield only minute quantities compared with ABH antigens, for example, in glandular secretions, in ovarian cysts, and in epithelia. Therefore, the first successful purification of ABH substances was from mucin and, later on, ABH-associated glyosphingolipids or membrane proteins bound to polylactosaminoglycanes derived from tissues. At that point investigators were prompted by their observations to propose the term "histo-blood group (HBG) antigens".

In most cases, the expression of all erythroid polymorphic structures that represent blood group antigens, common or rare, is compatible with a normal physiologic function. A rather broad literature has emerged on ABO antigens that represent receptor structures for pathogens, for example, viruses such as norovirus.[5] In most cases, the absence of an erythroid gene product (serologic null phenotype) does not cause disease; at this time, information is lacking as to whether the same is true for products, or lack of products, of nonerythroid alleles. Nevertheless, alleles of erythroid genes that express a common blood group phenotype may also be associated with disease.[6] Because the Duffy blood group protein is a *Plasmodium vivax* receptor, the majority of African and American black people do not express the antigen on their RBCs, rendering them resistant to *P. vivax* invasion and with an advantage in surviving infection. Besides the erythroid system, this Duffy antigen receptor for chemokines (DARC) is expressed in microvascular endothelial and epithelial cells of different nonerythroid tissues, including brain tissues.[7]

The erythroid phenotypes can be assessed readily by serology. Hence, documentation of their incidence and distribution exists for a large number of world populations. The resulting information is fragmented, as many populations have not been tested, particularly for the presence of the rare alleles. Although serological analysis remains a powerful tool for identifying variant individuals to examine and to study their variant alleles, genotyping becomes an important option for identification of many new alleles, as in the ABO and RH systems.

The expression of all polymorphic erythroid forms, and certainly those present in solid tissues (FIG. 2), is independent of nongenetic factors such as age and environment.

ALLOIMMUNE HISTO-BLOOD GROUP ANTIGENS

Deducing the existence of HBG antigens from Landsteiner's discovery of ABO, discovery of further systems on the basis of existing isoagglutinins with specificities other than ABO would have been logical. One may be startled by the fact that the ABO HBG remains the only HBG system with naturally occurring antibodies against non-self. Therefore, discovery of further systems would have remained intricate had allogeneic blood transfusion not become a standard treatment for acute or therapy-resistant chronic anemias, such as thalassemia or hemophilia. In addition to hemophiliacs, such as Mr. Duffy, childbearing women like Mrs. Kellacher produced alloantibodies that prompted the discovery of the respective blood group systems on

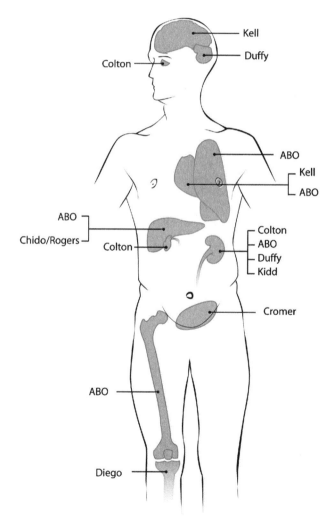

FIGURE 2. Organ distribution of the histo-blood groups. A schematic representation for the distribution of histo-blood group systems in human tissues is shown. The histo-blood group systems are selected based on their possible importance for solid organ transplantation, and their major organ allocations are depicted.

the basis of inefficient transfusions and hemolytic disease of the newborn. With hemolysis, the alloantigens easily reach organized lymphatic tissue and secondary lymphoid organs, with ensuing complement-activating alloantibody synthesis of the IgG class.

With many of the HBG systems being expressed in tissues (FIG. 2), anti-HBG alloantibodies may play a role in solid organ transplantation. The passenger lymphocytes transplanted along with resident solid organs of preterminally hypertransfused or alloimmunized cadaveric organ donors may continue to produce alloantibody in the recipient and contribute to hemolysis[8] or organ damage. In addition, ABO incompatibility may lead to polyclonal B cell activation that spurs formation of autoantibodies, for example, islet cell autoantibodies.[9]

HISTO-BLOOD GROUP ANTIGENS IN ALLOTRANSPLANTATION

The major polymorphic antigen system thus far attributed with the greatest importance in allotransplantation is the human leukocyte antigen (HLA) system, originally found on peripheral blood leukocytes.[10] The HLA complex on chromosome 6 comprises over 200 genes, more than 40 of which encode leukocyte antigen class I genes expressed by most somatic cells, although the level of expression varies in different tissues.[11] Whereas HLA class II antigens mainly serve to present peptides to CD4[+] lymphocytes,[12] and hence are predominantly represented on antigen-presenting cells, the proteins encoded by the class III region are found on the membrane surfaces of such diverse cells as lymphoid and epithelial cells, fibroblasts, and hepatocytes, as well as on the cells of many organs such as adrenal gland, liver, and testis, and can be induced ubiquitously by heat shock stimuli.[13]

The fate of expression of further HBGs (TABLE 2, FIG. 2) after transfusion has drawn little attention, given the fact that with disappearance of transfused RBCs the introduced HBGs disappear as well. Certainly, hypertransfusion of one given allo-antigen often induces antibodies, but the fate of the antigen is concealed. In contrast, transplanted solid organs may give rise to different dynamics insofar as their associated HBGs, an aspect thus far largely ignored by the transplant community. Depending on the protein or carbohydrate nature of the HBGs, the former antigens may continue to be expressed as they were in the donor body, as the cells expressing them are part and parcel of the transplanted organ. However, in the case of carbohydrate antigens, the glycosysltransferases, such as FUT1 (encodes H), FUT2 (encodes secretor phenotype), and FUT3 (encodes Lewis), are the gene products, and the blood group antigen is the synthesized sugar. Hence, the transplanted organ is exposed to the glycosyltransferase environment of the recipient, which may well affect the transplant's HBG phenotype.

The role of the ABO system in allotransplantation has now been expanded by the possibility that ABO-incompatible transplants may escape rejection and undergo adaptation.[14] This view is supported by two lines of evidence, namely accidental and elective ABO-incompatible transplants, the latter mainly occurring with living-donor kidneys. For example, a B→O heart transplantation in 1997 led the HBG type of the allograft to change to that of the recipient by the year 2000.[15] In infants, such ABO conversion from donor to recipient following ABO-incompatible heart transplantation in the context of a trial was not apparent, and donor antigen persistence lasted for as long as four years after B→O transplantation.[16] Such situations, so far accidental in adults, might be safeguarded by IVIG-bolus and plasmapheresis to reduce the cytotoxicity of anti-A/B;[17] we expect further examples of ABO change to be reported in the coming years.

AUTOIMMUNE HISTO-BLOOD GROUP ANTIGENS

The prime example of HBG antigen drifting towards autoimmunity is auto-immune hemolytic anemia (AIHA). It occurs either as an elusive side event to under-lying autoimmune disease, for example, systemic lupus erythematosus, or on its own. Explanations for such an event by various immunologists have attempted to ad-dress the sudden transgression of quantitative and temporal thresholds that normally preclude progression from physiologic autoimmunity to aggressive, clinically overt autoimmunity, as well as the loss of immune surveillance. An explanation may be derived at least in part from peptide sequence similarities between HBGs and infec-tious antigens, or by interactions of certain drugs with the red blood cell membrane that result in antibody production against the RBC, causing hemolytic anemia. Although molecular mimicry of RBC antigens by drugs has not been found so far, penicillin-type immune hemolysis involves penicilloyl fixation to RBCs and formation of a neoantigen, antibodies against which lead to reduced survival time of penicilloyl-coated RBCs. The myelosuppressive effect of infection is induced by bacterial products and/or viral assault of hematopoietic progenitors. Parvovirus B19 induces aplastic anemia via recruitment of autoreactivity against hematopoietic cells.[18] Sim-ilarities between peptide sequences of the infectious agent and of self-antigens lead to the concept that the highly specific T cell recognition fails to distinguish between the infectious agent and self, the T cell thus becoming a victim of molecular mimicry, that is, T cell receptor cross-reactivity involving peptides from an infectious agent and a self-antigen.[19] This is even more important, because autoantibodies present autoantigens to autoaggressive T cells in the form of immune complexes,[20] and con-sequently may trigger or enhance autoimmune disease. Identification of immuno-dominant regions in autoantigens by means of epitopic footprinting reveals autoantigen immunogenicity, either by a costimulatory viral peptide or by bystander T cell help. This has been suggested recently using human thyroperoxidase antigens as an example relevant in human autoimmune thyroiditis.[21,22] Prevailing peptide se-quences associated with anion channel band 3 protein have been identified that bear the helper epitope in hemolytic anemia in NZB mice.[22] The loss of immunological tolerance in adults against RBC antigens has been discussed recently elsewhere.[23]

THE IMMUNE SYSTEM PREVENTS AUTOIMMUNE DISEASE AS EXEMPLIFIED BY ANTI-GLYCOTOPE ANTIBODIES

Since 1969. naturally occurring anti-A and anti-B antibodies of IgM and IgG type have been known to be induced by, for example, *Escherichia coli*–associated ABO and H glycotopes that immunize the gut-associated lymphoid system (GALT).[24] This occurs despite the various bacterial species comprising normal intestinal flora having some capacity to provoke mucosal inflammation. In fact, normally, regulatory

T cells may drive nonresponsiveness to commensal enteric baceria.[25] Tolerance to self-antigens is more complete in T than in B lymphocytes, and low-affinity auto-antibodies, usually germ-line encoded, are frequently detected in normal individuals. The appearance of anti-A and anti-B antibodies in the circulation of those individuals not expressing the cognate antigen thus have a bacterial etiology. At present, we disregard whether anti-A and anti-B antibodies are not among the natural antibodies produced by B1 lymphocytes, albeit their formation no doubt occurs permanently during life in the absence of T cell help. CD5+ helpers and ABO-type oligosaccharides also induce Ig isotypes other than IgM, probably because these antigens stimulate cytokine production. For instance, in humans, the dominant antibody class against pneumoccocal capsular polysaccharide is IgG_2 and the anti-carbohydrate antibodies in humans extend to such specificities as *Salmonella, Klebsiella,* and *Clostridia.*[26] Once class switch recombination (CRS) and somatic hypermutation (SHM) have resulted in a "one and only" specific lymphocytic cell clone, such cells form part of a storage compartment endowed with memory. The memory pool is composed of part of the progeny of antigen-stimulated B and T cells that have never differentiated into effector cells, that is, quiescent memory lymphocytes.

We have analyzed anti-A and anti-B antibodies as part of a naturally occurring pool, that is, those referred to as being synthesized during the whole of life owing to the perpetual presence of *E. coli* in the gut. One might be astonished with the consistency of individual antibody production patterns. Applying the relatively simple technique of spectrotype analysis using immune electropheresis/affinity immuno-blotting, we were able to reveal the spectrotypes of anti-A, anti-B, and gal α1-3gal antibodies[27] (anti-Gal). Whereas the naturally occurring IgM displayed a similar, if not identical, pattern among different blood donors, the naturally occurring IgG pattern showed wide interindividual variability, reflecting the individual constitution of the CSR and SHM mechanisms among the donors. In serum samples taken from the same normal donor six months apart, the banding pattern of anti-Gal IgM/IgG remained unchanged.

Detection of the spectrotypes of anti-Gal IgM kappa and lambda chains revealed more or less individually distinctive banding patterns with polyclonal bands at pH 4.5 to 7. The VH_2f gene family involvement in the generation of anti-Gal, which is also involved in the generation of antibodies against bacterial pathogens, could mean that spontaneous autoimmunity against ABH antigens on RBCs is extremely rare.[27] The continuous presence of large amounts of *E. coli* and the carbohydrate composition of the ABO and H antigens do not explain on their own their inability to induce autoimmunity. Rather, the explanation of the noninitiating immunopathogenicity of self-reactive anti-A and anti-B antibodies has had to wait some years, and is based today on two major pillars—(i) *Self-tolerance at the B cell level*: Using the potent EL4 thymoma cells for B cell stimulation, we were able to show that either a highly resistant anergic state or clonal deletion of self-A/B histo-blood group–specific human B cells accounts for the downregulation of potentially self-reactive anti-A/B.[28] In agreement with this finding, it was recently shown that ABO-incompatible heart transplantation during infancy results in B cell tolerance to A/B antigens as well.[16] (ii) *Anti-idiotypic inhibition of self-reactive anti-A/B*: It was shown that IgG antibodies reactive with autologous ABO purified by affinity chromatography from IgG of individuals of blood group A exhibited an affinity for A trisaccharide antigen and agglutinated A red cells. Whereas autoantibodies reactive with self-A and self-B antigens are readily detected in purified IgG and IgM fractions, their expression is restricted in whole serum as a result of complementary interactions between variable regions of antibodies.[29] Such anti-idiotypic downregulation is a very potent mechanism, as appropriate pooling of A, B, and AB plasma results in a plasma pool with antiA/B titers < 1:4 and can be exploited at least in part for the production of Uniplas, a plasma product that is universally transfusable irrespective of the ABO type of the recipient. These observations indicate that tolerance to autologous ABO blood group antigens becomes suppressed by the above-described second pillar, that is, an anti-idiotype–mediated peripheral control of antibody autoreactivity. Preventing autoimmunity against these antigens in the pathogenetic version is mediated by regulatory T cells.

HISTO-BLOOD GROUP ANTIGENS IN AUTOIMMUNE DISEASE

Rarely does a series of epitopes lend itself so ideally to the study of autoimmunity as in the case of blood group antigens because of their overtly exposed expression on RBCs. AIHA is an example offering two major types of reactants: warm- or cold-reactive autoantibodies, the former being RBC-directed immune responses that are maximally reactive at 37°C. Typical specificities of this type of autoantibody are anti-e, anti-E, anti-C, and anti-D, that is, directed mostly at proteinaceous rhesus-type antigens that occur exclusively on RBCs but not in tissue. Such antibodies are poor inducers of clinically overt anemia; rather, they accompany autoimmune conditions such as lupus or idiopathic thrombocytopenic purpura, and malignant hematologic neoplasms. In their animal counterpart, NZB/W lupus-prone mice start their disease with autoimmune hemolytic anemia, then develop proteinuria.[30] With Evans syndrome, the autoantibody is also directed against platelets. In contrast to warm-reactive antibodies, the cold-reactive ones, cold agglutinins, predominantly react with carbohydrate-type RBC antigens, that is, Ii, MN, and P. The P-reactive cold agglutinins recognize either the P1 antigen or the Pr cryptantigen exposed on RBCs more readily after papain treatment. In fact, treatment of RBCs with this enzyme is known to remove sialic acid–rich compounds from the surface, including T antigen. Thus, the sialic acid–binding immunoglobulin superfamily lectins (Siglecs) have allowed confirmation of the sialic acid dependency of the binding of certain (auto)antibodies.[31] This makes such antibodies resemble the protective antibodies induced by vaccination with some bacterial polysaccharides (see above). Bacterial pathogens evade immune surveillance by decorating their surfaces with polysaccharides that share extensive structural homology with human tissue antigens, again provoking molecular mimicry.[32]

ACKNOWLEDGMENTS

We acknowledge the artwork by Beatrice Boog (AUM–Division of Instructional Media, University of Bern) and Christian Langenegger (Inselspital Bern, FGZ).

W. A. Flegel shared the 2004 Philip Levine–Prize for his work on the molecular genetics of the rhesus blood group system.

REFERENCES

1. STARZL, T.E., T.L. MARCHIORO, J.J. HOLMES, et al. 1964. Renal homografts in patients with major donor-recipient blood group incompatibilities. Surgery **55:** 195–200.
2. GORDON, R.D., S. IWATSUKI, C.O. ESQUIVEL, et al. 1986. Liver transplantation across ABO blood groups. Surgery **100:** 342–348.
3. DANIELS, G.L., A. FLETCHER, G. GARRATTY, et al. 2004. Blood group terminology 2004: from the International Society of Blood Transfusion committee on terminology for red cell surface antigens. Vox Sang. **87:** 304–316.
4. CARTRON, J.P. & Y. COLIN. 2001. Structural and functional diversity of blood group antigens. Transfus. Clin. Biol. **8:** 163–199.
5. HUTSON, A.M., R.L. ATMAR, D.M. MARCUS & M.K. ESTES. 2003. Norwalk virus-like particle hemagglutination by binding to h histo-blood group antigens. J. Virol. **77:** 405–415.
6. NYDEGGER, U.E., W.A. WUILLEMIN, F. JULMY, et al. 2003. Association of ABO histo-blood group B allele with myocardial infarction. Eur. J. Immunogenet. **30:** 201–206.
7. CHAUDHURI, A., G. YUEN, F. FANG & J. STORRY. 2004. Development of Duffy transgenic mouse: in vivo expression of human Duffy gene with 33T→C promoter mutation in non-erythroid tissues. Br. J. Haematol. **127:** 356–360.
8. FUNG, M.K., H. SHEIKH, B. EGHTESAD & I. LOPEZ-PLAZA. 2004. Severe hemolysis resulting from D incompatibility in a case of ABO-identical liver transplant. Transfusion **44:** 1637–1639.
9. ELFVING, A.M., B.A. LINDBERG, M. LANDIN-OLSSON, et al. 2003. Islet cell autoantibodies in cord blood from children with blood group incompatibility or hyperbilirubinemia. Autoimmunity **36:** 111–115.
10. OPELZ, G. & T. WUJCIAK. 1994. The influence of HLA compatibility on graft survival after heart transplantation. The Collaborative Transplant Study. N. Engl. J. Med. **330:** 816–819.
11. KLEIN, J. & A. SATO. 2000. The HLA system. First of two parts. N. Engl. J. Med. **343:** 702–709.
12. ZINKERNAGEL, R.M. 1997. Cellular immune recognition and the biological role of major tranplantation antigens. Scand. J. Immunol. **46:** 421–436.
13. MILNER, C.M., B. AGUADO & R.D. CAMPBELL. 1998. HLA class III region. In Encyclopedia of Immunology, 2nd edn. Vol. 2, pp. 1114–1121. Academic Press. San Diego.
14. GALILI, U. 2004. Immune response, accommodation, and tolerance to transplantation carbohydrate antigens. Transplantation **78:** 1093–1098.
15. KOESTNER, S.C., A. KAPPELER, T. SCHAFFNER, et al. 2004. Histo-blood group type change of the graft from B to O after ABO mismatched heart transplantation. Lancet **363:** 1523–1525.
16. FAN, X., A. ANG, S.M. POLLOCK-BARZIV, et al. 2004. Donor-specific B-cell tolerance after ABO-incompatible infant heart transplantation. Nat. Med. **10:** 1227–1233.
17. MARIOKA, D., H. SEKIDO, K. KUBOTA, et al. 2004. Antibody-mediated rejection after adult ABO-incompatible liver transplantation remedied by gamma-globulin bolus infusion combined with plasmapheresis. Transplantation **78:** 1225–1228.
18. SEVERIN, M.C. & Y. SHOENFELD. 2004. Parvovirus B19 infection and its association with autoimmune disease. In Infection and Autoimmunity. Elsevier. Amsterdam.
19. WUCHERPFENNIG, K.W. 2004. Implications of T cell receptor crossreactivity for the pathogenesis of autoimmune diseases. In Infection and Autoimmunity, pp. 7–18. Elsevier. Amsterdam.
20. NYDEGGER, U.E. 2004. Immune complexes. In Kelley's Textbook of Rheumatology. Vol. 1, pp. 332–341. Elsevier/Saunders. Philadelphia.
21. BRESSON, D., M. PUGNIERE, F. ROQUET, et al. 2004. Directed mutagenesis in region 713-720 of human thyroperoxidase assigns 713KFPED717 residues as being involved in the B domain of the discontinuous immunodominant region recognized by human autoantibodies. J. Biol. Chem. **279:** 39058–39067.
22. SHEN, C.R., A.R. YOUSSEF, A. DEVINE, et al. 2003. Peptides containing a dominant T-cell epitope from red cell band 3 have in vivo immunomodulatory properties in NZB mice with autoimmune hemolytic anemia. Blood **102:** 3800–3806.

23. FAGIOLO, E. 2004. Immunological tolerance loss vs. erythrocyte self antigens and the cytokine network disregulation in autoimmune hemolytic anemia. Autoimmun. Rev. **3:** 53–59.
24. SPRINGER, G.F. & R.E. HORTON. 1969. Blood group isoantibody stimulation in man by feeding blood group-active bacteria. J. Clin. Invest. **48:** 1280–1291.
25. CONG, Y., C.T. WEAVER, A. LAZENBY & C.O. ELSON. 2002. Bacterial-reactive T regulatory cells inhibit pathogenic immune responses to the enteric flora. J. Immunol. **169:** 6112–6119.
26. NYDEGGER, U. 2004. Nature bundles immunoglobulin iso-allo and idiotype to target adaptive immune response. Transfus. Med. Hemother. **31:** 143–150.
27. TINGUELY, C., M. SCHALLER, T. CARREL & U.E. NYDEGGER. 2002. Spectrotype analysis and clonal characteristics of human anti-Gal alpha1-3Gal antibodies. Xenotransplantation **9:** 252–259.
28. RIEBEN, R., A. TUCCI, U.E. NYDEGGER & R.H. ZUBLER. 1992. Self tolerance to human A and B histo-blood group antigens exists at the B cell level and cannot be broken by potent polyclonal B cell activation in vitro. Eur. J. Immunol. **22:** 2713–2717.
29. SPALTER, S.H., S.V. KAVERI, E. BONNIN, *et al.* 1999. Normal human serum contains natural antibodies reactive with autologous ABO blood group antigens. Blood **93:** 4418–4424.
30. HELYER, B.J. & J.B. HOWIE. 1963. Spontaneous auto-immune disease in NZB/W mice. Br. J. Hematol. **9:** 119–131.
31. BRINKMAN-VAN DER LINDEN, E.C. & A. VARKI. 2003. Probing masked and unmasked siglecs on cell surfaces. Methods Enzymol. **363:** 113–120.
32. MACKENZIE, C.R. & H.J. JENNINGS. 2003. Characterization of polysaccharide conformational epitopes by surface plasmon resonance. Methods Enzymol. **363:** 340–354.

The Mechanism of Molecular Redundancy in Autoimmune Inflammation in the Context of CD44 Deficiency

DAVID NAOR,[a] SHLOMO NEDVETZKI,[a] NATHALIE ASSAYAG,[a] ROBIN L. THURMOND,[b] JING-FENG HUANG,[b] AND EVA A. TURLEY[c]

[a]The Lautenberg Center for General and Tumor Immunology, Hebrew University–Hadassah Medical School, Jerusalem, Israel

[b]Johnson & Johnson, Pharmaceutical Research and Development, L. L. C., San Diego, California, USA

[c]London Regional Cancer Center, University of Western Ontario, London, Ontario, Canada

ABSTRACT: Molecular redundancy refers to the ability of genes to back up damaged genes or gene loss. Although this term is widely discussed in many scientific circles, the process is still ill-defined, as shown by reviewing examples from the literature. Exploring the collagen-induced arthritis model in the context of CD44 knockout mice, we suggest a mechanistic explanation for molecular redundancy that depends neither on upregulation of the compensating molecule nor on structural similarity between the original molecule and the replacement molecule. The backup process is dependent, however, on two key properties shared by the two molecules: ligand binding and support of cell trafficking.

KEYWORDS: CD44; molecular redundancy; collagen; gene; inflammation

INTRODUCTION

Molecular redundancy is a term assigned to the ability of multiple ligands, substrates, or transcription factors to interact with a single receptor, enzyme, or DNA recognition element and vice versa. Thus, the product of the damaged gene can be replaced by the redundant molecule and the relevant biological function is preserved. It has been assumed that a simple Darwinian "evolutionary rationale" stands behind this concept, providing a backup for vital genes undergoing a "loss of function" mutation. It has been suggested that duplication of "life-supporting genes" is the appropriate evolutionary response to this challenge. However, there is no reason to retain identical duplicated genes through the course of evolution, because survival pressure can be maintained only if mutations occur simultaneously in both genes.

Address for correspondence: David Naor, The Lautenberg Center for General and Tumor Immunology, Hebrew University–Hadassah Medical School, Jerusalem 91120, Israel. Voice: +972-2-6758722; fax: +972-2-6424653.
naord@md.huji.ac.il

Ann. N.Y. Acad. Sci. 1050: 52–63 (2005). © 2005 New York Academy of Sciences.
doi: 10.1196/annals.1313.007

Because this is an extremely infrequent event, genetic drift would eventually eliminate the redundant gene.[1] On the other hand, a "gain of function" mutation may generate, in the duplicated redundant gene, a new essential function, additional to the original one (now designated a cross-reactive function). Hence, the "new" function would protect the redundant gene from genetic drift, whereas the "old" cross-reactive function would provide a backup for the original gene.[1,2] If this is the case, the redundant gene should be structurally and functionally related to the original gene, with some sequence modification associated with acquisition of the new function, that is, the redundant gene and the original gene must be included in the same gene family.

EXAMPLES OF MOLECULAR REDUNDANCY

Molecular redundancy is widely distributed among families of cytokines and cytokine receptors.[3] For example, redundant molecules include IL-2 and IL-15 receptors (both transduce signals for T cell growth), type I and type II receptors of IL-4 (both transduce signals for Th2 differentiation), as well as IL-4 and IL-13 receptors (both transduce signals for Th2 differentiation and IgE production via activation of Stat-6). The molecular basis of these and other cytokine receptors has not been thoroughly clarified. However, sequence similarity has been reported for redundant IL-4 receptor chains, as well as for IL-7 and thymic stromal lymphopoietin (TSLP) receptors, which share some functions (e.g., support of T cell growth), but diverge in others. The IL-3 receptor, which transduces broad signaling for hematopoiesis, displays in the mouse two related redundant molecules.[3] In many receptors (e.g., receptors for IL-3, IL-5, and GM-CSF), the α chain dictates cytokine specificity, whereas the β chain shares common signal transducing components of the receptor, which explains, at least in part, the functional redundancy of cytokines.[4]

As in cytokines and their receptors, much redundancy and interaction promiscuity are detected among chemokines and their receptors. Many of the chemokine genes arose through gene duplication, as indicated by their chromosome clustering and functional similarity, for example, attraction of neutrophils or monocytes to inflammation sites. This also suggests that they emerged relatively late in evolution. Hence, a single receptor can signal for several chemokines, whereas a single chemokine may interact with several receptors. For example, CXCL1, CXCL2, CXCL3, CXCL5 (ENA-78), CXCL6 (GCP-2), CXCL7 (NAP-2), and CXCL8 (IL-8) are all clustered on the same chromosome and interact with the CXCR2 receptor. CXCL6 and CXCL8 also interact with the CXCR1 receptor. Similarly, CXCL9 (Mig), CXCL10 (IP-10), and CXCL11 (I-TAC) (again, clustered on the same chromosome) interact with the CXCR3 receptor.[5] Some relevant questions may be raised following analysis of, for example, the redundancy of chemokines such as CCL4 and CCL4L1. These chemokines competed similarly with radiolabeled CCL4 for binding to a human embryonic kidney cell line expressing the relevant CCR5 chemokine receptor, and they showed almost identical chemotactic effects in the transwell migration assay. Only minor, insignificant differences were detected in their ability to inhibit HIV replication.[6] In view of the discussion above, this redundancy may imply that the duplication event occurred too late in evolution to allow genetic drift, or alternatively that the new function of the duplicated gene has not been identified. Linkage disequilibrium with an essential third party gene is yet another possibility.

Greater attention has been focused on molecular redundancy since the development of knockout mouse technology over the past ten years. This technology is based on gene deletion in embryonic stem cells by homologous recombination and subsequent transplantation of mouse blastocytes containing these stem cells into pseudopregnant females, resulting in mutant descendants. Knockout technology has been developed in an attempt to define the function of the deleted gene *in vivo*, as reflected in the phenotype of the mutant animal. However, in many cases a defective phenotype has not been detected following gene targeting, ultimately raising the possibility of gene compensation by a redundant gene.

Follistatin,[7,8] noggin,[9,10] and chordin,[11,12] are sequence-unrelated, but functionally similar genes that apparently can compensate for one another to induce neural tissue formation during early vertebrate embryonic development.[1] This notion is based on the observation that each one of these proteins can interrupt the activity of the TGF-β superfamily of molecules, which antagonize neural development, thus directly or indirectly enabling the formation of the nervous system. This interaction has been conserved phylogenetically, as shown by the short gastrulation (sog) gene and its countermolecule, the TGF-β-like decapentaplegic (dpp) gene, which dictate similar functions in drosophila.[13] However, murine knockout of follistatin,[14] noggin,[15] or chordin,[16] as well as chordin and noggin in combination[17] (double knockout) generated defective mutants, indicating that deletion of each one of these genes cannot be compensated by its apparently redundant counterparts. Therefore, we must assume that, at least in the mouse, each one of these proteins is essential, but not sufficient, to back up the functions of the others. Another rationalization, which better reconciles with the Xenopus experiments,[1] but does not fully agree with the redundancy concept, is that the follistatin, noggin, and chordin genes all play roles in the initial phase of neural induction, but subtly different ones. Therefore, individuals with all genes functional are superior to individuals in which any of them are inactive.

Retinoic acid (RA, also known as vitamin A) signaling is mediated by two distinct classes of receptors, RA receptors (RARs) and retinoid X receptors (RXRs). The two families of nuclear receptors are, in fact, transcription factors that activate target genes by binding to promoter elements. Activation of the RA receptor by retinoic acid is associated with prenatal and postnatal development, including growth, morphogenesis, and epithelial homeostasis. Each family includes three genes: RARα, RARβ, and RARγ, or RXRα, RXRβ, and RXRγ. Every gene of the RAR family expresses several isoforms, for example, RARα1 and RARα2, RARβ1, RARβ2, RARβ3, etc., suggesting that they display, in addition to overlapping functions, exclusive functions that have been conserved in the course of evolution.[18–21] However, knockout mice with disrupted RARα1,[18,19] RARβ2,[20] or RARγ2[21] do not display an unusual phenotype, that is, the animal appears normal, suggesting that the deleted genes are compensated for by the redundant RAR isoforms. On the other hand, upregulation of RARα2, for example, was not detected in RARα1 knockout mice.[18] In contrast, knockout of all RARα[19] or RARγ[21] subfamily molecules caused early postnatal death. Collectively, these findings suggest that RAR isoforms overlap functions that back up one another, but each one of them also has its own essential activity, thereby avoiding genetic drift. On the other hand, each one of the RAR subfamily genes (e.g., RARα, RARβ) encodes a life-supporting function that cannot be replaced by a gene product of the other subfamilies (e.g., RARγ). Cellular retinoic acid binding protein I and II (CRAB1 and

CRAB2) are related proteins that regulate the activity of retinoic acid receptors at all stages of embryonic development. Although CRAB1-knockout mice are normal, CRAB2 expression in these mice is not upregulated, indicating, as cited by researchers, that CRAB1 does not play a critical role in the RA signaling pathway.[22] Later, we will see that there may be a different interpretation of this finding.

Hck, fgr, lyn, and *yes* encode Src family protein kinases involved in the terminal differentiation of myelomonocytic cells or in specific functions of mature effector cells of innate immunity. Hematopoiesis appears to proceed normally in *hck-* and *fgr*-deficient mice, as well as in *hck-fgr* double knockout mice. Furthermore, macrophages from the doubly homozygous animals normally retain many functions,[23] suggesting gene compensation by other *src* family members. *Fgr*[23] or *yes*[24] knockout mice do not display any overt phenotype. On the other hand, phagocytosis is attenuated in *hck*-deficient macrophages, and the doubly *hck-fgr* mutant animals exhibit augmented susceptibility to infection by *Listeria monocytogenes*. Lyn protein kinase is increased in *hck*-deficient macrophages, suggesting that Lyn compensates for *hck* deficiency.[23] In general, crossing of Src family mutants with each other leads to more severe phenotypes than observed in single mutants.[24] This suggests that Src family members back up other members of the family, generating a redundant network of genes to ensure protection of both the individual and the species.

The *ras* genes encode a family of highly related proteins that transmit extracellular signals for cellular proliferation and differentiation. However, *N-ras* knockout mice do not show any overt phenotype.[25] Thus, the authors suggest that "function of *N-ras* gene is dispensable for normal mouse development, growth and fertility", possibly because it is compensated for by a product of a redundant gene from the *ras* family.

Intermediate filament (IF) proteins are components of the cytoskeleton and nuclear envelope of eukaryotic cells, including cells of mesenchymal origin that express the IF vimentin,[26] or astrocytes of the central nervous system (CNS), which express the IF glial fibrillary acidic protein (GFAP).[27,28] Despite the apparently essential function of IFs, vimentin knockout mice[26] or GFAP knockout mice[27,28] display normal development, including normal CNS function. Interestingly, immuno-histochemical analysis revealed that the loss of GFAP is not compensated for by the upregulation of other intermediate filament proteins, such as vimentin,[28] leaving an open question: What gene products replace IF in IF knockout mice? Later, we shall see that the compensating molecule may not necessarily occur within the original family of molecules, but in structurally unrelated molecules as well.

Tenascin is one of the most abundant extracellular maxtrix (ECM) proteins of the brain, but knocking out this molecule did not reveal its function because no overt phenotype was detected in the gene-deficient mice. Upregulation of other tenascins was not identified,[29] suggesting that redundancy may be found in unrelated molecules.

Finally, type x collagen, which had been considered to be involved in long-bone growth and development, was found to be dispensable in type x collagen knockout mice.[30] However, because mice and humans with dominant-acting type x collagen mutations display bone abnormalities, it has been suggested[30] that only the presence of abnormal type x collagen influences bone development. Furthermore, the absence of collagen x must be compensated for by a redundant protein from the collagen family or from outside the family. Otherwise, if collagen x is not required for bone growth and development, as well as for other functions, how did it survive in the course of evolution?

A DIFFERENT OUTLOOK ON MOLECULAR REDUNDANCY IN THE CONTEXT OF COLLAGEN-INDUCED ARTHRITIS

Molecular redundancy is widely discussed in many scientific circles, but the mechanism of this process is ill-defined. Three concepts are generally accepted, as shown previously, but not always supported by experimental data: (1) The redundant gene compensates for the life-supporting gene, which is essential to the development of the embryo. However, many such genes are not backed up by redundant genes, as their deletion results in prenatal death. Why are some genes compensated for by other genes, whereas others are not? (2) The redundant gene is upregulated when the relevant original gene is deleted. The inability to detect such upregulation sometimes leads to the conclusion that the missing targeted gene is not essential for survival. But for at least some genes, the question may be raised: How have these genes survived during evolution? (3) The redundant gene is a member of the same family as the deleted gene, with functions overlapping those of the missing gene. As we will see later, this is not always the case.

We have exploited the mouse model of collagen-induced arthritis (CIA) to elucidate several aspects of the elusive molecular redundancy in the context of CD44 deficiency. Alternative splicing, as well as differential glycosylation and attachment of glycosaminoglycan chains, generate multiple structural and functional versions of CD44. Proinflammatory activities, such as cell-cell and cell-matrix interaction, as well as support of cell migration, are part of the CD44 functional list.[31–33] Hyaluronic acid (HA),[34] the principal ligand of CD44, mediates extravasation and movement in the extracellular matrix (ECM) of $CD44^{+/+}$ leukocytes[35] and is expressed by activated endothelial cells of small blood vessels.[36] CD44 is a member of the link module of the superfamily of the HA binding proteins (HABPs) or hyaladherins.[37] The receptor for hyaluronan-mediated motility (RHAMM) is also a hyaladherin, but it lacks a link module. RHAMM is expressed on the cell surface (where it is designated CD168) and in the cytoplasm, as well as in the cytoskeleton and nucleus. As with CD44, RHAMM engages in alternative splicing,[38–41] particularly during and after neoplastic conversion and tissue repair.[41] Upon interaction with HA, RHAMM delivers signals for cell migration and proliferation in both malignant and normal cells.[39,41–43]

We previously found that disruption of CD44 function by anti-CD44 monoclonal antibodies (mAbs)[44,45] or hyaluronidase[45,46] reduces the pathological activities in experimental autoimmune diseases such as CIA in DBA/1 mice[44,46] and insulin-dependent diabetes in NOD mice,[45] as well as in lymphoma dissemination in BALB/c mice.[47,48] We concluded, therefore, that these experimental diseases are CD44-dependent, and predicted that, for example, injection of type II collagen into CD44 knockout mice could reasonably fail to induce autoimmune joint inflammation. To our surprise, we found that administration of collagen not only generated arthritis in CD44-deficient animals, but that the disease was even more severe than that found in arthritic or wild-type mice (ref. 46 and present communication). It was suggested, therefore, that the redundant gene product in CD44-deficient mice is more efficient in supporting CIA than the original gene. The ultimate aim of the study was to prove this notion and to identify the redundant gene.

CD44-deficient mice,[49] provided by Dr. Tak Mak (Ontario Cancer Institute, Ontario, Canada) were backcrossed for seven generations onto a DBA/1 background to establish a CD44 knockout mouse line susceptible to CIA. It has been reported[49–51] that CD44 knockout mice display an almost normal phenotype with only a few exceptions, for example, impaired lymphocyte homing to the lymph nodes and thymus.[50] Evidence for the absence of CD44 in the DBA/1 CD44 knockout mice was presented in our previous communication.[46] PCR analysis of DNA derived from the mouse tail was able to discriminate between CD44-deficient mice, wild-type mice, and heterozygous mice. Accordingly, we established three mouse lines.

CD44 knockout mice administered a single dose of type II collagen developed arthritis within 25 days. In contrast, wild-type mice administered a single dose of type II collagen did not develop arthritis even after 40 days. A second dose of collagen was required to induce arthritis within the next 5 days.[46] Histopathological examination revealed that not only was CIA accelerated in CD44-deficient mice, but that it was more aggravated than in wild-type mice. In this and all subsequent experiments, CIA, in both normal and knockout mice, was generated by two injections of collagen, three weeks apart. Tarsal/metarsal joints were removed 14 days after CIA onset, decalcified, fixed, and stained with hematoxylin and eosin. Wild-type mice showed severe erosion of bone and cartilage, although some cartilage remained intact. The joint space was still evident and the joint architecture was partially preserved. On the other hand, CD44-deficient mice showed severe erosion of bone and complete erosion of cartilage; the entire joint architecture, including joint spaces, disappeared.[46] Interestingly, histochemical examination of HA, using hyaluronic acid binding protein as a specific probe for this glycosaminoglycan, showed fourfold higher accumulation of HA in the joint tissue of CD44-deficient mice when compared with wild-type mice, as monitored by photoimaging. The HA accumulation was markedly reduced after injection of hyaluronidase. Because cell surface CD44 is required for binding, internalization, and intracellular digestion of HA, it is hardly surprising that HA tends to accumulate in the absence of CD44 (i.e., in CD44-deficient mice), thus intensifying the inflammatory cascade.

The aggravated inflammatory response in CD44$^{-/-}$ mice also is reflected by activation of genes involved directly or indirectly in inflammation, as shown by microarray analysis. Total RNA was extracted with RNazol from splenic T cells separated with anti-CD3 mAb-coated beads and a magnetic cell sorter. The T cells were obtained from arthritic and nonarthritic wild-type and CD44-deficient mice at disease onset. The T cell RNA samples were subjected to microarray analysis. cDNA microarrays containing ~13,000 mouse cDNA clones on three slides were used in this study. The cDNA clones were obtained from Research Genetics (I.M.A.G.E. Consortium, Huntsville, AL), Incyte Genomics (Palo Alto, CA), and internal sources. Each clone was printed in duplicate on a given chip. Printing, hybridization, scanning, and image analysis were carried out as described.[52] Each RNA sample from the purified T cells was hybridized with two cDNA microarray slides run in parallel, thus yielding quadruplicate data points for each RNA sample and gene combination. Data cleanup and normalization consisted of an initial normalization between hybridization replicates within a single sample, followed by a secondary normalization across all the samples within a project.[53] Within each normalization step, a nonlinear, smoothing spline method was used after 75th percentile linear normalization. Normalized data were then used to compare differences in gene expression between T cells from CD44 knockout mice and wild-type mice. RNA hybridization with cDNA clones that showed at least twofold changes in expression were considered differentially expressed transcripts.

The number of transcripts that changed upon induction of arthritis was much greater in CD44$^{-/-}$ mice than in wild-type mice (170 vs. 47). When arthritic wild-type mice and CD44$^{-/-}$ mice were compared, 53 changes in transcript expression were observed, of which at least 18 were associated with upregulation of genes directly or indirectly involved in inflammation, for example, IL-1β, IL-8 receptor β, c-jun, Fos, Syk, c-c chemokine receptor 4 (CCR4), and TNFRp75 (CD120b).[46] These findings are compatible with the concept that CD44 deficiency synergizes with the arthritic activity induced by collagen, thereby increasing the number of upregulated inflammation-involved transcripts (including migration-supporting genes, such as IL-8 receptor β). This process results in perpetuation of the disease and increased joint deterioration. Notably, microarray analysis of CD44$^{-/-}$ cDNA detected increased expression of jun and fos, as well as increased expression of proinflammatory genes regulated by AP-1, which is formed from jun and fos dimers. Hence, the processes involved in the enhancement of joint destruction in the absence of CD44 are associated with altered HA metabolism and upregulation of inflammatory mediators, particularly those linked to cell migration and AP-1 formation.

Collectively, our findings suggest that molecular redundancy in CD44-deficient mice generates more aggravated CIA than in wild-type mice. What is the identity of the redundant molecule? We first showed that injection of anti-CD44 mAb at the onset of collagen-induced arthritis and then every other day for 10 days markedly reduced CIA in wild-type and heterozygous mice, when compared with that in similarly treated wild-type mice administered isotype-matched control mAb.[46] The reduced arthritic activity was evaluated by measuring footpad swelling of the inflamed paws with a microcaliper, as described in our previous article.[44] In contrast, using the same protocol we found that injection of anti-CD44 mAb did not change the course of the joint disease in CD44 knockout mice. As we could reproduce the ability to decrease CIA activity in wild-type mice by injecting hyaluronidase (but not heparinase) upon initiation of the disease and then every other day for five weeks, it was suggested that the interaction between cell surface CD44 and the HA of the extracellular matrix promotes the development of joint inflammation. Furthermore, injection of hyaluronidase, according to the same treatment protocol, reduced CIA to nearly the same extent in CD44-deficient, wild-type, and heterozygous mice,[46] implying that the molecule compensating for CD44 in CD44 knockout mice recognizes HA. This supposition is supported by the finding that CD44-deficient and wild-type splenocytes bound to almost the same extent to immobilized HA, regardless of whether they were derived from arthritic or nonarthritic mice. Of the many molecules that can interact with HA, we found, after electronic screening of the literature, that RHAMM not only binds, like CD44, to HA, but also supports, again like CD44, cell motility. We asked, therefore, whether RHAMM compensates for CD44 in supporting CIA in CD44-deficient mice.

Western blot and flow cytometry analysis with anti-RHAMM polyclonal antibodies revealed that RHAMM was not upregulated on the cell surface of CD44-deficient spleen cells or joint-infiltrating cells,[46] as well as on intracellular compartments of CD44-deficient spleen cells (FIG. 1), when compared with wild-type cells, regardless of whether they were derived from arthritic or nonarthritic mice. This finding was confirmed further by microarray analysis, which showed no difference in RHAMM transcript expression between wild-type and CD44-deficient mice, regardless of whether they were arthritic or not.

Enhancement of inflammatory cell motility in CD44-deficient mice could be a major factor in their aggravated CIA. Indeed, the transwell migration assay revealed that arthritic CD44-deficient spleen cells migrate through HA-coated filters towards a chemoattractant more intensively (i.e., at higher numbers) than do nonarthritic CD44-deficient spleen cells or arthritic and nonarthritic wild-type spleen cells. Furthermore, the migration of arthritic and nonarthritic CD44-deficient splenocytes through HA-coated filters was inhibited by anti-RHAMM antibodies, but not by anti-CD44 antibodies. Under the same conditions, the migration of arthritic and non-

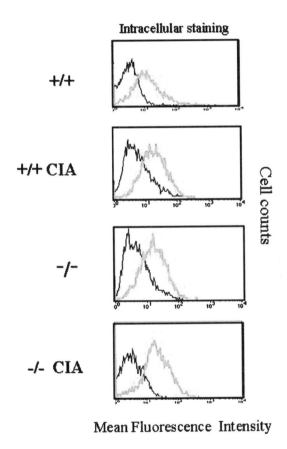

Intracellular staining

+/+

+/+ CIA

Cell counts

-/-

-/- CIA

Mean Fluorescence Intensity

FIGURE 1. Flow cytometry analysis of intracellular RHAMM in CD44-deficient and wild-type splenocytes derived from arthritic and nonarthritic mice. A quantity of 10^5 spleen leukocytes was incubated with formaldehyde, using a Cytofix/Cytoperm Plus kit, washed, and stained with polyclonal anti-RHAMM antibody for 45 min on ice. After extensive rinsing, the cells were incubated with fluorescence-labeled secondary anti-immunoglobulin antibody (Jackson ImmunResearch) for 30 min on ice. The cells were then washed and analyzed by flow cytometry. The left histogram in each panel shows the nonspecific binding of the second antibody alone. Flow cytometry data were collected for viable cells according to side scatter and forward scatter.

arthritic wild-type splenocytes was slightly, albeit significantly, inhibited by both anti-RHAMM and anti-CD44 mAbs.[46] These results show that RHAMM supports migration of leukocytes to a much greater extent when they are deficient in CD44. Can this observation find support in an *in vivo* study?

Using standard protocols,[46] injection of anti-RHAMM mAb or soluble RHAMM conjugated to GST (RHAMM-GST) did not influence CIA activity in wild-type mice, but markedly reduced this activity in CD44-deficient mice, as monitored by footpad swelling. Injection of isotype-matched IgG1 or GST alone did not influence the course of this inflammatory joint disease.

CONCLUSIONS

How does one piece together a complete and reasonable picture from all of these mosaic stones? A schematic, possibly oversimplified, description is shown in FIGURE 2. In the presence of CD44, that is, in wild-type mice, cell surface CD44 successfully competes with cell surface RHAMM for binding to HA of arthritic joint tissue. Successful competition may simply be related to a quantitative effect—there are more cell surface CD44 molecules than cell surface RHAMM molecules. However, as cell surface CD44 is involved in intracellular HA cleavage,[54] the joint tissue contains relatively small amounts of HA in $CD44^{-/-}$ mice. Therefore, the invasion of joint-infiltrating destructive cells is reduced in wild-type mice, as this migratory cell invasion is dependent on HA-CD44 interaction. The outcome of this sequence of events is limited activation of inflammatory genes and moderate CIA. On the other

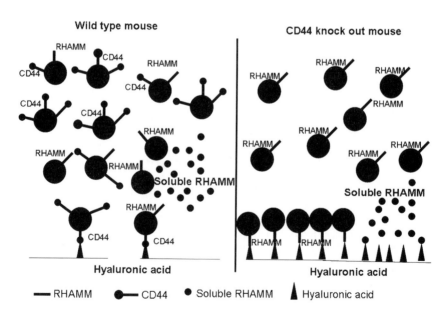

FIGURE 2. Schematic interpretation of molecular redundancy in CD44 knockout mice. For explanation, see text.

hand, in the absence of CD44, as in CD44 knockout mice, cell surface RHAMM is free to interact with excess joint tissue HA (which is not exposed to CD44-dependent degradation), resulting in greater activation of inflammatory genes, enhanced cell motility, and more aggravated CIA. Under such circumstances, however, soluble RHAMM can compete with cell surface RHAMM for HA binding, resulting in inhibition of CIA.[46]

We previously reported[44] that injection of anti-CD44 mAb into wild-type mice reduced their CIA activity. Why does CD44 targeting by antibody in adulthood not free cell surface RHAMM to induce aggravated CIA, as embryonic genetic deletion of CD44 does? Because CD44 is essential to embryo development, we suggest that the continuous pressure to replace CD44 in CD44-deficient mice modifies the RHAMM gene (in a still unknown manner), allowing it to compensate for CD44, while retaining its original functions. This effect cannot be reproduced by targeting CD44 during adulthood. Alternatively, or in addition, the continuous CD44 deficiency in knockout mice allows substantial accumulation of HA, rendering the animal more susceptible to inflammation.[55] This effect cannot be obtained after a limited regimen of anti-CD44 antibody injections in adulthood.

In conclusion, we present here a mechanistic explanation for molecular redundancy that does not depend on gene duplication, gene product upregulation, or phylogenetic evolution of a redundant gene. This different interpretation of molecular redundancy is not mutually exclusive of the other explanations cited in this communication, as several backup strategies may exist.

ACKNOWLEDGMENTS

This work was supported by grants from the Society of Research Associates of the Lautenberg Center and the Foundation for Research into Diseases of Aging (Bala Cynwyd, PA).

REFERENCES

1. COOKE, J., M.A. NOWAK, M. BOERLIJST & J. MAYNARD-SMITH. 1997. Evolutionary origins and maintenance of redundant gene expression during metazoan development. Trends Genet. **13:** 360–364.
2. NOWAK, M.A., M. BOERLIJST, J. COOKE & J.M. SMITH. 1997. Evolution of genetic redundancy. Nature **10:** 167–171.
3. OZAKI, K. & W.J. LEONARD. 2002. Cytokine and cytokine receptor pleiotropy and redundancy. J. Biol. Chem. **277:** 29355–29358.
4. HADDAD, J.J. 2002. Cytokines and related receptor-mediated signaling pathways. Biochem. Biophys. Res. Commun. **297:** 700–713.
5. ZLOTNIK, A. & O. YOSHIE. 2000. Chemokines: a new classification system and their role in immunity. Immunity **12:** 121–127.
6. HOWARD, O.M., J.A. TURPIN, R. GOLDMAN & W.S. MODI. 2004. Functional redundancy of the human CCL4 and CCL4L1 chemokine genes. Biochem. Biophys. Res. Commun. **30:** 927–931.
7. NAKAMURA, T., K. SUGINO, K. TITANI & H. SUGINO. 1991. Follistatin, an activin-binding protein, associates with heparan sulfate chains of proteoglycans on follicular granulosa cells. J. Biol. Chem. **266:** 19432–19437.

8. HEMMATI-BRIVANLOU, A., O.G. KELLY & D.A. MELTON. 1994. Follistatin, an antago-nist of activin, is expressed in the Spemann organizer and displays direct neuralizing activity. Cell **77:** 283–295.
9. LAMB, T.M. *et al.* 1993. Neural induction by the secreted polypeptide noggin. Science **262:** 713–718.
10. ZIMMERMAN, L.B., J.M. DE JESUS-ESCOBAR & R.M. HARLAND. 1996. The Spemann organizer signal noggin binds and inactivates bone morphogenetic protein 4. Cell **86:** 599–606.
11. SASAI, Y., B. LU, H. STEINBEISSER & E.M. DE ROBERTIS. 1995. Regulation of neural induction by the Chd and Bmp-4 antagonistic patterning signals in Xenopus. Nature **376:** 333–336.
12. PICCOLO, S., B. LU, Y. SASAI & E.M. DE ROBERTIS. 1996. Dorsoventral patterning in Xenopus: inhibition of ventral signals by direct binding of chordin to BMP-4. Cell **86:** 589–598.
13. BIEHS, B., V. FRANCOIS & E. BIER. 1996. The Drosophila short gastrulation gene pre-vents Dpp from autoactivating and suppressing neurogenesis in the neuroectoderm. Genes Dev. **10:** 2922–2934.
14. MATZUK, M.M. *et al.* 1995. Multiple defects and perinatal death in mice deficient in follistatin. Nature **374:** 360–363.
15. MCMAHON, J.A. *et al.* 1998. Noggin-mediated antagonism of BMP signaling is required for growth and patterning of the neural tube and somite. Genes Dev. **12:** 1438–1452.
16. BACHILLER, D. *et al.* 2003. The role of chordin/Bmp signals in mammalian pharyngeal development and DiGeorge syndrome. Development **130:** 3567–3578.
17. BACHILLER, D. *et al.* 2000. The organizer factors Chordin and Noggin are required for mouse forebrain development. Nature **403:** 658–661.
18. LI, E. *et al.* 1993. Normal development and growth of mice carrying a targeted disruption of the alpha 1 retinoic acid receptor gene. Proc. Natl. Acad. Sci. USA **90:** 1590–1594.
19. LUFKIN, T. *et al.* 1993. High postnatal lethality and testis degeneration in retinoic acid receptor alpha mutant mice. Proc. Natl. Acad. Sci. USA **90:** 7225–7229.
20. MENDELSOHN, C. *et al.* 1994. Retinoic acid receptor beta 2 (RAR beta 2) null mutant mice appear normal. Dev. Biol. **166:** 246–258.
21. LOHNES, D. *et al.* 1993. Function of retinoic acid receptor gamma in the mouse. Cell **73:** 643–658.
22. GORRY, P. *et al.* 1994. The cellular retinoic acid binding protein I is dispensable. Proc. Natl. Acad. Sci. USA **91:** 9032–9036.
23. LOWELL, C.A., P. SORIANO & H.E. VARMUS. 1994. Functional overlap in the src gene family: inactivation of hck and fgr impairs natural immunity. Genes Dev. **8:** 387–898.
24. STEIN, P.L., H. VOGEL & P. SORIANO. 1994. Combined deficiencies of Src, Fyn, and Yes tyrosine kinases in mutant mice. Genes Dev. **8:** 1999–2007.
25. UMANOFF, H., W. EDELMANN, A. PELLICER & R. KUCHERLAPATI. 1995. The murine N-ras gene is not essential for growth and development. Proc. Natl. Acad. Sci. USA **92:** 1709–1713.
26. COLUCCI-GUYON, E. *et al.* 1994. Mice lacking vimentin develop and reproduce without an obvious phenotype. Cell **79:** 679–694.
27. GOMI, H. *et al.* 1995. Mice devoid of the glial fibrillary acidic protein develop normally and are susceptible to scrapie prions. Neuron **14:** 29–41.
28. PEKNY, M. *et al.* 1995. Mice lacking glial fibrillary acidic protein display astrocytes devoid of intermediate filaments but develop and reproduce normally. EMBO J. **14:** 1590–1598.
29. STEINDLER, D.A. *et al.* 1995. Tenascin knockout mice: barrels, boundary molecules, and glial scars. J. Neurosci. **15:** 1971–1983.
30. ROSATI, R. *et al.* 1994. Normal long bone growth and development in type X collagen-null mice. Nat. Genet. **8:** 129–135.
31. NAOR, D. *et al.* 2002. CD44 in cancer. Crit. Rev. Clin. Lab. Sci. **39:** 527–579.
32. LESLEY, J., R. HYMAN & P.W. KINCADE. 1993. CD44 and its interaction with extracellular matrix. Adv. Immunol. **54:** 271–335.

33. NAOR, D., R. VOGT SIONOV & D. ISH-SHALOM. 1997. CD44: structure, function, and association with the malignant process. Adv. Cancer Res. **71:** 241–319.
34. TAMMI, M.I., A.J. DAY & E.A. TURLEY. 2002. Hyaluronan and homeostasis: a balancing act. J. Biol. Chem. **277:** 4581–4584.
35. DEGRENDELE, H.C., M. KOSFISZER, P. ESTESS & M.H. SIEGELMAN. 1997. CD44 activation and associated primary adhesion is inducible via T cell receptor stimulation. J. Immunol. **159:** 2549–2553.
36. MOHAMADZADEH, M. *et al.* 1998. Proinflammatory stimuli regulate endothelial hyaluronan expression and CD44/HA-dependent primary adhesion. J. Clin. Invest. **101:** 97–108.
37. DAY, A. J. & G.D. PRESTWICH. 2002. Hyaluronan-binding proteins: tying up the giant. J. Biol. Chem. **277:** 4585–4588.
38. ZHANG, S. *et al.* 1998. The hyaluronan receptor RHAMM regulates extracellular-regulated kinase. J. Biol. Chem. **273:** 11342–11348.
39. AKIYAMA, Y. *et al.* 2001. Hyaluronate receptors mediating glioma cell migration and proliferation. J. Neuro-Oncol. **53:** 115–127.
40. LYNN, B.D., E.A. TURLEY & J.I. NAGY. 2001. Subcellular distribution, calmodulin interaction, and mitochondrial association of the hyaluronan-binding protein RHAMM in rat brain. J. Neurosci. Res. **65:** 6–16.
41. TURLEY, E.A., P.W. NOBLE & L.Y.W. BOURGUIGNON. 2002. Signaling properties of hyaluronan receptors. J. Biol. Chem. **277:** 4589–4592.
42. MOHAPATRA, S. *et al.* 1996. Soluble hyaluronan receptor RHAMM induces mitotic arrest by suppressing Cdc2 and cyclin B1 expression. J. Exp. Med. **183:** 1663–1668.
43. CHEUNG, W.F., T.F. CRUZ & E.A. TURLEY. 1999. Receptor for hyaluronan-mediated motility (RHAMM), a hyaladherin that regulates cell responses to growth factors. Biochem. Soc. Trans. **27:** 135–142.
44. NEDVETZKI, S. *et al.* 1999. CD44 involvement in experimental collagen-induced arthritis (CIA). J. Autoimmun. **13:** 39–47.
45. WEISS, L. *et al.* 2000. Induction of resistance to diabetes in non-obese diabetic mice by targeting CD44 with a specific monoclonal antibody. Proc. Natl. Acad. Sci. USA **97:** 285–290.
46. NEDVETZKI, S. *et al.* 2004. RHAMM, a receptor for hyaluronan-mediated motility, compensates for CD44 in inflamed CD44-knockout mice: a different interpretation of redundancy. Proc. Natl. Acad. Sci. USA **101:** 18081–18086.
47. ZAHALKA, M.A. *et al.* 1995. Lymph node (but not spleen) invasion by murine lymphoma is both CD44- and hyaluronate-dependent. J. Immunol. **154:** 5345–5355.
48. WALLACH-DAYAN, S.B. *et al.* 2001. CD44-dependent lymphoma cell dissemination: a cell surface CD44 variant, rather than standard CD44, supports *in vitro* lymphoma cell rolling on hyaluronic acid substrate and its in vivo accumulation in the peripheral lymph nodes. J. Cell Sci. **114:** 3463–3477.
49. SCHMITS, R. *et al.* 1997. CD44 regulates hematopoietic progenitor distribution, granuloma formation, and tumorigenicity. Blood **90:** 2217–2233.
50. PROTIN, U., T. SCHWEIGHOFFER, W. JOCHUM & F. HILBERG. 1999. CD44-deficient mice develop normally with changes in subpopulations and recirculation of lymphocyte subsets. J. Immunol. **163:** 4917–4923.
51. STOOP, R. *et al.* 2001. Increased resistance to collagen-induced arthritis in CD44-deficient DBA/1 mice. Arthritis Rheum. **44:** 2922–2931.
52. BONAVENTURE, P. *et al.* 2002. Nuclei and subnuclei gene expression profiling in mammalian brain. Brain Res. **943:** 38–47.
53. SHAW, K.J. *et al.* 2003. Comparison of the changes in global gene expression of Escherichia coli induced by four bactericidal agents. J. Mol. Microbiol. Biotechnol. **5:** 105–122.
54. KNUDSON, W., G. CHOW & C.B. KNUDSON. 2002. CD44-mediated uptake and degradation of hyaluronan. Matrix Biol. **21:** 15–23.
55. TEDER, P. *et al.* 2002. Resolution of lung inflammation by CD44. Science **296:** 155–158.

Functional Genomics in Early Autoimmunity

EVIE MELANITOU

Immunopathology Unit, Department of Molecular Medicine, Pasteur Institute, Paris, France

ABSTRACT: The molecular mechanisms initiating the autoimmune process in type 1 diabetes mellitus (T1DM) remain unknown, and studies aiming to address this question have been compromised by the difficulty of predicting the disease at an early age both in humans and in animal models. An additional hindrance in selecting individuals at an early age has been the complex genetic inheritance of autoimmune diabetes, implicating not only several genes but also environmental factors. We have previously demonstrated the predictive value of insulin autoantibodies (IAAs) at an early age, between three to five weeks in the NOD mouse. Animals positive for early appearance of IAAs (E-IAAs) develop autoimmune diabetes earlier. We showed a correlation between the presence of IAAs in the mothers during pregnancy, E-IAAs in the litters, and the early appearance of T1DM. NOD mice, E-IAA–positive, within litters from IAA-positive mothers during pregnancy, develop diabetes earlier and at a much greater rate than animals that are IAA-negative and from IAA-negative mothers. The molecular mechanisms responsible for this early autoimmune subphenotype were addressed by a global approach to differential gene expression analysis in the pancreatic lymph nodes (PaLNs). Although the data analysis is currently in progress, gene expression signatures were observed that are characteristic for PaLNs with regard to the presence or absence of IAAs. Overall, these data are consistent with the hypothesis of an early environmental influence from the autoimmune maternal environment on the genetic predisposition of the offspring, characterized by specific gene signatures leading to autoimmune disease.

KEYWORDS: autoimmunity; type 1 diabetes mellitus; insulin autoantibodies; maternal; pancreatic lymph nodes; transcriptome

INTRODUCTION

Little is known concerning the early molecular steps of autoimmune destruction, mainly because of the complexity of the autoimmune process and the involvement of several genes with mostly low or incomplete penetrance.[1–4]

Type 1A diabetes mellitus (T1DM) is one of the most well-studied autoimmune diseases, owing in part to the existence of animal models mimicking the human condition.[5] It is an organ-specific disease, resulting from the self-destruction of the insulin-producing β cells in the pancreatic islets of Langerhans.[6]

Insulin autoantibodies (IAAs) in human as well as in NOD mouse sera represent a well-characterized marker for the later appearance of insulitis and/or diabetes.[7,8]

Address for correspondence: Evie Melanitou, Immunopathology Unit, Department of Molecular Medicine, Pasteur Institute, 25 rue du Dr Roux, 75724 Paris Cedex 15, France.
eviemel@pasteur.fr

Ann. N.Y. Acad. Sci. 1050: 64–72 (2005). © 2005 New York Academy of Sciences.
doi: 10.1196/annals.1313.008

Among all autoantibodies, IAAs appear to be unique, as it has been shown that their presence is predictive of the later appearance of the disease, and their levels are dramatically and inversely correlated with the age at which type 1 diabetes develops in the NOD mouse as well as in humans.[8]

In an attempt to study the early stages of the diabetes phenotype, just before the peri-insulitis/insulitis lesions appear, we have used this marker at as early as three weeks of age in the NOD mouse. We have thus shown that IAAs are found in the NOD mouse model at three weeks of age (at weaning) and, interestingly, that presence of IAAs is a quantal by litter phenotype.[9] Although transplacental transmission of these autoantibodies seems to be excluded, however, at least two reports have demonstrated that maternal autoantibody status influences this early phenotype.[9,10] Data reported herein show that E-IAA–positive animals of litters from IAA-positive antepartum mothers develop E-IAAs with a significantly higher incidence than E-IAA–negative animals from IAA-negative mothers. Histologic examination of the pancreas shows no correlation between E-IAAs and insulitis, arguing in favor of IAAs as an early marker of autoimmunity in the NOD mouse.[9]

With the aim of deciphering the early molecular events preceding an autoimmune condition, we used this early diabetes subphenotype and selected autoimmune-prone animals at an early age, five weeks. Subsequently, we assessed whether specific gene transcripts involved in known pathways are changed in the pancreatic lymph nodes according to the presence or absence of early expression of insulin autoantibodies. We used oligonucleotide microarrays (Affymetrix, Santa Clara, CA) to compare between the global patterns of transcriptional changes occurring in the two subphenotypes. Gene expression profiles specific to the pancreatic lymph nodes (PaLNs) have thus been established, as we believe that this tissue reflects immune changes occurring in the pancreas. The first data analysis shows that gene expression signatures discriminate between presence and absence of E-IAAs in the NOD mouse.

These data suggest that the early molecular mechanisms responsible for the breakdown of self-tolerance are subjected not only to the physiological status of the mother, possibly representing an environmental component for disease, but also to molecular changes, as reflected by gene expression differences between the two subphenotypes studied. This latter observation underlines the genetic component predisposing to T1DM and brings to light the molecular mechanisms involved in the initiation process.

MATERIALS AND METHODS

Mice

Mice were purchased from Taconic Farms (NOD/*tac*), Germantown, NY, and housed in specific pathogen-free conditions. Experimental protocols conformed to guidelines from the Institutional Animal Care and Use Committee. Pregnant females were tested one week before delivery for the presence of IAAs.

Animals were tested for the presence of IAAs as previously described.[9] Briefly, sera from three- (at weaning), four-, and five-week-old NOD mice were assessed for the presence of IAAs. The last sera for IAA detection, taken at the time the animals were sacrificed at five weeks of age for RNA preparation, represent another checkpoint for the presence or absence of IAAs. Our established phenotypic requirement dictates that the presence of IAAs, when detected, must be confirmed at least twice within one-week intervals. Animals remaining IAA-positive for two consecutive assays, together with their IAA-negative controls, were sacrificed by cervical dislocation after light anesthesia. The pancreas from each animal was taken and separated in half, one sample for RNA preparation and the other for histology. This was not the case for the PaLNs, which, due to their small size, could be used for RNA preparation or for histology only, but not for both.

IAA Assay

IAAs were measured by a radioimmunoassay incorporating competition with unlabeled insulin and precipitation with Protein A/G sepharose in a 96-well filtration plate, as previously described.[8,9]

RNA Preparation for Microarrays

After sacrifice of the animals, PaLNs were immediately placed in RNAlater reagent (Qiagen) and processed for total RNA preparation on the same day. Total RNA was prepared with the Qiagen mini- or midi-RNA kit following the manufacturer's protocol; 500 ng of total RNA was assessed for quality using an Agilent Bioanalyzer (Agilent Technologies). High-quality RNA samples (4.5 μg) from E-IAA–positive (four mice) and E-IAA–negative (five mice) were reverse transcribed and, after biotinylated labeling of cRNA, were hybridized to an Affymetrix (Santa Clara, CA) first array MG-U74Av2 GeneChip, according to standard Affymetrix protocols. The first array in the set (MG-U74Av2) represents the majority of sequences (~6000) in the Mouse UniGene database that have been functionally characterized. In addition, ~6000 EST clusters are also represented on this single array. In total, the MG-U74AV2 GeneChip contains probe sets representing 12,488 transcripts. MicroChip scanning and data capture were also used according to standard Affymetrix methods (http://www.affymetrix.com/support/technical/manual/expression_manual.affx).

Normalization, filtering, and sorting of the data were undertaken using Affymetrix Data Mining Tool software, preliminary explorative analyses were carried out in GeneSpring (Sillicon Genetics), and statistics were assessed in Excel (Microsoft). For statistical analysis, data were log_2 transformed and, because this was a first exploratory analysis, a Welch's t-test, which does not assume that variances are equal, with a P value cutoff of .10, was applied to identify the most statistically significant changes in gene expression between E-IAA–positive and E-IAA–negative samples. The Benjamini and Hochberg[11] false discovery rate as the multiple testing correction method was used because this does not require an equal number of samples in each group.[12] Gene functions were assessed with GO (Gene Ontology tool, http://www.geneontology.org).

RESULTS AND DISCUSSION

Maternal Autoimmune Environment Affects Diabetes Subphenotypes and Final Disease Onset in the Offspring

The aim of this work was to establish the early molecular events preceding an autoimmune condition. Previously, we established the implications of IAAs as an

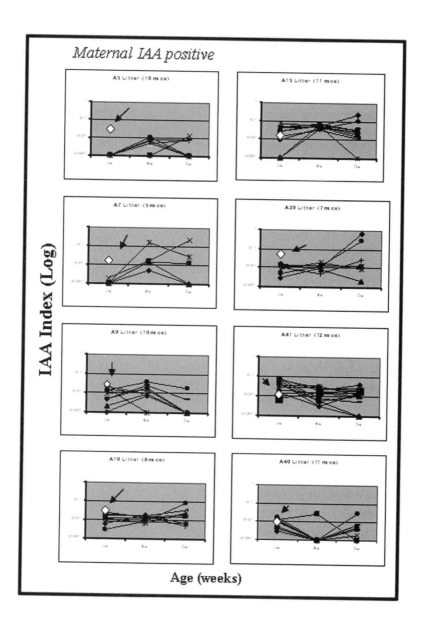

FIGURE 1A. Maternal IAA levels influence the overall level of IAAs in the litters. Presence of insulin autoantibodies (IAA index) in sera of individual litters from NOD mice at three, four, and five weeks of age. *Arrows* indicate maternal IAA levels antepartum for each litter.

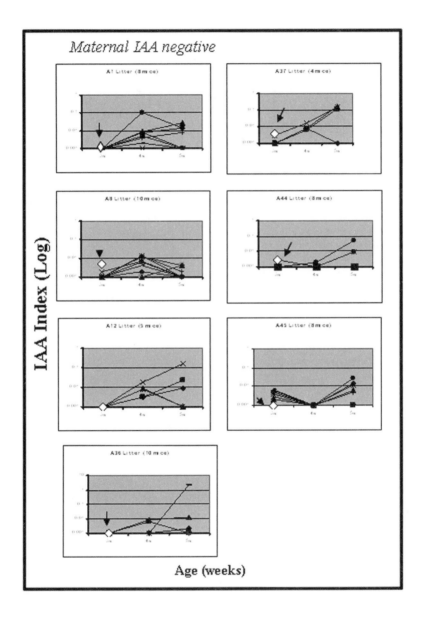

FIGURE 1B. Maternal IAA levels influence the overall level of IAAs in the litters. Presence of insulin autoantibodies (IAA index) in sera of individual litters from NOD mice at three, four, and five weeks of age. *Arrows* indicate maternal IAA levels antepartum for each litter.

TABLE 1. Comparison of insulin autoantibody levels in sera of 3- to 5-week-old mice between IAA-positive and IAA-negative mothers at antepartum

Age (weeks)	Maternal IAA−	Maternal IAA+	χ^2	P value
3	0/53	39/74	40.31	$P < .0001$
4	6/53	38/74	19.44	$P < .0001$
5	14/53	35/74	5.683	$P = .017$

early marker of T1DM in the NOD mouse.[9] Here, we report supplementary data providing additional evidence in support of the hypothesis that molecular changes take place very early in life in individuals genetically predisposed to develop autoimmune conditions. These molecular changes are influenced by environmental factors including, in this case, the presence of maternal IAAs antepartum. We used IAAs as a marker for autoimmunity and demonstrated that maternal immune imprinting is taking place *in utero* and that this correlates with later disease onset (FIGS. 1A and 1B).

IAAs are present as early as three weeks of age, and their appearance is a quantal subphenotype, as it runs by litters.[9] In addition, maternal IAA status has been found to affect the presence of IAAs in the offspring.[9] Maternal IAA-positive litters have increased numbers of offspring that are IAA-positive at between three and five weeks of age (FIG. 1A). In contrast, litters from IAA-negative mothers had a smaller number of offspring that were IAA-positive at the same ages. In the maternal IAA-negative litters, 20 of 53 animals showed positive levels of IAAs at all three ages studied (TABLE 1). Alternatively, in maternal IAA-positive litters, 35 of 74 were IAA-positive. These differences were significant ($P < .0001$) at three and four weeks of age, as well as at five weeks ($P = .017$; TABLE 1). Although the transplacental origin of E-IAAs cannot be completely excluded, it is noteworthy that the majority of animals that were IAA-positive at three weeks remained positive at later ages (FIG. 1A and TABLE 1). In addition, autoantibody levels were higher in the offspring than in the mothers as measured at one week antepartum (FIG. 1A; e.g., litters A15, A41). The presence of IAA-negative mice within litters that were, for the most part, IAA-positive also argues in favor of a nontransplacental origin for these autoantibodies (FIG. 1B). In another study, Greeley *et al.* also established maternal IAAs as a factor influencing development of T1DM in the offspring.[10] Indeed, depletion of maternal IAAs protects against diabetes in the NOD mouse.[10]

The mechanisms by which the maternal immune environment influences disease and how neonatal events might increase the risk for T1DM, in humans as well as in NOD mice, are not well understood. Several studies have addressed the relationship between islet autoantibodies during gestation and the later appearance of disease in children.[13,14] In a recent study, umbilical cord blood islet autoantibodies were measured and it was reported that these autoantibodies are not predictive of subsequent development of islet autoimmunity in humans.[15] It is tempting to speculate that the presence of maternal IAAs *in utero* in the NOD mouse may be a humoral marker of an autoimmune-prone environment predisposing the offspring to T1DM. However, so far the value of such a predictive marker in human disease is not clear.

In NOD mice, when the final diabetes phenotype is examined in offspring IAA-positive at three to five weeks of age from maternal IAA-positive litters, there is a clear difference in disease onset between autoantibody-positive and autoantibody-

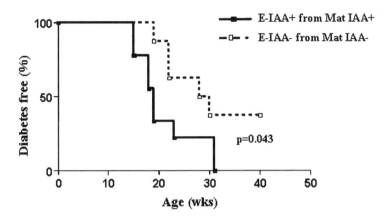

FIGURE 2. Life survival curves for E-IAA–positive animals from antepartum IAA-positive mothers (*solid lines*) and E-IAA–negative animals from antepartum IAA-negative mothers (*dashed lines*).

negative offspring. The majority of IAA-positive animals develop disease by 30 weeks of age, whereas IAA-negative animals do not ($P = .043$, FIG. 2). Taken together, these data establish that maternal influence in autoimmune changes takes place early, before the appearance of insulitis and before the onset of diabetes, and this can be traced by the presence of IAAs.

Is There a Molecular Signature Characteristic of Early Preinflammatory Stages Marked by the Presence of E-IAAs?

Numerous studies have contributed significantly to our knowledge of the immune-mediated mechanisms and the underlying genetic particularities of type 1 diabetes.[16,17] However, the initial molecular events that take place before the appearance of insulitis and predispose to the development of disease remain unknown. Despite the existence of a very well-characterized animal model, the NOD mouse, the low penetrance of genes implicated in this disease has compromised attempts to elucidate early molecular changes underlying the diabetes phenotype. Indeed, although NOD mice are inbred, not all develop the disease, with incidence ranging from 40% to 90% of female mice, depending on the colony. With the aim of identifying early changes related to autoimmune diabetes, we have demonstrated that the IAA sub-phenotype can be used as an early biological marker for the disease.[9] In addition, maternal IAAs affect final disease onset by predisposing the offspring to early appearance of T1DM, and may represent an environmental factor in disease incidence, without, however, excluding the possibility of an initiating effect on disease by the insulin autoantibodies or the insulin molecule itself as a primary autoantigen.

As our aim has been to identify the molecular changes of the early autoimmune processes, we have assessed, therefore, whether specific gene transcript variations, involved in known pathways, are changed in the pancreatic lymph node, according to the presence or absence of early expression of insulin autoantibodies. Auto-immune-prone molecular mechanisms have been suspected to take place around three weeks of age in the NOD mouse. These mechanisms might precede a local insult that causes the pancreatic endothelium to release antigens, attracting T cells from the periphery, with early priming in the pancreatic lymph nodes.[18] In this possible scenario, β cell antigens might trigger reactive T cells to invade the islets.[19] Therefore, we hypothesized that gene expression changes might take place in lymphoid tissue, and, in particular, in the lymphoid tissue closest to the pancreas, the PaLNs.

We used Affymetrix oligonucleotide arrays to compare transcriptional changes in the global patterns from the two phenotypes. Out of the over 12,900 genes present in the microchip, 125 genes were found to be differentially expressed in the two phenotypes, with 90 genes (72%) being upregulated in the RNA samples from E-IAA–positive mice and 35 genes downregulated. Our data are currently undergoing further analysis using additional transcriptome programs, as well as experimental biological confirmation, and will be described in detail in another report. However, the first exploratory analysis of the overall data revealed that at least 40 of the 90 upregulated genes showed high differential expression patterns, varying between 10- to 128-fold of relative expression differences. With the exception of 2 new genes corresponding to sequenced ESTs, all others have been described to have an immune function and to play a role in infection and inflammation (19 genes), or in cancer, neoplasia, and apoptosis (12 genes), including 4 genes with additional cellular functions and 7 genes that have been described to play a role in autoimmunity, whereas 4 of these are related to diabetes. Finally, 5 genes of this set might be implicated in cellular responses of the host during infection. Further analyses to confirm the transcriptome data and to assess the biological role of these genes experimentally are under way.

The relevance of the proposed findings to human disease is as follows: Our preliminary analysis of the transcriptome data indicate that deregulation of the immune system at an early state, in autoimmune-susceptible individuals, might parallel mechanisms that are similar to the ones implicated in immune system dysfunction during tumorigenesis and infection. The effect of infections on autoimmune diseases has been suspected previously without being demonstrated formally. Several of the identified genes have the potential to be used as biological markers for autoimmune diseases, such as type 1 diabetes. Additional prospective applications include potential diagnostic and prognostic markers for certain cancers and infection-mediated immune responses. These data are currently under additional evaluation to identify gene networks that might be implicated in the etiology of preinflammatory processes underlying not only autoimmunity, but also certain malignancies and infections.

In summary, our data show that the E-IAA humoral marker for early autoimmunity not only discriminates among NOD mice for onset of diabetes, but also reflects the molecular changes taking place early, prior to the initiation of the inflammatory process. It is shown herein that careful examination and selection of subphenotypes related to a final heterogeneous disorder can be valuable in selecting animals for temporal studies aiming to unravel the mechanisms characterizing specific disease checkpoints. Cautious application of functional genomic approaches represents a method of choice in deciphering gene expression involved in multifactorial diseases such as autoimmune diabetes.

ACKNOWLEDGMENTS

Special acknowledgments are due to Dr. George Eisenbarth, in whose laboratory at the Barbara Davis Center for Childhood Diabetes, Denver, CO, I initiated this work during my sabbatical. I am thankful for his constant support. I thank also Rebecca Brown for her help with the transcriptome data analysis.

REFERENCES

1. TODD, J.A. & L.S. WICKER. 2001. Genetic protection from the inflammatory disease type 1 diabetes in humans and animal models. Immunity 15: 387–395.
2. BACH, J.F. 1999. Etiology and pathogenesis of human insulin-dependent diabetes mellitus. In Contemporary Endocrinology: Autoimmune Endocrinopathies, pp. 293–307. Humana Press. Totowa, NJ.
3. BELL, J.I. 1993. Polygenic disease. Curr. Opin. Genet. Dev. 3: 466–469.
4. MELANITOU, E., P. FAIN & G.S. EISENBARTH. 2003. Genetics of type 1A (immune mediated) diabetes. J. Autoimmun. 21: 93–98.
5. LEITER, E.H., D.V. SERREZE & M. PROCHAZKA. 1990. The genetics and epidemiology of diabetes in NOD mice. Immunol. Today 11: 147–149.
6. LEITER, E.H. 1993. The NOD mouse: a model for analyzing the interplay between heredity and environment in development of autoimmune disease. ILAR News 35: 4.
7. AMERICAN DIABETES ASSOCATION. 1997. Report of the expert committee on the diagnosis and classification of diabetes mellitus. Diabetes Care 20: 1183–1197.
8. YU, L. et al. 2000. Early expression of antiinsulin autoantibodies of humans and the NOD mouse: evidence for early determination of subsequent diabetes. Proc. Natl. Acad. Sci. USA 97: 1701–1706.
9. MELANITOU, E. et al. 2004. Early and quantal (by litter) expression of insulin autoantibodies in the nonobese diabetic mice predict early diabetes onset. J. Immunol. 173: 6603–6610.
10. GREELEY, S.A. et al. 2002. Elimination of maternally transmitted autoantibodies prevents diabetes in nonobese diabetic mice. Nat. Med. 8: 399–402.
11. HOCHBERG, Y. & Y. BENJAMINI. 1990. More powerful procedures for multiple significance testing. Stat. Med. 9: 811–818.
12. LI, H. et al. 2004. Analysis of oligonucleotide array experiments with repeated measures using mixed models. BMC Bioinformatics 5: 209.
13. NASERKE, H.E., E. BONIFACIO & A.G. ZIEGLER. 2001. Prevalence, characteristics and diabetes risk associated with transient maternally acquired islet antibodies and persistent islet antibodies in offspring of parents with type 1 diabetes. J. Clin. Endocrinol. Metab. 86: 4826–4833.
14. LARSSON, K. et al. 2004. Genetic and perinatal factors as risk for childhood type 1 diabetes. Diabetes Metab. Res. Rev. 20: 429–437.
15. STANLEY, H.M. et al. 2004. Is presence of islet autoantibodies at birth associated with development of persistent islet autoimmunity? The Diabetes Autoimmunity Study in the Young (DAISY). Diabetes Care 27: 497–502.
16. BACH, J.F. et al. 2004. The role of innate immunity in autoimmunity. J. Exp. Med. 200: 1527–1531.
17. SERREZE, D.V. & E.H. LEITER. 2001. Genes and cellular requirements for autoimmune diabetes susceptibility in nonobese diabetic mice. Curr. Dir. Autoimmun. 4: 31–67.
18. ANDRE, I. et al. 1996. Checkpoints in the progression of autoimmune disease: lessons from diabetes models. Proc. Natl. Acad. Sci. USA 93: 2260–2263.
19. HOGLUND, P. et al. 1999. Initiation of autoimmune diabetes by developmentally regulated presentation of islet cell antigens in the pancreatic lymph nodes. J. Exp. Med. 189: 331–339.

IgE and FcεRI Regulation

DONALD MacGLASHAN, JR.

The Johns Hopkins Asthma and Allergy Center, Baltimore, Maryland, USA

ABSTRACT: A central feature of allergic reactions is the aggregation of the high-affinity IgE receptor, FcεRI, to initiate a change in the behavior of the cell expressing the receptor. It is now clear that a number of cell types can express this receptor, which broadens the biology that revolves around IgE antibody. It is also quite clear that the presence of monomeric IgE antibody alters the expression of FcεRI. There remains considerable uncertainty about the importance of independent regulation of the FcεRIβ subunit or its splice variant $β_T$, in terms of regulating both expression and function of FcεRI. There is also only primitive understanding of the role of various polymorphisms in the subunit genes on the atopic phenotype. There are, however, many efforts being made to resolve these issues and to discover other factors that regulate expression of this receptor. Of particular interest for understanding the variation in expression in atopy among patients, the role of this receptor on non-mast cell/basophils will be important to elucidate.

KEYWORDS: IgE; FcεRI; FcεRIβ subunit; antibody; function; receptor; role; regulation; variant

INTRODUCTION

A central feature of allergic reactions is the aggregation of the high-affinity IgE receptor, FcεRI, to initiate a change in the behavior of the cell expressing the receptor. Today, it is apparent that not only mast cells and basophils express this receptor on their cell surface but there is clear evidence that Langerhans cells,[1] monocytes[2] (or a subset of monocytes), and cells derived from monocytes, such as dendritic cells,[3] also express this receptor. There are more controversial reports that the receptor is also expressed on eosinophils,[4–6] neutrophils,[7] and platelets,[8] but this biology is not, as yet, as well defined. For example, our own evidence indicates the presence of the FcεRI α subunit inside of eosinophils but no measurable cell surface expression.[6] There may be conditions that allow surface expression,[9,10] but this possibility needs further exploration and/or confirmation. Despite these unsettled issues, it is now clear that a number of cell types can express this receptor, which broadens the biology that revolves around IgE antibody.

It is also quite clear that the presence of monomeric IgE antibody alters the expression of FcεRI. Studies by Malveaux and Lichtenstein in 1978 noted a correlation between cell surface FcεRI densities on peripheral blood basophils and the titer of

Address for correspondence: Donald MacGlashan, Jr., M.D., Ph.D., The Johns Hopkins Asthma and Allergy Center, 5501 Bayview Circle, Baltimore, MD 21224.
   dmacglas@jhmi.edu

Ann. N.Y. Acad. Sci. 1050: 73–88 (2005). © 2005 New York Academy of Sciences.
doi: 10.1196/annals.1313.009

serum IgE.[11] A similar result was obtained more recently in a study examining a wider range of diseases with elevated serum IgE.[12] Studies in the laboratory of Chaviva Isersky in the mid-1980s noted that inclusion of IgE in cultures of rat basophilic leukemia (RBL) cells increased expression of FcεRI.[13] This observation was not extended to nontumor cells for several years, possibly because there were other observations of FcεRI processing that distinguished RBL cells from normal human basophils and mast cells. Nevertheless, the possibility remained that IgE modulated FcεRI expression, and this was more directly addressed by studies in the early and mid-1990s, both in human basophils and mast cells and in murine mast cells.[14–17] The observation that the presence of IgE could upregulate expression of FcεRI and its absence downregulate expression has important implications for both the biology of atopy and therapeutic approaches that attempt control of this disease constellation.

REGULATION OF FCεRI EXPRESSION

FcεRI is a receptor that can be composed of three subunits, designated α, β, and γ. The stoichiometry of expression, when all three components are present, is one α, one β, and two disulfide-linked γ subunits. The α chain is responsible for binding IgE, and the X-ray crystal structure of the combined IgE and receptor extracellular domain has been resolved to 3.5 Å.[18] IgE binds to the receptor asymmetrically; there are two primary contact sites between FcεRIα and the Ce2-Ce3 domains of IgE whereby FcεRIα binds to each of the Ce3 chains of IgE at different sites.[18,19] This way of binding precludes more than one IgE binding to one FcεRIα. The large area of contact and the amino acid residues involved leads to a very high affinity interaction. In addition, Ce3 of IgE must change conformation during binding to optimize contact.[18,20,21] As yet, there is no known function for the cytoplasmic tail of the α subunit.

Both the β and γ chains contain ITAMs (immunoreceptor tyrosine activation motifs) that mediate interaction with closely associated kinases; the receptor subunits themselves have no enzymatic activity. In rodents, all three components must be expressed for placement of the receptor on the cell surface,[22,23] whereas in humans the receptor can be expressed in the absence of FcεRIβ.[22] It seems likely that this ability to express FcεRI even the absence of FcεRIβ explains the ability of non-mast cell/basophils in man to express FcεRI as the $\alpha\gamma_2$ species. In transgenic mice expressing human subunits, monocytes and Langerhans cells are able to express the human FcεRIαγ_2.[24] However, it should be noted that from one perspective this situation is not so different from rodents, where all three subunits are needed for surface expression. In man, the cells that do not express FcεRIβ, for reasons not yet fully understood, also only express very low densities of FcεRI, up to 100-fold less receptor than basophils. For example, it is not uncommon to observe 500,000 FcεRI on circulating basophils of atopics and a maximum of 5000 receptors (and sometimes considerably less) on their monocytes. Because the expression of the receptors on monocytes and dendritic cells is also under the influence of circulating IgE (this form of regulating receptor expression seems intact[2,25–28]), it is possible that the absence of FcεRIβ restricts the cell's ability to load its cell surface with high densities of FcεRI. Studies with transfected cell lines demonstrate that coexpression of FcεRIβ leads to lines that express higher densities of FcεRI, although these studies would not suggest such a marked difference in expression levels in cells expressing $\alpha\gamma_2$ versus $\alpha\beta\gamma_2$. Notably, the stable transfectants with heterotrimer, $\alpha\gamma_2$, expressed only 3- to 6-fold lower densities of surface FcεRI than stable transfectants expressing the heterotetramer, $\alpha\beta\gamma_2$.[2,29] There are additional implications for differential FcεRIβ expression,[30] and these will be examined further below. However, it seems likely that there are at least two conditions that have a strong influence on the expression of FcεRI, expression of FcεRIβ and the local concentration of IgE antibody. Modulation of receptor expression can also follow exposure of mast cells to IL-4[17,31,32] (but not basophils), although the extent to which this mechanism is direct or indirect through effects on maturation or phenotype plasticity is not clear.

Gene Regulation

The genomic organization of the FcεRI subunits is well described, but the *cis*- and *trans*-acting factors that regulate the promoters of these genes are only poorly understood. FIGURE 1 shows the available evidence for genomic structure. It is notable that expression of the receptor coincides (at least within the temporal discrimination currently examined in cell culture studies) with the expression of other proteins associated with mast cell maturation (at least those proteins that are associated with identifiable mast cells).[33] Therefore, it seems likely that some of the *trans*-acting factors, such as GATA-1 or GATA-2 (which have been associated with upregulation of other mast cell-associated genes), may play a role in turning on expression of this receptor.[34,35] Because FcεRIβ appears to play an important role in the expression and activity of this receptor, the regulation of its expression attracts special attention. Notably, the gene for FcεRIβ is located in humans in the region of 11q13, a region that has been associated in a variety of studies with various aspects of atopic disease.[36] (This region also contains a variety of related 4-transmembrane spanning proteins now identified as MS4A, with FcεRIβ designated as MS4A2.) More recently, polymorphisms of the FcεRIβ gene have been associated with atopy,[37,38] total IgE levels,[39] asthma,[40] bronchial hyperresponsiveness,[41] allergic rhinitis,[42] and atopic dermatitis.[43] In particular, three polymorphisms in the coding region, I181L, V183L, and E237G, show linkage with atopy, but to date efforts to find a change in the behavior of FcεRIβ with these changes incorporated have not revealed significant differences from the canonical FcεRIβ.[44] Whether there are other functions of FcεRIβ that are affected by these polymorphisms remains an open question. Several single nucleotide polymorphisms (SNPs) have also been identified in an extended region of the FcεRIβ gene: 38 sequence variants were identified from a population of 12 individuals, 35 were SNPs, 2 were simple dinucleotide repeats, and one a 3-base deletion.[45] The authors of this study predict that this survey captured, with 99% probability, alleles with a frequency greater than 0.1. Surprisingly, this survey did not detect the I181L and V183L polymorphisms, although it did detect the E237G variant. Of the 38 polymorphisms, only the E237G variant is found in the coding region. Other than the E237G variant, none of these polymorphisms has been tested for modifications in the regulation of its expression. A more recent study found that there was an association between expression of the E237G variant and expression of FcεRI on circulating basophils.[46] However, for reasons still unclear, this SNP also is associated with a higher IgE level, and this may account for the higher receptor expression. More interestingly, this same study found that two other SNPs in the promoter of the FcεRIβ gene were tightly linked to the E237G SNP and that these polymorphisms did lead to more promoter activity by mechanisms unknown.

There is a recently identified splice variant of FcεRIβ that may influence the cell surface expression of FcεRI.[47] This splice variant, designated β_T, includes the fifth intron of the FcεRIβ gene and, because this intron contains a stop codon, a truncated version of FcεRIβ is generated as a protein. Recent studies using stable and transient transfectants of FcεRIβ and FcεRIβ$_T$ indicate that the normal chaperone functions of FcεRIβ are disrupted by the presence of FcεRIβ$_T$. In the current model of FcεRI synthesis, FcεRIα contains an ER retention sequence that is modulated by the presence of either FcεRIβ or FcεRIγ in humans. This allows FcεRI to progress to the Golgi for further glycosylation and migration to the plasma membrane. When FcεRIβ$_T$ associates with FcεRIα in the ER, it apparently does not mask this retention signal and the complex becomes targeted for destruction, resulting in suppression of FcεRI expression at the cell surface. Transcripts for FcεRIβ$_T$ have been detected in cultured human mast cells and circulating basophils, although a detailed analysis of its presence in the general population, or those with atopic diseases, and its influence on expression levels of FcεRI has not been conducted.

Some of the dynamics of FcεRIβ expression have been studied. One question that arises when considering the ability of FcεRI to be expressed with or without FcεRIβ is whether the ratio of FcεRIβ to FcεRIα is constant among cells that can express the tetrameric form of FcεRI (i.e., basophils or mast cells). The most accessible cell is the basophil, so this cell was examined for the above ratio using donors with known

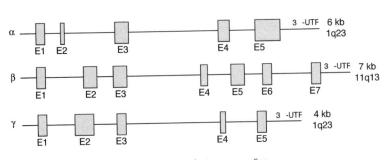

α: 4 known sequence variants, none coding
β: 38 known sequence variants, most non-coding
γ: 1 known sequence variant, non-coding

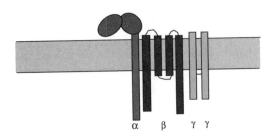

FIGURE 1. Schematic of the genomic structure of the three subunits of the high-affinity IgE receptor (FcεRI).

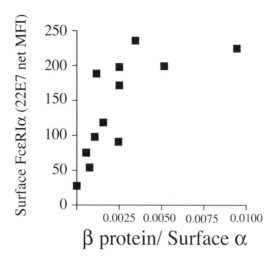

FIGURE 2. Relationship between the ratio of FcεRIβ to FcεRIα and cell surface expression of FcεRI on peripheral blood basophils.

differences in cell surface FcεRI density. Surprisingly, this ratio was considerably variable, ranging nearly 100-fold.[48] FIGURE 2 shows the relationship between the ratio and total cell surface FcεRI; greater ratios were associated with greater FcεRI density and if the data is taken at face value, the relationship appears to saturate (these data have not been "adjusted" to account for differences in total serum IgE concentration). The same studies found that IL-3 could upregulate the steady-state expression of mRNA for FcεRIβ, and unpublished studies suggest that IL-3 does not alter mRNA degradation so that the change in steady state is likely the result of increased transcription. FcεRIβ protein also increases in culture with IL-3. Only a couple studies of promoter regulation have been done. A study of the murine FcεRIβ promoter suggests a role for GATA-1 (which may be sensitive to the presence of IL-3),[49] and a study of the human promoter concluded that OCT-1 *cis*-acting elements have a role in FcεRIβ gene transcription.[50]

In one study of SNPs in the FcεRIα gene, only three SNPs were identified; none were in the coding region, but all were located in the 5' flanking region.[51] One SNP was found to have an association with serum total IgE levels in an asthmatic population. A second study has identified a SNP in the promoter of the FcεRIα gene.[52] This SNP appears to increase transcription frequency by adding an additional GATA-1 site to the promoter, and in a Japanese population allergic donors were more likely to be homozygous for the "T" variant that confers higher transcription rates.

The γ subunit of FcεRI is shared among several immunoreceptors, FcεRI, FcγRIα, and FcγRIIIα. This shared status raises the interesting possibility that competition for this common resource among Fc receptors present in the same cell may influence their expression.[53] The FcεRIγ gene is located on human chromosome 1q23 and it is a member of the TCRζ family of signaling molecules. As shown in FIGURE 1, this gene appears to have five exons, with the leader sequence of the protein occurring in exon 1, the very short extracellular domain starting within exon 2, and the critical ITAM spanning exons 4 and 5. Although Genbank appears to include several possible sequence variants for the coding region of this gene, these variants may be sequencing artifacts, because a recent study failed to find the various mutations in a screen of 146 different donors.[54] Only one polymorphism was found in one donor and it coded for a valine to methionine mutation in a noncoding region. Although this is a relatively small gene, the absence of SNPs in the coding region is surprising (the average gene having one SNP per kilobase pairs). A search of the broader population may turn up additional polymorphisms.

Like the β subunit, the γ subunit has two potential roles, regulating the expression of the α subunits by protecting them from premature shunting into a degradative pathway in the ER, and providing the cell surface receptor with all-important ITAMs. Each γ subunit has one ITAM, therefore FcεRI has at least two ITAMs if the receptor is heterotrimeric and three ITAMS if heterotetrameric. The γ ITAMs are known to provide a docking site for syk SH2 domains (for which there are two in tandem that can bind to both γ ITAMs). These ITAMs are critical for the function of the receptor.[55,56]

IgE-Dependent Regulation

The addition of IgE to a culture of purified human basophils results in the upregulation of cell surface FcεRI. The upregulation is caused by the interaction of IgE with the receptor itself and not with accessory cells or other receptors that may bind IgE.[57] There is an unexpected concentration dependence for upregulation; the EC_{50} for upregulation is approximately 250 ng/mL (~1 nM) of IgE, 30- to 100-fold higher than the anticipated concentration for 50% occupancy of the receptor.[58] When cell surface receptor increases, so too does the total FcεRIα content of the cell. Likewise, removal of IgE results in loss of both cell surface receptor and total cellular FcεRIα.[58] These results suggest that there is no major preformed store of receptor that shuttles from the inside to the outside of the cell (or vice versa). The model which best fits this and other observations on the behavior of the system with respect to IgE is one where FcεRIα is constitutively synthesized and IgE controls the loss of receptor from the cell surface once it appears on the surface of the cell.[59] The mechanism of loss remains unknown, but IgE clearly protects the receptor from loss.[60] If endogenously present IgE is removed from the cell by treatment with a slightly acidic buffer, the receptor is lost with a half-life of approximately 24 h (reloading these treated cells with IgE completely prevents loss).[59] No changes in the steady-state concentrations of mRNA for FcεRIα, FcεRIβ, or FcεRIγ have been observed to follow culture with IgE, nor is the synthetic rate of FcεRIα altered by the presence of IgE.[59] The unexpected EC_{50} for upregulation results from the slow forward rate constant of IgE binding to the receptor. This makes sense because receptor is only protected from loss if IgE is bound, and higher concentrations of IgE are needed to compensate for the relatively slow forward binding constant of the reaction (as newly formed receptor appears on the cell surface). There is a familiarity to this situation. CD23 (FcεRII) expression is also dependent on IgE.[61–63] For this receptor, IgE protects its loss by a proteolytic mechanism. However, for FcεRI, drugs that inhibit the proteases cleaving CD23 do not inhibit loss of FcεRI in the absence of IgE.[59]

A second unexpected outcome of *in vitro* studies of IgE interaction with the receptor is that the dissociation constant is considerably slower than estimates based on transfected cell lines. The *in vitro* studies suggest that 10 days are required for 50% dissociation, even if an IgE trap is included in the culture (a trap such as Xolair/ E25 or Tanox's Hu901).[58] This result suggests that the affinity of IgE for FcεRI in a natural setting is quite high, closer to 1×10^{11}. The consequence of this higher affinity is that dissociation of IgE from cells *in vivo* may take many weeks, a point discussed in further detail below.

The studies of IgE-dependent regulation of FcεRI expression provided the first indication that monomeric IgE could provide some sort of signal to the receptor (it should be noted that dimeric IgE actually results in suppression of upregulation). Although the "signal" for IgE-mediated retention of FcεRI may be the passive presence of bound IgE, the possibility of monomeric IgE signaling through the receptor led to a variety of studies in which monomeric IgE has a wide variety of effects on mast cell function. The initial studies of this phenomenon noted a variety of signaling steps being activated by IgE (enriched for monomeric species by HPLC). Indeed, with the exception of degranulation and arachidonic acid metabolite release, there was little distinction between monomeric IgE-induced activation and aggregation of FcεRI with antigen.[64] Given the long history of studies that begin with sensitization of the cells with antigen-specific IgE, these results were confusing. The EC_{50} for the activation of signaling by putatively monomeric IgE is quite high, ~1 μg/mL. The data suggested a radical rethinking of the consequences of IgE binding to its receptor. However, it now appears that there is something more subtle operating in these *in vitro* conditions that may or may not have application *in vivo*. The key experiment that reveals this subtlety derives from the nature of the IgE used to demonstrate the effect. Thus far, the IgE that most readily demonstrates strong signaling is a mouse monoclonal IgE specific for conjugated dinitrophenyl (DNP) haptens. Inclusion of monovalent hapten with the IgE prevents the signaling induced by the putatively monomeric IgE. This result suggests that the antigen-binding portion of the monomeric IgE is interacting with its ligand to induce a reaction similar to aggregation. The nature of this interaction remains unclear, but it is apparent that not all monomeric IgE molecules can induce this kind of signaling. Kawakami and his colleagues have labeled IgE species as highly cytokinergic or poorly cytokinergic (HC vs. PC).[65] There remains considerable debate about the frequency of HC IgEs, but this problem has not been examined in the context of natural systems. The anti-DNP IgE that most readily induces overt signaling is commercially available as SPE-7. The ligand binding site of SPE-7 has been shown to bind to possibly three very different ligands.[66] The hypothesis has been proposed that SPE-7 represents a type of IgE that may interact weakly with some extracellular structure, not necessarily DNP-like, inducing a hybrid form of aggregate on the cell surface. There is evidence from studies in the early 1980s by Daeron and his colleagues that aggregation of FcεRI with cell surface structures leads to signaling and mediator release.[67] Further, studies by McConnell in the mid-1980s demonstrated that even transiently associating receptors whose densities were quite high could induce signaling.[68–70] More recently, Metzger and associates have shown that signaling dynamics may follow a process termed kinetic proofreading (the ability of a signal to progress through the entire cascade being dependent on the transience of the first signal, in this case aggregation), but that certain steps can escape kinetic proofreading. In experimental studies of this escape mechanism, a more transient signal could still induce cytokine/chemokine release.[71] Putting these pieces of information together leads to the hypothesis that IgE interacting weakly with cell surface structures may generate weak signals that drive only certain aspects of cell function. The studies by Kawakami and associates suggest that at least one such process is survival of mast cells.[72] Because even IgE-induced survival requires the same early signaling components as normal aggregation-induced secretion,[73] it seems possible that transient weak signals are driving survival. If this viewpoint is correct, then one of the central questions that needs answering is as follows: how often does one find antigen-specific IgE that can engage in this behavior, and what are the requirements for the effects to occur (IgE concentration and the density of unoccupied FcεRI)? It should be noted that it is unlikely that IgE protects loss of FcεRI through a similar mechanism. Treatment of human basophils with an inhibitor of src family kinases—which should completely inhibit the initiation of normal signaling—does not inhibit the protection afforded by IgE bound to receptor. Using mast cells derived from mice not expressing syk kinase (see below), monomeric IgE continues to result in upregulation of FcεRI, whereas its effects on survival are blocked.[73]

One prediction of a model where IgE does not influence the synthesis of FcεRI but only protects its loss, once expressed, is that there will be a steady state reached even in the absence of IgE.[59] This is found in experimental studies, and it appears that the natural steady state is somewhere between 5000 to 10,000 receptors per cell.[58,59,74] At concentrations of IgE that allow the lowest steady state to occur, the occupancy of the receptor is quite low. For example, at 5 ng/mL of IgE, receptor occupancy is less than 20%. As will be seen, even this level of occupancy (and low density) might be sufficient for partial function of the cell.

The *in vitro* studies of IgE dissociation from human basophils suggest slow dissociation with a half-life of approximately 10 days. Recent studies of changes in mast cell receptor densities following treatment of patients with an anti-IgE antibody (omalizumab) suggest a long half-life as well.[75] Although it is possible that conditions in the skin of patients (where the biopsies for mast cell receptor density were taken) do not allow rapid loss of IgE from the mast cell, the results are compatible with *in vitro* data. In contrast, the apparent rapid loss of receptor (and IgE) on circulating basophils in the same patients[74] seems to contradict *in vitro* studies. However, one possible explanation for the discrepancy relates to the rapid turnover of basophils in circulation.[76] When considering how anti-IgE antibody acts on the system and making some assumptions about the lifespan of circulating basophils, the data become consistent with what is known about IgE dissociation times. Indeed, this analysis also leads to the conclusion that the apparent loss of IgE and receptor from circulating basophils is (counterintuitively) a measure of the rate that receptors are loaded onto basophils during maturation and the length of time that basophils mature, that is, from the time they begin expressing receptor to their appearance and disappearance from peripheral blood. Parenthetically, if this analysis is correct, then basophils in the bone marrow synthesize receptors faster than observed *in vitro*.

SIGNALING AND REQUIREMENTS FOR FUNCTION

The traditional view of immediate hypersensitivity is that there is first an immune response, skewed in such a way that IgE antibody is generated, IgE binds to circulating basophils or tissue-bound mast cells or Langerhans cells, and antigen re-enters the system sometime later and by inducing aggregation of surface-bound specific IgE initiates a signal in the IgE-bearing cells. For mast cells and basophils, one functional consequence is the secretion of a variety of mediators. Some of these are preformed and stored in granules, for example, histamine, and some mediators are newly formed, such as the leukotrienes or prostaglandins (mast cells). Histamine and arachidonic acid products such as LTC4 are released rapidly, but later in the reaction the cells also synthesize cytokines and chemokines. Detailed studies of human basophils and less detailed studies of tissue mast cells indicate that only approximately 2000 antigen-specific IgE molecules need be aggregated to result in 50% of the cells' maximal response.[77,78] This sensitivity differs among individuals, notably some individuals' basophils require less than 300 antigen-specific IgE molecules to reach the 50% response point.[79] Because the typical atopic patient has 250,000 receptors, reducing the cellular response requires significant reductions in circulating IgE. Because receptor expression decreases with decreases in free IgE, there is synergy in the reduction of cell surface IgE, but the synergy works in reverse with increases in IgE. In addition, the minimum steady state achievable (see above) limits the effects of synergy at the low end of free-IgE concentrations. In large part, only the occupancy of receptor continues to be reduced with further reductions in free IgE. The system responds to the total IgE concentration, that is, these numbers apply when considering all IgE. However, for any given patient, antigen-specific IgE represents a fraction of the total IgE. If this fraction is low enough, even modest reductions in total IgE may reduce cell function. In contrast, if antigen-specific IgE represents an appreciable fraction of the total IgE, it could be very difficult to achieve a reduction in the cell response. This possibility has not been examined directly, although preliminary data in a phase I trial of omalizumab[74] suggest that the ratio of antigen-specific IgE to total IgE is a predictor of the final suppression of the basophil response.

Phase I trials also demonstrated that at therapeutic doses of omalizumab, the basophil and mast cell responses were at a threshold. Slight reductions in omalizumab dose resulted in a near return to normal function. FIGURE 3 illustrates this result. Note that prior to the start of therapy, both IgE and FcεRI density on circulating basophils average approximately 250,000 per basophil, that is, near total occupancy, with serum free-IgE concentrations of approximately 400 ng/mL (~2 nM). After 3 months with circulating free IgE reduced to 4 ng/mL, receptor expression was reduced to approximately 10,000 per cell and IgE to less than 1500 per cell, that is, less than 15% occupancy. Histamine release from isolated basophils stimulated with optimal or suboptimal concentrations of dust mite antigen was reduced, on average, about 90%. At 6 months, the dose of omalizumab was reduced by 3- to 20-fold, resulting in an increase in serum free IgE of 3-fold and an increase in receptor expression of 3-fold. Although the increase in receptor expression and loading with IgE was relatively subtle, there was a nearly complete return of antigen-induced histamine release to levels observed prior to treatment.[80]

As noted above, one parameter of cellular responsiveness is sensitivity, the number of antigen-specific IgE molecules per cell required for a half-maximal response. Knowledge of this parameter of cell function helps in understanding what is needed for cells to respond. To determine the average value of 2000 molecules per cell, human basophils were tested for histamine release. We have also examined other end-

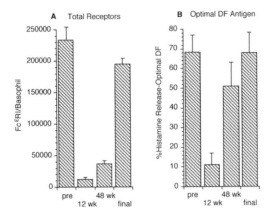

FIGURE 3. Loss and recovery of antigen-induced histamine release from peripheral blood basophils during treatment with anti-IgE antibody relative to changes FcεRI expression.

points of secretion; a similar value applies to the secretion of LTC4 and IL-4.[79,81] However, this may not be true for mast cells. Although human mast cells have not been examined for LTC4 or cytokine secretion (but histamine release is similar to basophils), studies in cultured mouse mast cells suggest that cytokine release requires high densities of antigen-specific IgE.[82] A similar parameter has not been developed for activation of other $\alpha\gamma_2$-FcεRI-bearing cells. For example, it is not known how much IgE must be bound to dendritic or Langerhans cells to initiate substantial antigen presentation. Furthermore, the relationship between IgE concentration and expression of FcεRI on these cells is not well understood, although it is apparent that the relationship exists.[2,25–27] Therefore, a prediction of how changes in IgE might alter the response of these cells cannot be made at this time.

When considering the consequences of reducing circulating IgE in man, the reduction in basophil and mast cell secretion and, possibly, the reduction in function of dendritic and Langerhans cells may regulate another important feedback loop. The cytokines secreted by basophils and mast cells are likely to regulate the allergic inflammatory status of their environment, and likely to regulate the immune response characteristics that lead to IgE synthesis. For example, there is mounting evidence that basophils are a primary source of IL-4 and IL-13.[83–86] In humans, it has not yet been possible to demonstrate IL-4 protein secretion from tissue mast cells and even in cultured mast cells, but this continues to be a controversial issue. However, basophils secrete quantities similar to T cells, and because the frequency of basophils (with their panspecific IgE) is much greater than that of antigen-specific T cells, on balance, basophils may generate most of the IL-4 present in tissues (at certain times). Recent studies in mice support a prominent role for basophils.[87–90] Hence, significant reductions in IL-4 and IL-13 secretion from basophils during a reduction in circulating IgE (e.g., with omalizumab) could have long-term consequences to the synthesis of IgE. The longer-term feedback loop therefore further favors a reduction in the atopic diathesis.

There is evidence that IgE synthesis occurs, in large part, in mucosal tissues.[91-93] Indeed, there are examples of patients where serum IgE is unmeasurable while IgE can be found in mucosal tissues. The feedback loop involving IgE upregulation of FcεRI, upregulated receptor inducing greater IL-4 secretion (with antigen present), and this IL-4 inducing further B cell switching for IgE synthesis is an interesting possibility. One study suggests that although mast cells and basophils may express CD40L, only basophils can provide a full signal (IL-4 and CD40L) to local B cells to drive the IgE switch.[94] However, one might expect that this potentially strong positive-feedback loop should have some braking mechanism. There are indications that aggregation of mIgE or CD23a on B cells acts to inhibit IgE generation.[95,96] However, this negative feedback loop operates at IgE concentrations that are 100- to 1000-fold higher than the positive feedback loop noted above. Therefore, the braking action of this negative feedback loop takes place only at higher concentrations of IgE. Further regulation may come from the cytokines in these local environments that are also thought to regulate receptor expression.

SUMMARY

There is rapidly expanding interest in the factors that regulate expression of FcεRI. There remains considerable uncertainty about the importance of independent regulation of the FcεRIβ subunit or its splice variant β_T, in terms of regulating both expression and function of FcεRI. There is also only primitive understanding of the role of various polymorphisms in the subunit genes on the atopic phenotype. There are, however, many efforts being made to resolve these issues and to discover other factors that regulate expression of this receptor. Of particular interest for understanding the variation in expression in atopy among patients, the role of this receptor on non-mast cell/basophils will be important to elucidate.

REFERENCES

1. WANG, B., A. RIEGER, O. KILGUS, *et al.* 1992. Epidermal Langerhans cells from normal human skin bind monomeric IgE via FcεRI. J. Exp. Med. **175:** 1353–1365.
2. MAURER, D., E. FIEBIGER, B. REININGER, *et al.* 1994. Expression of functional high affinity immunoglobulin E receptors (FcεRI) on monocytes of atopic individuals. J. Exp. Med. **179:** 745–750.
3. MAURER, D., S. FIEBIGER, C. EBNER, *et al.* 1996. Peripheral blood dendritic cells express Fc epsilon RI as a complex composed of Fc epsilon RI alpha- and Fc epsilon RI gamma-chains and can use this receptor for IgE-mediated allergen presentation. J. Immunol. **157:** 607–616.
4. KITA, H., M. KANEKO, K.R. BARTEMES, *et al.* 1999. Does IgE bind to and activate eosinophils from patients with allergy? J. Immunol. **162:** 6901–6911.
5. GOUNNI, A.S., B. LAMKHIOUED, K. OCHIAI, *et al.* 1994. High-affinity IgE receptor on eosinophils is involved in defence against parasites. Nature **367:** 183–186.
6. SEMINARIO, M.C., S.S. SAINI, D.W. MACGLASHAN, JR. & B.S. BOCHNER. 1999. Intracellular expression and release of FcεRIα by human eosinophils. J. Immunol. **162:** 6893–6900.
7. GOUNNI, A.S., B. LAMKHIOUED, L. KOUSSIH, *et al.* 2001. Human neutrophils express the high-affinity receptor for immunoglobulin E (FcεRI): role in asthma. FASEB J. **15:** 940–949.

8. JOSEPH, M., A.S. GOUNNI, J.P. KUSNIERZ, et al. 1997. Expression and functions of the high-affinity IgE receptor on human platelets and megakaryocyte precursors. Eur. J. Immunol. 27: 2212–2218.
9. BJERKE, T., H.J. HOFFMANN, E.I. CHRISTENSEN, et al. 1999. Regulation of FcεARI synthesis in human eosinophils. Int. Arch. Allergy Immunol. 118: 440–442.
10. TERADA, N., A. KONNO, Y. TERADA, et al. 1995. IL-4 upregulates FcεRIα-chain messenger RNA in eosinophils. J. Allergy Clin. Immunol. 96: 1161–1169.
11. MALVEAUX, F.J., M.C. CONROY, N.F.J. ADKINSON & L.M. LICHTENSTEIN. 1978. IgE receptors on human basophils: relationship to serum IgE concentration. J. Clin. Invest. 62: 176–181.
12. SAINI, S.S., A.D. KLION, S.M. HOLLAND, et al. 2000. The relationship between serum IgE and surface levels of FcεR on human leukocytes in various diseases: correlation of expression with FcεRI on basophils but not on monocytes or eosinophils. J. Allergy Clin. Immunol. 106: 514–520.
13. FURUICHI, K., J. RIVERA & C. ISERSKY. 1985. The receptor for immunoglobulin E on rat basophilic leukemia cells: effect of ligand binding on receptor expression. Proc. Natl. Acad. Sci. USA 82: 1522–1525.
14. HSU, C. & D. MACGLASHAN, JR. 1996. IgE antibody up-regulates high affinity IgE binding on murine bone marrow-derived mast cells. Immunol. Lett. 52: 129–134.
15. TORU, H., C. RA, S. NONOYAMA, et al. 1997. Induction of high affinity IgE receptor on human mast cells by IL-4. J. Allergy Clin. Immunol. 99: S103.
16. LANTZ, C.S., M. YAMAGUCHI, H.C. OETTGEN, et al. 1997. IgE regulates mouse basophil Fc epsilon RI expression in vivo. J. Immunol. 158: 2517–2521.
17. YAMAGUCHI, M., K. SAYAMA, K. YANO, et al. 1999. IgE enhances Fcεreceptor I expression and IgE-dependent release of histamine and lipid mediators from human umbilical cord blood-derived mast cells: synergistic effect of IL-4 and IgE on human mast cell Fcε receptor I expression and mediator release. J. Immunol. 162: 5455–5465.
18. GARMAN, S.C., B.A. WURZBURG, S.S. TARCHEVSKAYA, et al. 2000. Structure of the Fc fragment of human IgE bound to its high-affinity receptor FcεRIα. Nature 406: 259–266.
19. HENRY, A.J., J.P. COOK, J.M. MCDONNELL, et al. 1997. Participation of the N-terminal region of Cε3 in the binding of human IgE to its high-affinity receptor FcεRI. Biochemistry 36: 15568–15578.
20. GARMAN, S.C., S. SECHI, J.P. KINET & T.S. JARDETZKY. 2001. The analysis of the human high affinity IgE receptor FcεRIα from multiple crystal forms. J. Mol. Biol. 311: 1049–1062.
21. WURZBURG, B.A., S.C. GARMAN & T.S. JARDETZKY. 2000. Structure of the human IgE-Fc C epsilon 3-C epsilon 4 reveals conformational flexibility in the antibody effector domains. Immunity 13: 375–385.
22. MILLER, L., U. BLANK, H. METZGER & J.P. KINET. 1989. Expression of high-affinity binding of human immunoglobulin E by transfected cells. Science 244: 334–337.
23. HIRAOKA, S., Y. FURUMOTO, H. KOSEKI, et al. 1999. Fc receptor β subunit is required for full activation of mast cells through Fc receptor engagement. Int. Immunol. 11: 199–207.
24. FUNG-LEUNG, W.P., J. DE SOUSA-HITZLER, A. ISHAQUE, et al. 1996. Transgenic mice expressing the human high-affinity immunoglobulin (Ig) E receptor α chain respond to human IgE in mast cell degranulation and in allergic reactions. J. Exp. Med. 183: 49–56.
25. REISCHL, I.G., G.R. DUBOIS, S. PEIRITSCH, et al. 2000. Regulation of FcεRI expression on human monocytic cells by ligand and IL-4. Clin. Exp. Allergy 30: 1033–1040.
26. DUBOIS, G.R., I.G. REISCHL, S. PEIRITSCH, et al. 1999. Regulation of FcARI expression on monocytic cell lines. Int. Arch. Allergy Immunol. 118: 294–295.
27. SIHRA, B.S., O.M. KON, J.A. GRANT & A.B. KAY. 1997. Expression of high-affinity IgE receptors (Fc epsilon RI) on peripheral blood basophils, monocytes, and eosinophils in atopic and nonatopic subjects: relationship to total serum IgE concentrations. J. Allergy Clin. Immunol. 99: 699–706.
28. FOSTER, B., D.D. METCALFE & C. PRUSSIN. 2003. Human dendritic cell 1 and dendritic cell 2 subsets express FcεRI: correlation with serum IgE and allergic asthma. J. Allergy Clin. Immunol. 112: 1132–1138.

29. DONNADIEU, E., M.H. JOUVIN & J.P. KINET. 2000. A second amplifier function for the allergy-associated Fc(epsilon)RI-beta subunit. Immunity 12: 515–523.
30. LIN, S., C. CICAIA, A.M. SCHARENBERG & J.P. KINET. 1996. The Fc(epsilon)RIbeta subunit functions as an amplifier of Fc(epsilon)RIgamma-mediated cell activation signals. Cell 85: 985–995.
31. TORU, H., C. RA, S. NONOYAMA, et al. 1996. Induction of the high-affinity IgE receptor (Fc epsilon RI) on human mast cells by IL-4. Int. Immunol. 8: 1367–1373.
32. XIA, H.Z., Z. DU, S. CRAIG, et al. 1997. Effect of recombinant human IL-4 on tryptase, chymase, and Fc epsilon receptor type I expression in recombinant human stem cell factor-dependent fetal liver-derived human mast cells. J. Immunol. 159: 2911–2921.
33. THOMPSON, H.L., D.D. METCALFE & J.P. KINET. 1990. Early expression of high-affinity receptor for immunoglobulin E (Fc epsilon RI) during differentiation of mouse mast cells and human basophils. J. Clin. Invest. 85: 1227–1233.
34. ZON, L.I., M.F. GURISH, R.L. STEVENS, et al. 1991. GATA-binding transcription factors in mast cells regulate the promoter of the mast cell carboxypeptidase A gene. J. Biol. Chem. 266: 22948–22953.
35. NISHIYAMA, C., T. YOKOTA, K. OKUMURA & C. RA. 1999. The transcription factors Elf-1 and GATA-1 bind to cell-specific enhancer elements of human high-affinity IgE receptor α-chain gene. J. Immunol. 163: 623–630.
36. COOKSON, W.O., P.A. SHARP, J.A. FAUX & J.M. HOPKIN. 1989. Linkage between immunoglobulin E responses underlying asthma and rhinitis and chromosome 11q. Lancet 1(8650): 1292–1295.
37. SHIRAKAWA, T., A. LI, M. DUBOWITZ, et al. 1994. Association between atopy and variants of the beta subunit of the high-affinity immunoglobulin E receptor. Nat. Genet. 7: 125–129.
38. SANDFORD, A.J., T. SHIRAKAWA, M.F. MOFFATT, et al. 1993. Localisation of atopy and beta subunit of high-affinity IgE receptor (Fc epsilon RI) on chromosome 11q. Lancet 341: 332–334.
39. PALMER, L.J., P.D. PARE, J.A. FAUX, et al. 1997. Fc epsilon R1-beta polymorphism and total serum IgE levels in endemically parasitized Australian aborigines. Am. J. Hum. Genet. 61: 182–188.
40. SHIRAKAWA, T., X.Q. MAO, S. SASAKI, et al. 1996. Association between atopic asthma and a coding variant of Fc epsilon RI beta in a Japanese population. Hum. Mol. Genet. 5: 2068.
41. LAPRISE, C., L.P. BOULET, J. MORISSETTE, et al. 2000. Evidence for association and linkage between atopy, airway hyper-responsiveness, and the β subunit Glu237Gly variant of the high-affinity receptor for immunoglobulin E in the French-Canadian population. Immunogenetics 51: 695–702.
42. NAGATA, H., H. MUTOH, K. KUMAHARA, et al. 2001. Association between nasal allergy and a coding variant of the FcεRIβ gene Glu237Gly in a Japanese population. Hum. Genet. 109: 262–266.
43. COX, H.E., M.F. MOFFATT, J.A. FAUX, et al. 1998. Association of atopic dermatitis to the beta subunit of the high affinity immunoglobulin E receptor. Br. J. Dermatol. 138: 182–187.
44. DONNADIEU, E., W.O. COOKSON, M.H. JOUVIN & J.P. KINET. 2000. Allergy-associated polymorphisms of the FcεRIβ subunit do not impact its two amplification functions. J. Immunol. 165: 3917–3922.
45. TRAHERNE, J.A., M.R. HILL, P. HYSI, et al. 2003. LD mapping of maternally and non-maternally derived alleles and atopy in FcεRI-β. Hum. Mol. Genet. 12: 2577–2585.
46. NISHIYAMA, C., Y. AKIZAWA, M. NISHIYAMA, et al. 2004. Polymorphisms in the FcεRIβ promoter region affecting transcription activity: a possible promoter-dependent mechanism for association between FcεRIβ and atopy. J. Immunol. 173: 6458–6464.
47. DONNADIEU, E., M.H. JOUVIN, S. RANA, et al. 2003. Competing functions encoded in the allergy-associated F(c)εRIβ gene. Immunity 18: 665–674.
48. SAINI, S., J.J. RICHARDSON, C. WOFSY, et al. 2001. Expression and modulation of FcεRIα and FcεRIβ in human blood basophils. J. Allergy Clin. Immunol. 107: 832–841.

49. MAEDA, K., C. NISHIYAMA, T. TOKURA, *et al.* 2003. Regulation of cell type-specific mouse FcεRI β-chain gene expression by GATA-1 via four GATA motifs in the promoter. J. Immunol. **170:** 334–340.
50. AKIZAWA, Y., C. NISHIYAMA, M. HASEGAWA, *et al.* 2003. Regulation of human FcεRIβ chain gene expression by Oct-1. Int. Immunol. **15:** 549–556.
51. SHIKANAI, T., E.S. SILVERMAN, B.W. MORSE, *et al.* 2002. Sequence variants in the FcεRI alpha chain gene. J. Appl. Physiol. **93:** 37–41.
52. HASEGAWA, M., C. NISHIYAMA, M. NISHIYAMA, *et al.* 2003. A novel -66T/C polymorphism in FcεRI α-chain promoter affecting the transcription activity: possible relationship to allergic diseases. J. Immunol. **171:** 1927–1933.
53. DOMBROWICZ, D., V. FLAMAND, I. MIYAJIMA, *et al.* 1997. Absence of FcεRI αchain results in upregulation of FcγRIII-dependent mast cell degranulation and anaphylaxis: evidence of competition between FcεRI and FcγRIII for limiting amounts of FcR β and γ chains. J. Clin. Invest. **99:** 915–925.
54. WU, J., J.C. EDBERG, A.W. GIBSON & R.P. KIMBERLY. 2002. Conservation of FcεRI gamma chain coding region in normals and in SLE patients. Lupus **11:** 42–45.
55. SHIUE, L., J. GREEN, O.M. GREEN, *et al.* 1995. Interaction of p72syk with the γ and βsubunits of the high-affinity receptor for immunoglobulin E, FcεRI. Mol. Cell. Biol. **15:** 272–281.
56. WILSON, B.S., N. KAPP, R.J. LEE, *et al.* 1995. Distinct functions of the FcεR1 γ and β subunits in the control of FcεR1-mediated tyrosine kinase activation and signaling responses in RBL-2H3 mast cells. J. Biol. Chem. **270:** 4013–4022.
57. MACGLASHAN, D.W., JR., L.M. LICHTENSTEIN, J. MCKENZIE-WHITE, *et al.* 1999. Upregulation of FcεRI on human basophils by IgE antibody is mediated by interaction of IgE with FcεRI. J. Allergy Clin. Immunol. **104:** 492–498.
58. MACGLASHAN, D.W., JR., J. MCKENZIE-WHITE, K. CHICHESTER, *et al.* 1998. In vitro regulation of FcεRIα expression on human basophils by IgE antibody. Blood **91:** 1633–1643.
59. MACGLASHAN, D.W., JR., H.Z. XIA, L.B. SCHWARTZ & J.P. GONG. 2001. IgE-regulated loss, not IgE-regulated synthesis, controls expression of FcεRI in human basophils. J. Leukoc. Biol. **70:** 207–218.
60. BORKOWSKI, T.A., M.H. JOUVIN, S.Y. LIN & J.P. KINET. 2001. Minimal requirements for IgE-mediated regulation of surface FcεRI. J. Immunol. **167:** 1290–1296.
61. DAERON, M. & K. ISHIZAKA. 1986. Induction of Fc epsilon receptors on mouse macrophages and lymphocytes by homologous IgE. J. Immunol. **136:** 1612–1619.
62. LEE, W.T. & D.H. CONRAD. 1986. Murine B cell hybridomas bearing ligand-inducible Fc receptors for IgE. J. Immunol. **136:** 4573–45780.
63. LEE, W.T., M. RAO & D.H. CONRAD. 1987. The murine lymphocyte receptor for IgE. IV. The mechanism of ligand-specific receptor upregulation on B cells. J. Immunol. **139:** 1191–1198.
64. KALESNIKOFF, J., M. HUBER, V. LAM, *et al.* 2001. Monomeric IgE stimulates signaling pathways in mast cells that lead to cytokine production and cell survival. Immunity **14:** 801–811.
65. KITAURA, J., J. SONG, M. TSAI, *et al.* 2003. Evidence that IgE molecules mediate a spectrum of effects on mast cell survival and activation via aggregation of the FcεRI. Proc. Natl. Acad. Sci. USA **100:** 12911–12916.
66. JAMES, L.C., P. ROVERSI & D.S. TAWFIK. 2003. Antibody multispecificity mediated by conformational diversity. Science **299:** 1362–1367.
67. DAERON, M. & G.A. VOISIN. 1979. Mast cell membrane antigens and Fc receptors in anaphylaxis. I. Products of the major histocompatibility complex involved in alloantibody-induced mast cell activation. Immunology **38:** 447–458.
68. WEIS, R.M., K. BALAKRISHNAN, B. SMITH & H.M. MCCONNELL. 1982. Stimulation of fluorescence in a small contact region between rat basophil leukemia cells and planar lipid membrane targets by coherent evanescent radiation. J. Biol. Chem. **257:** 6440–6445.
69. COOPER, A.D., K. BALAKRISHNAN & H.M. MCCONNELL. 1981. Mobile haptens in liposomes stimulate serotonin release by rat basophil leukemia cells in the presence of specific immunoglobulin E. J. Biol. Chem. **256:** 9379–9381.

70. BALAKRISHNAN, K., F.J. HSU, A.D. COOPER & H.M. MCCONNELL. 1982. Lipid hapten containing membrane targets can trigger specific immunoglobulin E-dependent degranulation of rat basophil leukemia cells. J. Biol. Chem. **257:** 6427–6433.

71. LIU, Z.J., H. HALEEM-SMITH, H. CHEN & H. METZGER. 2001. Unexpected signals in a system subject to kinetic proofreading. Proc. Natl. Acad. Sci. USA **98:** 7289–7294.

72. ASAI, K., J. KITAURA, Y. KAWAKAMI, et al. 2001. Regulation of mast cell survival by IgE. Immunity **14:** 791–800.

73. KITAURA, J., W. XIAO, M. MAEDA-YAMAMOTO, et al. 2004. Early divergence of Fcε receptor I signals for receptor up-regulation and internalization from degranulation, cytokine production, and survival. J. Immunol. **173:** 4317–4323.

74. MACGLASHAN, JR., D.W., B.S. BOCHNER, D.C. ADELMAN, et al. 1997. Down-regulation of Fc(epsilon)RI expression on human basophils during in vivo treatment of atopic patients with anti-IgE antibody. J. Immunol. **158:** 1438–1445.

75. BECK, L.A., G.V. MARCOTTE, D. MACGLASHAN, et al. 2004. Omalizumab-induced reductions in mast cell FcεRI expression and function. J. Allergy Clin. Immunol. **114:** 527–530.

76. MACGLASHAN, D. 2004. Loss of receptors and IgE in vivo during treatment with anti-IgE antibody. J. Allergy Clin. Immunol. **114:** 1472–1474.

77. MACGLASHAN, D.W., JR. 1993. Releasability of human basophils: cellular sensitivity and maximal histamine release are independent variables. J. Allergy Clin. Immunol. **91:** 605–615.

78. MACGLASHAN, D.W., JR. & L.M. LICHTENSTEIN. 1987. Basic characteristics of human lung mast cell desensitization. J. Immunol. **139:** 501–505.

79. MACGLASHAN, D.W., JR., S.P. PETERS, J. WARNER & L.M. LICHTENSTEIN. 1986. Characteristics of human basophil sulfidopeptide leukotriene release: releasability defined as the ability of the basophil to respond to dimeric cross-links. J. Immunol. **136:** 2231–2239.

80. SAINI, S.S., D.W. MACGLASHAN, JR., S.A. STERBINSKY, et al. 1999. Down-regulation of human basophil IgE and FCεRIα surface densities and mediator release by anti-IgE-infusions is reversible in vitro and in vivo. J. Immunol. **162:** 5624–5630.

81. MACGLASHAN, D.W., JR. & J.T. SCHROEDER. 2000. Functional consequences of FcεRIα up-regulation by IgE in human basophils. J. Leukoc. Biol. **68:** 479–486.

82. YAMAGUCHI, M., C.S. LANTZ, H.C. OETTGEN, et al. 1997. IgE enhances mouse mast cell FcεRI expression in vitro and in vivo: evidence for a novel amplification mechanism in IgE-dependent reactions. J. Exp. Med. **185:** 663–672.

83. DEVOUASSOUX, G., G. FOSTER, L.M. SCOTT, et al. 1999. Frequency and characterization of antigen-specific IL-4- and IL-13-producing basophils and T cells in peripheral blood of healthy and asthmatic subjects. J. Allergy Clin. Immunol. **104:** 811–819.

84. SCHROEDER, J., L. LICHTENSTEIN, E. ROCHE, et al. 2001. IL-4 production by human basophils found in the lung following segmental allergen challenge. J. Allergy Clin. Immunol. **107:** 265–271.

85. KASAIAN, M.T., M.J. CLAY, M.P. HAPP, et al. 1996. IL-4 production by allergen-stimulated primary cultures: identification of basophils as the major IL-4-producing cell type. Int. Immunol. **8:** 1287–1297.

86. MITRE, E., R.T. TAYLOR, J. KUBOFCIK & T.B. NUTMAN. 2004. Parasite antigen-driven basophils are a major source of IL-4 in human filarial infections. J. Immunol. **172:** 2439–2445.

87. LUCCIOLI, S., D.T. BRODY, S. HASAN, et al. 2002. IgE(+), Kit(–), I-A/I-E(–) myeloid cells are the initial source of Il-4 after antigen challenge in a mouse model of allergic pulmonary inflammation. J. Allergy Clin. Immunol. **110:** 117–124.

88. KHODOUN, M.V., T. OREKHOVA, C. POTTER, et al. 2004. Basophils initiate IL-4 production during a memory T-dependent response. J. Exp. Med. **200:** 857–870.

89. MIN, B., M. PROUT, J. HU-LI, et al. 2004. Basophils produce IL-4 and accumulate in tissues after infection with a Th2-inducing parasite. J. Exp. Med. **200:** 507–517.

90. VOEHRINGER, D., K. SHINKAI & R.M. LOCKSLEY. 2004. Type 2 immunity reflects orchestrated recruitment of cells committed to IL-4 production. Immunity **20:** 267–277.

91. DURHAM, S.R., L. SMURTHWAITE & H.J. GOULD. 2000. Local IgE production. Am. J. Rhinol. **14:** 305–307.

92. SMURTHWAITE, L., S.N. WALKER, D.R. WILSON, *et al.* 2001. Persistent IgE synthesis in the nasal mucosa of hay fever patients. Eur. J. Immunol. **31:** 3422–3431.
93. WILSON, D.R., T.G. MERRETT, E.M. VARGA, *et al.* 2002. Increases in allergen-specific IgE in BAL after segmental allergen challenge in atopic asthmatics. Am. J. Respir. Crit. Care Med. **165:** 22–26.
94. GAUCHAT, J.F., S. HENCHOZ, G. MAZZEI, *et al.* 1993. Induction of human IgE synthesis in B cells by mast cells and basophils. Nature **365:** 340–343.
95. LAMERS, M.C. & P. YU. 1995. Regulation of IgE synthesis. Lessons from the study of IgE transgenic and CD23-deficient mice. Immunol. Rev. **148:** 71–95.
96. PAYET, M. & D.H. CONRAD. 1999. IgE regulation in CD23 knockout and transgenic mice. Allergy **54:** 1125–1129.

Interspecific Structural Differences in Nucleosome as Revealed by Heteroimmunization in Mice with Human Nucleosome

Y. KANAI,[a,b] M. WATANABE,[c] AND T. KUBOTA[c]

[a]Fukushimura Institute of Health and Medical Services for the Aged, Toyohashi, Japan

[b]Laboratory Animal Research Center, Institute of Medical Science, University of Tokyo, Tokyo, Japan

[c]Tokyo Medical and Dental University, Tokyo, Japan

ABSTRACT: Although mounting evidence suggests the association of anti-nucleosome (NS) antibodies with lupus nephropathy in humans, the influence of interspecific differences in NS structure on the diagnosis has not been studied fully. Thus, we investigated the interspecific differences in NS structure by immunizing normal BALB/c mice with human nucleosomes (hNS). We purified hNS and mouse nucleosomes (mNS) from individual established cell lines. Purified NS was of high-pressure liquid chromatography grade and contained less than 1% dinucleosome, if any. Immune responses to NS were tested by an enzyme-linked immunosorbent assay. Of 6 mice, 2 responded to both hNS and mNS. However, antibodies produced in individual mice had higher affinity to mNS than to hNS. IgG response to hNS was IgG1 and IgG2b in subclass, whereas that to mNS was restricted to IgG1. Coincident with this response difference, agarose gel electrophoresis showed a mobility difference between hNS and mNS: the former was slower than the latter. In conclusion, immunodifferentiation *in vivo* in mice of autologous from heterologous NS together with their mobility difference in agarose gel suggest the presence of interspecific differences in NS. In humans, 2 out of 14 randomly tested patients with systemic lupus erythematosus preferred hNS over mNS; the IgG subclass in one was IgG1, and in the other IgG4. Taken together, interspecific differences in NS will provide a new area of study not only in biochemistry but also in immunology and/or autoimmunity.

KEYWORDS: nucleosome; high-pressure liquid chromatography; IgG subclass; epitope spreading

INTRODUCTION

The nucleosome (NS) concept, proposed 30 years ago by Kornberg that each subunit of chromatin is composed of approximately 200 DNA base pairs (bp) wrapped

Address for correspondence: Dr. Yoshiyuki Kanai, M.D., Ph.D., Laboratory Animal Research Center, Institute of Medical Science, University of Tokyo, 4-6-1 Shirokanedai, Minato-Ku, Tokyo 108-8639, Japan.

kanai@ims.u-tokyo.ac.jp

Ann. N.Y. Acad. Sci. 1050: 89–96 (2005). © 2005 New York Academy of Sciences.

doi: 10.1196/annals.1313.010

around a repeating core unit of 8 histone molecules, has paved the way to subsequent research on chromatin.[1,2] For this study, procedures were used ensuring that NS were kept in their native state as much as possible. The fundamental procedure for NS preparation developed by Kornberg *et al.*[3] involves isolation of nuclei, micrococcal nuclease (MN) digestion, and sucrose density ultracentrifugation (SDU). A number of methods for the isolation of NS have been reported; however, the critical step of NS purification is separation of monoNS from poly- or oligoNS after MN digestion of chromatin, irrespective of whether it contains histone H1 or not. For this purpose, SDU and chromatography using a Sepharose 6B or a Superdex 200 column have been used.[4,5] The focus on NS in the study of autoimmunity is because of the availability of NS *in vivo* as autoantigens associated with apoptosis in peripheral leukocytes/lymphocytes.[6,7] Anti–double-stranded DNA (dsDNA) antibody has primarily been considered a hallmark of systemic lupus erythematosus (SLE),[8] but recently the significance of anti-NS antibodies in SLE has been highlighted not only for its early diagnostic value but also for its etiopathogenic role.[9–11] In this respect, our concern is whether NS usually used in studies is really monoNS or not, because diNS possibly contained in the NS preparation may enhance the anti-dsDNA antibody response via 60-bp linker DNAs. Under these circumstances, first, we developed an innovative rapid purification method for monoNS of high-grade purity from cultured human and mouse cells,and second, we investigated the interspecific differences of NS in terms of both immunobiology and biochemistry.

PREPARATION OF NUCLEOSOMES

Cell Preparation/Isolation of Nuclei/MN Digestion of Chromatin/HPLC

All chemicals used were of analytical grade. Hypotonic buffer (buffer A) for nuclear isolation was composed of 0.25 M sucrose, 50 mM Tris (pH 7.4), 50 mM KCl, 0.5 mM $MgCl_2$, and 0.5 mM 2-mercapthoetanol (ME). Reaction buffer (buffer B) for chromatin digestion with MN (Sigma) was composed of sucrose-depleted buffer A and 2.5 mM $CaCl_2$. Tris-buffered saline (pH 7.4) (buffer C) was composed of 25 mM Tris and 250 mM NaCl. In all buffers, NaN_3 was added to 0.04%. To prevent unnecessary degradation of chromatin or NS, 100 µM 4-(2-aminoethyl)-benzenesulfonyl fluoride (AEBSF) was added together with manufacturer-recommended amounts of protease-inhibitor cocktail (PIC) (Boehringer Mannheim) to all buffers used in the steps after isolation of nuclei except for chromatography, for which 5 mM $NaHSO_4$ was added in place of AEBSF (Sigma) and PIC. HL-60 cells (promyelocytic leukemia cell origin) were cultured in DMEM supplemented with 5% fetal bovine serum (Hyclone), 2 mM L-glutamine, 0.1 mM nonessential amino acids, 50 µM 2-ME, 100 µg/mL streptomycin, and 100 U/mL penicillin in a humidified air/CO_2 (19:1) atmosphere at 37°C. When confluency was reached, cells were harvested by centrifugation (500g) at 4°C. Pelleted cells were washed once with Tris-buffered saline (TBS: 25 mM Tris, 140 mM NaCl, 0.04% NaN_3, pH 7.4). Washed cells were stored at −70°C until use. KML_1-7 cells originating from an MRL/lpr mouse inguinal lymph node[12] were cultured and treated under the same conditions as those for HL-60 cells. A quantity of 2×10^8 HL-60 cells was suspended in 15 mL buffer A and homogenized in a Potter-Elvehjem homogenizer for 20 strokes with a Teflon pestle at 4°C. Naked nuclei were pelleted by centrifugation as above and were washed once with buffer A by centrifugation. Nuclei of KML_1-1 cells were isolated under the same conditions as those for HL-60 cells. Pellets of nuclei from either HL-60 or KML_1-7 cells were suspended in 1 mL buffer B with the addition of 1 unit MN per 1 mL reaction mixture and incubated at 37°C. Digestion was terminated by the addition of 5 mM EGTA (Dojindo, Kumamoto, Japan), and the insoluble chromatin pellets were spun down and resuspended in buffer C. Soluble fractions obtained after vortex mixing followed by centrifugation were subjected to high-pressure liquid chromatography (HPLC) on a Superdex 200 column (Amersham Pharmacia Biotech) that had been equilibrated with buffer C. HPLC was manipulated by a 321 pump (Gilson, Middleton, WI). A single peak eluted at around 10.5 to 11.0 min (corresponding to three tubes, each containing 0.5 mL) was collected and concentrated 10 times with Amicon Ultra (Millipore). An aliquot of the concentrate was rechromatographed on Superdex 200 to confirm purity as well as integrity.

CHARACTERIZATION OF PURIFIED NUCLEOSOMES

DNA Extraction and Agarose Gel Electrophoresis

DNA was extracted from monoNS according to the modified method of Ishizawa *et al.*[13] Briefly, HPLC-purified NS was digested with proteinase K (Wako, Tokyo, Japan) in the presence of 1% SDS at 37°C. After heating at 60°C for 15 min in denaturing solution (sodium iodide, sodium-*N*-lauroyl sarcosine, Tris, EDTA, and glycogen, pH 7.8), solubilized DNA was precipitated with 50% isopropyl alcohol. DNA was rehydrated in TE buffer (10 mM Tris, 1 mM EDTA, pH 7.4) and was subjected to 2% agarose gel electrophoresis under a constant voltage of 100 V (Mupid, Cosmobio, Tokyo, Japan) in the presence of ethidium bromide.

Electrophoretic Analysis of Histones in NS

MonoNS treated with sample buffer (final concentration, 62.5 mM Tris, 10% glycerol, pH 6.8) with or without 2-ME plus heating was subjected to 15% SDS-PAGE at room temperature. Proteins were stained by Coomassie Brilliant Blue R-250 (Nakarai Tesque, Kyoto, Japan).

Physicochemical Treatment of NS

In order to compare the stability of hNS and mNS, both were treated in buffer C with proteinase K, by freeze-thawing, and by 30-min heating at 56°C.

CHARACTERISTICS OF PURIFIED NUCLEOSOMES

Nucleosomes are said to be very unstable and easily degraded by freeze-thawing. Accordingly, storage of NS is usually made in liquid condition at 4°C in the presence of preservatives.[3,14] Under such conditions, native configuration cannot be maintained more than 2 weeks. In fact, both hNS and mNS obtained by our method were susceptible to freeze-thawing. However, both NS were resistant to heat treatment at

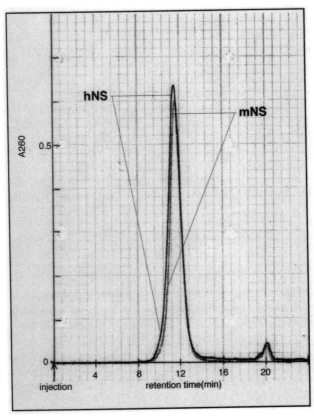

FIGURE 1. Comparison between Superdex 200 HPLC column profiles of mNS and hNS. At first glance, there seems to be no significant difference in retention time. However, as described in the text, the retention time difference (~15 s) between mNS and hNS was significant, because the lag in injecting individual samples to the column was repeatedly within 5 s. It should be noted that di- or oligoNS is not seen ahead of the single sharp peak with either hNS or mNS.

65°C for 30 min, and the native configuration could be maintained for over 8 weeks in liquid in the presence of 2-ME and PIC, as judged by both HPLC and agarose gel electrophoresis. The main reason for the improved stability of our NS in liquid phase may be the rapidity of preparation, which was completed within 4 h after the isolation of nuclei. The stability of NS from both mice and humans was essentially the same, but slight differences could be detected in their configurations. For example, retention time of hNS in HPLC is shorter than that of mNS (FIG. 1), and mNS moved faster than hNS on agarose gel electrophoresis (FIG. 2). It should be mentioned that differences between hNS and mNS in either HPLC or electrophoretic pattern as shown in FIGURE 1 and FIGURE 2 were reproducible in samples used within 8 weeks after their preparation. These findings suggest that the hNS is larger and/or more complicated in the structure than the mNS.

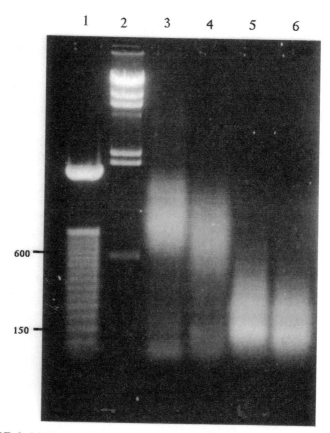

FIGURE 2. Mobility difference between hNS and mNS on agarose gel electrophoresis. Mobility of mNS (lane 4) is faster than that of hNS (lane 3), indicating that the configuration of hNS is more complicated or larger, as is suggested by the HPLC retention time difference. Faster bands seen ahead of both NS appear to be DNA separated from NS during electrophoresis. Mono- and diNS DNA are shown in lane 5 and lane 6, respectively, and these bands correspond in size to 150 and 300 bp, as shown in the lane 1 ladder marker. Mobility of both mNS and hNS is shown to be significantly retarded as compared with that of 150-bp monoNS DNA (lanes 5 and 6), indicating the so-called mobility shift.[16] Lanes: (1) ladder marker; (2) λHindIII marker; (3) hNS; (4) mNS; (5) hdiNS DNA; (6) mdiNS DNA.

IMMUNE RESPONSES TO NUCLEOSOMES

Immunization

Female BALB/c mice were purchased from Charles River, Japan and were maintained in the Animal Research Center of Tokyo Medical and Dental University under certification by the Institutional Animal Care and Use Committee. A first injection of 50 μg hNS in Freund's complete adjuvant was administered subcutaneously at age 10 weeks. The same amounts of hNS in Freund's incomplete adjuvant were injected at age 15, 22, and 31 weeks. Blood samples were collected from the tail vein 10 days after the last immunization. Sera were stored at −30°C.

Enzyme-Linked Immunosorbent Assay

Immulon 2HB plates were coated with hNS or mNS in buffer C overnight and were blocked with 2% skim milk in buffer C. Enzyme-linked immunosorbent assay (ELISA) plates completed by washing with Tris-buffered saline (TBS-PLUS: 25 mM Tris, 140 mM NaCl, 1 mM EDTA, 1 mM EGTA, 0.04% NaN_3, pH 7.4). Mouse sera were diluted 1:100 in TBS-PLUS containing 2% bovine serum albumin and 0.5% skim milk. Alkaline phosphatase (AP)-conjugated anti–mouse IgG (γ-chain specific) goat antibodies (Zymed) were used as a second antibody. Bound anti-hNS or anti-mNS antibodies were measured by an autoreader and expressed as A_{405} units using p-nitrophenyl phosphate as a substrate. For mouse IgG antibody subclass determination, subclass-specific goat antibodies labeled with biotin were used (Zymed). Bound biotin-tagged second antibodies were detected with streptoavidin-conjugated AP (Zymed). IgG antibody subclasses, that is, IgG1, IgG2a, IgG2b, and IgG3, were expressed similarly as in the case of IgG isotype antibody. The ELISA plates were washed after each step with TBS-PLUS containing 0.05% Tween 20.

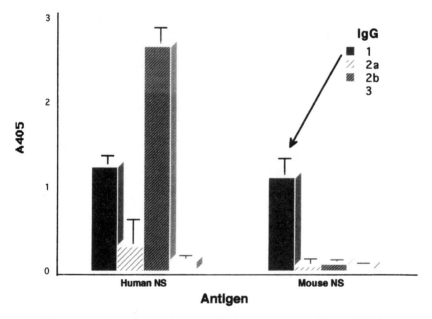

FIGURE 3. Profiles of IgG subclass antibody responses to mNS and hNS in a mouse immunized with mNS. Immunization protocol is described in the text. The immune response pattern of another mouse (data not shown) is essentially the same as this pattern. Both IgG1 and IgG2b responses against hNS are seen, but IgG1 response alone (*arrow*) is seen against mNS.

Immune Response of Mice to NS

Experimental induction of autoimmunity to mNS in mice by immunization with hNS has been considered difficult because the constituents of mNS are essentially the same as those in hNS. Actually, experimental induction of autoimmunity to mNS in mice has not been reported, to the best of our knowledge. In our study as well, only two of six mice immunized extensively with hNS produced moderate levels of IgG antibodies to hNS as well as mNS, as tested by ELISA. However, their apparent affinity seemed different between hNS and mNS: affinity for the former was lower than that for the latter. In order to exclude the possibility that the mouse response to hNS was a cross-reaction to mNS, we investigated IgG subclass differences between anti-hNS and anti-mNS antibodies and found that the IgG response to hNS was IgG1 and IgG2b in subclass, whereas that to mNS was restricted to IgG1 (FIG. 3). Dissociation of IgG subclass could exclude the possibility that antibody responses to mNS are not the result of cross-reaction to mNS, but, rather, would suggest so-called epitope spreading[15] to mNS from hNS. Studies on the shift of subclass with time following immunization would contribute to unveiling the mechanism of epitope spreading. If the configuration or structure of mNS is completely the same as that of hNS, epitope spreading would not be seen. Coincident with the mobility difference on agarose gel electophoresis as well as a slight difference in retention time on HPLC, immunodifferentiation *in vivo* of autologous from heterologous NS suggests the presence of interspecific NS differences.

Immune Responses to NS in Patients with SLE

As to the binding of antibodies to either hNS or mNS in humans, 2 preferred hNS and 2 preferred mNS out of 14 randomly selected SLE patients. Among these, with strong preference to hNS was shown by IgG1. The significance of these findings should be evaluated by further studies; however, these antibodies more or less suggest the presence of conformational epitopes of NS specific for different species rather than individual components such as core histones or DNA.

CONCLUSIONS

We have not always taken into account the interspecific differences in either eukaryotic nucleic acids or histones in regards to autoimmunity. This has been the case for NS. However, heteroimmunization of mice with hNS has revealed that immune responses of mice can differentiate the structure of hNS from mNS. The differences, although small, will provide a new area of study on NS, not only in biochemistry but also in autoimmunity.

REFERENCES

1. KORNBERG, R.D. 1974. Chromatin structure: a repeating unit of histones and DNA. Science **184**: 868–871.
2. KORNBERG, R.D. 1999. Twenty-five years of the nucleosome, fundamental particle of the eukaryote chromosome. Cell **98**: 285–294.

3. KORNBERG, R.D., J.R. LAPOINTE & Y. LORCH. 1989. Preparation of nucleosomes and chromatin. Methods Enzymol. **170:** 3–14.
4. KOUTOUZOV, S. *et al.* 1996. Binding of nucleosomes to a cell surface receptor: redistribution and endocytosis in the presence of lupus antibodies. Eur. J. Immunol. **26:** 472–486.
5. CABRESPINES, A. *et al.* 1998. Isolation and characterization of apoptotic nucleosomes, free and complexed with lupus autoantibody generated during hybridoma B-cell apoptosis. J. Autoimmun. **11:** 19–27.
6. MOUNTZ, J.D., J. WU, J. CHENG & T. ZHOU. 1994. Autoimmune disease: a problem of defective apoptosis. Arthritis Rheum. **37:** 1415–1420.
7. UTZ, P.J. & P. ANDERSON. 1998. Posttranslational protein modifications, apoptosis, and the bypass of tolerance to autoantigens. Arthritis Rheum. **41:** 1152–1160.
8. TAN, E.M. 1989. Antinuclear antibodies: diagnostic markers for autoimmune diseases and probes for cell biology. Adv. Immunol. **44:** 93–151.
9. AMOURA, Z. *et al.* 1994. Nucleosome–restricted antibodies are detected before anti-dsDNA and/or antihistone antibodies in serum of MRL-Mp lpr/lpr and +/+ mice with proteinuria. Arthritis Rheum. **37:** 1684–1688.
10. CHABRE, H. *et al.* 1995. Presence of nucleosome-restricted antibodies in patients with systemic lupus erythematosus. Arthritis Rheum. **38:** 1485–1491.
11. AMOURA, Z. *et al.* 2000. Presence of antinucleosome antibodies in a restricted set of connective tissue diseases: antinucleosome antibodies of the IgG3 subclass are markers of renal pathogenicity in systemic lupus erythematosus. Arthritis Rheum. **43:** 76–84.
12. KANAI, Y. *et al.* 1986. An established MRL/Mp-lpr/lpr cell line with null cell properties produces a B cell differentiation factor(s) that promotes anti-single-stranded DNA antibody production in MRL spleen cell culture. Int. Arch. Allergy. Appl. Immunol. **81:** 92–94.
13. KANAI, Y., S. KYUWA, K. MIURA & Y. KUROSAWA. 1995. Induction and natural occurrence of serum nucleosomal DNA in autoimmune MRL/lpr/lpr mice: its relation to apoptosis in the thymus. Immunol. Lett. **46:** 207–214.
14. LUTTER, L.C. 1978. Kinetic analysis of deoxyribonuclease I cleavages in the nucleosome core: evidence for a DNA superhelix. J. Mol. Biol. **124:** 391–420.
15. UMESH, S. 2003. Mechanisms of autoantibody diversification to SLE-related autoantigens. Ann. N.Y. Acad. Sci. **987:** 91–98.
16. XIAN, J., M.G. HARRINGTON & E.H. DAVIDSON. 1996. DNA-binding assays from a single sea urchin egg: a high-sensitivity capillary electrophoresis method. Proc. Natl. Acad. Sci. USA **93:** 86–90.

Differential Regulation of the IL-10 Gene in Th1 and Th2 T Cells

KYU-HO KANG AND SIN-HYEOG IM

Department of Life Science, Gwangju Institute of Science and Technology, Gwangju, Korea

ABSTRACT: Interleukin-10 (IL-10), an immunoregulatory cytokine, modulates the function of various immune and nonimmune cells, yet little information is available on the molecular mechanism of transcriptional regulation at the chromatin level. During T cell differentiation from naive T cells into Th1 and Th2 cells, the expression of IL-10 in Th1 cells slowly disappears, whereas Th2 cells produce more IL-10. We examined the chromatin structural changes associated with *IL-10* gene transcription by naive and differentiated murine Th1 and Th2 cells. Naive T cells lack DNase I hypersensitivity (HS) sites in the vicinity of the *IL-10* gene, whereas differentiated T cells display a strong 3′ constitutive HS site as well as several inducible sites. In committed Th1 cells, the mechanism of *IL-10* gene silencing is associated with a closed chromatin structure, the lack of an HS site at the promoter region, and the development of repressive histone modification near the *IL-10* promoter and introns 3 and 4. We confirm that the majority of HS sites coincide with conserved noncoding sequences (CNSs) identified by comparative genomic sequence alignment between human and mouse genomes. Potential transcription factor binding sites were located by comparing CNSs with the TRANSFAC database. Predicted *in vivo* binding of specific factors on the CNS locus were confirmed by chromatin immunoprecipitation assays. Our results suggest that the combination of HS site and comparative genomic approaches allows identification of regulatory elements involved in differential *IL-10* gene expression between Th1 and Th2 cells during T cell differentiation.

KEYWORDS: IL-10; comparative genomics; Th1; Th2; chromatin remodeling

INTRODUCTION

Interleukin-10 (IL-10) is a pluripotent cytokine with potent effects on numerous cell populations, in particular circulating and resident immune cells as well as epithelial cells. IL-10 is produced by many cell types, such as T cells (Th2 cells, recently differentiated Th1 cells, regulatory T cells), B cells, monocytes, macrophages, and dendritic cells. IL-10 stimulates functions of innate immunity (NK cell activity) and

Address for correspondence: Dr. Sin-Hyeog Im, Department of Life Science, Gwangju Institute of Science and Technology, 1 Oryong-dong, Puk-ku, Gwangju 500-712, Korea. Voice: +82-62-970-2503; fax: +82-62-970-2484.
imsh@gist.ac.kr

Ann. N.Y. Acad. Sci. 1050: 97–107 (2005). © 2005 New York Academy of Sciences.
doi: 10.1196/annals.1313.011

Th2-related immunity (B cell), but it suppresses inflammation-associated immune responses (Th1, cytokine proinflammatory secretion by macrophages).[1,2] IL-10–deficient mice develop severe chronic enterocolitis (inflammatory bowel disease, IBD), emphasizing the protective role of this cytokine in inflammatory and auto-immune conditions. Paradoxically, however, IL-10 stimulates polyclonal B cell activation and thus has a pathogenic role in systemic lupus erythematosus (SLE). During development of naive $CD4^+$ T helper (Th) cells into cytokine-producing effector cells in response to antigen stimulation, Th cells differentiate into distinct Th1 or Th2 cells characterized by differential expression of cytokine genes. Naive T cells differentiate to Th1 cells in the presence of IL-12 and interferon gamma (IFNγ), or differentiate to Th2 cells in the presence of IL-4. Th1 cells produce IL-2, IFNγ, and lymphotoxin, and promote cellular immune responses by activating macrophages or $CD8^+$ cytotoxic T cells, but do not produce IL-4 or IL-13. Th2 cells produce IL-4, IL-5, IL-6, IL-10, and IL-13, and promote humoral immunity, but do not produce IFNγ.[3,4] These mutually exclusive patterns of cytokine production are mainly observed in fully committed Th1 and Th2 cells. Recent studies on exclusive cytokine expression profiles of Th1 (IFNγ) and Th2 (IL-4) demonstrated opposing chromatin modification depending on the direction of polarization.[5,6] Th1 and Th2 cells develop an active chromatin configuration on the IFNγ and IL-4 genes, respectively. In Th1 cells, the *IFNγ* gene locus, like the *IL-4* locus in Th2 cells, displays an open chromatin configuration characterized by increased DNase I hypersensitivity (HS) and histone acetylation. But Th1 cells develop a strongly silenced chromatin configuration at the *IL-4* gene, as do Th2 cells at the *IFNγ* gene. Unlike IL-4, IL-10 is produced in both recently differentiated primary Th1 and Th2 cells, although Th2 cells produce much higher levels (10 to 50 times, depending on Th2 phenotype) than Th1 cells. This phenomenon is unique, compared with the exclusive expression profile of IFNγ and IL-4 in Th1 and Th2 cells, respectively. As naive T cells differentiate to Th1 and Th2 cells, Th1 cells slowly lose their ability to express IL-10 after the first week of differentiation, whereas Th2 cells increase IL-10 production and maintain high IL-10 levels. These results suggest dynamic chromatin remodeling at the *IL-10* locus during T cell differentiation. Although the immunoregulatory role of IL-10 has been studied extensively for decades, little information is available on the molecular mechanism of its transcriptional regulation, especially at the chromatin level. To locate and identify the regulatory elements involved in *IL-10* gene regulation, we combined two different methods, namely combination of conventional DNase I HS analysis and *in silico* analysis of orthologous genomic sequences. We examined the development of DNase I HS patterns in and around the *IL-10* gene in naive and differentiated T cells. We show that naive T cells lack any HS sites within a 22-kb region containing the *IL-10* gene, whereas differentiated T cells display a strong constitutive HS site just 3′ of the gene, as well as several inducible sites. In parallel, we performed bioinformatic analysis of the *IL-10* locus of the human and mouse genomic sequences and located the strongly conserved noncoding sequence (CNS) regions. Overlay of HS analysis data and CNS profiles shows remarkable correspondence between the positions of experimentally determined DNase I HS regions in the *IL-10* gene and CNSs identified by sequence comparisons of mammalian genomes. Our results suggest that the combination of HS site and comparative genomic approaches allows identification of the regulatory elements involved in lineage-dependent differential gene expression at the chromatin level (FIG. 1).

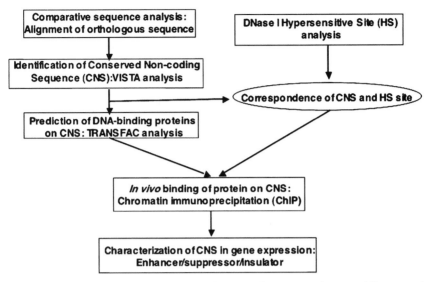

FIGURE 1. Multiple processes for identification of regulatory elements. Alignment of evolutionarily related sequences allows identification of conserved noncoding sequences (CNSs) between species. The identified CNSs correspond to DNase I hypersensitive (HS) sites in IL-10, IL-4, IL-5, IL-2, IFNγ, and GM-CSF, suggesting that comparative sequence alignment is a reliable tool to identify possible regulatory elements in target genes.[16,30,31] Candidate regulatory elements can be predicted by PipMaker, VISTA/TRANSFAC analysis. The predicted binding of DNA-binding proteins on CNSs *in vivo* may be examined by chromatin immunoprecipitation (ChIP) with antibodies to predicted proteins. The role of regulatory elements in gene expression can be characterized further to elucidate their function as enhancers, matrix attachment regions, insulators/boundary elements, and sites of relief from transcriptional attenuation.

MATERIALS AND METHODS

Bioinformatics: VISTA (Visualization Tool for Alignment) and rVista (Regulatory Vista) Analysis

The mouse and human *IL-10* DNA sequences were aligned and the extent of homology was computed with a Web-based program, VISTA (http://www-gsd.lbl.gov/vista/).[7,8] Regions at least 100 bp in length that showed at least 75% sequence identity at each segment of the alignment between successive gaps were identified as CNSs. Transcription factor binding sites (TFBS) on CNSs were predicted using rVista 2.0 (http://rvista.dcode.org/). rVista analysis of alignments spanning ~50 kb including the *IL-10* gene locus was performed using TFBS matrices for available transcription factors. The TFBS search with a 0.85 matrix similarity cut-off identified matches that are highly conserved in the human–mouse alignment. The stretches with over 90% identity within CNSs have been used to screen the TRANSFAC database (http://www.gene-regulation.com/pub/databases.html#transfac) to determine whether they have already been described as transcription factor binding sites in similar or different biological contexts.[9]

Analysis of DNase I Hypersensitivity (HS)

Th1 and Th2 clones and *in vitro* differentiated Th1 and Th2 cells were stimulated for 4 h, and nuclei were isolated and incubated with DNase I.[10] Purified genomic DNAs were completely digested with Bam HI and resolved on a 0.6% agarose gel, transferred to Nytran membranes, and hybridized with IL-10 exon 1, exon 3, or exon 5 probes labeled by random priming.

Chromatin Immunoprecipitation (ChIP) Assays

ChIP analysis was carried out essentially as described.[11] Cloned Th1 (D5) or Th2 (D10) cells (1×10^8) were either left unstimulated or were stimulated for 20 min with PMA (10 nM) plus ionomycin (2 μM), then cross-linked using formaldehyde. This time point was chosen based on the early kinetics of *IL-10* gene transcription (peak transcript levels attained at 30 min in both the D10 clone and primary Th2 cells). Nuclei were isolated and sonicated four times for 10 s each at the maximal setting, with 1 min cooling on ice in between. The average fragment size of sonicated DNA was ~0.5 kb. The chromatin was immunoprecipitated using anti-NFAT1 (anti-67.1 and anti–NFAT1-C antibodies specific for the family member NFAT1-C).[12] Following reversal of cross-links, the presence of selected DNA sequences was assessed by polymerase chain reaction (PCR).

RESULTS AND DISCUSSION

Analysis of DNase I Hypersensitivity Sites in the IL-10 Locus

The DNase I HS assay identifies regions of the genome with an open nucleosome structure that are therefore readily degraded by the DNase I. Such regions are potentially available as transcription factor binding sites and mark nucleosome-poor regions that tend to be located near protein-bound regulatory elements. HS site analysis reveals binding sites for key transcription factors and it correlates with critical regulatory regions of the gene, inducible or tissue-specific enhancers, locus control regions, matrix attachment regions, insulators/boundary elements, and sites of relief from transcriptional attenuation.[13] Mapping of HS sites in the *IL-10* locus provides the first indication of transcription competency versus the silent state and helps to locate long-range mapping of potentially important regulatory regions. We compared the chromatin structure of the *IL-10* gene in Th1 and Th2 cells by using two fully differentiated T cell clones, the D5 (Th1) clone[14] and the D10 (Th2) clone,[15] as well as primary differentiated Th1 and Th2 cells. D5 cells showed no expression of IL-10 mRNA, regardless of stimulation, whereas D10 cells expressed low basal levels of IL-10 transcripts under resting conditions and rapidly induced IL-10 transcription upon stimulation (up to 500 times more IL-10 production than the D5 clone). Using exon 1, 3, and 5 probes we examined the DNase I hypersensitivity pattern in the 5' and 3' regions as well as intronic regions of the *IL-10* gene in the D5 and D10 clones and in the *in vitro* primary differentiated Th1 and Th2 cells. Resting

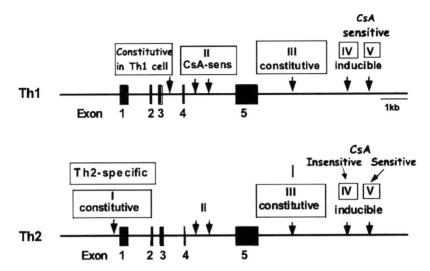

FIGURE 2. Summary of DNase I hypersensitivity (HS) sites in the *IL-10* gene locus in Th1 and Th2 cells and correspondence of HS sites to conserved noncoding sequence regions. The *arrows* above the *IL-10* locus denote the approximate locations of HS sites identified as CNSs (not shown), and emphasize the close correspondence of HS sites and CNS regions.

Th2 cells showed a strong HS site at the proximal *IL-10* promoter that was not apparent in resting Th1 cells. This difference is consistent with basal expression versus silencing of the IL-10 gene in the D10 and D5 clones, respectively (FIG. 2). We also identified intronic HS sites II by using an exon 3 probe. We used an exon 5 probe to monitor hypersensitivity patterns in the 3′ region of the *IL-10* gene (FIG. 2). Under resting conditions, both Th1 and Th2 cells displayed a strong constitutive HS site, designated HS site III. This result implies that the 3′ constitutive DNase I HS site binds lineage-specific transcription factors rather than inducible transcription factors that mediate acute transcription of the *IL-10* gene.[16] Both cell types also displayed weakly inducible site IV and site V. Both site IV and site V were lost upon cyclosporine A (CsA) treatment in Th1 cells (see FIG. 2), whereas in Th2 cells, the site V band was CsA-sensitive but site IV was CsA-insensitive. Very similar patterns of DNase I hypersensitivity were observed in primary T cells (data not shown). We also examined IL-10 transcription and HS patterns in primary Th1 and Th2 cells. Naive CD4 T cells showed no evidence of any HS sites on the *IL-10* gene, using either the exon 5 or the exon 1 probe (data not shown). The cells were differentiated under Th1 or Th2 conditions for 1 week, then restimulated with phorbol ester (PMA) plus calcium ionophore (ionomycin) in the presence or absence of CsA for 4 h. In contrast to the silencing of the *IL-10* gene observed in the committed D5 clone, recently differentiated Th1 cells showed strong induction of IL-10 transcripts upon stimulation, and this induction was completely blocked by CsA. The DNase I hypersensitivity pattern of primary Th1 cells was similar to that observed in D5 cells (data not shown). Recently differentiated Th2 cells expressed a low basal level of IL-10 transcripts and showed strong induction of IL-10 transcripts upon stimulation. In contrast to the strong CsA-sensitivity of Th1 IL-10 transcription, however, IL-10 production by Th2 cells was almost insensitive to CsA. The pattern of DNase I hypersensitivity sites observed on the *IL-10* gene in primary Th2 cells was identical to that observed in D10 cells.

Together, these data show that Th1 and Th2 cells differ not only in the signals they utilize to regulate *IL-10* gene transcription, but also in their patterns of DNase I hypersensitivity on the *IL-10* gene. In Th1 cells, both IL-10 expression and HS site induction were strongly inhibited by CsA; in contrast, in Th2 cells, the CsA-insensitivity of *IL-10* gene expression was most closely correlated with the CsA-insensitive induction of HS site IV (FIG. 2).

Comparative Genomic Approach to Identify the Regulatory Region in the IL-10 Locus

Although the DNase I HS assay is a powerful tool for identifying regulatory elements in a specific gene, it is an unguided, labor-intensive, time-consuming wet method. Recently, comparative genomic approaches have been focused on the computational analysis of large genome databases.[17] Cross-species sequence comparisons have been used to identify noncoding sequences that have a reasonable possibility of having gene regulatory properties. This is possible because noncoding sequences that mediate gene expression tend to be conserved between species.[18,19] A comparative genomic approach by a web-based program, VISTA (Visualization Tools for Alignment)[8] is very useful for finding *cis*-acting regulatory elements of the *IL*-10 gene (FIG. 1 and TABLE 1). The majority of DNase I HS sites in the *IL-10* gene coincide with CNSs (TABLE 1). We also used rVista (regulatory Vista)[20] to recognize specific CNSs that are potential transcription factor binding sites among the many CNS regions. The rVista program compares CNSs with TRANSFAC,[9] the most widely used database for transcription factor binding sites. In the *IL-10* locus, the transcription factor NFAT binding sites were predicted by rVista analysis (TABLE 2), and *in vivo* NFAT binding on CNSs was confirmed by chromatin immunoprecipitation (ChIP) assays.[16] The rVista analysis not only showed several transcription factor

TABLE 1. Correlation of CNSs with DNase I hypersensitivity (HS) sites

DNase I HS site	CNS regions – mouse chr1 (human chr1)	Size (bp)	Identity
IL-10 promoter	130889572 (203334693) – 130889850 (203334419)	284	77.8%
HS site I/intron 3	130891794 (203332529) – 130891984 (203332340)	195	76.4%
HS site II/intron 4	130892815 (203331471) – 130893136 (203331149)	330	73.9%
	130893195 (203331039) – 130893362 (203330876)	168	73.8%
	130893483 (203330765) – 130893582 (203330671)	100	72.0%
HS site III	130896242 (203328258) – 130896392 (203328104)	155	82.6%
HS site IV	130897781 (203326939) – 130897887 (203326835)	107	72.0%

NOTE: Chromosomal location, size, and percent identity for each aligned CNS were determined by VISTA Browser 2.0.

TABLE 2. Localization of functionally characterized NFAT1 binding site to conserved blocks

Hypersensitivity (HS) site	Location	base (mouse) second (human)	Element sequence	NFAT(%ID)
IL-10 promoter	+ 221-232 109-120	base second	220 230 TCTGCCTCAGGAAAT-CAACTTT |:::||:||||||| |||||| TTCTCCCCAGGAAATTCAACTTT 120 110	90.00
HS site II / Intron 4	+ 257-268 598-609	base second	260 270 GTGACATAGGAAACAGAAAGTACA |||||:||||||||||||||| GTGACAAAGGAAACAGAAAGTACA 610 600 590	100.00

NOTE: This table represents functionally characterized NFAT binding sites. Element position is indicated in reference to the beginning of the 5' UTR of the gene. NFAT binding sites were independently identified using the TRANSFAC database and compared with the published sequences. Conserved NFAT binding sites are in bold (Online Web version displays these as blue). Percent identity (%ID) for each aligned NFAT binding sites was determined by rVista 2.0.

binding sites in the *IL-10* CNS regions, but also revealed specific transcription factor binding sequences. However, a comparative genomic approach alone cannot establish whether given CNS regions are really used by specific cell types or specific developmental stages. Therefore, combined approaches of comparative genomics and DNase I HS analysis are more effective in identifying regulatory elements in the locus of a specific gene of interest.

Chromatin Remodeling and Epigenetic Regulation Mechanism of the IL-10 Gene

The mechanisms that permit cellular specification are associated with changes in gene structure, known as epigenetic chromatin remodeling. The term epigenetic implies a specific and heritable pattern of gene expression in progeny of differentiating cells, without changing the genome sequence.[21] By contrast, the term chromatin remodeling can be used in reference to acute, reversible, time-dependent changes in the chromatin structure of a promoter. Beyond chromatin remodeling, the acute transcriptional induction of subset-specific genes can be mediated by transcription factors that are either activated or expressed selectively in one subset, but that can induce transcription of remodeled gene targets only.[22] Chromatin remodeling may be required to induce competence for gene expression or transcription, and is mediated by histone modifications, of which the best studied are acetylation, methylation, and phosphorylation. The functions of acetylation, methylation, and phosphorylation are complex and may vary depending on the specific histone residue that is being modified.[23,24] How chromatin states (active or silent) are begun, maintained, changed, and inherited are now fertile areas of investigation.

Analysis of DNase I HS sites and location of CNSs by a comparative genomic approach revealed the presence of a Th2-specific constitutive HS site at the *IL-10* promoter region (FIG. 2), suggesting that the promoter is poised for activation of transcription in Th2 cells but silenced in Th1 cells. This hypothesis was confirmed by the ChIP technique, a method for detection of *in vivo* binding of specific transcription factors on specific regions of the target genome. Like the *IL-4* promoter, the *IL-10* promoter was hyperacetylated on histone H4 in Th2 cells even prior to stimulation. Both promoters showed basal occupancy by RNA polymerase II, confirming their poised status.[16] *IL-4* and *IL-10* promoters became accessible to NFAT1 after stimulation, correlating with the rapid increase in IL-4 and IL-10 production by stimulated Th2 cells. In contrast, Th1 cells, which do not produce either IL-4 or IL-10, showed hypoacetylation, no RNA polymerase II occupancy, and no NFAT1 binding at *IL-4* and *IL-10* promoters, whereas the IFNγ promoter showed constitutive hyperacetylation, constitutive RNA polymerse II occupancy, and inducible NFAT1 binding, consistent with their competence to produce IFNγ upon stimulation.[16] In addition, DNase I HS site II (intron 4) of the *IL-10* gene occurs despite a "silenced" chromatin configuration characterized by decreased histone H4 acetylation, decreased H3K4 methylation, and constitutive association with histone deacetylase (HDAC) 1.[16] HDAC recruitment by NFAT may also contribute to the silencing of a subset of many genes. Analyses of cDNA microarrays revealed genes whose expression is decreased by calcium/calcineurin signaling.[25] In the *IL-10* gene locus, HDAC1 is constitutively associated with both DNase I HS site on intron 3 and DNase I HS site II on intron 4 in Th1 cells, but NFAT1 binds inducibly only to DNase I HS site II. This result suggests the possibility of NFAT-mediated silencing of *IL-10* gene expression in Th1 cells. Ca^{2+}/calcineurin-NFAT-mediated signaling pathways are involved in diverse cellular reactions by regulating gene expression either positively or negatively. Recently studies show that the transcriptional activity of NFAT proteins can be either activating or deactivating depending on which binding partners are involved.[26] Interaction of NFAT with AP-1 turns on the genes involved in active immune responses, whereas NFAT without cooperative binding of AP-1 turns on a T cell anergy program and blocks T cell activation and proliferation.[27] In addition, interaction of NFAT with HDAC proteins may induce gene silencing. This finding suggests that the coordinated binding of a specific combination of transcription factors is more important than the functions of the specific transcription factors alone.[26]

Importance of IL-10 Regulation Studies on Clinical Applications

The effective immunoregulatory properties of IL-10 and its dysregulated expression levels are associated with many diseases, such as autoimmune disorders, AIDS progression, HCV infection, advanced alcoholic liver disease, Epstein-Barr virus infection, gastric cancer, cervical cancer, multiple myeloma, cutaneous malignant melanoma, increased risk of hepatocellular carcinoma, and resistance to antiviral therapy.[28] On the other hand, delivery of IL-10 showed anti-inflammatory effects on the course of several inflammatory diseases in experimental models as well as clinical trials. Recently, human recombinant IL-10 has been tested in healthy volunteers, in patients with Crohn's disease, rheumatoid arthritis, psoriasis, or hepatitis C infection, and in patients undergoing organ transplantation.[28] Improper IL-10 expression seems to have considerable pathophysiological impact. Not only overexpression (e.g., in lymphoma, SLE, intensive care unit patients) but also IL-10 deficiency (e.g., in inflammatory bowel disease, psoriasis) are likely to have pathophysiological significance. Therefore, neutralization of the cytokine could be a promising approach to treat diseases from the first group, whereas application of IL-10 itself could be helpful for diseases from the second group. One major concern in manipulating the levels of IL-10 clinically is its critical role in immune homeostasis. In addition, IL-10 can induce the formation of regulatory T cells, with major impact on immune regulation.[29] Enriched IL-10–expressing regulatory T cells could prevent inflammatory disease. Therefore, efforts to manipulate *IL-10* gene expression at the chromatin level could contribute to the development of more effective therapies for diseases related to abnormal IL-10 expression.

CONCLUSIONS AND OUTLOOK

IL-10 is a pleiotropic cytokine and is considered a major regulator of the balance between immunity and tolerance. Regardless of the importance of IL-10 in immune regulation, little information is available as yet on the molecular mechanism of IL-10 regulation. The results of our studies on IL-10 regulation in Th1 and Th2 cells provide important insights into the surprising diversity of mechanisms used to regulate gene expression at the chromatin level. We characterized the DNase I HS patterns of the *IL-10* gene in naive and differentiated T cells. This analysis revealed that the majority of DNase I HS sites correspond to conserved noncoding genomic regions identified by sequence comparisons of mammalian genomes. We have described a novel promoter-mediated silencing mechanism in Th1 cells that is a completely closed chromatin structure and not accessible to binding by any factor for IL-10 expression. Currently, we are extending our studies on the mechanism of IL-10 regulation at the chromatin level from T cells to B cells and other IL-10–producing immune cells. This study will seek to identify and characterize inducible, distal regulatory regions, and to investigate factors and pathways for regulatory signal transduction in *IL-10* gene expression in different immune cells. But practically speaking, to identify and locate the regulatory region of a specific gene of interest is quite difficult. DNase I HS analysis is a powerful tool, as it reflects perturbations introduced by protein binding to nucleosomal DNA. However, it has several drawbacks, such as the need for large cell numbers (up to 1×10^8 cells), technical difficulties in titration of DNase I activity, and labor-intensive Southern blot analysis. Recently, human and rodent (mouse and rat) genomic sequences have been obtained. In addition, most of the proteins in humans and rodents have similar functions and expression profiles, suggesting the possibility that conserved regulatory loci may exist. Indeed, recent studies on the IL-10, IFNγ, and IL-4 loci revealed the correspondence of DNase I HS sites and computer-predicted CNSs.[16,30,31] VISTA and TRANSFAC analysis revealed possible regulatory elements,[18,32] but this *in silico* analysis itself is not enough to give any detailed information, such as lineage specificity (Th1, Th2, B cells, antigen-presenting cells), relationship with degree of gene expression level, and specific factor binding. The combination of HS site analysis and comparative genomic approaches during lineage development, and the appearance of specific HS sites or CNSs during lymphocyte development will allow elucidation of the *in vivo* function of regulatory regions (HS or CNS). Our studies on IL-10 regulation identified a series of CNS/HS sites within ~50 kb of the *IL-10* locus. Still, we need to characterize further the biological function of HS/CNS sites by identification of specific CNS-binding transcription factors and their relationship to the specific appearance of HS/CNS loci during Th1 and Th2 cell differentiation from naive T cells. Additionally, in general, BALB/c mice easily induce Th2 responses, whereas C57BL/6 mice strongly induce Th1 responses.[33] The existing DNase I HS site analysis data is from primary T cells of Th2-prone BALB/c genetic background.[16] Therefore, further DNase I HS site mapping is necessary for primary T cells from Th1-prone C57BL/6 mice. Studies on single nucleotide polymorphisms (SNPs) of the *IL-10* gene in different diseases has revealed that, indeed, dysregulated IL-10 expression is seen in different immune disorders associated with autoimmunity, cancer, and viral infection. Most SNP studies focused mainly on the promoter region of *IL-10*. However, in addition to the promoter region, other loci such as introns and regions 5' upstream or 3' downstream of the *IL-10* locus may be more important in IL-10 regulation. Once the key regulatory locus (HS or CNS) in IL-10 regulation is identified, SNP studies on the site will reveal the relationships between different dysregulated IL-10-associated diseases. This result will serve as a marker to diagnose specific disease. In conclusion, by a combination of HS site analysis and bioinformatics analysis we revealed the loci involved in differential IL-10 regulation in Th1 and Th2 cells. Furthermore, we showed *in vivo* binding of NFAT on the CNS locus identified by rVista. Our results indicate that the combination of HS site analysis and comparative genomic approaches is a useful and powerful tool to identify the regulatory elements of a gene of interest involved in differential gene expression between cells of different lineage.

ACKNOWLEDGMENTS

This work was supported by KISPEP Grant No. 2004-01843 to S-H. Im.

REFERENCES

1. MOORE, K.W. *et al.* 2001. Interleukin-10 and the interleukin-10 receptor. Annu. Rev. Immunol. **19:** 683–765.
2. PESTKA, S. *et al.* 2004. Interleukin-10 and related cytokines and receptors. Annu. Rev. Immunol. **22:** 929–979.
3. ABBAS, A.K., K.M. MURPHY & A. SHER. 1996. Functional diversity of helper T lymphocytes. Nature **383:** 787–793.
4. PAUL, W.E. & R.A. SEDER. 1994. Lymphocyte responses and cytokines. Cell **76:** 241–251.
5. AGARWAL, S. & A. RAO. 1998. Modulation of chromatin structure regulates cytokine gene expression during T cell differentiation. Immunity **9:** 765–775.
6. AVNI, O. *et al.* 2002. T(H) cell differentiation is accompanied by dynamic changes in histone acetylation of cytokine genes. Nat. Immunol. **3:** 643–651.
7. DUBCHAK, I. *et al.* 2000. Active conservation of noncoding sequences revealed by three-way species comparisons. Genome Res. **10:** 1304–1306.
8. MAYOR, C. *et al.* 2000. VISTA: visualizing global DNA sequence alignments of arbitrary length. Bioinformatics **16:** 1046–1047.
9. WINGENDER, E. *et al.* 2000. TRANSFAC: an integrated system for gene expression regulation. Nucleic Acids Res. **28:** 316–319.
10. COCKERILL, P.N. *et al.* 1993. The granulocyte-macrophage colony-stimulating factor/interleukin 3 locus is regulated by an inducible cyclosporin A-sensitive enhancer. Proc. Natl. Acad. Sci. USA **90:** 2466–2470.
11. SHANG, Y. *et al.* 2000. Cofactor dynamics and sufficiency in estrogen receptor-regulated transcription. Cell **103:** 843–852.

12. WANG, D., P. MCCAFFREY & A. RAO. 1995. The cyclosporin-sensitive transcription factor NFATp is expressed in several classes of cells in the immune system. Ann. N.Y. Acad. Sci. **766:** 182–194.
13. GROSS, D.S. & W.T. GARRARD. 1988. Nuclease hypersensitive sites in chromatin. Annu. Rev. Biochem. **57:** 159–197.
14. RAO, A., S.J. FAAS & H. CANTOR. 1984. Activation specificity of arsonate-reactive T cell clones. J. Exp. Med. **159:** 479–494.
15. KAYE, J. *et al.* 1983. Both a monoclonal antibody and antisera specific for determinants unique to individual cloned helper T cell lines can substitute for antigen and antigen-presenting cells in the activation of T cells. J. Exp. Med. **158:** 836–856.
16. IM, S-H. *et al.* 2004. Chromatin-level regulation of the IL10 gene in T cells. J. Biol. Chem. **279:** 46818–46825.
17. KOLBE, D. *et al.* 2004. Regulatory potential scores from genome-wide three-way alignments of human, mouse, and rat. Genome Res. **14:** 700–707.
18. FRAZER, K.A. *et al.* 2003. Cross-species sequence comparisons: a review of methods and available resources. Genome Res. **13:** 1-12.
19. HARDISON, R.C. 2000. Conserved noncoding sequences are reliable guides to regulatory elements. Trends Genet. **16:** 369–372.
20. LOOTS, G.G. *et al.* 2002. rVista for comparative sequence-based discovery of functional transcription factor binding sites. Genome Res. **12:** 832–839.
21. ANSEL, K.M., D.U. LEE & A. RAO. 2003. An epigenetic view of helper T cell differentiation. Nat. Immunol. **4:** 616–623.
22. MURPHY, K.M. & S.L. REINER. 2002. The lineage decisions of helper T cells. Nat. Rev. Immunol. **2:** 933–444.
23. SMALE, S.T. & A.G. FISHER. 2002. Chromatin structure and gene regulation in the immune system. Annu. Rev. Immunol. **20:** 427–462.
24. GEORGOPOULOS, K. 2002. Haematopoietic cell-fate decisions, chromatin regulation and ikaros. Nat. Rev. Immunol. **2:** 162–174.
25. FESKE, S. *et al.* 2001. Gene regulation mediated by calcium signals in T lymphocytes. Nat. Immunol. **2:** 316–324.
26. IM, S-H. & A. RAO. 2004. Activation and deactivation of gene expression by Ca^{2+}/calcineurin-NFAT-mediated signaling. Mol. Cells **18:** 1–9.
27. MACIAN, F. *et al.* 2002. Transcriptional mechanisms underlying lymphocyte tolerance. Cell **109:** 719–731.
28. ASADULLAH, K., W. STERRY & H.D. VOLK. 2003. Interleukin-10 therapy—review of a new approach. Pharmacol. Rev. **55:** 241–269.
29. LEVINGS, M.K. *et al.* 2001. IFN-alpha and IL-10 induce the differentiation of human type 1 T regulatory cells. J. Immunol. **166:** 5530–5539.
30. NARDONE, J. *et al.* 2004. Comparative genomics for discovering transcriptional regulatory regions in DNA. Nat, Immunol. In press.
31. LEE, D.U., O. AVNI, L. CHEN & A. RAO. 2004. A distal enhancer in the interferon-gamma (IFN-gamma) locus revealed by genome sequence comparison. J. Biol. Chem. **279:** 4802–4810.
32. MARGULIES, E.H. *et al.* 2003. Identification and characterization of multi-species conserved sequences. Genome Res. **13:** 2507–2518.
33. KURODA, E. & U. YAMASHITA. 2003. Mechanisms of enhanced macrophage-mediated prostaglandin E2 production and its suppressive role in Th1 activation in Th2-dominant BALB/c mice. J. Immunol. **170:** 757–764.

Central Memory and Effector Memory Subsets of Human CD4+ and CD8+ T Cells Display Differential Sensitivity to TNF-α-Induced Apoptosis

SUDHIR GUPTA, RUIFEN BI, AND SASTRY GOLLAPUDI

Cellular and Molecular Immunology Laboratories, Division of Basic and Clinical Immunology, University of California, Irvine, California, USA

ABSTRACT: Upon activation by antigen, naive T cell subsets undergo prolifer-ation and differentiation into effector cells, followed by the generation of a pool of memory T cells. Based upon migration pattern and functions, they are clas-sified into central memory (predominantly homing to the lymph nodes) and effector memory (predominantly homing to extralymphoid sites) subsets. These subsets are defined phenotypically by a set of cell surface molecules. In this investigation, we demonstrate that naive and central memory CD4+ and CD8+ T cells in humans undergo tumor necrosis factor-α (TNF-α)–induced apoptosis, whereas effector memory CD4+ and CD8+ T cells are relatively resistant to TNF-α-induced apoptosis. We also provide evidence for the molecular mecha-nisms underlying the differential sensitivity of naive and different sets of memory T cells to TNF-α-induced apoptosis.

KEYWORDS: CD4+; CD8+; T cells; memory; tumor necrosis factor-α (TNF-α); apoptosis; sensitivity

INTRODUCTION

Upon interaction with an antigen, naive T cells undergo a series of proliferative and differentiation steps to generate a pool of long-lasting memory T cells.[1] During initial stages of the immune response, naive T cells undergo clonal expansion into effector T cells to clear the antigen. This phase of immune expansion is followed by a phase of contraction in which most of the effector T cells are removed by apoptosis, and a small pool of effector cells is retained as memory T cells. Recently, based upon homing pattern and functions, memory T cells have been divided further into central memory (TCM, predominantly migrating to lymphoid tissues) and effector memory (predominantly migrating to extralymphoid tissue) subpopulations, which are iden-

Address for correspondence: Sudhir Gupta, M.D., Ph.D., Medical Sci. I, C-240, University of California, Irvine, CA 92697. Voice: 949-824-5818; fax: 949-824-4362.
sgupta@uci.edu

Ann. N.Y. Acad. Sci. 1050: 108–114 (2005). © 2005 New York Academy of Sciences.
doi: 10.1196/annals.1313.012

tified by a number of cell surface markers.[1-8] The effector memory T cells are subdivided further into CD45RA– (TEM) and CD45RA+ (TEMRA). The presence of the CD8+ TEMRA subset is well established; however, there is debate as to whether the CD4+ TEMRA subset exists. Our data suggest that CD4+ TEMRA cells do exist, albeit as a very small population (1–2% of CD4+ cells); however, this subpopulation is increased in aged humans.[9]

The biological activity of tumor necrosis factor-α (TNF-α), a proinflammatory cytokine, is mediated via two distinct receptors, TNF receptor I (TNFR-I) and TNFR-II. TNFRs belong to the TNFR/nerve growth factor receptor superfamily. The two TNFRs differ from each other in that TNFR-I contains a death domain (DD) motif in its cytoplasmic tail, whereas TNFR-II lacks a DD.[10] As a result, TNFR-I mediates both death and survival signals, whereas TNFR-II predominantly mediates a survival signal.[11-13]

The relative sensitivity to TNF-α-induced apoptosis of the above-mentioned different subsets of CD4+ and CD8+ T cells has not been examined in detail. In this investigation, we summarize our data on the relative sensitivity of naive, central memory, and effector memory CD8+ and CD4+ T cell subsets to TNF-α-induced apoptosis. Naive and central memory CD4+ and CD8+ T cells are sensitive to TNF-α-induced apoptosis, whereas effector memory subsets are relative resistant.

MATERIALS AND METHODS

Peripheral blood was obtained from healthy young volunteers (ages 18 to 30 years) under a protocol approved by the Institutional Review Board (Human) of the University of California, Irvine.

Anti–TNFR-I and anti–TNFR-II monoclonal antibodies and isotype controls were purchased from Caltag Laboratories (Burlingame, CA). Monoclonal antibodies against CD8 and CD45RA and their isotype controls were obtained from BD Biosciences (San Diego, CA), and anti-CCR7 monoclonal antibody and isotype control were purchased from R & D Systems (Minneapolis, MN). Antibodies to Bcl-2, Bax, and phospho-IκB were obtained from Transduction Laboratory (San Diego, CA). Fluorescein-labeled peptide substrates that bind to activated caspase-8 (FAM-IETD-FMK) and activated caspase-3 (FAM-DEVD-FMK) were purchased from Serological Corporation (Norcross, GA).

Naive, central memory, and effector memory CD4+ and CD8+ T cells were analyzed using monoclonal antibodies and multicolor flow cytometry. Naive (CD8+ or CD4+ CD45RA+CCR7+), central memory (CD8+ or CD4+ CD45RA–CCR7+), effector memory (CD8+ or CD4+ CD45RA–CCR7–), and CD45RA+ effector memory (CD8+ or CD4+ CD45RA+CCR7–) subsets were defined.

Peripheral blood mononuclear cells were stimulated with anti-CD3 monoclonal antibody for 48 h at 37°C, followed by culture for an additional 4 days in medium containing IL-2 (10 ng/mL). At the end of incubation, cells were washed and treated with TNF-α for an additional 48 h, and apoptosis and caspase-8 and caspase-3 activation were measured by TUNEL and cytofluorometric assays, respectively.

Expression of Bcl-2, Bax, cIAP, and phospho-IκB was determined by Western blotting. NF-κB activity was measured by ELISA.

RESULTS AND DISCUSSION

TNF-α exerts its biological activity by binding to TNFR-I and TNFR-II and activating several signaling pathways.[10–13] TNFR-I contains a cytoplasmic death domain, whereas TNFR-II lacks a DD. Therefore, TNFR-I induces both cell survival and cell death signals, whereas TNFR-II primarily mediates a cell survival signal. However, recent data suggest that TNFR-II might potentiate death signals mediated by TNFR-I. Both cell survival and cell death signals mediated by TNF-α require distinct sets of adapters and other downstream signaling molecules.

Upon ligation with TNF-α, TNFR-I undergoes trimerization of its receptor death domain, which in turn recruits an adapter protein, TNFR-associated death domain (TRADD) protein. TRADD then may recruit another adapter molecule, the Fas-associated death domain (FADD) protein. FADD protein then recruits procaspase-8, which becomes active on dimerization. Alternatively, TRADD may recruit distinct sets of adapter proteins, TRAF-2 (TNFR-associated factor-2) and receptor inter-active protein (RIP). TRAF-2 and RIP stimulate pathways leading to activation of MAP kinase and NF-κB.

In this study, we show that naive and TCM CD4+ T cells (TCM > naive) are sensitive to TNF-α-induced apoptosis, whereas TEM CD4+ and TEMRA CD4+ T cells are resistant to TNF-α-induced apoptosis (FIG. 1). This differential apoptosis is associated with increased activation of both caspase-8 and caspase-3 (FIG. 2) in naive and TCM CD4+ T cells, and no activation or minimal activation in TEM and TEMRA CD4+ T cells. Similar patterns of differential sensitivity to TNF-α-induced apoptosis and caspase-8 and caspase-3 activation have been observed with naive and memory

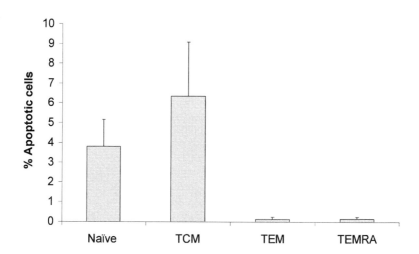

FIGURE 1. TNF-α-induced apoptosis in CD4+ naive, central memory (TCM), CD45RA– effector memory (TEM), and CD45RA+ effector memory (TEMRA) subsets. Mononuclear cells were activated with anti-CD3 for 2 days followed by an additional 3 days of incubation in IL-2-containing medium. At the end of culture, cells were treated with TNF-α for 48 h, and apoptosis was measured by TUNEL assay using multicolor flow cytometry. Data are expressed as percent (mean ± SD) of each subset undergoing apoptosis.

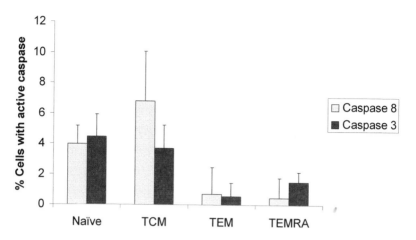

FIGURE 2. Activation of caspase-8 and caspase-3 in naive and memory CD4+ T cell subsets during TNF-α-induced apoptosis. Data are expressed as mean ± SD.

subsets of CD8+ T cells.[14] To determine whether the differential sensitivity to apoptosis among various subsets is the result of differences in TNFR expression, TNFR-I and TNFR-II expression was examined by multicolor flow cytometry. There was no difference in the expression of TNFR-I or TNFR-II (FIG. 3) among subpopulations of CD4+ T cells. Similar data have been observed with naive, TCM, TEM, and TEMRA CD8+ T cells.[14]

These observations suggest that the differential sensitivity of naive and various memory cell subsets to TNF-α-induced apoptosis is due to signals downstream of TNFRs. We have observed that both anti–TNFR-I and anti–TNFR-II inhibitory monoclonal antibodies partially block TNF-α-induced apoptosis in both naive and TCM CD4+ and CD8+ T cells (unpublished data). This suggests that a molecule common to both TNFR-I and TNFR-II signaling may be involved. NF-κB is one such molecule that is activated via both TNFRs.

Studies in mice and humans have shown that NF-κB is a repressor of apoptosis.[15–17] NF-κB exists as either a heterodimer or homodimer of a subfamily of the Rel family of proteins. The predominant form of NF-κB is a heterodimer composed of p50 (NF-κB1) and p65 (RelA). In unstimulated cells, NF-κB is kept in the cytoplasm through interaction with an inhibitory protein termed IκB (inhibitor κB).[16–19] When cells are exposed to TNF-α, IκB is phosphorylated at two specific serine residues,[20–22] which is a signal for ubiquitination and degradation of IκB by the 26S proteosome.[21] Free NF-κB dimers are released and translocated to the nucleus, where they activate transcription of target genes. We have observed that TNF-α-induced NF-κB activation is significantly lower in CD8+CD28+ T cells (both naive and TCM) as compared with CD8+CD28− T cells (both TEM and TEMRA), which may explain the increased sensitivity of naive and TCM T cells to TNF-α-induced apoptosis. Furthermore, we observed less IκB phosphorylation in CD8+CD28+ T cells as compared with the CD8+CD28− population. The protein kinase complex that phosphorylates IκB in response to TNF-α contains two catalytic subunits, IKKα

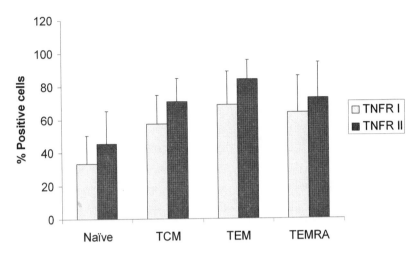

FIGURE 3. Expression of TNFR-I and TNFR-II in naive and in different memory CD4+ T cell subsets. Mononuclear cells were activated as above. At day 5 (prior to the addition of TNF-α), cells were stained with TNFR-I and TNFR-II monoclonal antibodies among various subsets, using multicolor flow cytometry. Data are expressed as percent (mean ± SD) of each subset positive for TNFR-I or TNFR-II.

and IKKβ, and a regulatory subunit, IKKγ.[18,19] IKKβ is essential for the activation of IKK by TNF-α. Furthermore, it has been demonstrated that IKKβ is essential for protecting cells from apoptosis, including protecting T cells from TNF-α-induced apoptosis.[23,24] It is likely that IKKβ activity is lower in naive and TCM T cells as compared with TEM and TEMRA T cell subsets. We have observed decreased IKKβ expression and activity in aged T cells that is associated with decreased IκB phosphorylation and decreased NF-κB activation.[9]

The suppression of apoptosis by NF-κB depends on the induction of a number of genes whose products inhibit apoptosis. NF-κB induces the expression of a number of antiapoptotic genes, including cIAPs (inhibitor of apoptosis proteins), Bcl-2, and Bcl-xL.[18,19] Inhibition of NF-κB is also associated with upregulation of Bax, suggesting that Bax is negatively regulated by NF-κB.[25] We have observed decreased expression of Bcl-2 and cIAP1 and increased expression of Bax in CD8+CD28– T cells (naive and TCM) as compared with CD8+CD28– T cells (TEM and TEMRA).

Taken together, it appears that NF-κB activity plays a major role in the differential sensitivity of naive and memory T cell subsets to TNF-α-induced apoptosis. Both TNFR-I and TNFR-II and NF-κB appear to be involved in differential sensitivity to apoptosis. A molecule upstream of NF-κB, that is IκB, and IKKβ, which is activated via both TNFR-I and TNFR-II, is receptor interacting protein (RIP). Pimentel-Muinos and Seed[26] have demonstrated that TNFR-II triggers apoptosis in the presence of RIP, whereas TNFR-II activates NF-κB in the absence of RIP. However, RIP knockout mice show increased sensitivity to TNF-α-induced apoptosis.[27] These discrepancies may be explained by the presence and activity of a family of RIP kinases. RIP is a family of serine/threonine kinases. A number of homologs, including RIP2,

3, 4, and 5, have been described.[28–30] RIP3 and RIP5 interact with RIP and inhibit its activity and NF-κB activation, and therefore induce apoptosis. Recently, it has been demonstrated that RIP also plays a crucial role in oxidative stress–induced apoptosis.[31] Interestingly, we have also observed that naive and TCM CD4+ and CD8+ T cells are sensitive to oxidative stress–induced apoptosis, whereas TEM and TEMRA CD4+ and CD8+ T cells are resistant to apoptosis.[32]

In summary, naive and TCM (TCM > naive) CD4+ and CD8+ T cells are sensitive to apoptosis, whereas TEM and TEMRA subsets are resistant to apoptosis. Decreased NF-κB activity and associated decreased antiapoptotic target molecules (Bcl-2, cIAP) and increased proapoptotic Bax (negatively regulated by NF-κB) appear to play an important role in differential sensitivity to apoptosis. The role of RIP kinases remains to be investigated.

ACKNOWLEDGMENTS

Part of the work cited was supported by USPHS Grant No. AG 18313.

REFERENCES

1. KAECH, S.M. & R. AHMED. 2001. Memory CD8+ T cell differentiation: initial antigen encounter triggers a developmental program in naive cells. Nat. Immunol. **2:** 415–422.
2. MOSER, B. & P. LOETSCHER. 2001. Lymphocyte traffic control by chemokines. Nat. Immunol. **2:** 123–128.
3. SCHLUNS, K.S. & L. LEFRANCOIS. 2003. Cytokine control of memory T-cell development and survival. Nat. Rev. Immunol. **3:** 269–279.
4. MASOPUST, D., V. VEZYS, A.L. MARZO & L. LEFRANCOIS. 2001. Preferential localization of effector memory cells in nonlymphoid tissue. Science **291:** 2413–2417.
5. SALLUSTO, F., D. LENIG, R. FORSTER, *et al.* 1999. Two subsets of memory T lymphocytes with distinct homing potentials and effector functions. Nature **401:** 708–712.
6. WENINGER, W., M.A. CROWLEY, N. MANJUNATH & U.H. VON ANDRIAN. 2001. Migratory properties of naive, effector, and memory CD8(+) T cells. J. Exp. Med. **194:** 953–966.
7. TOMIYAMA, H., T. MATSUDA & M. TAKIGUCHI. 2002. Differentiation of CD8+ T cells from a memory to memory/effector phenotype. J. Immunol. **168:** 5538–5550.
8. GUPTA, S., R. BI, K. SU, *et al.* 2004. Characterization of naive, memory and effector CD8+ T cells: effect of age. Exp. Gerontol. **39:** 545–550.
9. GUPTA, S. & S. GOLLAPUDI. 2005. Molecular mechanisms of TNF-α-induced apoptosis in aging human T cell subsets. Int. J. Biochem. Cell Biol. **37:** 1034–1042.
10. LOCKSLEY, R.M., N. KILLEEN & M.J. LENARDO. 2001. The TNF and TNF receptor superfamilies: integrating mammalian biology. Cell **104:** 487–501.
11. GUPTA, S. 2000. Molecular steps of death receptor and mitochondrial pathways of apoptosis. Life Sci. **69:** 2957–2964.
12. GUPTA, S. 2001. Molecular steps of tumor necrosis factor receptor-mediated apoptosis. Curr. Mol. Med. **1:** 299–306.
13. GUPTA, S. 2002. A decision between life and death during TNF-α-induced signaling. J. Clin. Immunol. **22:** 270–278.
14. GUPTA, S., R. BI & S. GOLLAPUDI. 2005. Differential sensitivity of naive and memory subsets of human CD8+ T cells to TNF-α-induced apoptosis. J. Immunol. Submitted.
15. BEG, A.A. & D. BALTIMORE. 1996. An essential role for NF-κB in preventing TNF-α-induced cell death. Science **274:** 782–784.
16. GHOSH, S., M.J. MAY & E.B. KOPP. 1998. NF-κB and Rel proteins: evolutionarily conserved mediators of immune responses. Annu. Rev. Immunol. **16:** 225–260.
17. BALDWIN, A.S. 1996. The NF-κB and IκB proteins: new discoveries and insights. Annu. Rev. Immunol. **14:** 649–681.

18. KARIN, M. & A. LIN. 2002. NF-κB at the crossroads of life and death. Nat. Immunol. **3:** 221–227.
19. GHOSH, S. & M. KARIN. 2002. Missing pieces in the NF-κB puzzle. Cell **109:** S81–S96.
20. ZANDI, E., Y.I. CHEN & M. KARIN. 1998. Direct phosphorylation of IκB by IKKα and IKKβ: discrimination between free and NF-κB-bound substrate. Science **281:** 1360–1363.
21. BROWN, K., S. GERSTBERGER, L. CARLSON, et al. 1995. Control of IκB-a proteolysis by site-specific, signal-induced phosphorylation. Science **281:** 1360–1363.
22. PAHL, H.L. 1999. Activators and target genes of Rel/NF-κB transcription factors. Oncogene **18:** 6855–6866.
23. LI, Z.W., W.M. CHU, Y.L. HU, et al. 1999. The IKKβ subunit of IκB kinase (IKK) is essential for nuclear factor κB activation and prevention of apoptosis. J. Exp. Med. **189:** 1839–1845.
24. SENFTLEBEN, U., Z-W. LI, V. BAUD & M. KARIN. 2001. IKKβ is essential for protecting T cells from TNFα-induced apoptosis. Cell **14:** 217–230.
25. BENTIRES-ALJ, M., E. DEJARDIN, P. VIATOUR, et al. 2001. Inhibition of the NF-κB transcription factor increases Bax expression in cancer cell lines. Oncogene **20:** 2805–2813.
26. PIMENTEL-MUINOS, F.X. & B. SEED. 1999. Regulated commitment of TNF receptor signaling: a molecular switch for death or activation. Immunity **11:** 783–793.
27. KELLIHER, M.A., S. GRIMM, Y. ISHIDA, et al. 1998. The death domain kinase RIP mediates the TNF-induced NF-kappa B signal. Immunity **8:** 297–303.
28. YANG, Y., J. MA, Y. CHEN & M. WU. 2004. Nucleocytoplasmic shuttling of receptor-interacting protein 3 (RIP3): identification of novel nuclear export and import signals in RIP3. J. Biol. Chem. **279:** 38820–38829.
29. ZHA, J., O. ZHOU, L.G. XU, et al. 2004. RIP5 is a RIP-homologous inducer of cell death. Biochem. Biophys. Res. Commun. **319:** 298–303.
30. MEYLAN, E., F. MARTINON, M. THOME, et al. 2002. RIP4 (DIK/PKK), a novel member of the RIP kinase family, activates NF-κB and is processed during apoptosis. EMBO Rep. **3:** 1201–1208.
31. SHEN, H-M., Y. LIN, S. CHOKSI, et al. 2004. Essential role of receptor-interacting protein and TRAF2 in oxidative stress-induced cell death. Mol. Cell. Immunol. **24:** 5914–5922.
32. YOUNG, T., S. GOLLAPUDI, S. AGRAWAL & S. GUPTA. 2005. Oxidative stress-induced apoptosis in naive, central memory, and effector memory CD4+ and CD8+ T cells. FASEB J. **19:** A959.

Non-Antigen-Specific CD8+ T Suppressor Lymphocytes in Diseases Characterized by Chronic Immune Responses and Inflammation

G. FILACI,[a,b,c] M. RIZZI,[a,b] M. SETTI,[b] D. FENOGLIO,[a,b] M. FRAVEGA,[a] M. BASSO,[b] G. ANSALDO,[d] P. CEPPA,[d] G. BORGONOVO,[d] G. MURDACA,[b] F. FERRERA,[a] A. PICCIOTTO,[b] R. FIOCCA,[d] G. TORRE,[d] AND F. INDIVERI[a,b]

[a]Center of Excellence for Biomedical Research (CEBR), University of Genoa, Genoa, Italy

[b]Department of Internal Medicine, University of Genoa, Genoa, Italy

[c]Center for Advanced Biotechnology (CBA), Genoa, Italy

[d]Department of Surgical and Morphological Disciplines and Integrated Methodologies, University of Genoa, Genoa, Italy

ABSTRACT: Recent studies on regulatory lymphocytes demonstrate that CD8+ T suppressor (Ts) cells may have great relevance in controlling immune system homeostasis and avoiding development of chronic inflammatory diseases. Among the three subpopulations of CD8+ Ts cells so far recognized in humans, the type 2 (non-antigen-specific) cell is characterized by the capacity to inhibit both T cell proliferation and cytotoxic T lymphocyte activity through secretion of soluble factors. Previous work has shown the impairment of *in vitro* generation of type 2 CD8+ Ts cells from the peripheral blood of relapsed patients with multiple sclerosis, systemic lupus erythematosus, or systemic sclerosis. Here, similar findings are demonstrated for patients with human immunodeficiency virus or chronic hepatitis C virus infection. Furthermore, the presence of type 2 CD8+ Ts cells infiltrating diseased tissues in patients with autoimmune thyroiditis or cancer is shown. Collectively, these findings suggest that type 2 CD8+ Ts cells may be involved in the control of pathologic chronic immune responses, contributing in some cases to the pathogenesis of the disease.

KEYWORDS: suppressor lymphocytes; IL-10; HIV; HCV; thyroiditis; tumor-infiltrating lymphocytes

INTRODUCTION

The matter concerning CD8+ T suppressor (Ts) lymphocytes is quite long and particular. It began in the early 1970s when Gershon and Kondo, in experiments on tolerance transfer, found evidence of the existence of a subset of suppressor cells within the population of CD8+ T lymphocytes.[1] Unfortunately, technology at that

Address for correspondence: Gilberto Filaci, Center of Excellence for Biomedical Research (CEBR), University of Genoa, Genoa, Italy. Voice: +39-010-3538984; fax: +39-010-3533025. gfilaci@unige.it

Ann. N.Y. Acad. Sci. 1050: 115–123 (2005). © 2005 New York Academy of Sciences. doi: 10.1196/annals.1313.013

time was not adequately sophisticated to allow isolation and functional characterization of these cells. For this reason, most immunologists remained skeptical of the existence of suppressor lymphocytes.[2] It required more than a decade to acquire data clearly demonstrating the presence and functional relevance of CD8+ T cell clones mediating suppressor activity in experimental animal models.[3,4] These findings prompted studies in humans that have led in the last fifteen years to the isolation and characterization of CD8+ Ts cells from the peripheral blood of healthy donors.[5,6] In particular, three subtypes of CD8+ Ts cells have been recognized so far in humans: type 1, which acts through the transfer of inhibitory signals to antigen-presenting cells (APC) by direct cell-to-cell contact after antigen recognition;[6,7] type 2, which acts via cytokine secretion without antigen activation and/or restriction;[5,8,9] and type 3, which are stimulated by antigen recognition and induce suppression through IL-10 secretion.[10] Many researchers have attempted to uncover the *in vivo* biological relevance of CD8+ Ts cells through analysis of the phenotypic and functional features of these lymphocytes, as well as through the demonstration of their presence and activity in patients with diseases whose pathogenesis could be related to the abnormal activity of suppressor cell subpopulations. In particular, three kinds of diseases have been under investigation: (a) immune-dependent inflammatory diseases; (b) infectious diseases; and (c) cancer. Concerning the first category of diseases, Suciu-Foca and coworkers, who are actively investigating the functions of type 1 CD8+ Ts cells, identified rejection of allograft transplantation as a disease model to explore the relevance of these cells *in vivo*.[11–13] Their finding of an indirect correlation between the circulating concentration of type 1 CD8+ Ts cells and the frequency of organ transplant rejection is a strong argument in favor of the important role played by this T cell regulatory subset in processes allowing induction and maintenance of tolerance against alloantigens. In our laboratory research has been focused on the *in vivo* involvement of type 2 CD8+ Ts cells in diseases for which chronic immune responses and chronic inflammation represent the main biologic features.[8,14] Thus, analyses have been performed in patients with viral infectious diseases with agents such as human immunodeficiency virus (HIV) and hepatitis C virus (HCV); systemic or organ-specific autoimmune diseases; and cancer. The present report summarizes the most recent findings in these areas. For simplicity, from this point onward CD8+ Ts cells will indicate type 2 CD8+ Ts cells.

MATERIALS AND METHODS

Patients

Twenty-two HIV-infected patients at different stages of disease and 9 HCV chronically infected patients were enrolled at the Department of Internal Medicine, University of Genoa.

Three patients affected by Hashimoto thyroiditis and two patients with Graves' disease as well as 16 cancer patients with advanced disease (stage 4), affected by colon ($n = 6$), gastric ($n = 3$), kidney ($n = 2$), pancreas ($n = 1$), breast ($n = 1$), head/neck ($n = 1$), melanoma ($n = 1$), sarcoma ($n = 1$) cancers, were diagnosed and selected for the study at the Department of Surgical and Morphological Disciplines and Integrated Methodologies, University of Genoa.

Generation of CD8+ Ts Cells

CD8+ Ts cells were generated from the peripheral blood of HIV- or HCV-infected patients as described.[8] Briefly, peripheral blood mononuclear cells (PBMCs) were isolated by centrifugation on a Ficoll-Hypaque gradient for 30 min at 1800 rpm. PBMCs were incubated in RPMI 1640 culture medium (Sigma, Milan, Italy) with 10% fetal calf serum (Sigma), 2% glutamine (Sigma), and penicillin 100 U/mL–streptomycin 0.1 mg/mL (Sigma, Milan) in culture flasks (Corning Costar, Cambridge, MA) at 37°C overnight. After removal of nonadherent cells, monocytes were collected by gentle scraping with a cell lifter (Corning Costar) and irradiated (2500 rad). Purification of CD8+CD28– T cells was performed by magnetic bead cell sorting. Positive purification of CD8+ lymphocytes was achieved using Dynabeads M-450 CD8 and the CD8 Detachbead (Dynal Inc., Great Neck, NY). Negative purification of CD8+CD28– T cells was achieved by preincubation of CD8+ T cells with the anti-CD28 9.3 monoclonal antibody (mAb), followed by incubation with magnetic rat anti-mouse conjugated with an anti–mouse IgG monoclonal antibody (IgG Microbeads, Miltenyi Biotec GmbH, Bergish Gladbach, Germany). The procedure was repeated until the cell population was highly enriched in CD8+CD28– T cells (>95%) as demonstrated by flow cytometric analysis. CD8+CD28– T lymphocytes (1×10^5 cells/well) were incubated with autologous irradiated monocytes (2.5×10^4 cells/well) in 96-well flat-bottomed plates (Corning Costar) in RPMI medium containing 20 U/mL IL-2 (Chiron, Emeryville, CA) and 10 ng/mL GM-CSF (Roche, Milan, Italy) at 37°C up to 7 days. At the end of the incubation, nonadherent cells were collected and the CD8+CD28– T cell population was further purified as above. Each single CD8+ T cell preparation was used for one single experiment.

Purification and Function of CD8+ Ts Cells

The presence of CD8+ Ts cells was analyzed in the peripheral blood and thyroids of patients with thyroiditis, and in the peripheral blood, primitive tumor mass, and satellite lymph nodes from cancer patients, according to the clinical conditions of the patients and the availability of surgical samples. PBMCs were obtained by centrifugation on a Ficoll-Hypaque gradient for 30 min at 1800 rpm. Thyroid-infiltrating lymphocytes, tumor-infiltrating lymphocytes, and lymphocytes from satellite lymph nodes were obtained from surgical specimens by mincing freshly resected thyroid, tumor, or lymph nodes, filtering the cell suspension through sterile gauze, and running the filtrate on discontinuous Ficoll gradients (from 75% to 100%) to separate lymphocytes from other cell types.

Because CD8+ Ts cells do not express CD28 antigen,[2] we purified CD8+CD28– T cells from PBMCs and surgical samples, and then analyzed their suppressor activity. Cell purification was performed as outlined above.

Analysis of Suppressor Activity of In Vitro Generated and Ex Vivo Purified CD8+ Ts Cells

The suppressor activity of CD8+ Ts cells generated *in vitro* or purified *ex vivo* was analyzed as follows: PBMCs were seeded in a 96-well flat-bottomed plate (1×10^5 cells/well) with the anti-CD3 UCHT-1 mAb (5 µg/mL), and cultured for 5 days in the presence or absence of irradiated *in vitro* generated CD8+ Ts cells or *ex vivo* purified CD8+CD28– T lymphocytes (8×10^4 cells/well). The experiment was performed in a Transwell system (Corning Costar), seeding anti-CD3–stimulated PBMCs and suppressor lymphocytes on the opposite sides of a pored membrane to avoid direct cell-to-cell contact. The proliferative activity of stimulated T cells was analyzed by measuring the incorporation of ^{3}H-thymidine (0.5 μCi/well) added to the wells 12 h before the end of the assay. We arbitrarily considered a suppressor activity of 25% as significant. This cutoff was chosen because in repeated preliminary experiments CD8+CD28– T cells purified from the peripheral blood of healthy subjects never caused suppression of autologous PBMC proliferation 10%. Thus, the finding of a rate of inhibition of proliferation 25% is, in our hands, atypical for CD8+CD28– T lymphocytes not induced to differentiate *in vitro* into suppressor cells, and, hence, must be considered a property specifically acquired and expressed by suppressor lymphocytes.

Immunofluorescence Analyses

Incubations with monoclonal antibodies were performed at 4°C for 30 min in the dark. The percentage of CD8+CD28– T cells in peripheral blood and in cell preparations after tissue isolation was analyzed as follows: 1×10^5 PBMCs resuspended in 100 μL of Hanks' balanced salt solution (HBSS, Sigma) were stained with an anti-CD28PE mAb (Coulter Immunotech, Miami, FL) and an anti-CD8 FITC mAb (Caltag Laboratories, Burlingame, CA) and then washed with PBS. Cells were then analyzed by a FACSCalibur flow cytometer (Beckton-Dickinson). The concentration of CD8+CD28– cells was >95% in each experiment.

Statistical Analyses

The existence of statistically significant differences between means of values was analyzed by the Mann-Whitney *t*-test for nonparametric values. The existence of statistically significant correlation between values was analyzed by the Spearman test for nonparametric data. All calculations were performed using the GraphPad PrismTM Version 3.0 software.

RESULTS

Generation of CD8+ Ts Cells in Patients with HIV Infection

Previous work demonstrated that circulating CD8+CD28– T cells contain the precursors for CD8+ Ts cells.[9] Thus, the concentration of these cells in the peripheral blood of HIV-infected patients as well as their capacity to generate CD8+ Ts cells *in vitro* were analyzed in comparison with those of healthy subjects. In our series of HIV-infected patients the percentages of circulating CD8+CD28– T lymphocytes (mean = 43 ± 12) were statistically comparable to those of healthy subjects (mean = 47 ± 15, $P = .6$) (TABLES 1A and 1B). In contrast, generation of CD8+ Ts cells from circulating CD8+CD28– T cells revealed a strong impairment in HIV-infected patients with respect to healthy subjects (TABLES 1A and 1B). In fact, a statistically significant difference was found between the mean percent suppression by CD8+ Ts cells generated *in vitro* from HIV-infected patients (10 ± 18) and that from

TABLE 1. Circulating CD8+CD28– T cells and suppression activity of generated CD8+ Ts cells

Subject no.	Percentage of circulating CD8+CD28– T cells	Percent suppression activity of generated CD8+ Ts cells
(A) Healthy subjects		
1	50	88
2	75	92
3	51	76
4	67	68
5	40	94
6	52	81
7	34	66
8	37	79
9	22	71
10	42	80
(B) HIV-infected patients		
1	31	0
2	35	0
3	52	27
4	66	0
5	45	0
6	58	0
7	43	0
8	45	0
9	52	0
10	39	10
11	25	0
12	34	0
13	29	33
14	58	0
15	39	0
16	47	75
17	46	0
18	50	14
19	61	2
20	55	24
21	30	0
22	17	34

TABLE 1. *(continued)* **Circulating CD8+CD28– T cells and suppression activity of generated CD8+ Ts cells**

Subject no.	Percentage of circulating CD8+CD28– T cells	Percent suppression activity of generated CD8+ Ts cells
(C) HCV-infected patients		
1	85	50
2	29	58
3	13	0
4	12	40
5	11	0
6	50	40
7	6	60
8	40	10
9	55	0

healthy subjects (79 ± 9) ($P < .001$). This finding suggests that circulating precursors for CD8+ Ts cells are markedly diminished in HIV-infected patients as a result of a real cell disappearance mediated by unknown mechanisms or of tissue compartmentalization. The impaired generation of CD8+ Ts cells in HIV-infected patients was independent from factors such as clinical stage, number of circulating CD4+ T cells, concentration of circulating virus RNA, and therapy, as no statistically significant correlation was found with any of these parameters (data not shown).

Generation of CD8+ Ts Cells in Patients with HCV Infection

Percentages of circulating CD8+CD28– T cells and generation of CD8+ Ts cells from peripheral blood were also tested in nine untreated patients chronically infected with HCV (TABLE 1C) and compared with those of a control population. The percentages of circulating CD8+CD28– T cells did not vary significantly between patient (mean = 33 ± 26) and control (mean = 47 ± 15) groups ($P = .1$). In contrast, a decreased percent suppressor activity of CD8+ Ts cells generated from peripheral blood was observed in the patient group (28 ± 25) compared with healthy donors (79 ± 9) ($P = .0001$). Such impairment was particularly relevant in 4 of 9 HCV-infected patients examined. However, no statistically significant correlation could be found between CD8+ Ts cell suppressor activity and factors such as percentage of circulating CD8+CD28– T cells, circulating HCV RNA concentration, and response to treatment with interferon and ribavirin (data not shown).

CD8+ Ts Cells Infiltrate Inflammatory and Cancer Tissues

Studies analyzing the *in vitro* generation of CD8+ Ts cells from circulating CD8+CD28– T cell precursors in patients affected by autoimmune diseases [e.g., multiple sclerosis,[5] systemic lupus erythematosus (SLE),[8] systemic sclerosis[14]] or by chronic infectious diseases (e.g., HIV, HCV, as above) demonstrate an impairment of CD8+ Ts cell generation with respect to healthy individuals. One possible

TABLE 2. Suppression activity of CD8+CD28– T cells from patients with thyroiditis

Patient no.	Disease	Percent suppression activity of CD8+CD28– cells from peripheral blood	Percent suppression activity of CD8+CD28– cells from thyroid
1	Hashimoto	18	25
2	Hashimoto	39	45
3	Hashimoto	49	60
4	Graves	25	40
5	Graves	25	27

TABLE 3. Detection of suppressor CD8+CD28– T cells in cancer patients

PBMC	Primitive tumor	Metastatic satellite lymph node	Nonmetastatic satellite lymph node
11/15 (73%)	6/6 (100%)	13/15 (86%)	0/2 (0%)

NOTE: Data are expressed as the number of positive detections of suppressor CD8+CD28– T cells out of the total number of examined patients; the relative percentage of positivity is shown in parentheses. The cutoff for considering the suppressor activity as positive has been arbitrarily fixed at 25%.

explanation for this observation could be tissue compartmentalization of CD8+ Ts cells and/or their precursors. To test such a possibility we began studying the presence of infiltrating CD8+ Ts cells in pathologic tissues from patients with thyroid inflammatory diseases and cancer. Hence, CD8+CD28– T cells were extracted and purified from thyroid (and from peripheral blood for comparison) of three patients with Hashimoto thyroiditis and two patients with Graves' disease. The suppressor activity of these lymphocytes was analyzed in tests of inhibition of PBMC proliferation and the results are summarized in TABLE 2. In all patients, tissue-derived CD8+CD28– T cells showed suppressor function. Notably, this was also the case with cells purified from the peripheral blood. Such a finding is remarkable because in our experience no relevant suppressor function (always ≤10%) is expressed by CD8+CD28– T lymphocytes from the peripheral blood of healthy subjects.

Similar findings were observed in cancer patients. In fact, in 16 patients so far analyzed, suppressor CD8+CD28– T cells from primitive cancer lesions were detected in 100% of tested cases and in 80% of metastatic satellite lymph nodes (TABLE 3). Furthermore, suppressor CD8+CD28– T cells were also observed in the peripheral blood in 80% of these patients. Interestingly, low or absent suppressor activity was shown by CD8+CD28– T cells from two nonmetastatic satellite lymph nodes.

DISCUSSION

The main results of this work show that (a) impaired generation of CD8+ Ts cells from peripheral blood lymphocytes is generally present in patients with chronic infectious diseases such as HIV and HCV virus infections; (b) CD8+ Ts cells infiltrate tissues that are affected by diseases characterized by chronic immune responses and inflammation, including autoimmune thyroiditis and cancer.

Markedly impaired generation of CD8+ Ts cells from the peripheral blood of HIV- or HCV-infected patients was observed, similar to what has been found in relapsed patients with chronic inflammatory diseases such as multiple sclerosis,[4] SLE,[8] and systemic sclerosis.[14] These findings may reflect two opposite conditions: the physical elimination of CD8+ Ts cell precursors (caused by unknown mechanisms) or the compartmentalization of these cells and CD8+ Ts cells in tissues. Although it is impossible to assess at the moment which of the two hypotheses is real, both conditions may be associated with pathogenic effects. (Future studies analyzing the eventual CD8+ Ts cell and/or relative precursor infiltration of either lymph nodes in HIV-infected patients or the liver in HCV-infected patients will be useful to clarify this point.) In fact, in the former case, the impaired CD8+ Ts cell function consequent to their disappearance could lead to a reduced efficiency in regulatory control by these lymphocytes on T cell responses of virus-infected patients. In HIV-infected patients this condition could favor the entrance of CD4+ T cells into an activated state and, consequently, predispose them to HIV infection and relative cytopathic effects.[15] Accordingly, a progressive increase in the percentage of CD4+ T cells expressing markers of activation (CD38, HLA-DR) during HIV disease progression has been demonstrated.[16] In HCV-infected patients the same condition might explain the establishment of a chronic intraliver cytopathic immune response. In contrast, in the latter case, recruitment of CD8+ Ts cells from the periphery to the site of developing immune responses could represent a further mechanism contributing to establishment of immunodeficiency in HIV-infected patients. In patients with HCV infection this condition may correspond to an attempt by the immune system to autoregulate the chronically persistent anti-virus immune reaction. The recent demonstration of antigen-specific CD8+ T suppressor cell lines infiltrating the livers of patients with chronic HCV infection[17] supports this hypothesis.

The finding of impaired generation of CD8+ Ts cells from the blood of patients with autoimmune diseases or with chronic virus infections has prompted new research aimed at exploring the presence of CD8+ Ts cells in organs affected by diseases characterized by chronic immune responses and inflammation. In particular, thyroid autoimmune diseases and cancer have been chosen as experimental targets due to the consideration that they represent the "two sides of the coin", being characterized by exaggerated and hypoeffective immune responses, respectively. Furthermore, surgical specimens may be obtained easily for both types of diseases. CD8+ Ts cells were found to infiltrate affected organs in both autoimmune thyroiditis and cancer. This finding supports the view that CD8+ Ts cells generally are recruited at the site of inflamed tissues. In the case of autoimmune thyroiditis such a phenomenon likely constitutes a mechanism by which the immune system tries to autoregulate overwhelming responses. Thus, it has a protective function. In contrast, in the case of cancer, the presence of CD8+ Ts cells probably manifests a pathogenic role for these cells, as they may participate in silencing *in situ* anti-tumor immune responses and in establishing and spreading tumor-associated immune deficiency. It remains to be clarified whether tissue-infiltrating CD8+ Ts cells are generated *in situ* or whether they originate in lymphoid organs and then migrate in response to chemoattractants and are recruited to diseased organs. The observation of circulating CD8+ Ts cells in the peripheral blood of patients but not of healthy subjects may support the latter hypothesis.

In conclusion, type 2 CD8+ T suppressor cells appear to be involved in the pathogenic and/or physiopathologic processes underlying diseases characterized by chronic stimulation of the immune system and chronic inflammation. Hence, more detailed information on their phenotypic and functional features will likely allow us to understand how to modulate their activity and set new protocols for cell-mediated immunotherapy.

ACKNOWLEDGMENTS

This study was supported by grants from Ministero della Sanità–Istituto Superiore di Sanità, Programma Nazionale di Ricerche sull'AIDS 2000 (No. 40D.45), from MURST National Program "Meccanismi Umorali e Cellulari di Modulazione dell'Immunoflogosi" (No. 9706117821-001), and from Compagnia di San Paolo, Torino.

REFERENCES

1. GERSHON, R.K. & K. KONDO. 1971. Infectious immunological tolerance. Immunology **21:** 903–914.
2. MOLLER, G. 1988. Do suppressor T cells exist? Scand. J. Immunol. **27:** 247–250.
3. SERCARZ, E.E. & U. KRZYCH. 1991. The distinctive specificity of antigen-specific suppressor T cells. Immunol. Today **12:** 111–118.
4. SUN, D. *et al.* 1988. Suppression of experimentally induced autoimmune encephalomyelitis by cytolytic T-T cell interactions. Nature **332:** 843–845.
5. BALASHOV, K.E., S.J. KHOURY, D.A. HAFLER & H.L. WEINER. 1995. Inhibition of T cell responses by activated human CD8+ T cells is mediated by interferon-γ and is defective in chronic progressive multiple sclerosis. J. Clin. Invest. **95:** 2711–2719.
6. LIU, Z., S. TUGULEA, R. CORTESINI & N. SUCIU-FOCA. 1998. Specific suppression of T helper alloreactivity by allo-MHC class I-restricted CD8+CD28− T cells. Int. Immunol. **10:** 775–783.
7. CHANG, C.C. *et al.* 2002. Tolerization of dendritic cells by Ts cells: the crucial role of inhibitory receptors ILT3 and ILT4. Nat. Immunol. **3:** 237–243.
8. FILACI, G. *et al.* 2001. Impairment of CD8+ T suppressor cell function in patients with active systemic lupus erythematosus. J. Immunol. **166:** 6452–6457.
9. FILACI, G. *et al.* 2004. Nonantigen specific CD8+ T suppressor lymphocytes originate from CD8+CD28− T cells and inhibit both T cells proliferation and CTL function. Hum. Immunol. **65:** 142–156.
10. GILLIET, M. & Y-J. LIU. 2002. Generation of human CD8 T regulatory cells by CD40 ligand-activated plasmacytoid dendritic cells. J. Exp. Med. **195:** 695–704.
11. CIUBOTARIU, R. *et al.* 2001. Detection of T suppressor cells in patients with organ allografts. Hum. Immunol. **62:** 15–20.
12. CORTESINI, R. *et al.* 2002. Tailoring of immunosuppression in renal and liver allograft recipients displaying donor specific T-suppressor cells. Hum. Immunol. **63:** 1010–1018.
13. COLOVAI, A.I. *et al.* 2003. Regulatory CD8+CD28− T cells in heart transplant recipients. Hum. Immunol. **64:** 31–37.
14. FILACI, G. *et al.* 2004. Non-antigen specific CD8+ T suppressor lymphocytes. Clin. Exp. Med. **4:** 86–92.
15. ZACK, J.A. *et al.* 1990. HIV-1 entry into quiescent primary lymphocytes: molecular analysis reveals a labile, latent viral structure. Cell **61:** 213–222.
16. CHOREMI-PAPADOPOULOU, H. *et al.* 1994. Downregulation of CD28 surface antigen on CD4+ and CD8+ T lymphocytes during HIV-1 infection. J. Acquir. Immune Defic. Syndr. **7:** 245–253.
17. ACCAPEZZATO, D. *et al.* 2004. Hepatic expansion of a virus-specific regulatory CD8+ T cell population in chronic hepatitis C virus infection. J. Clin. Invest. **113:** 963–972.

Long-Lived Plasma Cells and Their Contribution to Autoimmunity

BIMBA F. HOYER,[a,b] RUDOLF A. MANZ,[b] ANDREAS RADBRUCH,[b]
AND FALK HIEPE[a,b]

[a]Department of Medicine (Rheumatology and Clinical Immunology),
Charité–University Hospital Berlin, Berlin, Germany

[b]German Rheumatism Research Center, Berlin, Germany

ABSTRACT: The current view holds that chronic autoimmune diseases are driven by the continuous activation of autoreactive B and T lymphocytes. However, despite the use of potent immunosuppressants, the production of autoantibodies may persist and contribute to the autoimmune pathology. We recently demonstrated in autoimmune mice that both short-lived plasmablasts and long-lived plasma cells are involved in autoantibody production. While anti-proliferative immunosuppressive therapy and monoclonal anti-CD20 antibody deplete short-lived plasmablasts, long-lived plasma cells survive and continue to produce (auto)antibodies. Thus, strategies for targeting long-lived plasma cells may provide potent new treatment modalities.

KEYWORDS: antibody; autoantibody; autoimmune; B cells; humoral; long-lived; plasma cells; plasmablasts; survival

Plasma cells are terminally differentiated B cells that produce antibodies to provide immediate and long-term protection against pathogens; hence, they play a critical role in humoral immunity.[1–3] However, under certain conditions, B cells specific for self-antigens may become activated and differentiate into autoreactive plasma cells that cause autoimmune diseases. Although important for understanding humoral immunity, little is known about these cells, which are often considered to be short-lived end stages of B-cell development.[4–6] This view was recently challenged. Several investigators have shown that a substantial fraction of plasma cells can survive and continue to secrete antibodies for extended periods of time in the absence of any detectable memory B cells and antigen stimulation.[7–9]

Address for correspondence: Falk Hiepe, M.D., Ph.D., Department of Medicine (Rheumatology and Clinical Immunology), Charité–University Hospital Berlin, Schumannstr. 20/21, D-10117 Berlin, Germany. Voice: +49-30-450-513012; fax: +49-30-450-513922.
falk.hiepe@charite.de

Ann. N.Y. Acad. Sci. 1050: 124–133 (2005). © 2005 New York Academy of Sciences.
doi: 10.1196/annals.1313.014

LONG-LASTING PERSISTENCE OF (AUTO)ANTIBODIES DESPITE IMMUNOSUPPRESSION INDICATES THE EXISTENCE OF LONG-LIVED PLASMA CELLS

Antibodies secreted by autoreactive plasma cells are a common feature of systemic and organ-specific autoimmune diseases.[10,11] They can contribute to the pathogenesis of these autoimmune diseases either directly, by classic effector mechanisms, or indirectly, through the extensive formation and deposition of immune complexes.[12,13]

Several clinical findings suggest that long-lived plasma cells may play a role in autoimmune diseases. Persistent autoantibody titers are often observed in the serum of patients with certain autoimmune diseases despite continuous treatment with immunosuppressive drugs. In a retrospective longitudinal study in patients with systemic sclerosis, stable titers of anti-topoisomerase I (Scl-70) autoantibodies persisted for up to 16 years, as was demonstrated by ELISA.[14] Scleroderma-associated autoantibodies can even be detected after autologous stem cell transplantation.[15]

Anti-Ro/SSA and anti-La/SSB autoantibody titers were monitored in patients with primary Sjögren's syndrome (SS) and systemic lupus erythematosus (SLE) for periods between 15 and 128 months. In the majority of these patients, the anti-Ro/SSA and anti-La/SSB levels did not change.[16]

In a 3-year prospective follow-up study of 42 patients with biopsy-confirmed glomerulonephritis, the prevalence of thyroid peroxidase antibodies remained unchanged in both females and males (47% and 15%, respectively), although the majority of patients had been treated with immunosuppressants. The prevalence of thyroglobulin antibodies was unaffected, as was that of antinuclear antibodies (ANA) in the group of males and females combined. Even in males, the prevalence of ANA tended to be higher at follow-up.[17] Allogeneic bone marrow transplantation in a patient with aplastic anemia also failed to prevent mild hemolysis due to the long-term production of preexisting alloantibodies to E and c.[18] Antimitochondrial antibodies, the classical serologic markers of primary biliary cirrhosis (PBC), were monitored in the sera of patients for 7 to 28 years. Despite this long follow-up, there was no evidence of a significant change in AMA levels, which also were not influenced by drug therapy during the period of observation.[19] Persistence of gastric parietal cell antibodies in gastritis and of islet-specific autoantibodies in type 1 diabetes following immunosuppression was also described.[20,21]

Autoantibodies directed against double-stranded DNA characteristically found in murine and human forms of SLE correlate with disease activity.[12,22] They can cause severe organ manifestations such as lupus nephritis and may remain stable in severe cases refractory to aggressive cyclophosphamide therapy.[23,24] In all 7 of our SLE patients treated with immunoablation and subsequent autologous stem cell transplantation, anti-dsDNA antibody levels have persisted until now in spite of monthly intravenous cyclophosphamide therapy.

Protective antibodies can also be very resistant to immunosuppression. In patients treated for autoimmune diseases or hematological disorders, persistence not only of autoantibodies, but also of some protective antibodies has been observed. Despite high-dose myeloablative treatment in conjunction with allogeneic stem cell transplantation or marrow transplantation, antibody titers for polio, tetanus, and Hemophilus influenzae did not change after transplantation.[25]

LONG-LIVED PLASMA CELLS CONTRIBUTE
TO HUMORAL AUTOIMMUNITY

To prove their existence, we analyzed the role of long-lived plasma cells in autoimmune pathology in a murine model of SLE.[26] Bromodeoxyuridine (BrdU), which is incorporated into the DNA of dividing cells, was added to the drinking water of 5-month-old NZB/W mice with anti-dsDNA autoantibodies for a period of up to 12 weeks. We then used a plasma cell marker (CD138) in order to distinguish cytometrically between proliferating (short-lived) and nonproliferating (long-lived) cells in plasma cell compartments of the spleen (FIG. 1). About 60% of all CD138+ cells became BrdU-positive within 10 days of BrdU feeding. The other 40% remained unlabeled and therefore BrdU-negative for the entire 12 weeks of BrdU feeding, indicating that these cells are long-lived, nondividing plasma cells (FIGS. 2 and 3). The

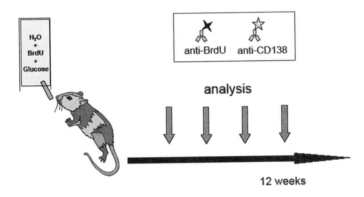

FIGURE 1. Life span analysis of plasma cells in NZB/W mice.

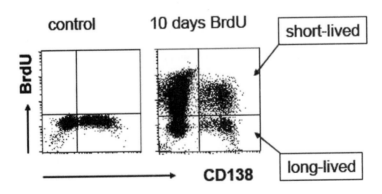

FIGURE 2. Cytometric differentiation between BrdU-positive, short-lived plasmablasts and BrdU-negative, long-lived plasma cells in plasma cell compartments of the spleen of NZB/W mice after 10 days of BrdU feeding.

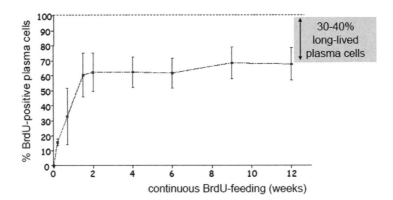

FIGURE 3. Kinetics of BrdU incorporation in splenic plasma cells from NZB/W mice as observed by FACS analysis.

total number of BrdU-negative CD138+ plasma cells did not change during these 3 months. All long-lived BrdU-negative plasma cells expressed little MHC II.

Our discovery of an unusually prominent, long-lived splenic plasma cell population in NZB/W mice made us wonder whether these cells are responsible for treatment-resistant (auto)antibody titers. In NZB/W mice treated experimentally with cyclophosphamide, the generation of short-lived plasmablasts is blocked efficiently, but long-lived plasma cells survive. This cyclophosphamide-resistant, long-lived plasma cell population contained a significant fraction of anti-DNA antibody-secreting cells, as identified by ELISPOT.

In NZB/W mice transgenic for the DNA-specific D42 antibody heavy chain, the frequencies of short-lived plasmablasts and long-lived plasma cells in the spleen were very similar to those observed in nontransgenic NZB/W mice, according to our BrdU incorporation data. After 12 weeks of BrdU feeding, the compartment of BrdU-negative, long-lived plasma cells contained about 20% of D42 transgene-bearing plasma cells. This is direct evidence that autoreactive cells are contained within the compartment of long-lived plasma cells.

In these mice, both long-lived autoreactive plasma cells and short-lived, constantly *de novo* generated plasmablasts and plasma cells contribute to autoantibody levels at a ratio of 1:3, as evidenced for dsDNA-specific antibody-secreting cells.[26]

SURVIVAL NICHES FOR LONGEVITY OF PLASMA CELLS

Whether autoantibody-secreting cells can become long-lived plasma cells may depend on the time and mode of their generation. The mechanisms by which the survival and migration of plasma cells are regulated are not completely understood. Recent findings suggest that plasma cell longevity is not (only) an intrinsic capacity, but depends on a supportive environment, that is, specific survival niches, which can be found in bone marrow, inflamed tissue and in the autoimmune spleen.[27] It has been shown that, after immunization of NZB/W mice, antigen-specific antibody-secreting cells migrate not only to the bone marrow, but in similar numbers also to the chronically inflamed kidneys.[28] Very recently, autoreactive plasma cells with specificity for glomerular antigens have been demonstrated to be markedly higher in lupus kidneys than in the spleen and peripheral blood.[29] Anti-Ro/SSA and anti-La/SSB autoantibodies are produced and are present in lymphocyte infiltrates of inflamed salivary glands from patients with SS.[30,31] These findings suggest a potential involvement of locally produced autoantibodies in organ injury.

The fact that many more plasma cells are generated during an adaptive immune response than finally survive and become long-lived suggests that only a selected fraction of plasma cells enter the pool of long-lived plasma cells. Competition of plasma cells for survival niches thus presumably controls the establishment of humoral immunity and immunopathology.[32]

It is remarkable that the spleens of NZB/W mice provide such niches for about ten times more long-lived plasma cells than those of normal mice. Factors involved in plasma cell survival include cytokines IL-5, IL-6, TNF-α, BAFF/BLys, and stromal cell–derived factor 1α (CXCL12), as well as signaling via CD44 and BCMA expression on plasma cells. Chemokines addressing the chemokine receptors, CXCR3 and CXCR4, control not only the survival of plasma cells, like CXCL12, but also their migration.[33–37]

The assumption that there is competition for survival niches is supported by the recent findings of Odendahl et al., who surprisingly detected a high number of non-tetanus-specific plasma cells with a very mature plasma cell phenotype and resembling bone marrow–derived plasma cells in addition to tetanus-specific plasmablasts in the peripheral blood at 1 week after secondary immunization with tetanus toxoid. We speculate that the enormous masses of newly formed plasma cells competed with the preexisting plasma cells for survival niches, and that some of the "older" plasma cells, identified by the low expression of MHC class II, moved from the niches to appear in the circulation.[38]

In the NZB/W model for lupus, however, long-lived plasma cells and recently generated short-lived plasmablasts apparently do not compete for plasma cell survival niches. In established diseases, the long-lived plasma cells generated early in disease are not replaced by more recently generated plasmablasts/plasma cells. Whether this reflects different intrinsic properties of early and late generated plasmablasts or separate compartments remains to be shown.

B-CELL DEPLETION WITH ANTI-CD20 ANTIBODY HAS NO IMPACT ON LONG-LIVED PLASMA CELLS

B-cell depletion using monoclonal anti-CD20 antibodies (rituximab) was recently introduced in the treatment of several autoimmune diseases such as rheumatoid arthritis and SLE.[39] Of note, this effective treatment does not result in the disappearance of autoantibodies and protective antibodies. In a phase I/II trial of rituximab in 8 SLE patients with effective B-cell depletion in the peripheral blood and elevated levels of anti-dsDNA at baseline, serum antibody titers did not change significantly after 1 year of treatment. On closer inspection, 4 patients did show a decrease in serum anti-dsDNA at 1 year posttreatment.[40] This variability contrasts with the persistence of protective antibody levels such as anti-tetanus and anti-pneumococcal

TABLE 1. Features of B cells and (auto)antibody producing cells[46-49]

	Activated B cells	Plasmablasts	Plasma cells
Proliferation	++	++	–
Surface Ig	High	Low	No
Intracellular Ig	No	High	High
Antibody secretion	No	Yes	Yes
CD138	No	High	High
CD38	No	High	High
CD20	High	No	No
CD19	High	Intermediate	Low
CD22	High	No	No
CD27	Intermediate	High	High
CD45	High	Intermediate	Low
CD95	High	High	Low
Bcl-2		Low	High
MHC class II	High	High	Low
Blimp-1	No	Intermediate	High
Migration competent	Yes	Yes	No
Response to immuno-suppression	Yes	Yes	No
Location	Secondary lymphoid organs, peripheral blood	Secondary lymphoid organs, peripheral blood, inflamed tissue	Bone marrow, secondary lymphoid organs, inflamed tissue

IgG. In this context, it should be restated that plasma cells and B cells are not the same cells with identical functions, but that plasma cells are terminally differentiated B cells. Antibodies are produced by plasmablasts and plasma cells, but not by B cells. Additionally, the development stages of B cells and plasmablasts are distinguishable by different expression of lineage, differentiation, and activation markers. Expression of CD20, the molecule targeted by rituximab, is high in B cells, but does not occur in plasmablasts and plasma cells (TABLE 1). Consequently, rituximab cannot target antibody-secreting cells, but interrupts the release of newly generated plasmablasts from memory B cells, which are depleted by the drug. Patients with active SLE were shown to have high frequencies of plasmablasts,[41] which contribute to autoantibody production[42,43] and are the product of recent B-cell activation.[38] The reduction of autoantibody levels may therefore reflect discontinuation of the generation of new antibody-secreting cells. It means further that the reduced or disappearing autoantibodies were produced by plasmablasts and short-lived plasma cells. Another possibility is that B-cell depletion may injure the survival niches of long-lived plasma cells in inflamed tissues. The possibility that some of the autoantibody-secreting cells may express CD20 also cannot be completely excluded. Thus, several findings suggest that autoantibodies and protective antibodies that persist after rituximab treatment are produced by CD20-negative, long-lived plasma cells. However, regarding autoantibody production, it is possible that precursor B cells may be incompletely depleted by rituximab, thus providing a reservoir for the continuous production of autoreactive plasma cells.[40]

Since autoantibodies may not necessarily disappear after rituximab treatment, it is important to address the question of which role autoantibodies play in the pathogenesis of autoimmune diseases. Of course, not all autoantibodies are in fact pathogenic. One could speculate that the treatment results in a preferred elimination of pathogenic autoantibodies, or that the depletion of B cells alone has an enormous impact on the inflammatory effector mechanisms. The role of autoreactive plasma cell memory in initiating relapses of disease after reconstitution of B cells seems to be an important question.

TARGETS FOR LONG-LIVED PLASMA CELLS

Since long-lived plasma cells can contribute to the development of autoimmune diseases by producing pathogenic autoantibodies, strategies for targeting these cells may provide potent new treatment modalities. In principal, there may be several ways to effectively act on long-lived plasma cell compartments. One is to target factors of plasma cell survival, such as chemokines and cytokines. BAFF/BLys is an important determining factor in the longevity of plasma cells. BAFF/BLys inhibition using soluble receptor-Ig constructs, for example, TACI-Ig or BCMA-Ig, or antibodies to BAFF/BLys may successfully suppress autoantibody production and disease in mouse models of systemic lupus.[44,45] The first clinical trials have commenced.

Immunoablation with antithymocyte globulin plus autologous stem cell transplantation (ASCT) seems to be a drastic way to impact on long-lived plasma cell compartments. On the one hand, it alters the survival niches by targeting T cells and dendritic cells and, on the other hand, it may directly eliminate B cells and plasma cells. Using this method, we have observed the complete disappearance of autoantibodies in patients with refractory SLE after ASCT. ASCT conditioning regimens, including immunoablation by antithymocyte globulin, may therefore be effective modalities for targeting the long-lived plasma cell compartment.

OUTLOOK

There is clear evidence that long-lived plasma cells that do not express CD20 can contribute to humoral autoimmunity. The rising awareness of the importance of long-lived plasma cells for the maintenance of protective and autoimmune humoral memory should stimulate our future research efforts to gain more insight into the biology and clinical relevance of long-lived plasma cells, including their appearance, migratory behavior, location, and survival mechanisms. New therapies involving B-cell depletion, immunoablation plus autologous stem cell transplantation, and the targeting of survival factors like BAFF/BLys will help us to better understand the role of plasma cell memory from the clinical perspective. The identification of novel cellular and molecular targets is a challenge that could lead to curative therapies for autoimmunity, allergies, and transplant rejection in cases where pathogenic antibodies of long-lived plasma cells play a role.

ACKNOWLEDGMENTS

The work was supported by Deutsche Forschungsgemeinschaft through Grant Nos. SFB 421 and MA 2273.

REFERENCES

1. AHMED, R. & D. GRAY. 1996. Immunological memory and protective immunity: understanding their relation. Science **272:** 54–60.
2. CALAME, K.L. 2001. Plasma cells: finding new light at the end of B cell development. Nat. Immunol. **2:** 1103–1108.
3. MANZ, R.A., A.E. HAUSER, F. HIEPE & A. RADBRUCH. 2004. Maintenance of serum antibody levels. Annu. Rev. Immunol. In press.
4. HO, F., J.E. LORTAN, I.C. MACLENNAN & M. KHAN. 1986. Distinct short-lived and long-lived antibody-producing cell populations. Eur. J. Immunol. **16:** 1297–1301.
5. SMITH, K.G., T.D. HEWITSON, G.J. NOSSAL & D.M. TARLINTON. 1996. The phenotype and fate of the antibody-forming cells of the splenic foci. Eur. J. Immunol. **26:** 444–448.
6. TALBOT, P.J. & M.J. BUCHMEIER. 1987. Catabolism of homologous murine monoclonal hybridoma IgG antibodies in mice. Immunology **60:** 485–489.
7. MANZ, R.A., A. THIEL & A. RADBRUCH. 1997. Lifetime of plasma cells in the bone marrow. Nature **388:** 133–134.
8. MANZ, R.A., M. LOHNING, G. CASSESE *et al.* 1998. Survival of long-lived plasma cells is independent of antigen. Int. Immunol. **10:** 1703–1711.
9. SLIFKA, M.K., R. ANTIA, J.K. WHITMIRE & R. AHMED. 1998. Humoral immunity due to long-lived plasma cells. Immunity **8:** 363–372.
10. DAVIDSON, A. & B. DIAMOND. 2001. Autoimmune diseases. N. Engl. J. Med. **345:** 340–350.
11. TAN, E.M. 1991. Autoantibodies in pathology and cell biology. Cell **67:** 841–842.
12. HAHN, B.H. 1998. Antibodies to DNA. N. Engl. J. Med. **338:** 1359–1368.
13. MARTIN, F. & A.C. CHAN. 2004. Pathogenic roles of B cells in human autoimmunity; insights from the clinic. Immunity **20:** 517–527.
14. HILDEBRANDT, S., G. JACKH, S. WEBER & H.H. PETER. 1993. A long-term longitudinal isotypic study of anti-topoisomerase I autoantibodies. Rheumatol. Int. **12:** 231–234.
15. MCSWEENEY, P.A., R.A. NASH, K.M. SULLIVAN *et al.* 2002. High-dose immunosuppressive therapy for severe systemic sclerosis: initial outcomes. Blood **100:** 1602–1610.
16. WAHREN, M., P. TENGNER, I. GUNNARSSON *et al.* 1998. Ro/SS-A and La/SS-B antibody level variation in patients with Sjogren's syndrome and systemic lupus erythematosus. J. Autoimmun. **11:** 29–38.
17. WESTMAN, K.W., P.G. BYGREN, U.B. ERICSSON *et al.* 1998. Persistent high prevalence of thyroid antibodies after immunosuppressive therapy in subjects with glomerulonephritis: a prospective three-year follow-up study. Am. J. Nephrol. **18:** 274–279.
18. IZUMI, N., I. FUSE, T. FURUKAWA *et al.* 2003. Long-term production of pre-existing alloantibodies to E and c after allogenic BMT in a patient with aplastic anemia resulting in delayed hemolytic anemia. Transfusion **43:** 241–245.
19. BENSON, G.D., K. KIKUCHI, H. MIYAKAWA *et al.* 2004. Serial analysis of antimitochondrial antibody in patients with primary biliary cirrhosis. Clin. Dev. Immunol. **11:** 129–133.
20. DE BLOCK, C.E., I.H. DE LEEUW, R.P. ROOMAN *et al.* 2000. Gastric parietal cell antibodies are associated with glutamic acid decarboxylase-65 antibodies and the HLA DQA1*0501-DQB1*0301 haplotype in type 1 diabetes mellitus: Belgian Diabetes Registry. Diabet. Med. **17:** 618–622.

21. DECOCHEZ, K., J. TITS, J.L. COOLENS *et al.* 2000. High frequency of persisting or increasing islet-specific autoantibody levels after diagnosis of type 1 diabetes presenting before 40 years of age: the Belgian Diabetes Registry. Diabet. Care **23:** 838–844.

22. BRUNS, A., S. BLÄSS, G. HAUSDORF *et al.* 2000. Nucleosomes are major T and B cell autoantigens in systemic lupus erythematosus. Arthritis Rheum. **43:** 2307–2315.

23. ROSEN, O., A. THIEL, G. MASSENKEIL *et al.* 2000. Autologous stem-cell transplantation in refractory autoimmune diseases after *in vivo* immunoablation and *ex vivo* depletion of mononuclear cells. Arthritis Res. **2:** 327–336.

24. TRAYNOR, A.E., J. SCHROEDER, R.M. ROSA *et al.* 2000. Treatment of severe systemic lupus erythematosus with high-dose chemotherapy and haemopoietic stem-cell transplantation: a phase I study. Lancet **356:** 701–707.

25. STOREK, J., F. VIGANEGO, M.A. DAWSON *et al.* 2003. Factors affecting antibody levels after allogeneic hematopoietic cell transplantation. Blood **101:** 3319–3324.

26. HOYER, B.F., K. MOSER, A.E. HAUSER *et al.* 2004. Short-lived plasmablasts and long-lived plasma cells contribute to chronic humoral autoimmunity in NZB/W mice. J. Exp. Med. **199:** 1577–1584.

27. MANZ, R.A., S. ARCE, G. CASSESE *et al.* 2002. Humoral immunity and long-lived plasma cells. Curr. Opin. Immunol. **14:** 517–521.

28. CASSESE, G., S. LINDENAU, B. DE BOER *et al.* 2001. Inflamed kidneys of NZB/W mice are a major site for the homeostasis of plasma cells. Eur. J. Immunol. **31:** 2726–2732.

29. SEKINE, H., H. WATANABE & G.S. GILKESON. 2004. Enrichment of anti-glomerular antigen antibody-producing cells in the kidneys of MRL/MpJ-Fas(lpr) mice. J. Immunol. **172:** 3913–3921.

30. SALOMONSSON, S., M.V. JONSSON, K. SKARSTEIN *et al.* 2003. Cellular basis of ectopic germinal center formation and autoantibody production in the target organ of patients with Sjögren's syndrome. Arthritis Rheum. **48:** 3187–3201.

31. TENGNER, P., A.K. HALSE, H.J. HAGA *et al.* 1998. Detection of anti-Ro/SSA and anti-La/SSB autoantibody-producing cells in salivary glands from patients with Sjögren's syndrome. Arthritis Rheum. **41:** 2238–2248.

32. MANZ, R.A., S. ARCE, G. CASSESE *et al.* 2002. Humoral immunity and long-lived plasma cells. Curr. Opin. Immunol. **14:** 517–521.

33. CASSESE, G., S. ARCE, A.E. HAUSER *et al.* 2003. Plasma cell survival is mediated by synergistic effects of cytokines and adhesion-dependent signals. J. Immunol. **171:** 1684–1690.

34. HAUSER, A.E., G.F. DEBES, S. ARCE *et al.* 2002. Chemotactic responsiveness toward ligands for CXCR3 and CXCR4 is regulated on plasmablasts during the time course of a memory immune response. J. Immunol. **169:** 1277–1282.

35. MINGES WOLS, H.A., G.H. UNDERHILL, G.S. KANSAS & P.L. WITTE. 2002. The role of bone marrow–derived stromal cells in the maintenance of plasma cell longevity. J. Immunol. **169:** 4213–4221.

36. MUEHLINGHAUS, G., L. CIGLIANO, S. HUEHN *et al.* 2005. Regulation of CXCR3 and CXCR4 expression during terminal differentiation of memory B cells into plasma cells. Blood. In press.

37. O'CONNOR, B.P., V.S. RAMAN, L.D. ERICKSON *et al.* 2004. BCMA is essential for the survival of long-lived bone marrow plasma cells. J. Exp. Med. **199:** 91–98.

38. ODENDAHL, M., H. MEI, B.F. HOYER *et al.* 2005. Generation of migratory antigen-specific plasmablasts and mobilization of resident plasma cells in a secondary immune response. Blood **105:** 1614–1621.

39. SILVERMAN, G.J. & S. WEISMAN. 2003. Rituximab therapy and autoimmune disorders: prospects for anti-B cell therapy. Arthritis Rheum. **48:** 1484–1492.

40. ANOLIK, J.H., J. BARNARD, A. CAPPIONE *et al.* 2004. Rituximab improves peripheral B cell abnormalities in human systemic lupus erythematosus. Arthritis Rheum. **50:** 3580–3590.

41. ODENDAHL, M., A. JACOBI, A. HANSEN *et al.* 2000. Disturbed peripheral B lymphocyte homeostasis in systemic lupus erythematosus. J. Immunol. **165:** 5970–5979.

42. JACOBI, A.M., M. ODENDAHL, K. REITER *et al.* 2003. Correlation between circulating CD27high plasma cells and disease activity in patients with systemic lupus erythematosus. Arthritis Rheum. **48:** 1332–1342.

43. ODENDAHL, M., R. KEITZER, U. WAHN *et al.* 2003. Perturbations of peripheral B lymphocyte homeostasis in children with systemic lupus erythematosus. Ann. Rheum. Dis. **62:** 851–858.
44. MACKAY, F. & S.G. TANGYE. 2004. The role of the BAFF/APRIL system in B cell homeostasis and lymphoid cancers. Curr. Opin. Pharmacol. **4:** 347–354.
45. MELCHERS, F. 2003. Actions of BAFF in B cell maturation and its effects on the development of autoimmune disease. Ann. Rheum. Dis. **62**(suppl. 2): ii25–ii27.
46. ARCE, S., E. LUGER, G. MUEHLINGHAUS *et al.* 2004. CD38 low IgG-secreting cells are precursors of various CD38 high–expressing plasma cell populations. J. Leukocyte Biol. **75:** 1022–1028.
47. KALLIES, A., J. HASBOLD, D.M. TARLINTON *et al.* 2004. Plasma cell ontogeny defined by quantitative changes in blimp-1 expression. J. Exp. Med. **200:** 967–977.
48. MCHEYZER-WILLIAMS, L.J. & M. MCHEYZER-WILLIAMS. 2004. Antigen-specific memory B cell development. Annu. Rev. Immunol. In press.
49. MEDINA, F., C. SEGUNDO, A. CAMPOS-CARO *et al.* 2002. The heterogeneity shown by human plasma cells from tonsil, blood, and bone marrow reveals graded stages of increasing maturity, but local profiles of adhesion molecule expression. Blood **99:** 2154–2161.

What Makes an Autoantigen an Autoantigen?

CHIH-TE WU, M. ERIC GERSHWIN, AND PAUL A. DAVIS

Division of Rheumatology, Allergy, and Clinical Immunology, Department of Internal Medicine, School of Medicine, University of California, Davis, California 95616, USA

ABSTRACT: Multiple classes of proteins are modified to tailor them for specific physiological roles. The nature of these posttranslational modifications of proteins, as well as the relationships between them including those of the immune system proteins themselves, and immune system responses are reviewed. Aspects of protein posttranslational modification and their relationship to the pathogenesis of several autoimmune diseases and primary biliary cirrhosis are highlighted.

KEYWORDS: posttranslational modification; protein function; immune system; autoimmunity; primary biliary cirrhosis; antigens

INTRODUCTION

In eukaryotic cells, protein synthesis is regulated by multiple mechanisms. First, specific genes are selected for transcription typically by the interaction of initiation complexes, which then assemble the necessary machinery to produce the RNA. The RNA then undergoes a process of modification, called maturation, which enables it to become a functional mRNA and then is translocated to the cytoplasm. The export of mRNA requires that newly synthesized precursor mRNAs undergo several processing steps, which include 5'-end capping, splicing, 3'-end cleavage, and polyadenylation. The formation of an export competent mRNP complex involves complex series of rearrangements of protein–protein and protein–RNA interactions, removal of the nuclear retention factors, and addition of signals necessary for the interaction with the nuclear export machinery. Once in the cytosol, the mRNA then can be translated into proteins, albeit only with the active assistance of a host of cytoplasmic factors. Translation initiation has been divided into three steps: first, binding of the specific initiator Met–tRNA (iMet) to the small ribosomal subunit; second, binding of the resulting complex to the mRNA and locating the initiation codon; and third, joining of the large ribosomal subunit to generate a translation-competent ribosome. All three steps are facilitated by soluble proteins termed translation initiation factors. However, protein synthesis does not end when the ribosomally bound product is released there. Many newly synthesized proteins go through additional modifications to become fully functional. For example, some enzymes require the addition of phos-

Address for correspondence: Paul A. Davis, Division of Rheumatology, Allergy, and Clinical Immunology, Department of Internal Medicine, GBSF Suite 6510, 451 E. Health Sciences Drive, University of California, Davis, CA 95616. Voice: 530-754-7852.

padavis@ucdavis.edu

Ann. N.Y. Acad. Sci. 1050: 134–145 (2005). © 2005 New York Academy of Sciences.
doi: 10.1196/annals.1313.015

phate groups (phosphorylation) to become active. Posttranslational modification of proteins not only "fine-tunes" the newly synthesized protein, but is also involved in many pathological conditions. Furthermore, posttranslational modification provides the cells with a rapid responding mechanism to cope with the constantly changing environment. Through the addition or deletion of a specific group, individual protein acquires different functional characteristics, which will enable it to react with other downstream molecules to get an appropriate response. In this review, we focus on the various ways that proteins can be modified as well as physiological and pathological consequences. We will also discuss the relationship between posttranslational modification of proteins and the immune system. Finally, we will discuss the role played by posttranslational modification toward the pathogenesis of several autoimmune diseases and primary biliary cirrhosis specifically.

POSTTRANSLATIONAL MODIFICATION OF STRUCTURAL PROTEINS

Structural proteins, the building blocks of various cellular organelles, represent the majority of the newly synthesized proteins. For example, the structural protein tubulin is involved in diverse processes such as cell motility, cell division, and metastasis in cancerous cells. After its synthesis, tubulin undergoes several modifications to regulate its assembly and function. In many eukaryotes, a conserved carboxyl-terminal tyrosine of tubulin is removed posttranslationally. However, this modification is reversible through the action of tubulin tyrosine ligase (TTL). The balance between tyrosination/detyrosination is regulated by TTL and carboxypeptidase,[1] which is thought to serve as a control point for the activity of microtubules.[2] TTL catalyzes the addition of tyrosine residue to the carboxyl terminus of the α-tubulin. Kato *et al.* analyzed the TTL mRNA expression in 74 primary neuroblastomas by quantitative real-time RT-PCR. They found that high expression of TTL was associated with low-stage disease as well as favorable prognosis.[3] TTL expression was also induced by the addition of bone morphogenetic protein 2 (BMP2) or all-*trans*-retinoic acid during neuronal differentiation. This means that during neuronal differentiation TTL expression is increased. In conclusion, decreased TTL expression will render the neuroblastoma in a more undifferentiated stage and indicate a poor prognosis. These results suggest that tubulin tyrosination through TTL is important in neuronal differentiation and metastasis of neuroblastoma, implying that by manipulating TTL expression, the neuroblastoma attains the ability to metastasize to distant sites and becomes more resistant to immunological attack.

High mobility group (HMG) proteins are nonhistone DNA binding proteins which are important in the regulation of chromatin structures. HMG has also been implicated in cancer cell metastasis potential.[4] Edberg *et al.* analyzed three human breast cancer cell lines with different metastasis potential. Using MALDI-TOF mass spectrometry, they identified dimethylation on specific arginine and lysine residues of HMG in metastatic cancer cells but not in nonmetastatic cell lines.[5] The HMG proteins from metastatic cell lines were also more acetylated than that from nonmetastatic cells. This suggests that posttranslational modification of HMG protein by methylation and/or acetylation can alter cell behavior, for example, metastatic potential or helping the malignant cells to evade immune surveillance.

In the Gram-negative bacteria *Nisseria gonorrhoeae* and *Nisseria meningitides*, protein filaments called type IV pili (Tfp) are important for attachment to host cells. Tfp is shown to react with a monoclonal antibody which recognizes a phosphocholine epitope.[6] Further evidence of posttranslational modification of Tfp comes from the study by Hegge and colleagues.[7] They were able to show that the mobility of the Tfp subunit in SDS-PAGE is decreased when it is not associated with phosphocholine.[7] Using mass spectrometry, they identified another posttranslational modification of Tfp by phosphoethanolamine. It is possible that through different modification of the Tfp (phosphocholine vs. phosphoethanolamine) the antigenicity of *Nisseriae* is changed, which will help the bacteria evade the detection by the host immune system.

Similarly, the lytic-phase protein gp42 of Epstein-Barr virus (EBV) can also undergo posttranslational modification. gp42 is shown to be able to bind to class II MHC molecules and hinder the interaction of class II MHC molecules with T cell receptor (TCR). gp42 occurs in two forms: a full-length transmembranous form and a truncated soluble form. During EBV lytic infection, the soluble form of gp42 is generated by proteolytic cleavage of the full-length, transmembrane form at the endoplasmic reticulum and is released. It is possible that the soluble form of gp42 plays an important role in the undetected spreading of EBV by hampering the interaction of class II MHC molecule with the TCR.[8]

In neurodegenerative diseases such as Alzheimer's disease, pathological protein inclusion bodies within the neurons can be found in the lesion. One of the most prominent proteins is the tau protein.[9] Tau is a microtubule-binding protein which is important for microtubule assembly and stability. It has been shown that hyperphosphorylation of tau has a negative effect on its ability to bind to microtubules.[10] This will result in an increase in the cytoplasm of unbound tau proteins, which eventually leads to the formation of inclusion body. Similarly, it has been demonstrated that the neural cell adhesion molecule (N-CAM) undergoes posttranslational modification with the addition of two sialic acids on α-2 and -8 positions.[11] Enzymatic cleavage of these sialic acids had an adverse effect in learning associated with altered cell adhesion.[12]

On the other hand, posttranslational modification is also an integral part of normal physiological processes. For example, α-melanocyte stimulating hormone (α-MSH) is secreted by the hypothalamus. Its receptor, the melanocortin 4 receptor (MC4R), is also located within the hypothalamus. Binding of α-MSH to MC4R will activate downstream regulators such as leptin and regulate energy balance.[13] It has been found that leptin can stimulate the formation of *N*-acetyl-α-MSH through the activation of α-MSH *N*-acetyltransferase in the hypothalamus.[14] The *N*-acetylated α-MSH is more potent than α-MSH in reducing food intake. This suggests that leptin exerts a negative effect in food intake via posttranslational modification of α-MSH.

In conclusion, proteins undergo a multiplicity of different types as well as extent of posttranslational modifications. Posttranslational modification plays an important part in the regulation of normal, physiological processes. TABLE 1 summarizes the posttranslational modifications discussed in this article. Alongside normal functions, pathogenic microorganisms and cancer cells utilize posttranslational modification in an effort to avoid either the detection or attack of the host immune system. Through these alterations, pathogenic microorganisms and cancer cells can rapidly take or terminate normal cell functions by modifying the proteins already present so as to

TABLE 1. Examples of posttranslational modification of structural proteins and their effects

Example	Modification	Effects
α-Tubulin	Tyrosylation/detyrosylation	Clinical stage and prognosis of neuroblastoma
High mobility group (HMG) protein	Methylation Acetylation	High metastasis potential
Type IV pili (Tfp)	Phosphocholination Phosphoethanolamination	Change in antigenicity
α-Melanocyte stimulating hormone	N-Acetylation	Reducing food intake
Tau	Phosphorylation	Inability to bind to microtubules Formation of inclusion body
Neural cell adhesion molecule (N-CAM)	Sialation	Proper neural cell adhesion

benefit these pathological entities. Some modifications can confer decreased differentiation and increased metastatic potential, others may alter antigenicity to evade host immune system, and still others may be associated with specific pathological conditions.

POSTTRANSLATIONAL MODIFICATION OF ENZYMES AND OTHER REGULATOR PROTEINS

Many enzymes are synthesized and secreted in an inactive form, that is, zymogens. Before becoming the active enzymes, the zymogens must first be processed and cleaved to release the inhibitory sections. For example, chymotrypsinogen, the precursor of the digestive enzyme trypsin synthesized and secreted from the pancreas, is totally devoid of enzymatic activity. Chymotrypsinogen must be cleaved to release the active form of the enzyme, the α-trypsin.[15] Similarly, in the human complement system, the precursor zymogens (C1s and C3b) are synthesized and secreted. At the site of inflammation or infection, these zymogens are cleaved to generate an active serine protease, leading to a cascade of cleavage and activation of downstream complement components.

Cleavage is not the sole means of activating enzyme precursor. The enzyme phospholipase C-γ (PLC-γ) is a crucial component in the signal transduction pathway. It cleaves the membrane lipid phosphatidylinositol bisphosphate (PIP$_2$) into inositol triphosphate (IP$_3$) and diacylglycerol (DAG). IP$_3$ and DAG, in turn, activate and recruit downstream intracellular molecules to transfer the signal from the cell membrane surface into the cell. For all these downstream events to happen, PLC-γ must first be phosphorylated on a tyrosine residue to become active.

Matrix metalloproteinases (MMPs) are a class of enzymes having cleavage activities against many matrix proteins including collagen. Membrane type 1 MMP (MT1-MMP) is found to undergo posttranslational modification by O-glycosylation.[16]

Glycosylation is able to regulate the substrate targeting of MT1-MMP. For example, pro-matrix metalloproteinase-2 (proMMP-2) is normally a substrate of MT1-MMP. However, without glycosylation, MT1-MMP is unable to activate proMMP-2 because of the failure of MT1-MMP to bind proMMP-2 to form an active complex.

The mitochondrial respiratory chain enzyme, cytochrome c, also is susceptible to posttranslational modification. For example, Nakagawa et al. found that treatment of cytochrome c with peroxynitrite resulted in mononitration at the tyrosine residue. Even though the tyrosine nitrated cytochrome c had similar redox capacity to its unnitrated counterparts, it does appear more susceptible to oxidation reaction by hydrogen peroxide. Furthermore, this nitrated cytochrome c also lost the ability to transfer electrons in the mitochondrial respiratory chain. Similarly, glutathione-S-transferase (GST) which is present in the liver is responsible for the detoxification of harmful electrophiles before their excretion. Treatment of GST with either peroxynitrite or tetranitromethane inhibited the activity of GST.[17] This inhibition was only partially reversible. Using HPLC, modification as increased level of nitrotyrosine was found. This suggests that modification with peroxynitrite or other oxidative stress has the potential to deprive the cell of its energy supply and, as a result, more susceptible to death or apoptosis. Additionally, some posttranslational modifications such as tyrosine nitration may not be reversible. Giulivi and coworkers have speculated that mitochondrial nitration of proteins in the liver is used to ensure adequate oxygen supply to those cells at the periphery of the liver by preventing the liver cells closest to oxygen delivery from monopolizing it through uptake and utilization.[18]

In summary, most of the enzymes need to be activated first before they acquire their catalytic activity. Posttranslational modification provides one mechanism, which is fast, effective, and easily controlled to achieve this goal. However, posttranslational modification also can interfere with or inhibit the activity of enzymes as illustrated in the case of tyrosine nitration of cytochrome c. Thus, it is of interest to understand these processes given that mitochondria are the energy source, and it is clear that mitochondrial energy production affects cell function with respect to whether the cell will die (either apoptosis or necrosis). This, in turn, is likely to have a profound effect on organ function, the immune system, and other cellular processes.

Other regulatory proteins also undergo posttranslational modification. For example, the nuclear protein Ki-67 is present in all proliferating cells in their active cell cycles (G1, S, G2, and M), but not in cells in resting cycle (G0).[19] Further analysis indicated that the temporal pattern of Ki-67 activity is associated with posttranslational modification. In resting cells, Ki-67 is phosphorylated and redistributed from the interior of the nucleus to the periphery of the condensed chromosomes.[20] On the other hand, dephosphorylation of Ki-67 readily enabled the cells to enter active cell cycle.

In eukaryotic cells, posttranslational modification of proteins with fatty acids is very common. Several different reactions have been found that are catalyzed by different enzymes. Among them, N-myristoylation, S-palmitoylation, N-palmitoylation, and fatty acylation are most important and have been studied.[21] One of the functions of fatty acid modification is that it promotes membrane association of otherwise soluble proteins. Palmitoylation also targets the protein to lipid rafts, a region on the plasma membrane that is rich in sphingolipids and cholesterol.[22] It has been shown that localization of signal proteins in lipid rafts is important for transduction of the signal into the cell. In T cells, non-receptor tyrosine kinase (NRTK) is S-acylated on Cys3 and Cys5 in addition to myristoylation on Gly2. Mutation of S-acylation sites

TABLE 2. Examples of posttranslational modification of enzymes/regulatory proteins and their effects

Example	Modification	Effects
Chymotrypsinogen	Cleavage	Activation
Complement C1s and C3b	Cleavage	Activation
Phospholipase C-γ	Phosphorylation	Activation
Matrix metalloproteinase	*O*-Glycosylation	Change of substrate profile
Cytochrome *c*	Nitration	Susceptibility to oxidation Inability to transfer electrons
Glutathione-S-transferase	Nitration	Inactivation
Nuclear protein Ki-67	Phosphorylation	Regulation of cell cycle
Rab	Prenylation	Association with membranes and effector proteins

rendered NRTK unable to target to the cell membrane and phosphorylate CD8-ζ chain, which, in turn, resulted in decreased T cell response upon antigen exposure.[23]

Rab proteins, which belong to the Ras DTPase superfamily, also have been found to undergo posttranslational modification with lipid moieties. The main function of the Rab proteins involves membrane trafficking and secretory pathways. Two cysteine-containing motifs are located at the carboxyl terminus of the Rab proteins, which are conjugated to different lipid moieties.[24] It has been found that Rab needs to be posttranslationally modified at these two cysteine residues with geranyl-geranyl moieties to be functionally active and be able to associate with membranes stably. Switching the two geranyl-geranyl moieties with other lipid moieties, such as one farnesyl group or one geranyl-geranyl group, results in nonfunctional Rab.[25] Furthermore, Yip1p, one of the effector proteins of Rab, loses its ability to interact with these mutant Rabs. This suggests that the addition of the lipid moieties is specific and functionally important.

In conclusion, posttranslational modification of enzymes and regulatory proteins through their effects on diverse downstream events such as activation/inactivation of catalytic activity, change of substrate spectrum, and regulation of cell cycles is integral to normal cell function (see TABLE 2).

POSTTRANSLATIONAL MODIFICATION AND THE IMMUNE SYSTEM

The immune system also utilizes posttranslational modification to control its function. Essentially, all immunoglobulins (Ig) contain carbohydrates attached to various sites. For example, *N*-linked carbohydrates are attached to the CH_2 region of the IgG molecule.[26] The absence of carbohydrate in the CH_2 region of IgG produces decreased complement activation, decreased half-life, and impaired binding to the Fcγ receptor.[27] IgA is the main class of immunoglobulins present on the mucosal surface. IgA is synthesized as a monomer, which will be assembled into dimer through the action of J chain. The dimerized IgA then binds to the poly-Ig receptor to be transported across the epithelial cell and secreted into the mucosal surface. An enzymatic cleavage frees the dimeric IgA which is still attached to part of the poly-Ig receptor (now called secretory piece).[28] Through the addition of J chain, two IgA molecules can be dimerized and bound to poly-Ig receptor. The addition of secretory piece confers resistance of the IgA to enzymatic digestion and inactivation on the mucosal surface.

Posttranslational modification of TCRs has also been documented. For example, different glycosyl groups on the TCR are associated with different development stages.[29] Peanut agglutinin can bind to Gal β(1→3) N-acetylgalactosamine (GalNAc) moiety, but loses the ability when this glycan moiety is sialated. Using peanut agglutinin as a probe, Reisner and colleagues[29] found that as double-positive immature T cells differentiate into single-positive mature T cells they also lose the ability to bind peanut agglutinin.

Posttranslational modification can also be found in human IL-2. Different glycosylation patterns at threonine residues have been identified using mass spectrometry.[30] However, despite this heterogeneous population of IL-2, all of the IL-2 is functional active. IL-6 also undergoes similar N-glycosylation, O-glycosylation, and phosphorylation, although no functional difference has been found.[31] The significance of the existence of diverse, functionally active cytokines may be multifactorial. First, it represents the redundancy of a specific cytokine. With the presence of multiple modification pathways, inhibition of one specific pathway will not stop the synthesis of other functionally active products. Second, cytokines are pleiotropic. Cytokine is able to interact with different cell types through the addition of various organic and inorganic compounds at different locations. It is likely more efficient and faster than making a brand new one.

Recently, it has been found that the antigenic peptides can undergo modifications before they are presented to the CD8+ T cells.[32,33] Typically antigens are degraded by proteases to smaller peptides, and these then are presented to the immune system. However, recently, an additional pathway, called peptide splicing, has been elucidated wherein specific proteasomes cleave some internal amino acids residues from a polypeptide and then reunite the newly formed amino-terminal and carboxyl-terminal residues.[32,33] The level of this activity and its implication in normal physiology conditions or pathological conditions remains unclear. Theoretically, this form of peptide splicing enables the immune system to generate a far more diverse array of antigenic peptides from a given protein molecule. However, if peptide splicing were to occur after T cell maturation within the thymus, then the neoantigen so produced might result in the generation of potential autoreactive T cells.

In T helper cells, T cell receptor signaling has been found to increase the expression of the enzyme arginine methyltransferase (PRMT). PRMT methylates the arginine residues located on the amino terminus of NIP45, the cofactor protein of the nuclear factor of activated T cells (NFAT).[34] The net result is increased cytokine production including IFN-γ and IL-4. Treatment of T helper cells with methyltransferase inhibitor 5′-methylthioadenosine impairs the ability of the T cells to produce cytokine. Thus, arginine methylation provides a rapid means for the T cells to react to external stimuli via cytokine production, thereby ensuring a timely response.

TABLE 3 summarizes some posttranslational modification occurring in the immune system.

TABLE 3. Examples of posttranslational modification of immune system components and their effects

Example	Modification	Effect
IgG	N-Glycosylation	Increase in complement activation Increase in half-life
IgA	Dimerization Addition of secretory piece	Secretion into mucosal surface Increase in half-life
T cell receptor	Sialation	T cell maturation
NIP45	Methylation	Binding to NFAT Increase in IFN-γ and IL-4 expression
IL-2	Glycosylation	Possible redundancy and pleiotropy
IL-6	Glycosylation	Possible redundancy and pleiotropy
Nonreceptor tyrosine kinase (NRTK)	S-Acylation Myristoylation	Decrease/loss in signal transduction Association with membranes

POSTTRANSLATIONAL MODIFICATION AND AUTOIMMUNITY

It has long been hypothesized that posttranslationally modified self-protein could act as a means to induce autoimmunity. After the modified self-protein is taken up, digested, and processed in antigen-presenting cells, potentially self-reactive T and B cells can recognize it, resulting in the breaking of tolerance and induction of autoimmunity. One explanation for the mechanism of loss of tolerance is that because the posttranslational modification happens after the negative selection processes during lymphocyte maturation, T cells and B cells exist that are able to recognize modified self-proteins. Through a process called epitope spreading, the immune response will be spread to unmodified self-protein and autoimmunity will take place and be maintained through the continuous supply of unmodified self-protein.

In support of this view, it has been demonstrated that posttranslational modifications do play an important role in autoimmunity. One example is illustrated in the case of rheumatoid arthritis. Both the antiperinuclear factor (APF) and anti-keratin antibodies (AKAs) are specific for the diagnosis of rheumatoid arthritis.[35] On immunohistochemistry, APF labels the keratohyalin granules of human buccal mucosa epithelium, whereas AKA labels the stratum corneum of various cornified epithelia. However, on Western blot, both of these antibodies targeted the epithelial protein filaggrin (**fil**ament **aggr**egating prote**in**). Filaggrins are posttranslationally modified by the enzyme peptidylarginine deiminase (PAD) which deiminates arginine to form citrulline.[36] *In vitro* deimination of a recombinant human filaggrin by PAD generated antifilaggrin autoantibody (AFA) epitopes on the protein. Further analysis showed that a citrulline was present in these epitopes, suggesting that citrulline is important in the recognition of filaggrin by AKA and APF.[37]

In another study by Myers *et al.*, they produced recombinant type II collagen (rCII) via a yeast expression system (rCII[pic]) or a baculovirus expression system (rCII[bac]).[38] Further analysis of rCII[pic], rCII[bac], and tissue-derived CII revealed that rCII[pic] is adequately hydroxylated at proline residues but unhydroxylated at lysine residues and has no glycosylation compared with tissue-derived CII. On the other hand, rCII[bac] also is adequately hydroxylated at proline residues but is underhydroxylated at lysine residues and underglycosylated compared with tissue-derived CII. When injected intradermally into DBA/1 mice, rCII^{pic} induced a lower incidence of arthritis than tissue-derived CII, whereas rCII^{bac} induced an intermediate level of arthritis. The induced arthritis is most severe in tissue-derived CII, followed by rCII^{bac}. It was least severe in mice immunized with rCII^{pic}. Similarly, T cell response as evaluated by T cell proliferative response and cytokine production also correlated with the degree of glycosylation (CII gives the strongest response and rCII^{pic} the lowest one). These results showed that posttranslational modification such as glycosylation is important in the arthrogenicity of type II collagen in collagen-induced arthritis.

Posttranslational modification of type II collagen also is important in the induction of self-tolerance. When the hydroxylated CII is expressed systematically, T cells are tolerant to the hydroxylated CII epitope.[39] To determine the mechanism of T cell tolerance, Yamada et al. measured the number of T cells expressing the specific hydroxylated CII epitope. Using FACS analysis, it was found that the number of specific T cells is significantly decreased, indicating that central deletion may be responsible for the establishment of T cell tolerance. On the other hand, when the expression of hydroxylated CII epitope is restricted to the cartilage, there was no sign of T cell tolerance, suggesting that the distribution of hydroxylated CII also played a role in the induction of T cell tolerance.

When B10.A mice are immunized with isoaspartate-modified cytochrome c peptide, strong B and T cell responses can be elicited. However, when native cytochrome c peptide containing aspartate residues is used, no such response is observed.[40] This indicates that antigenicity of the modified self-protein is dependent on what is conjugated to the protein as well as how it is done. Furthermore, these antibodies generated are cross-reactive to the naive cytochrome c molecule. Similarly, immunization of mice with an isoaspartate-modified autoantigen of human SLE results in strong B and T cell responses as well. Thus, posttranslationally modified proteins could serve as an immunological stimulus in the development of autoimmune disease.

However, note that a recent study also showed that T cell receptor recognition has limited plasticity when the amino acid residues of the contact region in the class II MHC bound epitope gpMBP72-85 are modified.[41] Different types of modification were applied to the amino acid residues within gpMBP72–85. These include glycosylation and replacing arginine residues with either citrulline or ornithine residues. It turned out that T cells specific for wild-type epitope did not recognize the modified peptides. Furthermore, T cell receptors that are specific for modified peptides did not recognize the wild-type epitope. It seems that the T cell receptor can discriminate between minute differences in amino acid resides within the epitope. How specific or degenerate a T cell receptor can be is still unclear, and further studies should be directed toward this question.

POSTTRANSLATIONAL MODIFICATION AND PRIMARY BILIARY CIRRHOSIS

In primary biliary cirrhosis, the immunodominant epitopes of the autoantigen E2 subunit of the pyruvate dehydrogenase complex (PDC-E2) contain posttranslational modified lipoic acids.[42] Further study showed that the lipoic acid was important for autoantibody recognition because unlipoated PDC-E2 did not bind effectively.[43] Further evidence for the importance of lipoic acid in the development of autoantibody in primary biliary cirrhosis comes from a study by Long *et al.*[44] in which they tested various halogenated organic compounds synthesized to mimic lipoic acid structurally. When these were tested with sera from primary biliary cirrhosis patients, several compounds reacted significantly better than the autoantigen PDC-E2 itself.[44] Upon injection into rabbits, these halogenated compounds were able to induce an antimitochondrial antibody response.[45] This suggests that lipoic acid is important for the induction of antimitochondrial antibody and that compounds mimic lipoic acid is able to break self-tolerance *in vivo*.

CONCLUSIONS

Posttranslational modification is crucial for the activity and regulation of proteins. Various pathways and enzymes are responsible for the modification. It represents a supplementary control mechanism of protein expression in addition to transcription and translation. As discussed above, posttranslational modification exists in structural protein, catalytic protein, as well as regulatory proteins in the cell cycle machinery and immune system. Further study is mandatory to explore this field of research to be able to have a fundamental understanding of physiological and pathological processes.

REFERENCES

1. BARRA, H.S., C.A. ARCE & C.E. ARGARANA. 1988. Posttranslational tyrosination/detyrosination of tubulin. Mol. Neurobiol. **2:** 133–153.
2. WESTERMANN, S. & K. WEBER. 2003. Post-translational modifications regulate microtubule function. Nat. Rev. Mol. Cell Biol. **4:** 938–947.
3. KATO, C., K. MIYAZAKI, A. NAKAGAWA, *et al.* 2004. Low expression of human tubulin tyrosine ligase and suppressed tubulin tyrosination/detyrosination cycle are associated with impaired neuronal differentiation in neuroblastomas with poor prognosis. Int. J. Cancer **112:** 365–375.
4. RAM, T.G., R. REEVES & H.L. HOSICK. 1993. Elevated high mobility group-I(Y) gene expression is associated with progressive transformation of mouse mammary epithelial cells. Cancer Res. **53:** 2655–2660.
5. EDBERG, D.D., J.E. BRUCE, W.F. SIEMS & R. REEVES. 2004. *In vivo* posttranslational modifications of the high mobility group A1a proteins in breast cancer cells of differing metastatic potential. Biochemistry **43:** 11500–11515.
6. WEISER, J.N., J.B. GOLDBERG, N. PAN, *et al.* 1998. The phosphorylcholine epitope undergoes phase variation on a 43-kilodalton protein in *Pseudomonas aeruginosa* and on pili of *Neisseria meningitidis* and *Neisseria gonorrhoeae*. Infect. Immunol. **66:** 4263–4267.
7. HEGGE, F.T., P.G. HITCHEN, F.E. AAS, *et al.* 2004. Unique modifications with phosphocholine and phosphoethanolamine define alternate antigenic forms of *Neisseria gonorrhoeae* type IV pili. Proc. Natl. Acad. Sci. USA **101:** 10798–10803.
8. RESSING, M.E., D. VAN LEEUWEN, F.A. VERRECK, *et al.* 2005. Epstein-Barr virus gp42 is posttranslationally modified to produce soluble gp42 that mediates HLA class II immune evasion. J. Virol. **79:** 841–852.
9. GOEDERT, M. 2001. The significance of tau and alpha-synuclein inclusions in neurodegenerative diseases. Curr. Opin. Genet. Dev. **11:** 343–351.

10. LEE, V.M., M. GOEDERT & J.Q. TROJANOWSKI. 2001. Neurodegenerative tauopathies. Annu. Rev. Neurosci. **24:** 1121–1159.
11. CUNNINGHAM, B.A., S. HOFFMAN, U. RUTISHAUSER, *et al.* 1983. Molecular topography of the neural cell adhesion molecule N-CAM: surface orientation and location of sialic acid-rich and binding regions. Proc. Natl. Acad. Sci. USA **80:** 3116–3120.
12. RUTISHAUSER, U., M. WATANABE, J. SILVER, *et al.* 1985. Specific alteration of NCAM-mediated cell adhesion by an endoneuraminidase. J. Cell Biol. **101:** 1842–1849.
13. CONE, R.D. 1999 The central melanocortin system and energy homeostasis. Trends Endocrinol. Metab. **10:** 211–216.
14. GUO, L., H. MUNZBERG, R.C. STUART, *et al.* 2004. *N*-Acetylation of hypothalamic alpha-melanocyte-stimulating hormone and regulation by leptin. Proc. Natl. Acad. Sci. USA **101:** 11797–11802.
15. DREYER, W.J. & H. NEURATH. 1955. The activation of chymotrypsinogen; isolation and identification of a peptide liberated during activation. J. Biol. Chem. **217:** 527–539.
16. WU, Y.I., H.G. MUNSHI, R. SEN, *et al.* 2004. Glycosylation broadens the substrate profile of membrane type 1 matrix metalloproteinase. J. Biol. Chem. **279:** 8278–8289.
17. WONG, P.S., J.P. EISERICH, S. REDDY, *et al.* 2001. Inactivation of glutathione S-transferases by nitric oxide-derived oxidants: exploring a role for tyrosine nitration. Arch. Biochem. Biophys. **394:** 216–228.
18. GIULIVI, C. 1998. Functional implications of nitric oxide produced by mitochondria in mitochondrial metabolism. Biochem. J. **332:** 673–679.
19. GERDES, J., H. LEMKE, H. BAISCH, *et al.* 1984. Cell cycle analysis of a cell proliferation-associated human nuclear antigen defined by the monoclonal antibody Ki-67. J. Immunol. **133:** 1710–1715.
20. ENDL, E. & J. GERDES. 2000. Posttranslational modifications of the KI-67 protein coincide with two major checkpoints during mitosis. J. Cell. Physiol. **182:** 371–380.
21. SMOTRYS, J.E. & M.E. LINDER. 2004. Palmitoylation of intracellular signaling proteins: regulation and function. Annu. Rev. Biochem. **73:** 559–587.
22. BROWN, D.A. & E. LONDON. 1998. Functions of lipid rafts in biological membranes. Annu. Rev. Cell Dev. Biol. **14:** 111–136.
23. KABOURIDIS, P.S., A.I. MAGEE & S.C. LEY. 1997. *S*-Acylation of LCK protein tyrosine kinase is essential for its signalling function in T lymphocytes. EMBO J. **16:** 4983–4998.
24. SEABRA, M.C. 1998. Membrane association and targeting of prenylated Ras-like GTPases. Cell. Signal. **10:** 167–172.
25. CALERO, M., C.Z. CHEN, W. ZHU, *et al.* 2003. Dual prenylation is required for Rab protein localization and function. Mol. Biol. Cell **14:** 1852–1867.
26. RADEMACHER, T.W., S.W. HOMANS, R.B. PAREKH & R.A. DWEK. 1986. Immunoglobulin G as a glycoprotein. Biochem. Soc. Symp. **51:** 131–148.
27. COLOMA, M.J., A. CLIFT, L. WIMS & S.L. MORRISON. 2000. The role of carbohydrate in the assembly and function of polymeric IgG. Mol. Immunol. **37:** 1081–1090.
28. BRANDTZAEG, P. & H. PRYDZ. 1984. Direct evidence for an integrated function of J chain and secretory component in epithelial transport of immunoglobulins. Nature **311:** 71–73.
29. REISNER, Y., M. LINKER-ISRAELI & N. SHARON. 1976. Separation of mouse thymocytes into two subpopulations by the use of peanut agglutinin. Cell. Immunol. **25:** 129–134.
30. ROBB, R.J., R.M. KUTNY, M. PANICO, *et al.* 1984. Amino acid sequence and post-translational modification of human interleukin 2. Proc. Natl. Acad. Sci. USA **81:** 6486–6490.
31. SANTHANAM, U., J. GHRAYEB, P.B. SEHGAL & L.T. MAY. 1989. Post-translational modifications of human interleukin-6. Arch. Biochem. Biophys. **274:** 161–170.
32. VIGNERON, N., V. STROOBANT, J. CHAPIRO, *et al.* 2004. An antigenic peptide produced by peptide splicing in the proteasome. Science **304:** 587–590.
33. HANADA, K., J.W. YEWDELL & J.C. YANG. 2004. Immune recognition of a human renal cancer antigen through post-translational protein splicing. Nature **427:** 252–256.
34. MOWEN, K.A., B.T. SCHURTER, J.W. FATHMAN, *et al.* 2004. Arginine methylation of NIP45 modulates cytokine gene expression in effector T lymphocytes. Mol. Cell **15:** 559–571.

35. SEBBAG, M., M. SIMON, C. VINCENT, *et al.* 1995. The antiperinuclear factor and the so-called antikeratin antibodies are the same rheumatoid arthritis-specific autoantibodies. J. Clin. Invest. **95:** 2672–2679.

36. GAN, S.Q., O.W. MCBRIDE, W.W. IDLER, *et al.* 1990. Organization, structure, and polymorphisms of the human profilaggrin gene. Biochemistry **29:** 9432–9440.

37. GIRBAL-NEUHAUSER, E., J.J. DURIEUX, M. ARNAUD, *et al.* 1999. The epitopes targeted by the rheumatoid arthritis-associated antifilaggrin autoantibodies are posttranslationally generated on various sites of (pro)filaggrin by deimination of arginine residues. J. Immunol. **162:** 585–594.

38. MYERS, L.K., J. MYLLYHARJU, M. NOKELAINEN, *et al.* 2004. Relevance of posttranslational modifications for the arthritogenicity of type II collagen. J. Immunol. **172:** 2970–2975.

39. YAMADA, H., B. DZHAMBAZOV, R. BOCKERMANN, *et al.* 2004. A transient post-translationally modified form of cartilage type II collagen is ignored by self-reactive T cells. J. Immunol. **173:** 4729–4735.

40. MAMULA, M.J., R.J. GEE, J.I. ELLIOTT, *et al.* 1999. Isoaspartyl post-translational modification triggers autoimmune responses to self-proteins. J. Biol. Chem. **274:** 22321–22327.

41. DE HAAN, E.C., J.P. WAGENAAR-HILBERS, R.M. LISKAMP, *et al.* 2005. Limited plasticity in T cell recognition of modified T cell receptor contact residues in MHC class II bound peptides. Mol. Immunol. **42:** 355–364.

42. SURH, C.D., R. COPPEL & M.E. GERSHWIN. 1990. Structural requirement for autoreactivity on human pyruvate dehydrogenase-E2, the major autoantigen of primary biliary cirrhosis: implication for a conformational autoepitope. J. Immunol. **144:** 3367–3374.

43. QUINN, J., A.G. DIAMOND, J.M. PALMER, *et al.* 1993. Lipoylated and unlipoylated domains of human PDC-E2 as autoantigens in primary biliary cirrhosis: significance of lipoate attachment. Hepatology **18:** 1384–1391.

44. LONG, S.A., C. QUAN, J. VAN DE WATER, *et al.* 2001. Immunoreactivity of organic mimeotopes of the E2 component of pyruvate dehydrogenase: connecting xenobiotics with primary biliary cirrhosis. J. Immunol. **167:** 2956–2963.

45. LEUNG, P.S., C. QUAN, O. PARK, *et al.* 2003. Immunization with a xenobiotic 6-bromo-hexanoate bovine serum albumin conjugate induces antimitochondrial antibodies. J. Immunol. **170:** 5326–5332.

DNA Lesions and Repair in Immunoglobulin Class Switch Recombination and Somatic Hypermutation

ZHENMING XU, ZSOLT FULOP, YUAN ZHONG, ALBERT J. EVINGER III, HONG ZAN, AND PAOLO CASALI

Center for Immunology, School of Medicine and School of Biological Sciences, University of California, Irvine, California 92697-4120, USA

ABSTRACT: Immunoglobulin (Ig) gene somatic hypermutation (SHM) and class switch DNA recombination (CSR) are critical for the maturation of the antibody response. These processes endow antibodies with increased antigen-binding affinity and acquisition of new biological effector functions, thereby underlying the generation of memory B cells and plasma cells. They are dependent on the generation of specific DNA lesions and the intervention of activation-induced cytidine deaminase as well as newly identified translesion DNA polymerases, which are expressed in germinal center B cells. DNA lesions include mismatches, abasic sites, nicks, single-strand breaks, and double-strand breaks (DSBs). DSBs in the switch (S) region DNA are critical for CSR, but they also occur in V(D)J regions and possibly contribute to the events that lead to SHM. The nature of the DSBs in the Ig locus, their generation, and the repair processes that they trigger and that are responsible for their regulation remain poorly understood. Aberrant regulation of these events can result in chromosomal breaks and translocations, which are significant steps in B-cell neoplastic transformation.

KEYWORDS: activation-induced cytosine deaminase (AID); class switch recombination (CSR); DNA lesion; double-strand break (DSB); error-prone DNA repair; lesion bypass or translesion DNA polymerase; pol ι; pol θ; pol ζ; somatic hypermutation (SHM); V(D)J recombination

INTRODUCTION

Antibody diversity is generated through processes occurring at sequential B-cell developmental stages: (1) rearrangement of different germline V (variable), D (diversity), and J (joining) genes to yield an enormous variety of V_HDJ_H gene segments in the heavy (H) chain locus; (2) rearrangement of V and J genes in the light (L) κ and λ chain loci, also giving rise to an enormous assortment of rearranged $V_\kappa J_\kappa$ or $V_\lambda J_\lambda$ segments; and finally (3) random pairing of rearranged V_HDJ_H and $V_\kappa J_\kappa$ or $V_\lambda J_\lambda$ chains. The staggering number of $V_HDJ_H/V_\kappa J_\kappa$ or $V_HDJ_H/V_\lambda J_\lambda$ pairs generated

Address for correspondence: Paolo Casali, Center for Immunology, 3028 Hewitt Hall, University of California, Irvine, CA 92697-4120. Voice: 949-824-4456.
pcasali@uci.edu

Ann. N.Y. Acad. Sci. 1050: 146–162 (2005). © 2005 New York Academy of Sciences.
doi: 10.1196/annals.1313.119

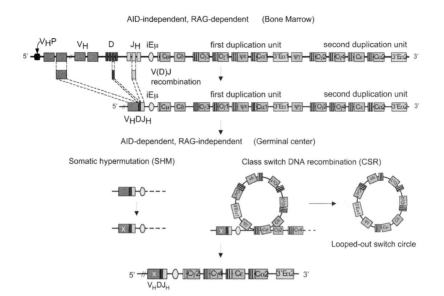

FIGURE 1. RAG and AID in B-cell differentiation. V(D)J recombination times B-cell development. It occurs in bone marrow and is dependent on the expression of RAG1 and RAG2, but not AID. Eventually, IgM$^+$ B cells will leave the bone marrow and colonize the peripheral lymphoid organs. They will be activated by encounter with antigen and undergo SHM and CSR. Both processes are dependent on AID expression, but not RAG1/RAG2. SHM inserts mainly point mutations in the variable region, whereas CSR changes the constant region of the IgH chain with a downstream C_H region, thereby "looping-out" the intervening DNA.

at any time (in excess of 10^9) underlies the high degree of diversity of the B-cell receptors (BCRs) for antigen and the primary antibody repertoire. This consists of IgM antibodies, in general, with a low to moderate affinity for antigens. All the gene rearrangement events that underlie the generation of the primary BCR repertoire depend on the expression of recombination-activating genes 1 (RAG1) and RAG2, which are critical for V(D)J gene rearrangement (FIG. 1).

The impact of antigen on the primary BCR repertoire results eventually in the production of antibodies of higher affinities and different classes, that is, IgG, IgA, and IgE. The shift to high-affinity and secondary isotypes is underpinned by two critical genetic processes: Ig somatic hypermutation (SHM)[1] and class switch DNA recombination (CSR)[2] (FIG. 1). Both SHM and CSR occur in the specialized micro-environment of the germinal center, and both contribute to the maturation of the antibody response, although in different ways. By diversifying the binding strength of the BCR, SHM provides the structural basis for clonal selection by antigen for higher affinity mutants and the affinity maturation of the antibody response. By changing the constant (C) region of the Ig H chain with a downstream C region, CSR changes the antibody effector functions, which will be better suited to the later stages of the antibody response. Ig V(D)J SHM is turned on at the germinal center centroblastic stage after mature B cells encounter antigen and in the presence of T-cell help. At the subsequent centrocytic stage of germinal center, B clones expressing BCRs with higher antigen-binding affinity undergo antigen-driven positive selection and develop into memory B cells or antibody-secreting plasma cells. Autoreactive B cells or low-affinity clones undergo negative selection through apoptosis, anergy, or receptor editing. Both *in vivo* and *in vitro* experiments have shown that SHM is induced in B cells that have received T-cell help and sustained BCR cross-linking, consistent with the role of T-cell and BCR engagement in germinal center formation.[3–5] Although different in their induction requirements, both SHM and CSR depend on the activity of a recently characterized cytidine deaminase, referred to as activation-induced deaminase (AID).[6,7] AID plays a central role in antigen-driven clonal expansion, selection, and differentiation of B cells in the peripheral lymphoid organs, eventually giving rise to memory B cells and plasma cells. Although dependent on AID, SHM and CSR are independent of RAG1 or RAG2.

DNA lesions include any alteration of the nucleotide composition of the double-strand that may lead to DNA informational or structural change. DNA lesions such as thymidine dimers, oxidized nucleotides, mismatches, and DNA strand breaks are caused by irradiation, oxidative chemicals, erroneous replication, and nucleolytic activities.[8] Double-strand breaks (DSBs) caused by irradiation, retroviral integration, transposition, or V(D)J recombination entail the loss of genetic information due to the deletion of significant stretches of DNA.[9,10] In general, DSBs are repaired through either non-homologous end joining (NHEJ) or homologous recombination (HR) in a faultless fashion. However, in hypermutating B cells, DNA lesions in the IgH as well as the κ and λ loci trigger a DNA repair process that is prone to insert mismatches, that is, mutations. DSBs are characteristic and critical DNA intermediates in CSR. These DNA breaks undergo processing by different protein complexes before being repaired. Some of the same protein factors and/or complexes may be involved in the repair of DSB occurring in the V(D)J region DNA, eventually leading to the insertion of mutations. Here, we discuss mechanisms of generation of DNA lesions in the Ig H locus, particularly DSBs, and the processes that are involved in their repair and that affect CSR and SHM.

DNA LESIONS AND REPAIR IN CSR

In the mouse, there are eight different Ig heavy chain constant region (C_H) genes downstream of the Ig VDJ region genes: Cμ, Cδ, Cγ3, Cγ1, Cγ2b, Cγ2a, Cε, and Cα. In the human, the H-chain locus underwent a phylogenetically semiconservative duplication, resulting in two tandem clusters of C_H genes separated by a duplicated 3′ enhancer (Eα): Cμ, Cδ, Cγ3, Cγ1, Cα1-Eα-Cγ2, Cγ4, Cε, and Cα2. In germinal center B cells, upon stimulation by CD40L expressed by activated CD4+ T cells and cytokines, the IgH locus undergoes CSR to juxtapose the VDJ region to a C_H gene downstream of Cδ. The DNA sequences mediating the CSR process are referred to as switch (S) regions, and an S region is present 5′ of each C_H gene with the exception of Cδ. In CSR, the 5′ portion of the upstream S region is joined to the 3′ portion of the downstream S region, thereby excising and circularizing the intervening genomic DNA (FIG. 1). The "looping-out" nature of CSR strongly suggests the existence of DNA DSB intermediates. CSR depends on transcription of the inter-

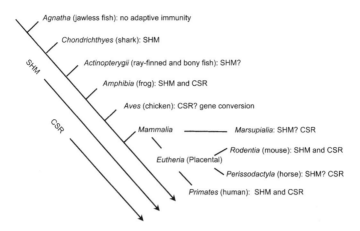

FIGURE 2. Phylogenetic emergence of SHM and CSR and development of adaptive immunity. From jawed fish to humans, SHM first emerges in cold-blooded vertebrates. CSR emerges first in amphibians. Both SHM and CSR are fully operational in mammals.

vening (I), S, and C regions of the upstream (donor) and downstream (acceptor) C_H loci, which is driven by the I_H promoter lying upstream of each I_H region and under both positive and negative regulations by switch regulatory elements (SREs).[11,12] Although variable in length, ranging from 1 (Sϵ) to 12 kb (Sγ1), all S regions contain highly repetitive GC-rich sequences. The 3-kb Sμ region consists of iterations of the [(GAGCT)$_n$(GGGGT)] sequence, which is believed to act as the recognition motif for the Sμ-Sx recombination. Interestingly, the *Xenopus laevis* Sμ region, which is AT-rich instead of GC-rich, also contains the "AGCT" repeats and can functionally replace the mammalian Sμ region,[13] suggesting that the repeated AGCT motif is important for an evolutionarily conserved targeting mechanism of CSR (FIG. 2). The palindromic nature of these repeated AGCT motifs raises the possibility that a complex and stable secondary structure may form during the Sμ region transcription. This structure may be a substrate of CSR recombinases itself or may serve as a scaffold to recruit important cofactors.[14] The Sϵ and Sα regions consist of the "RRGCT" repeats, a variation of the GAGCT repeats. Both (R)RGCT and (G)AGCT are different iterations of the RGYW/WRCY motif (R = A and G, Y = C and T, and W = A and T), the hypermutation "hot spot".[15–17] Indeed, more than 50% of the Sμ, Sϵ, and Sα DNA is accounted for by RGYW/WRCY sequences, and RGYW/WRCY is highly represented in Sγ regions (Sγ3, Sγ1, Sγ2b, and Sγ2a) as well, suggesting that CSR and SHM share a targeting mechanism and/or DNA intermediates. The top strand of all S-region DNA is G-rich, implying that there may exist another CSR targeting mechanism that entails the formation of stable RNA:DNA hybrid strands during the S-region transcription. The resulting single-stranded nontemplate DNA and possibly G-quartet structures formed within would be substrates of the CSR recombinase(s).[2,18]

Recent progress to identify factors involved in CSR has established an essential role for AID, which is expressed in B cells activated by antigen and CD4[+] helper

T cells.[6,7] AID is a sequelog[19] of the RNA-editing cytidine deaminase APOBEC1, suggesting that AID may edit an mRNA to code for a protein factor involved in CSR, possibly a DNA recombinase.[20–23] Although this hypothesis has been supported by the finding that *de novo* protein synthesis is required for the AID function in CSR,[20] it has recently lost much ground. A different but nonmutually exclusive possibility is that AID functions directly as a DNA deaminase, converting cytosine bases to uracil in germinal center B cells. This model is supported by the demonstration that AID can deaminate chromosomal DNA in *Escherichia coli* as well as cytosine bases in the WRCY motif in single-stranded DNA *in vitro*.[24,25] The resulting U:G mismatch is either replicated over to introduce transition mutations (C to T and G to A) or dealt with in two ways: (1) The U:G mismatch activates the mismatch repair (MMR) pathway, which involves the MutS homolog 2 (MSH2), MSH6, MutL homolog 1 (MLH1), postmitotic segregation protein 2 (PMS2), and exonuclease 1 (Exo1). Both MSH2 and Exo1 are critical for CSR, perhaps because of their role in

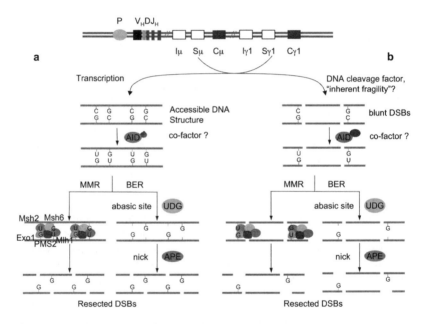

FIGURE 3. Generation of DSBs in S regions. **(a)** AID-dependent generation of DSBs: deamination of cytosine on both strands generates U:G mismatches, which will activate either the mismatch repair pathway (MMR) or the base excision pathway (BER). The MMR complex, consisting of Msh2, Msh6, Mlh1, Pms2, and Exo1, would generate gaps in opposite DNA strands and eventually DSBs. In the BER pathway, uracil DNA glycosylase (UDG) removes the uracil base to yield an abasic site, which in turn is cleaved off by apyrimidinic endonuclease to generate nicks and, when cleaving on opposite strands, DSBs. **(b)** AID-independent generation of DSBs and their processing by AID. DNA strands are cleaved to form blunt-ended DSBs by a yet to be defined endonuclease. AID-dependent processing of the blunt ends leads to the U:G mismatches, which eventually yield resected DSBs. In either **a** or **b**, whether upstream or downstream of blunt-ended DSBs, AID would be critical in generating resected free DNA ends.

generating and/or repairing DNA DSBs during the MMR.[26,27] (2) The U:G mismatch triggers the base excision repair (BER) pathway, which is dependent on UNG2, a uracil-DNA glycosylase (UDG). This removes the uracil base from the DNA to yield an abasic site, which is then excised by apyrimidinic endonuclease to generate a nick, resulting in a single-strand break. A similar nearby lesion on the opposite strand would generate a DSB, and DSBs in both an upstream and a downstream S region would lead to excision of the intervening DNA segment[28] (FIG. 3). Consistent with this AID-dependent DNA deamination and DNA lesion repair model, CSR is essentially abolished in $Msh2^{-/-}Ung2^{-/-}$ mice.[29] This model also entails the formation of RNA:DNA hybrid strands and exposed single-stranded DNA on the non-template strand (R-loop) as the potential AID substrate during the S-region transcription, which was also observed *in vivo*.[30–32]

Other trans-factors critical for CSR include Nijmegen breakage syndrome protein (Nbs1), Mre11, phosphorylated H2A histone family member X (γ-H2AX), ataxia-telangiectasia-mutated (ATM) kinase, p53-binding protein 1 (53BP1), and the Ku70/Ku80 heterodimer.[33–41] That these proteins all form complexes with other proteins and are involved in the DSB repair further strengthen the notion that DNA DSBs are important CSR intermediates and are processed and repaired by different protein complexes. DNA DSBs have been detected in the Sμ region in activated human B cells, whereas no DSB is detectable in the Cμ region.[42,43] In resting B cells, such Sμ region DSBs are blunt-ended; but in activated B cells undergoing CSR, Sμ DSBs are resected through an AID-dependent process.[42] The critical role of AID in processing blunt-end DSBs to yield resected ends is emphasized by the finding that in activated B cells from an AID[−/−] patient, DNA DSBs are still detected in the Sμ region[43] and such DSBs are blunt-ended (unpublished data). In this patient, failure to generate resected DSBs associates with failure to undergo CSR. This is consistent with the recent finding that the *c-Myc* gene is translocated to S regions at a similar frequency in AID-deficient mice as in wild-type mice, suggesting that the generation of S-region DSBs that are responsible for these translocations is independent of AID,[44] further favoring a model in which the "inherent fragility" of the Sμ region and *c-Myc* gene makes them substrates of yet to be determined DNA cleaving proteins to yield blunt-ended DSBs.[1,45] Our preliminary findings suggest that the upregulation and recruitment of AID to DSBs, possibly with a DNA helicase cofactor, lead to cytosine deamination near the free ends. The resulting U:G mismatches would activate the MMR and/or BER pathway, as described above, to generate resected DSBs (FIG. 3).

A critical implication inherent in a model entailing the occurrence of DSBs upstream of AID is that the blunt ends at different S regions are precluded from re-ligation of the intra-S region through NHEJ, a favored process because of the low energy requirement for directly ligating two adjacent ends. This re-ligation of blunt ends could partially be inhibited if AID is overexpressed in the nucleus. The current lack of quantitative study of AID expression in activated B cells makes it difficult to assess this possibility. Another question is how AID-generated staggered ends are tethered together for repair and ligation. It is possible that staggered-end generation and Sx-Sx region ligation are coupled and are effected within one large protein complex containing different enzymatic activities. However, this would pose significant spatial problems for the synapsis of different S regions. Alternatively, a post-resection complex, which may contain AID itself, could be recruited to prevent further end processing until it is later displaced by downstream recombinases while

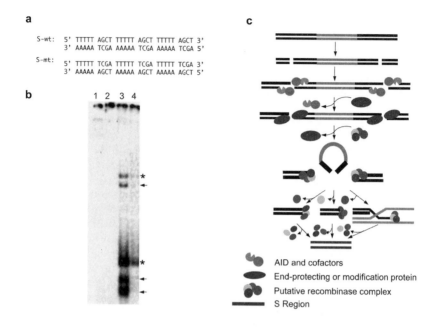

FIGURE 4. Protein factors bound to DNA DSBs. **(a)** The S-wt and S-mt oligonucleotide sequences. **(b)** The gel picture from an electrical mobility shift assay during which the ^{32}P-radiolabeled S-wt or S-mt was incubated without (*lanes 1 and 2*) or with (*lanes 3 and 4*) total CL-01 cell lysates on ice for 30 minutes. The DNA-protein complexes were separated through a 5% PAGE and then subjected to autoradiography. *Arrowheads* indicate three proteins or protein complexes specifically bound to the S-wt, but not S-mt; *Two proteins/protein complexes that are bound to both S-wt and S-mt. **(c)** Model depicting different proteins/protein complexes involved in DSB repair during CSR. Processing of blunt-end DSBs by AID and its cofactors yields resected ends. A putative end-protecting factor prevents religation of the ends intra-S regions until they are replaced by a recombinase complex while the intergenic region "loops out". The recombinase either fills in or further resects the ends to undergo an NHEJ process. Alternatively, the resected ends are repaired by HR.

the intervening region "loops out" (FIG. 4c). The putative post-resection complex may also modify DSB ends, which would then be repaired only by CSR-specific machinery. This mechanism is reminiscent of the hairpin intermediates during the V(D)J recombination. Such a hairpin is generated at the coding joint after RAG-mediated DNA cleavage and is subsequently opened by DNA-PK–activated Artemis.[46–48] The AID-dependent γ-H2AX foci formation at the CSR sites strongly suggests the recruitment of multiple protein factors to the proximity of the IgH gene[49] in response to AID-generated staggered ends. It is worthwhile to note that γ-H2AX foci formation does not necessarily reflect the generation of initial DSBs, but rather a later step in the DSB repair process,[50,51] and factors other than γ-H2AX may carry out the end-protecting and/or modification tasks.

To gain further insights into how the DSB ends are processed and into the temporal and spatial regulation of protein factors involved during CSR, we utilized an *in vitro* system to identify proteins specifically bound to those ends. The "S-wt" double-stranded oligonucleotide contains three repeats of palindromic AGCT, which is the most abundant RGYW motif in the Sμ region, separated by the TTTTT motifs. A control double-stranded oligonucleotide, S-mt, consists of a similar sequence, except that the AGCT repeat is replaced by its reverse TCGA, which is not an iteration of RGYW (FIG. 4a). Incubation with the total protein extracts from a subclone of B-lymphoma cell-line CL-01, which was selected for the high rate of spontaneous CSR, results in the formation of three S-wt–specific DNA-protein complexes, which shifted the mobility of the radiolabeled DNA oligo (FIG. 4b). These DNA-protein complexes may rely on different protein-DNA binding sites, in either the internal or the 3′-terminal AGCT motif. Since the S-wt and S-mt only differ in the presence or absence of the RGYW motif, these findings strongly suggest that the RGYW motifs play a role in targeting certain trans-factors to S regions. Specifically, these S-region RGYW motifs may function not only as the initial cleavage signal of endonucleases, but also as the recognition and binding sites for the end-protecting and processing complex(es) (FIG. 4c).

DSBs at the CSR sites would recruit Mre11/Rad50/Nbs1 complex and activate H2AX phosphorylation, which in turn catalyzes foci formation and the repair process. Free DNA ends can be rejoined with little or no regard for sequence homology by NHEJ or they can be "rejoined" through HR, a homologous template-directed recombination process. AID-dependent γ-H2AX foci formation in the IgH locus primarily occurs in the G1 phase,[49] suggesting that the repair process occurs through NHEJ, which also requires 53BP1 and Ku70/80. This is mechanistically different from V(D)J recombination. In V(D)J recombination, DNA-PKcs, Artemis, XRCC4, and DNA ligase IV, but not 53BP1, are necessary.[52] How staggered ends are resected by exonuclease or filled in by DNA polymerases to make ligation-compatible ends during CSR NHEJ is not clear. The frequent mutations found at the Sx-Sx junction suggest that an error-prone DNA polymerase is recruited to insert mismatched nucleotides and extends the strand to fill in the gap near the DSB ends (FIG. 4c). Although the available data strongly suggest that NHEJ is the major mechanism effecting Sx-Sx DNA repair, they do not rule out a possible role for HR in the resolution of S region DSBs. An abortive CSR repairing process can result in chromosomal breakage, which in turn can lead to chromosomal translocation involving protooncogenes, such as *Bcl-6*, *c-Myc*, and *Bcl-2*, as frequently occurring in germinal center B cells.

DNA LESIONS AND REPAIR IN SHM

IgV gene SHM entails the insertion of mainly point mutations with occasional insertions and deletions at a rate of approximately 10^{-3} changes/base/cell division, which is about one million-fold higher than the spontaneous somatic mutation rate of the genome at large.[53] Similar to CSR, SHM depends on AID upregulation and is linked to transcription.[6,54,55] It targets the V(D)J sequence immediately downstream of the IgV promoter, tapering off within the intronic DNA immediately upstream of Sμ while sparing the constant region,[56–58] and displays a striking preference for the RGYW/WRCY motif (mutational hot spot).[15–17] Ig V(D)J is not the only gene targeted by SHM, as DNA outside the Ig H and κ and λ light chain loci, such as *Bcl-6* in the human and *c-Myc* in both human and mice, are also targeted.[59–61] In antigen-selected antibodies, mutations are found mainly in the complementarity-determining regions (CDR). These regions dictate antibody specificity and comprise codons that are more inherently susceptible to replacement mutations than they would be for a random DNA sequence,[62] suggesting that their nucleotide composition possibly evolved as a mutational strategy for the generation of higher affinity antibodies.

Somatic mutations would be inserted during error-prone repair of DNA lesions involving SSBs or DSBs, as first hypothesized by Brenner and Milstein[63] in 1966. The existence of DSBs in a hypermutating V region was first inferred by the presence of TdT-accessible DNA ends embedded in the Ig V(D)J DNA of hypermutating B cells *in vitro* and later confirmed by the ligation-mediated polymerase chain reaction (LM-PCR) in human *ex vivo* germinal center B cells as well as human B-cell lines *in vitro*.[64–67] The occurrence of DSBs seems to be a highly specific function inherent only in the genes that can undergo SHM, such as those of the Ig locus, *Bcl-6* and *c-Myc*. By contrast, DSBs are not detectable in genes that cannot undergo SHM, including Cμ, PAX5, PIM1, and alpha-fetoprotein (AFP). In the same gene, DSBs change in nature when starting the SHM process. In nonhypermutating germline V genes, DSBs are blunt, while DSBs occurring in hypermutating rearranged V(D)J genes are resected to yield 3′ protruding free ends. Analysis of DNA from B cells at different stages of differentiation has shown that the resected DSBs appear at a germinal center stage when Ig V gene hypermutation is upregulated, but not in pre-germinal center or post-germinal center B cells, that is, memory B cells and plasma cells. Accordingly, in the same hypermutating B cell, blunt-ended DSBs occur in both germline and translocated *c-Myc* alleles, whereas resected DSBs occur only in the translocated and hypermutating *c-Myc* allele.[60,67] Hence, resected DSBs are characteristic of hypermutating genes and likely constitute crucial intermediates in the SHM process.[67] Processing of blunt-ended DSBs to generate resected ends would be mediated by AID. Indeed, although AID is dispensable for the generation of blunt-ended DSBs, it plays a critical role in the processing of blunt-ended DSBs to yield resected DSBs, possibly through deamination of cytosines within a few residues of free blunt ends. The appearance of U:G mismatches at these locations would trigger MMR or BER pathways, which would lead to the generation of staggered ends.

Staggered DSBs in hypermutating B cells appear predominantly in the S/G2 phase, suggesting that mutations are introduced during the DSB repair process through HR and involve error-prone DNA polymerases.[65] The role of resected DSB ends in strand invasion of sister chromatids and the subsequent events that lead to mismatches during HR have been further confirmed by ChIP assays, showing that γ-H2AX, Nbs1, Mre11, and Ku70/Ku80 are predominantly bound to the blunt ends. Rad 52 and Rad51, two Rad52 epistasis group proteins that are specific for HR, are bound only to resected DNA ends of rearranged $V_H DJ_H$ genes.[67] This implies that (1) the blunt ends of nonhypermutating germline or rearranged V_H genes recruit Ku70/Ku80 and are re-ligated through the NHEJ pathway, and (2) after the assembly of Rad51 nucleoprotein filament around the 3′-resected ends of the hypermutating rearranged V_H DNA, other factors, possibly including a chromatin remodeling protein and a DNA helicase, unwind the sister chromatids or homologous chromosomes to make them accessible for strand invasion (FIG. 5).

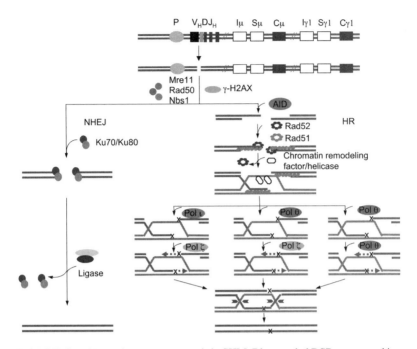

FIGURE 5. DSBs and error-prone repair in SHM. Blunt-ended DSBs generated in a re-arranged IgH variable region would recruit Mre11, Rad50, and Nbs1 as well as phosphorylated H2AX. They would be repaired by NHEJ through Ku70/Ku80 and DNA ligase. Alternatively, they would undergo AID processing to yield 3′ protruding ends, which recruit Rad51/Rad52 to initiate HR through invasion of sister chromatids or homologous chromosomes. A chromatin remodeling protein or a DNA helicase is likely involved in making the homologous region accessible. Different translesion DNA polymerases, upregulated in germinal center B cells, participate in the error-prone repairing process. Pol ι inserts incorrect single nucleotides, while polymerase ζ extends the DNA strand past the insertion. Pol θ could both insert mis-matched nucleotides and extend the terminus. However, the mismatched terminus generated by pol θ could also be extended by pol ζ.

The overwhelming segregation of DSBs within the RGYW/WRCY hypermutation hot spots suggests that during DSB repair a putative error-prone DNA polymerase inserts incorrect bases and extends the newly generated mismatched terminus. Error-prone translesion, or lesion bypass, polymerases have evolved to effect continued strand synthesis opposite DNA lesions that would otherwise stall a replication fork.[68,69] The growing family of recently identified or characterized polymerases adds to the high-fidelity DNA polymerases δ, ε, and α, which are responsible for DNA replication, and pol β, which performs faultless BER[68,70] (TABLE 1). Several studies have shown that the translesion DNA polymerases μ, λ, and κ are not essen-tial for SHM.[71–74] In patients with the *Xeroderma pigmentosum* variant (XPV) disease, who are deficient in DNA polymerase η (pol η), somatic mutations were found to be normal in frequency.[75–77] The profound downregulation of pol η by BCR cross-linking in actively hypermutating B cells suggests that this DNA poly-

TABLE 1. Eukaryotic DNA polymerases

DNA polymerase	Class[a]	Enzymatic activities	Fidelity[b]	Proposed functions
α	B	Initiation	10^{-5}–10^{-4}	Nuclear DNA primase
δ	B	Elongation, $3' \to 5'$ exonuclease	10^{-6}–10^{-5}	Nuclear DNA replication
ε	B	Elongation, $3' \to 5'$ exonuclease	10^{-6}–10^{-5}	Nuclear DNA replication
γ	A	Synthesis, $3' \to 5'$ exonuclease	10^{-6}–10^{-5}	Mitochondria DNA replication
σ	X	Terminal transferase, $3' \to 5'$ exonuclease	10^{-6}–10^{-4}	Sister chromatids cohesion
TdT	X	Terminal transferase		V(D)J-N insertion
λ	X	5'-Deoxyribose-5-phosphate lyase (dRP lyase)	10^{-5}–10^{-4}	NHEJ
μ	X	Terminal transferase	10^{-5}–10^{-4}	NHEJ
β	X	dRP lyase	10^{-5}–10^{-4}	High fidelity repair, base excision repair
REV1	Y	Inserting "C" across abasic sites		Translesion synthesis
κ	Y	Inserting "A" across abasic sites	10^{-4}–10^{-3}	Translesion synthesis, base substitution
η	Y		10^{-3}–10^{-2}	Translesion synthesis, UV damage repair
ι	Y	Inserting mismatches	$\sim 2 \times 10^{-1}$	Translesion synthesis, base excision repair, SHM
ζ	B	Extending mismatch terminus	10^{-5}–10^{-4}	Translesion synthesis, DSB repair, SHM
θ	A	Inserting "A" and other bases across AP sites	10^{-3}–10^{-2}	Translesion synthesis, DSB repair, SHM

[a]Eukaryotic DNA polymerases are classified into four main classes based on phylogenetic relationships with *E. coli* polymerase I (class A), *E. coli* polymerase II (class B), human polymerase β (class X), and *E. coli* UmuC/DinB and eukaryotic *RAD30/Xeroderma pigmentosum* variant (class Y).[91]
[b]Fidelity is defined as base substitution error frequency during nucleotide incorporation on intact single-strand template.

merase does not play a significant role in SHM.[78] Rather, DNA polymerases ι and ζ likely play an important role in SHM. DNA polymerase ι (pol ι) possesses a low processivity and is highly error-prone when copying undamaged DNA, whereas it efficiently incorporates single nucleotides opposing DNA lesions. DNA polymerase ζ (pol ζ) efficiently extends from a mismatched terminus to stabilize the mutation. The concerted and sequential action of polymerase ι and polymerase ζ would mediate DNA repair during HR, thereby introducing mismatches (mutations).[79] Gene inactivation of pol ι in the human Burkitt's lymphoma cell line BL2 abolished inducible SHM, but did not affect the background mutation frequency, suggesting that inducible hypermutation depends on pol ι.[80] BCR cross-linking, which is necessary to induce SHM, signals the upregulation of pol ζ, while blocking of pol ζ's REV3 catalytic subunit activity impairs Ig V(D)J and *Bcl-6* SHM without affecting cell cycle or viability.[74] Inhibition of human pol ζ REV3 expression, however, results in a profound decrease of damaged-induced DNA mutagenesis,[81] a function that is exquisitely mediated by this translesion polymerase in many cells of the body. This suggests that the machinery utilized by B cells for SHM, a sophisticated and highly specific function, is the same as that utilized to survive DNA damage, a critically basic process. The role of pol ζ in SHM has been verified *in vivo*. In transgenic mice generated to express antisense RNA to a portion of REV3, pol ζ REV3 is inhibited, and the accumulation of somatic mutations in the V_H genes of memory B cells is decreased and the generation of high-affinity antibodies is delayed.[82]

Another recently characterized human DNA polymerase, pol θ, which is encoded by the *pol* θ gene and belongs to the DNA polymerase A family,[83,84] possesses features that make it a good candidate in SHM. While an N-terminally truncated version of human pol θ has been shown to be a high-fidelity enzyme,[85] the full-length pol θ replicates undamaged DNA in an error-prone fashion. Interestingly, pol θ efficiently inserts "A", while strongly disfavoring "C", opposing an apurinic site, and effectually extends DNA synthesis, making it an efficient lesion bypass polymerase.[86] Because of its insertion and extension functions, its error-prone nature, and its upregulation in germinal center B cells,[87] pol θ may play a major role in the DNA lesion repair process that leads to SHM. Indeed, our recent data show that SHM is severely compromised in mice with either null *pol* θ alleles or mutated *pol* θ alleles, chaos 1,[88–90] strongly suggesting that pol θ inserts mismatches during Ig V DNA synthesis and the newly generated mismatch termini are extended by either pol θ itself or pol ζ.

The functional features of pol θ, pol ζ, and pol ι suggest that these DNA polymerases act in concert to introduce mismatches. Pol ι would insert incorrect single nucleotides, whereas pol ζ would extend the DNA strand past the mismatch. Pol θ could both insert mismatched nucleotides and extend the DNA terminus past the mismatch. The mismatch terminus generated by pol θ could also be extended by pol ζ (FIG. 5). Although the concerted action of pol ζ and pol θ would play a central role in generating mutations during the HR repair process of DSBs that underlies SHM, we cannot rule out the possibility that these polymerases introduce mismatches (mutations) while participating in a patch repair process outside main DNA regulation.

CONCLUSIONS AND PERSPECTIVES

Recent findings have defined the roles of DSBs, AID, and translesion DNA polymerases in CSR and SHM. The RGYW hot spot likely functions as the recognition and target sequence for the putative DNA enzyme involved in the generation of the DNA lesions that underlie CSR and SHM. Initial blunt-end DSBs are generated in Ig genes in an AID-independent fashion. AID-mediated resection of those blunt-end DSBs through cytosine deamination would yield U:G mismatches that trigger either the MMR or the BER pathway, which unfold through recruitment of multiple protein complexes. In CSR, synapsis of resected DSBs between upstream and downstream S regions and the subsequent DSB repair process, through either NHEJ or HR, lead to Sx-Sx DNA rejoining. In SHM, 3' free ends of such resected DSBs would initiate through Rad51 and Rad52 strand invasion to repair DSBs through HR in an error-prone fashion. Concerted activities of translesion pol ι, pol ζ, and pol θ would incorporate incorrect single nucleotides and extend the mismatched terminus that effectually introduces mutations in Ig genes. Aberrant regulation and repair of such DSBs can lead to chromosomal breaks and translocations, which are significant steps in B-cell neoplastic transformation (lymphomagenesis).

Important issues that still need to be addressed in CSR and SHM are (1) identification of the inherent DNA features, nature of nucleolytic activities, and molecular mechanisms that effect blunt DSBs; (2) identification of the AID cofactors to deaminate ssDNA or blunt-end DSBs and reconstitution of an *in vitro* system to generate AID-dependent resected DSBs; (3) identification of the DSB end-binding proteins, their spatial and temporal regulation in germinal center B cells, and their precise role in shepherding DNA lesions to the proper DNA repair pathway, either NHEJ or HR; and (4) characterization of the precise mechanism by which the NHEJ or HR resolves DSBs and the mechanism of error-prone DNA polymerases that introduce mutations. Genetic studies using such powerful tools as knockout mice have generated significant progress towards understanding these issues and will continue to unveil critical factors in SHM and CSR. Detailed biochemical studies will be instrumental in unfolding the precise mechanisms that underlie functions of those proteins. They will also be indispensable in identifying proteins with regulatory functions that fine-tune SHM and CSR, thereby unraveling the functioning of these central mechanisms of adaptive immunity.

ACKNOWLEDGMENTS

We thank Xiaoping Wu for insightful discussions and the sharing of unpublished data. This work was supported by National Institutes of Health Grant Nos. AR 40908 and AI 45011 (to P. Casali).

REFERENCES

1. WU, X. *et al.* 2003. Immunoglobulin somatic hypermutation: double-strand DNA breaks, AID, and error-prone DNA repair. J. Clin. Immunol. **23:** 235–246.
2. CHAUDHURI, J. & F.W. ALT. 2004. Class-switch recombination: interplay of transcription, DNA deamination, and DNA repair. Nat. Rev. Immunol. **4:** 541–552.
3. DENEPOUX, S. *et al.* 1997. Induction of somatic mutation in a human B cell line in vitro. Immunity **6:** 35–46.
4. MILLER, C. *et al.* 1995. Facultative role of germinal centers and T cells in the somatic diversification of IgVH genes. J. Exp. Med. **181:** 1319–1331.
5. ZAN, H. *et al.* 1999. Induction of Ig somatic hypermutation and class switching in a human monoclonal IgM+ IgD+ B cell line *in vitro*: definition of the requirements and modalities of hypermutation. J. Immunol. **162:** 3437–3447.
6. MURAMATSU, M. *et al.* 2000. Class switch recombination and hypermutation require activation-induced cytidine deaminase (AID), a potential RNA editing enzyme. Cell **102:** 553–563.

7. REVY, P. *et al.* 2000. Activation-induced cytidine deaminase (AID) deficiency causes the autosomal recessive form of the hyper-IgM syndrome (HIGM2). Cell **102**: 565–575.

8. LISBY, M. & R. ROTHSTEIN. 2004. DNA damage checkpoint and repair centers. Curr. Opin. Cell Biol. **16**: 328–334.

9. IZSVAK, Z. *et al.* 2004. Healing the wounds inflicted by sleeping beauty transposition by double-strand break repair in mammalian somatic cells. Mol. Cell **13**: 279–290.

10. VALERIE, K. & L.F. POVIRK. 2003. Regulation and mechanisms of mammalian double-strand break repair. Oncogene **22**: 5792–5812.

11. KIM, E.C. *et al.* 2004. The HoxC4 homeodomain protein mediates activation of the immunoglobulin heavy chain 3′ hs1,2 enhancer in human B cells: relevance to class switch DNA recombination. J. Biol. Chem. **279**: 42258–42269.

12. SCHAFFER, A. *et al.* 2003. Selective inhibition of class switching to IgG and IgE by recruitment of the HoxC4 and Oct-1 homeodomain proteins and Ku70/Ku86 to newly identified ATTT cis-elements. J. Biol. Chem. **278**: 23141–23150.

13. ZARRIN, A.A. *et al.* 2004. An evolutionarily conserved target motif for immunoglobulin class-switch recombination. Nat. Immunol. **5**: 1275–1281.

14. TASHIRO, J., K. KINOSHITA & T. HONJO. 2001. Palindromic but not G-rich sequences are targets of class switch recombination. Int. Immunol. **13**: 495–505.

15. ROGOZIN, I.B. & N.A. KOLCHANOV. 1992. Somatic hypermutagenesis in immunoglobulin genes. II. Influence of neighbouring base sequences on mutagenesis. Biochim. Biophys. Acta **1171**: 11–18.

16. WAGNER, S.D., C. MILSTEIN & M.S. NEUBERGER. 1995. Codon bias targets mutation. Nature **376**: 732.

17. FOSTER, S.J., T. DORNER & P.E. LIPSKY. 1999. Somatic hypermutation of VkappaJkappa rearrangements: targeting of RGYW motifs on both DNA strands and preferential selection of mutated codons within RGYW motifs. Eur. J. Immunol. **29**: 4011–4021.

18. DUQUETTE, M.L. *et al.* 2004. Intracellular transcription of G-rich DNAs induces formation of G-loops, novel structures containing G4 DNA. Genes Dev. **18**: 1618–1629.

19. VARSHAVSKY, A. 2004. "Spalog" and "sequelog": neutral terms for spatial and sequence similarity. Curr. Biol. **14**: R181–183.

20. DOI, T. *et al.* 2003. *De novo* protein synthesis is required for the activation-induced cytidine deaminase function in class-switch recombination. Proc. Natl. Acad. Sci. USA **100**: 2634–2638.

21. BEGUM, N.A. *et al.* 2004. Uracil DNA glycosylase activity is dispensable for immuno-globulin class switch. Science **305**: 1160–1163.

22. NAGAOKA, H. *et al.* 2005. DNA cleavage in immunoglobulin somatic hypermutation depends on de novo protein synthesis but not on uracil DNA glycosylase. Proc. Natl. Acad. Sci. USA **102**: 2022–2027.

23. TURELLI, P. & D. TRONO. 2005. Editing at the crossroad of innate and adaptive immunity. Science **307**: 1061–1065.

24. PETERSEN-MAHRT, S.K., R.S. HARRIS & M.S. NEUBERGER. 2002. AID mutates *E. coli* suggesting a DNA deamination mechanism for antibody diversification. Nature **418**: 99–103.

25. PHAM, P. *et al.* 2003. Processive AID-catalysed cytosine deamination on single-stranded DNA simulates somatic hypermutation. Nature **424**: 103–107.

26. BARDWELL, P.D. *et al.* 2004. Altered somatic hypermutation and reduced class-switch recombination in exonuclease 1-mutant mice. Nat. Immunol. **5**: 224–229.

27. EHRENSTEIN, M.R. & M.S. NEUBERGER. 1999. Deficiency in Msh2 affects the efficiency and local sequence specificity of immunoglobulin class-switch recombination: parallels with somatic hypermutation. EMBO J. **18**: 3484–3490.

28. DI NOIA, J. & M.S. NEUBERGER. 2002. Altering the pathway of immunoglobulin hyper-mutation by inhibiting uracil-DNA glycosylase. Nature **419**: 43–48.

29. RADA, C., J. M. DI NOIA & M.S. NEUBERGER. 2004. Mismatch recognition and uracil excision provide complementary paths to both Ig switching and the A/T-focused phase of somatic mutation. Mol. Cell **16**: 163–171.

30. RAMIRO, A.R. *et al.* 2003. Transcription enhances AID-mediated cytidine deamination by exposing single-stranded DNA on the nontemplate strand. Nat. Immunol. **4**: 452–456.

31. SHINKURA, R. *et al.* 2003. The influence of transcriptional orientation on endogenous switch region function. Nat. Immunol. **4:** 435–441.
32. YU, K. *et al.* 2003. R-loops at immunoglobulin class switch regions in the chromosomes of stimulated B cells. Nat. Immunol. **4:** 442–451.
33. REINA-SAN-MARTIN, B. *et al.* 2003. H2AX is required for recombination between immunoglobulin switch regions but not for intra-switch region recombination or somatic hypermutation. J. Exp. Med. **197:** 1767–1778.
34. REINA-SAN-MARTIN, B. *et al.* 2004. ATM is required for efficient recombination between immunoglobulin switch regions. J. Exp. Med. **200:** 1103–1110.
35. REINA-SAN-MARTIN, B. *et al.* 2005. Genomic instability, endoreduplication, and diminished Ig class-switch recombination in B cells lacking Nbs1. Proc. Natl. Acad. Sci. USA **102:** 1590–1595.
36. LUMSDEN, J.M. *et al.* 2004. Immunoglobulin class switch recombination is impaired in Atm-deficient mice. J. Exp. Med. **200:** 1111–1121.
37. LAHDESMAKI, A. *et al.* 2004. Delineation of the role of the Mre11 complex in class switch recombination. J. Biol. Chem. **279:** 16479–16487.
38. MANIS, J.P. *et al.* 2004. 53BP1 links DNA damage-response pathways to immunoglobulin heavy chain class-switch recombination. Nat. Immunol. **5:** 481–487.
39. KRACKER, S. *et al.* 2005. Nibrin functions in Ig class-switch recombination. Proc. Natl. Acad. Sci. USA **102:** 1584–1589.
40. WARD, I.M. *et al.* 2004. 53BP1 is required for class switch recombination. J. Cell Biol. **165:** 459–464.
41. ROONEY, S. *et al.* 2005. Artemis-independent functions of DNA-dependent protein kinase in Ig heavy chain class switch recombination and development. Proc. Natl. Acad. Sci. USA. Submitted.
42. RUSH, J.S., S.D. FUGMANN & D.G. SCHATZ. 2004. Staggered AID-dependent DNA double strand breaks are the predominant DNA lesions targeted to S mu in Ig class switch recombination. Int. Immunol. **16:** 549–557.
43. CATALAN, N. *et al.* 2003. The block in immunoglobulin class switch recombination caused by activation-induced cytidine deaminase deficiency occurs prior to the generation of DNA double strand breaks in switch mu region. J. Immunol. **171:** 2504–2509.
44. UNNIRAMAN, S., S. ZHOU & D.G. SCHATZ. 2004. Identification of an AID-independent pathway for chromosomal translocations between the IgH switch region and Myc. Nat. Immunol. **5:** 1117–1123.
45. CASALI, P. & H. ZAN. 2004. Class switching and Myc translocation: how does DNA break? Nat. Immunol. **5:** 1101–1103.
46. LEE, G.S. *et al.* 2004. RAG proteins shepherd double-strand breaks to a specific pathway, suppressing error-prone repair, but RAG nicking initiates homologous recombination. Cell **117:** 171–184.
47. LIEBER, M.R. *et al.* 2003. Mechanism and regulation of human non-homologous DNA end-joining. Nat. Rev. Mol. Cell Biol. **4:** 712–720.
48. MA, Y. *et al.* 2002. Hairpin opening and overhang processing by an Artemis/DNA-dependent protein kinase complex in nonhomologous end joining and V(D)J recombination. Cell **108:** 781–794.
49. PETERSEN, S. *et al.* 2001. AID is required to initiate Nbs1/gamma-H2AX focus formation and mutations at sites of class switching. Nature **414:** 660–665.
50. CELESTE, A. *et al.* 2003. Histone H2AX phosphorylation is dispensable for the initial recognition of DNA breaks. Nat. Cell Biol. **5:** 675–679.
51. CHUA, K.F., F.W. ALT & J.P. MANIS. 2002. The function of AID in somatic mutation and class switch recombination: upstream or downstream of DNA breaks. J. Exp. Med. **195:** F37–41.
52. POSEY, J.E., V.L. BRANDT & D.B. ROTH. 2004. Paradigm switching in the germinal center. Nat. Immunol. **5:** 476–477.
53. LEVY, N.S. *et al.* 1989. Early onset of somatic mutation in immunoglobulin VH genes during the primary immune response. J. Exp. Med. **169:** 2007–2019.
54. FUKITA, Y., H. JACOBS & K. RAJEWSKY. 1998. Somatic hypermutation in the heavy chain locus correlates with transcription. Immunity **9:** 105–114.

55. PETERS, A. & U. STORB. 1996. Somatic hypermutation of immunoglobulin genes is linked to transcription initiation. Immunity **4:** 57–65.

56. RADA, C. *et al.* 1994. The 5′ boundary of somatic hypermutation in a V kappa gene is in the leader intron. Eur. J. Immunol. **24:** 1453–1457.

57. LEBECQUE, S.G. & P.J. GEARHART. 1990. Boundaries of somatic mutation in rearranged immunoglobulin genes: 5′ boundary is near the promoter, and 3′ boundary is approximately 1 kb from V(D)J gene. J. Exp. Med. **172:** 1717–1727.

58. ROGERSON, B.J. 1994. Mapping the upstream boundary of somatic mutations in rearranged immunoglobulin transgenes and endogenous genes. Mol. Immunol. **31:** 83–98.

59. SHEN, H.M. *et al.* 1998. Mutation of BCL-6 gene in normal B cells by the process of somatic hypermutation of Ig genes. Science **280:** 1750–1752.

60. BEMARK, M. & M.S. NEUBERGER. 2000. The c-MYC allele that is translocated into the IgH locus undergoes constitutive hypermutation in a Burkitt's lymphoma line. Oncogene **19:** 3404–3410.

61. ZAN, H. *et al.* 2000. B cell receptor engagement and T cell contact induce Bcl-6 somatic hypermutation in human B cells: identity with Ig hypermutation. J. Immunol. **165:** 830–839.

62. CHANG, B. & P. CASALI. 1994. The CDR1 sequences of a major proportion of human germline Ig V_H genes are inherently susceptible to amino acid replacement. Immunol. Today **15:** 367–373.

63. BRENNER, S. & C. MILSTEIN. 1966. Origin of antibody variation. Nature **211:** 242–243.

64. SALE, J.E. & M.S. NEUBERGER. 1998. TdT-accessible breaks are scattered over the immunoglobulin V domain in a constitutively hypermutating B cell line. Immunity **9:** 859–869.

65. PAPAVASILIOU, F.N. & D.G. SCHATZ. 2000. Cell-cycle-regulated DNA double-stranded breaks in somatic hypermutation of immunoglobulin genes. Nature **408:** 216–221.

66. BROSS, L. *et al.* 2000. DNA double-strand breaks in immunoglobulin genes undergoing somatic hypermutation. Immunity **13:** 589–597.

67. ZAN, H. *et al.* 2003. AID-dependent generation of resected double-strand DNA breaks and recruitment of Rad52/Rad51 in somatic hypermutation. Immunity **18:** 727–738.

68. RATTRAY, A.J. & J.N. STRATHERN. 2003. Error-prone DNA polymerases: when making a mistake is the only way to get ahead. Annu. Rev. Genet. **37:** 31–66.

69. DIAZ, M. & P. CASALI. 2002. Somatic immunoglobulin hypermutation. Curr. Opin. Immunol. **14:** 235–240.

70. GOODMAN, M.F. 2002. Error-prone repair DNA polymerases in prokaryotes and eukaryotes. Annu. Rev. Biochem. **71:** 17–50.

71. SCHENTEN, D. *et al.* 2002. DNA polymerase kappa deficiency does not affect somatic hypermutation in mice. Eur. J. Immunol. **32:** 3152–3160.

72. LONGACRE, A. *et al.* 2003. Ig gene somatic hypermutation in mice defective for DNA polymerase delta proofreading. Int. Immunol. **15:** 477–481.

73. BERTOCCI, B. *et al.* 2002. Cutting edge: DNA polymerases mu and lambda are dispensable for Ig gene hypermutation. J. Immunol. **168:** 3702–3706.

74. ESPOSITO, G. *et al.* 2000. Mice reconstituted with DNA polymerase beta-deficient fetal liver cells are able to mount a T cell–dependent immune response and mutate their Ig genes normally. Proc. Natl. Acad. Sci. USA **97:** 1166–1171.

75. ROGOZIN, I.B. *et al.* 2001. Somatic mutation hotspots correlate with DNA polymerase eta error spectrum. Nat. Immunol. **2:** 530–536.

76. PAVLOV, Y.I. *et al.* 2002. Correlation of somatic hypermutation specificity and A-T base pair substitution errors by DNA polymerase eta during copying of a mouse immunoglobulin kappa light chain transgene. Proc. Natl. Acad. Sci. USA **99:** 9954–9959.

77. ZENG, X. *et al.* 2001. DNA polymerase eta is an A-T mutator in somatic hypermutation of immunoglobulin variable genes. Nat. Immunol. **2:** 537–541.

78. ZAN, H. *et al.* 2001. The translesion DNA polymerase zeta plays a major role in Ig and bcl-6 somatic hypermutation. Immunity **14:** 643–653.

79. JOHNSON, R.E. *et al.* 2000. Eukaryotic polymerases iota and zeta act sequentially to bypass DNA lesions. Nature **406:** 1015–1019.

80. FAILI, A. *et al.* 2002. Induction of somatic hypermutation in immunoglobulin genes is dependent on DNA polymerase iota. Nature **419:** 944–947.

81. GIBBS, P.E. *et al.* 1998. A human homolog of the *Saccharomyces cerevisiae* REV3 gene, which encodes the catalytic subunit of DNA polymerase zeta. Proc. Natl. Acad. Sci. USA **95:** 6876–6880.
82. DIAZ, M. *et al.* 2001. Decreased frequency of somatic hypermutation and impaired affinity maturation but intact germinal center formation in mice expressing antisense RNA to DNA polymerase zeta. J. Immunol. **167:** 327–335.
83. SEKI, M., F. MARINI & R. D. WOOD. 2003. POLQ (pol theta), a DNA polymerase and DNA-dependent ATPase in human cells. Nucleic Acids Res. **31:** 6117–6126.
84. SHARIEF, F.S. *et al.* 1999. Cloning and chromosomal mapping of the human DNA polymerase theta (POLQ), the eighth human DNA polymerase. Genomics **59:** 90–96.
85. MAGA, G. *et al.* 2002. DNA polymerase theta purified from human cells is a high-fidelity enzyme. J. Mol. Biol. **319:** 359–369.
86. SEKI, M. *et al.* 2004. High-efficiency bypass of DNA damage by human DNA polymerase Q. EMBO J. **23:** 4484–4494.
87. KAWAMURA, K. *et al.* 2004. DNA polymerase theta is preferentially expressed in lymphoid tissues and upregulated in human cancers. Int. J. Cancer **109:** 9–16.
88. SHIMA, N. *et al.* 2003. Phenotype-based identification of mouse chromosome instability mutants. Genetics **163:** 1031–1040.
89. SHIMA, N., R.J. MUNROE & J.C. SCHIMENTI. 2004. The mouse genomic instability mutation chaos 1 is an allele of pol θ that exhibits genetic interaction with Atm. Mol. Cell Biol. **24:** 10381–10389.
90. ZAN, H. *et al.* 2005. DNA polymerase theta plays a major role in immunoglobulin somatic hypermutation. Immunity. Submitted.
91. BURGERS, P.M. *et al.* 2001. Eukaryotic DNA polymerases: proposal for a revised nomenclature. J. Biol. Chem. **276:** 43487–43490.

Cross-Reactivity of IgM and IgG Anticardiolipin Antibodies with Oxidized–Low Density Lipoproteins

J. DAMOISEAUX, A. D. JEYASEKHARAN, R. THEUNISSEN, AND J. W. COHEN TERVAERT

Department of Clinical and Experimental Immunology, University Hospital Maastricht, Maastricht, the Netherlands

ABSTRACT: Anticardiolipin antibodies (aCLAs) and antibodies to oxidized–low density lipoproteins (oxLDL) are associated with two distinct diseases: the antiphospholipid syndrome and atherosclerosis. Because both diseases may be apparent in patients with systemic lupus erythematosus (SLE), it is important to establish the relationship between these two types of antibodies. In the present study, we examined whether sera containing IgM and/or IgG aCLAs also react with LDL that has been oxidized by conjugation with malondialdehyde (MDA-LDL) or by incubation with copper ions (Cu-LDL). Results revealed a clear correlation between IgM aCLAs and IgM anti-MDA-LDL antibodies, and a weak correlation between IgG aCLAs and IgG anti-Cu-LDL antibodies. Cross-reactivity between both antibodies seemed to be limited. Because aCLAs are heterogeneous, only a minor subset of these antibodies may cross-react with oxLDL. Therefore, identification of both antibodies may be relevant for determination of the prognosis of accelerated atherosclerosis in SLE patients.

KEYWORDS: antiphospholipid syndrome; autoantibodies; atherosclerosis

INTRODUCTION

Anticardiolipin antibodies (aCLAs) are a diagnostic marker for the antiphospholipid syndrome (APS). This syndrome is characterized clinically by arterial or venous thrombosis or (recurrent) fetal loss.[1] This disorder may occur alone (primary APS) or secondary to systemic lupus erythematosus (SLE; secondary APS).[2] Although the autoantibodies were originally thought to be directed to negatively charged phospholipids, they actually recognize protein cofactors, predominantly β_2-glycoprotein-I (β_2-GPI) and prothrombin.[3] Antibodies to oxidized–low density lipoproteins (oxLDL), on the other hand, have been associated with atherosclerosis and were found to be predictive of the progression of carotid atherosclerosis and myocardial infarction.[4–7] Several studies indicate that cross-reactivity exists between aCLAs and anti-oxLDL antibodies.[8,9] Sera of APS patients, as well as affinity-

Address for correspondence: Jan Damoiseaux, Ph.D., Department of Clinical and Experimental Immunology, University Hospital Maastricht, P. O. Box 5800, 6202 AZ Maastricht, the Netherlands. Voice: +31-43-3881433; fax: +31-43-3884164.
    jdam@limm.azm.nl

Ann. N.Y. Acad. Sci. 1050: 163–169 (2005). © 2005 New York Academy of Sciences.
doi: 10.1196/annals.1313.016

purified IgG aCLAs derived from their sera, bind exclusively to cardiolipin that has undergone lipid peroxidation, and not to a cardiolipin analogue unable to undergo lipid peroxidation. Later, it was demonstrated that these antibodies bind to protein cofactors, like β_2-GPI, only as a consequence of covalent adduct formation between oxidized phospholipids and these protein cofactors.[10] Opinion is divided as to whether pathogenic aCLAs are directed against the β_2-GPI/phospholipid complex, against a cryptic epitope revealed on β_2-GPI by binding to phospholipids, or whether they are of low affinity and require an increased density of immobilized β_2-GPI.[11] Interestingly, β_2-GPI also interacts with oxLDL,[12] and this interaction may generate similar immunogenic neoepitopes as obtained by complex formation between β_2-GPI and cardiolipin. It was demonstrated recently that ligands specific for β_2-GPI are oxidized forms of cholesteryl linoleate and that autoantibodies associated with arterial thrombosis in APS patients may be directed to the complex of oxLDL and β_2-GPI.

To further explore the relationship between aCLAs and anti-oxLDL antibodies, we determined in the present study whether sera containing IgM and/or IgG aCLAs also react with LDL that has been oxidized by conjugation with malondialdehyde (MDA-LDL) or by incubation with copper ions (Cu-LDL).

MATERIALS AND METHODS

Patient Samples

Samples from patients that were repeatedly tested for the presence of anticardiolipin antibodies were selected from our laboratory store based on the presence and/or absence of IgM and IgG aCLAs. A total of 65 samples were used in this study: 20 were double-negative, 14 were single-positive for IgM aCLAs, 16 were single-positive for IgG aCLAs, and 15 were double-positive (TABLE 1). Samples were selected irrespective of clinical diagnosis.

Anticardiolipin Antibodies

The presence of IgM and IgG aCLAs was measured by β_2-GP1–dependent ELISA (Varelisa Cardiolipin Antibody assay; Pharmacia & Upjohn Diagnostics, Freiburg, Germany) according to the instructions of the manufacturer. Results of IgM and IgG aCLAs are expressed in IgM antiphospholipid units (MPL) and IgG antiphospholipid units (GPL), respectively. Each unit corresponds to the binding activity of 1 μg/mL of aCLA that was purified from the Harris' standards (Louisville APL Diagnostics, Inc., Louisville, KY) by affinity chromatography. Cutoff values were 15 MPL for IgM aCLAs and 15 GPL for IgG aCLAs, based on information obtained from the analysis of 400 healthy controls by the manufacturer.

Anti-oxLDL Antibodies

LDL was isolated from the plasma of a healthy subject by ultracentrifugation in a potassium bromide discontinuous gradient according to Redgrave et al.[13] Potassium bromide and EDTA were removed by rapid filtration through disposable desalting columns (Econo-Pac 10 DG, Bio-Rad, Hercules, CA). The LDL protein content was determined according to Lowry et al.[14] Native LDL was either freshly used for preparation of oxLDL or stored at 4°C in PBS under N_2, with 1 mg/mL EDTA as a preservative. Two established forms of oxidation were used to generate oxLDL: malondialdehyde modification (MDA-LDL) with 100 µL of 0.5 M MDA for every mg of LDL for 3 h at 37°C,[15] and Cu oxidation (Cu-LDL) with $CuSO_4$ at a final concentration of 5 mM for 20 h at 37°C.[16]

Native LDL and oxidized LDL were diluted in PBS to 100 µg LDL/mL, and 100 µL per well (i.e., 10 µg/well) was incubated in microtiter plates (Nunc MaxiSorp, Nalge Nunc, Rochester, NY) overnight at 4°C. Wells were washed five times with a washing buffer containing 0.01 M Tris, 0.15 M NaCl, and 0.05% Tween 20 (pH 8.0). The wells were then incubated in triplicate with patient serum in a 1:100 dilution, 100 µL/well, in incubation buffer containing 0.1 M Tris, 0.3 M NaCl, and 0.05% Tween 20 (pH 8.0) and kept overnight at 4°C; a positive control was used on each plate to test for intra-assay variation. The next day, plates were washed five times with washing buffer and incubated with either alkaline phosphatase-conjugated goat F(ab′)₂ anti-human IgG (Fc)–specific conjugate (American Qualex, San Clemente, CA) or horseradish peroxidase conjugated to goat F(ab′)₂ anti-human IgM (Cappel, Durham, NC) for 1 h at 37°C. After washing five times with washing buffer, IgG anti-oxLDL antibodies were visualized by adding nitrophenyl phosphate as substrate. After 30 min on a shaking platform at room temperature, plates were read at 405 nm. For detection of IgM anti-oxLDL antibodies, orthophenylene diamine (OPD) was used as substrate and, after stopping the reaction at 15 min by adding 50 µL of 4 N H_2SO_4, the plates were read at 490 nm. Results are expressed as the ratio of anti-oxLDL to anti-LDL antibodies as described before.[17]

Statistical Analysis

All data are presented as median (range) unless stated otherwise. Because values for aCLAs and anti-oxLDL antibodies had a non-Gaussian distribution, all evaluations were nonparametric. Hence, the Spearman r value was calculated for correlation statistics with the continuous variables, and the Mann-Whitney U-test was used for determining a correlation with the aCLA status (i.e., positive vs. negative). Analyses were performed with GraphPad Prism version 3.00 (GraphPad Software Inc., San Diego, CA). A two-sided P value $< .05$ was considered to indicate statistical significance.

RESULTS

Of the 65 samples used in this study, the aCLA levels are presented in TABLE 1 as median (range) within the samples that were aCLA-negative, single-positive for IgM or IgG, and double-positive. In total, 29 samples were positive for IgM aCLAs (24 MPL; 15–100 MPL) and 31 were positive for IgG aCLAs (24 GPL; 16–100 GPL). TABLE 1 also contains the anti-oxLDL antibody ratios for MDA- and Cu-LDL. In the total cohort, the median MDA-LDL antibody ratios were 3.2 (1.5–14.6) and 2.4 (1.4–10.3) for IgM and IgG, respectively. The median Cu-LDL antibody ratios for IgM and IgG were 5.4 (1.8–9.4) and 1.5 (0.9–3.5), respectively. If cross-reactivity between aCLAs and anti-oxLDL antibodies involves the majority of these antibodies, it is to be expected that samples with IgM aCLAs, but not IgG aCLAs, have higher

TABLE 1. Anti-oxLDL antibody ratios in samples with different aCLA reactivity

IgM aCLA	IgG aCLA	N	IgM MDA-LDL	IgG MDA-LDL	IgM Cu-LDL	IgG Cu-LDL
Negative	Negative	20	2.5 (1.6–5.5)	2.3 (1.4–5.1)	5.1 (1.8–7.6)	1.4 (1.0–3.2)
Positive 26 (15–100)	Negative	14	3.3 (1.7–10.0)	2.5 (1.4–5.1)	6.2 (3.2–9.4)	1.4 (1.0–2.1)
Negative	Positive 23 (16–100)	16	2.9 (1.5–7.9)	2.6 (1.7–9.2)	4.7 (2.2–9.0)	1.6 (0.9–3.5)
Positive 24 (15–100)	Positive 32 (16–100)	15	7.3 (3.0–15.0)	2.7 (1.8–10.3)	6.1 (2.8–9.2)	1.6 (1.1–3.1)

NOTE: Results are presented as the median (range).
ABBREVIATIONS: aCLA, anticardiolipin antibodies; LDL, low density lipoproteins; Cu-LDL, copper-modified LDL; MDA-LDL, malondialdehyde-modified LDL; oxLDL, oxidized LDL.

TABLE 2. Correlation between aCLA and anti-oxLDL antibody ratio

	aCLA antibody level[a]	aCLA antibody status[b]
IgM aCLA & IgM MDA-LDL	0.52 ($P < .0001$)	$P = .0002$
IgM aCLA & IgM Cu-LDL	0.20 ($P = .10$; n.s.)	$P = .08$ (n.s.)
IgG aCLA & IgG MDA-LDL	0.26 ($P = .04$)	$P = .08$ (n.s.)
IgG aCLA & IgG Cu-LDL	0.27 ($P = .03$)	$P = .05$

ABBREVIATIONS: aCLA, anticardiolipin antibodies; LDL, low density lipoproteins; Cu-LDL, copper-modified LDL; MDA-LDL, malondialdehyde-modified LDL; n.s., not significant; oxLDL, oxidized LDL.
[a]Results of the correlation between aCLA antibody level and anti-oxLDL antibody ratio are presented as Spearman r value (P value).
[b]Results of the correlation between aCLA antibody status and anti-oxLDL antibody ratio are presented as P value (Mann-Whitney U-test).

IgM and lower IgG anti-oxLDL antibody ratios than samples with IgG aCLAs, but not IgM aCLAs. However, our results revealed that there was no difference in the four different anti-oxLDL antibody ratios between samples that were positive for IgM aCLAs ($n = 14$) or for IgG aCLAs ($n = 16$) (TABLE 1).

Next, we analyzed whether there was a correlation between aCLA levels and anti-oxLDL antibody ratios for IgM and IgG, respectively. A clear correlation was found between IgM aCLA levels and IgM anti-MDA-LDL antibody ratios (FIG. 1A). The Spearman r was 0.52 for these parameters ($P < .0001$). The correlation was also highly significant ($P = .0002$) when calculated on the basis of IgM aCLA status, that is, positive or negative (FIG. 1B). In addition, a weak association was observed between IgG aCLAs (level and status) and IgG anti-Cu-LDL antibody ratio (TABLE 2).

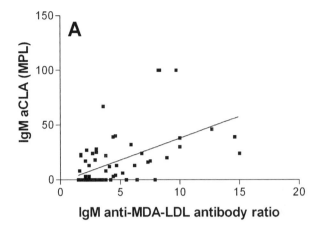

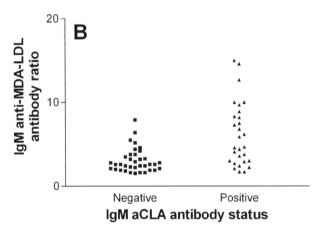

FIGURE 1. Correlation between IgM aCLAs and IgM anti-MDA-LDL antibody ratio. Both the IgM aCLA levels (**A**) as well as the IgM aCLA status (**B**) are correlated with the IgM anti-MDA-LDL antibody ratio. Correlation of the IgM aCLA levels gives a Spearman *r* value of 0.52 (*P* < .0001); the correlation of the IgM aCLA status is also statistically significant (*P* = .0002).

DISCUSSION

To establish the possibility of cross-reactivity between aCLAs and anti-oxLDL antibodies, we determined the presence of IgM and IgG anti-oxLDL antibodies in sera that were selected on the basis of the presence or absence of IgM and/or IgG aCLAs. Our data revealed a highly significant correlation between IgM aCLAs (both antibody level and status) and IgM anti-MDA-LDL antibody ratios. In addition, a weak association was observed between IgG aCLAs and IgG anti-Cu-LDL antibody ratios. However, IgM and IgG anti-oxLDL antibodies were not different between samples that were positive for either IgM or IgG aCLAs. The absence of such a difference suggests that cross-reactivity between aCLAs and anti-oxLDL antibodies is limited and, based on our correlation data, it concerns autoantibodies of the IgM isotype rather than the IgG isotype. Our results are not in agreement with previous studies that show that there is cross-reactivity. Indeed, it has been reported that binding of aCLAs to solid-phase cardiolipin is inhibited by oxLDL in 16 of 21 sera from SLE patients.[8] This discrepancy can be explained by the fact that no standard method is available for detection of anti-oxLDL antibodies.[18] In particular, the availability of β_2-GPI for binding to oxLDL may be a critical factor for detection of cross-reactivity between aCLAs and oxLDL. On the other hand, aCLAs are known to be very heterogeneous, and the patient population in our study is heterogeneous as well. Our results, therefore, do not exclude the possibility that a fraction of aCLAs, or aCLAs of a restricted patient population, does cross-react with oxLDL.

Although aCLAs are part of the classification criteria of APS,[1] anti-oxLDL antibodies have been associated with atherosclerosis.[4–7] Immunoassays for both autoantibodies are hampered by lack of standardization.[18,19] If there is substantial cross-reactivity between these antibodies, the clinical value of detection of both antibodies should be low. However, the limited association, as observed in our study, does not support this conclusion.

Cross-reactivity between aCLAs and anti-oxLDL antibodies may be important for understanding a possible link between arterial thrombosis and atherosclerosis. Recent reports have established that SLE patients undergo accelerated atherosclerosis.[20,21] Antibodies to oxLDL facilitate the formation of foam cells by receptor-mediated uptake of oxLDL by macrophages. This is particularly true for IgG antibodies; IgM anti-oxLDL antibodies may, however, be protective in atherosclerosis.[22] IgG antibodies to the complex of oxLDL and β_2-GPI also facilitate receptor-mediated phagocytosis of oxLDL,[12] and these antibodies are associated with arterial thrombosis, that is, myocardial infarction and cerebrovascular disease.[23] Therefore, it can be anticipated that SLE patients with secondary APS are at increased risk to develop accelerated atherosclerosis. However, the presence of aCLAs is not a risk factor for accelerated atherosclerosis in SLE.[20,21] Unfortunately, these studies did not discriminate between the presence of IgG and IgM aCLAs. This seems relevant because if cross-reactivity is present, the first may be pathogenic, whereas the latter may be protective. Furthermore, because only some aCLAs cross-react with anti-oxLDL antibodies, it can be postulated that only those antibodies that cross-react might be associated with accelerated atherosclerosis in SLE.

In conclusion, our data reveal that cross-reactivity between aCLAs and anti-oxLDL antibodies is rather limited. Therefore, these results do not support previous findings indicating that both antibodies have their own clinical value. Given the fact that aCLAs are heterogeneous and that a minor subset of these antibodies may cross-react with oxLDL, identification of these antibodies may be relevant for understanding the link between aCLAs and atherosclerosis.

REFERENCES

1. WILSON, W.A., A.E. GHARAVI, T. KOIKE, et al. 1999. International consensus statement on preliminary classification criteria for definite antiphospholipid syndrome: report of an international workshop. Arthritis Rheum. **42:** 1309–1311.

2. HUGHE, G.R. 1993. The antiphospholipid syndrome: ten years on. Lancet **342:** 341–344.
3. GALLI, M., P. COMFURIUS, C. MAASSEN, *et al.* 1990. Anticardiolipin antibodies (ACA) directed not to cardiolipin but to a plasma protein cofactor. Lancet **335:** 1544–1547.
4. SALONEN, J.T., S. YLA-HERTTUALA, R. YAMAMOTO, *et al.* 1992. Autoantibody against oxidised LDL and progression of carotid atherosclerosis. Lancet **339:** 883–837.
5. ARMSTRONG, V.W., E. WIELAND, F. DIEDRICH, *et al.* 1994. Serum antibodies to oxidised low-density lipoprotein in pre-eclampsia and coronary heart disease. Lancet **343:** 1570.
6. PUURUNEN, M., M. MANTTARI, V. MANNINEN, *et al.* 1994. Antibody against oxidized low-density lipoprotein predicting myocardial infarction. Arch. Intern. Med. **154:** 2605–2609.
7. BERGMARK, C., R. WU, U. DE FAIRE, *et al.* 1995. Patients with early-onset peripheral vascular disease have increased levels of autoantibodies against oxidized LDL. Arterioscler. Thromb. Vasc. Biol. **15:** 441–445.
8. VAARALA, O., G. ALFTHAN, M. JAUHIAINEN, *et al.* 1993. Crossreaction between antibodies to oxidised low-density lipoprotein and to cardiolipin in systemic lupus erythematosus. Lancet **341:** 923–925.
9. HORKKO, S., T. OLEE, L. MO, *et al.* 2001. Anticardiolipin antibodies from patients with the antiphospholipid antibody syndrome recognize epitopes in both beta(2)-glycoprotein 1 and oxidized low-density lipoprotein. Circulation **103:** 941–946.
10. HORKKO, S., E. MILLER, D.W. BRANCH, *et al.* 1997. The epitopes for some antiphospholipid antibodies are adducts of oxidized phospholipid and β2 glycoprotein 1 (and other proteins). Proc. Natl. Acad. Sci. USA **94:** 10356–10361.
11. GILES, I.P., D.A. ISENBERG, D.S. LATCHMAN, *et al.* 2003. How do antiphospholipid antibodies bind β2-glycoprotein I? Arthritis Rheum. **48:** 2111–2121.
12. KOBAYASHI, K., E. MATSUURA, Q. LIU, *et al.* 2001. A specific ligand for beta(2)-glycoprotein I mediates autoantibody-dependent uptake of oxidized low density lipoprotein by macrophages. J. Lipid Res. **42:** 697–709.
13. REDGRAVE, T.G., D.C. ROBERTS & C.E. WEST. 1975. Separation of plasma lipoproteins by density-gradient ultracentrifugation. Anal. Biochem. **65:** 42–49.
14. LOWRY, O.H., N.J. ROSEBROUGH, A.L. FARR, *et al.* 1951. Protein measurement with the Folin phenol reagent. J. Biol. Chem. **193:** 265–275.
15. PALINSKI, W., S. YLA-HERTTUALA, M.E. ROSENFELD, *et al.* 1990. Antisera and monoclonal antibodies specific for epitopes generated during oxidative modification of low density lipoprotein. Arteriosclerosis **10:** 325–335.
16. STEMME, S., B. FABER, J. HOLM, *et al.* 1995. T lymphocytes from human atherosclerotic plaques recognize oxidized low density lipoprotein. Proc. Natl. Acad. Sci. USA **92:** 3893–3897.
17. SWETS, B.P., D.A. BROUWER & J.W. COHEN TERVAERT. 2001. Patients with systemic vasculitis have increased levels of autoantibodies against oxidized LDL. Clin. Exp. Immunol. **124:** 163–167.
18. NARVANEN, O., A. ERKKILA & S. YLA-HERTTUALA. 2001. Evaluation and characterization of EIA measuring autoantibodies against oxidized LDL. Free Radic. Biol. Med. **31:** 769–777.
19. TINCANI, A., F. ALLEGRI, M. SANMARCO, *et al.* 2001. Anticardiolipin antibody assay: a methodological analysis for a better consensus in routine determinations—a cooperative project of the European Antiphospholipid Forum. Thromb. Haemost. **86:** 575–583.
20. ASANUMA, Y., A. OESER, A.K. SHINTANI, *et al.* 2003. Premature coronary-artery atherosclerosis in systemic lupus erythematosus. N. Engl. J. Med. **349:** 2407–2415.
21. ROMAN, M.J., B.A. SHANKER, A. DAVIS, *et al.* 2003. Prevalence and correlates of accelerated atherosclerosis in systemic lupus erythematosus. N. Engl. J. Med. **349:** 2399–2406.
22. SHAW, P.X., S. HORKKO, M.K. CHANG, *et al.* 2000. Natural antibodies with the T15 idiotype may act in atherosclerosis, apoptotic clearance, and protective immunity. J. Clin. Invest. **105:** 1731–1740.
23. MATSUURA, E., K. KOBAYASHI, T. KOIKE, *et al.* 2002. Autoantibody-mediated atherosclerosis. Autoimmun. Rev. **1:** 348–353.

The Anti-Alpha-Actinin Test Completes Anti-DNA Determination in Systemic Lupus Erythematosus

S. CROQUEFER,[a] Y. RENAUDINEAU,[a] S. JOUSSE,[b] P. GUEGUEN,[a] S. ANSART,[c] A. SARAUX,[b] AND P. YOUINOU[a]

[a]Laboratory of Immunology, [b]Unit of Rheumatology, [c]Unit of Internal Medicine, Brest University Medical School, Brest, France

ABSTRACT: In murine systemic lupus erythematosus (SLE) models, nephritogenic anti-dsDNA IgG has been shown to cross-react with a kidney antigen, alpha-actinin, and to be critical in renal pathogenesis. In humans, studies of anti-alpha-actinin antibodies (Abs) are scarce, and these antibodies remain to be evaluated. We have thus far tested sera from patients with SLE ($n = 103$), rheumatoid arthritis (RA, $n = 93$), and primary Sjögren syndrome (pSS, $n = 34$), and from healthy subjects ($n = 160$), for the presence of anti-alpha-actinin and anti-DNA Abs. The latter were tested using several methods [IIF on *Crithidia luciliae* (Crit) and ELISA using dsDNA]. Anti-alpha-actinin Abs were confirmed by Western blot. Sera from 23 of 103 SLE patients, 3 of 93 RA patients, 1 of 33 pSS patients, and 1 of 160 controls scored positive for anti-alpha-actinin Abs. In SLE, the positivity was significantly associated with anti-dsDNA reactivity (22 of 23): 19 of 23 sera were alpha-actinin-positive/dsDNA-positive and 13 were alpha-actinin-positive/Crit-positive. Few cases were alpha-actinin-positive/dsDNA-negative: 1 SLE, 3 RA, and 1 control. Furthermore, anti-alpha-actinin Abs have been detected at high level before or at the early stage of lupus nephritis when compared with active and inactive SLE without kidney manifestations.

KEYWORDS: systemic lupus erythematosus; anti-DNA; anti-alpha-actinin

INTRODUCTION

Systemic lupus erythematosus (SLE) is a systemic autoimmune disease characterized by the production of a multitude of autoantibodies (autoAbs) in conjunction with dysfunctional B cells.[1] Among these, antibodies to DNA are most frequently detected and have been used in the diagnosis and monitoring of individuals with SLE. These anti-DNA antibodies are known to be heterogeneous with respect to class specificity, DNA-precipitation capacity, and affinity. Thus, optimal screening procedures include anti-double-stranded (ds) DNA and anti-native (n) DNA deter-

Address for correspondence: Prof. Pierre Youinou, Laboratory of Immunology, Brest University Medical School Hospital, BP824, F29609 Brest, France. Voice: +(33)-2-98-22-33-84; fax: +(33)-2-98-22-38-47.

youinou@univ-brest.fr

Ann. N.Y. Acad. Sci. 1050: 170–175 (2005). © 2005 New York Academy of Sciences.
doi: 10.1196/annals.1313.017

minations using an ELISA and an immunofluorescence assay on *Crithidia luciliae*, respectively.

Cross-reactivity between anti-dsDNA monoclonal antibodies (mAbs) and glomerular antigens has been documented. These antigens include heparan sulfate,[2] phosphorylcholine,[3] ribosomal P protein,[4] translation factor EF-2,[5] laminin,[6] and alpha-actinin.[7,8] When administered to normal mice, anti-laminin/anti-dsDNA H241[6] and anti-actinin/anti-dsDNA R4A[7] mAbs deposit in glomeruli. However, administration of R4A mAb, but not H241 mAb, has been shown to induce glomerular damage and massive proteinuria. Consequently, anti-alpha-actinin Abs have been suspected to be involved in the induction of glomerular pathology.

To date, the prevalence of anti-alpha-actinin Abs and the association between anti-DNA and anti-alpha-actinin Abs have not been established in SLE or in other connective tissue diseases.

RESULTS AND DISCUSSION

Alpha-Actinin

In humans, four alpha-actinin genes encode highly homologous proteins that normally form head-to-tail homodimers. Although alpha-actinin 1 and 4 are ubiquitously expressed, alpha-actinin 2 and 3 are located predominantly in muscle. Interestingly, actinin 4 is detected solely in the kidney. It is found in podocytes, capillaries, and larger blood vessels, and is accessible on the surface of mesangial cells.[7,8] The best-defined function of alpha-actinin 4 is to cross-link and bundle actin filaments. Nevertheless, alpha-actinin 4 has also been found to interact with a large panel of other proteins.

Patients with alpha-actinin 4 mutations[9] and a null mice model[10] display glomerular disease, suggesting a fundamental role for alpha-actinin 4 in glomerular function.

Anti-DNA Antibodies Bind Directly to Glomerular Alpha-Actinin

Two different mechanisms have been proposed to explain the glomerular pathophysiology of anti-DNA. First, anti-DNA Abs may complex with nucleosomes before deposition in glomeruli (immune-complex theory). In the second hypothesis, anti-DNA Abs cross-react with kidney-specific antigens.

The prerequisite for the second theory includes the recognition of a glomerular kidney antigen by a subpopulation of anti-DNA Abs. This binding must be independent of nucleosomal immune complexes, which can be excluded by DNase treatment. Specific peptides should have the capacity to block binding of anti-DNA Abs to renal tissue *in vivo* and thus to block glomerular damage. This has been elegantly demonstrated in mice using anti-alpha-actinin/anti-dsDNA R4A mAb.[7,11]

Detection of Anti-Alpha-Actinin Antibodies

An anti-alpha-actinin assay was developed according to Mason *et al.*[12] with minor modifications. Plates were coated with chicken alpha-actinin in 0.1 M sodium carbonate, pH 9.6. The plates were left to evaporate overnight at 37°C. After three washes in phosphate-buffered saline (PBS), plates were saturated with 200 μL PBS

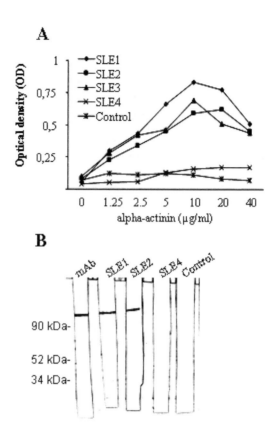

FIGURE 1. Anti-alpha-actinin Abs in SLE. (**A**) Determination of optimal alpha-actinin concentration in an anti-alpha-actinin ELISA. (**B**) Western blots for anti-alpha-actinin Abs. SLE1–3 are anti-alpha-actinin-positive/anti-dsDNA-positive; SLE4 is anti-alpha-actinin-negative/anti-dsDNA-positive; healthy control is anti-alpha-actinin-negative/anti-dsDNA-negative.

containing 2% bovine serum albumin (BSA) for 1 h at 37°C. Individual sera diluted 1:200 in PBS with 1% BSA were added and incubated for 90 min at 37°C. After washing, bound antibodies were detected using a goat anti-human IgG conjugated to alkaline phosphatase and subsequently developed with the substrate, *p*-nitrophenyl phosphate. Absorbance was read at 405 nm. Positive sera were used to determine the optimal concentration of alpha-actinin. Thus, a concentration of 10 µg/mL was used for the anti-alpha-actinin assay, as we observed an antibody-binding reduction at higher concentrations (FIG. 1). Absorbance values for antigen-free wells were systematically subtracted from those of alpha-actinin wells.

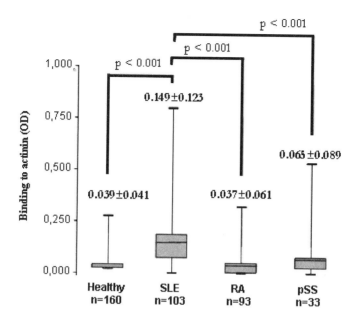

FIGURE 2. Box-plot of alpha-actinin-specific IgG levels as measured by ELISA. OD values in controls ($n = 160$) and in SLE ($n = 103$), RA ($n = 93$), and pSS ($n = 33$) patients are shown. Results are expressed as mean ± SD.

Prevalence of Anti-Alpha-Actinin Antibodies

The mean optical densities (OD ± SD) of anti-alpha-actinin Abs were 0.149 ± 0.123 for the SLE patients ($n = 103$); 0.039 ± 0.041 for the healthy controls ($n = 160$; $P < .001$, Student's test); 0.037 ± 0.061 for the 93 RA patients ($P < .001$ compared with SLE patients, and nonsignificant compared with controls); and 0.065 ± 0.089 for the 33 pSS patients ($P < .001$ compared with SLE patients, and nonsignificant compared with controls). (See FIG. 2.)

Positive sera (25 of 102 SLE, 2 of 160 controls, 4 of 93 RA, and 1 of 30 pSS) were tested for alpha-actinin reactivity after migration on SDS-PAGE. Therefore, the presence of anti-alpha-actinin Abs was confirmed by Western blotting (WB) for 23 SLE patients (22.5%), 1 healthy control (0.6%), 3 RA patients (3.1%), and 1 pSS patient (3.3%).

So far, in SLE, the anti-alpha-actinin assay has high specificity (99.4%), but poor sensitivity (21.6%), compared with healthy controls. The specificity decreased to 96.7% when the SLE population was compared with RA and pSS populations.

Correlation with Anti-DNA Antibodies in SLE

The correlation between anti-alpha-actinin and anti-DNA Abs was evaluated as follows: Double anti-alpha-actinin/anti-DNA Ab reactivity was detected in 22 of 23 SLE patients and 1 of 1 pSS patient, and absent in 3 of 3 RA patients and 1 of 1 healthy control. When both autoAbs were detected, specificity reached 100% and

TABLE 1. Correlation between anti-alpha-actinin, anti-dsDNA, and anti-nDNA in patients with SLE, along with the homogeneous aspect on HEp-2 cells

	Anti-dsDNA		Anti-nDNA		Homogeneous aspect	
	+	−	+	−	+	−
Anti-alpha-actinin						
Positive ($n = 23$)	19	4	13	10	13	10
Negative ($n = 80$)	16	64	12	68	22	58
	$P < .0001$		$P = .0001$		$P = .02$	

99.2% when SLE was compared with healthy controls and with RA and pSS populations, respectively.

Interestingly, in SLE, anti-alpha-actinin Abs were more likely to be associated with anti-dsDNA detected by ELISA (19 of 23) than with anti-nDNA using *Crithidia luciliae* (13 of 23). A homogeneous aspect on HEp-2 cells (13 of 23) was also correlated with anti-alpha-actinin detection (TABLE 1).

When regarding Ab titers, anti-dsDNA-positive/anti-alpha-actinin-positive sera were associated with high titers of anti-dsDNA Abs (0.848 ± 0.434), in contrast to anti-dsDNA-positive/anti-alpha-actinin-negative sera (0.304 ± 0.132). A similar correlation was also found with anti-nDNA-positive/anti-alpha-actinin-positive sera (titer $\geq$ 1:100) compared with anti-nDNA-positive/anti-alpha-actinin-negative sera (titer < 1:100).

High Levels of Anti-Alpha-Actinin Antibodies Observed in Nephritis Lupus

Clinical data were available for 15 of 22 anti-alpha-actinin-positive/anti-DNA-positive patients. They were divided into three subgroups: inactive SLE ($n = 5$), active SLE ($n = 5$), and SLE with nephritis or before onset of lupus nephritis ($n = 5$). The mean ODs for anti-alpha-actinin and anti-dsDNA Abs were 0.311 ± 0.072 and 0.322 ± 0.301 in inactive SLE, 0.297 ± 0.071 and 0.873 ± 0.552 in active SLE, and 0.456 ± 0.237 and 0.886 ± 0.560 in SLE with nephritis, respectively. So far, high levels of anti-dsDNA Abs seem to be associated with active SLE and SLE nephritis, although high levels of anti-alpha-actinin Abs are also associated with nephritis. This information must now be confirmed in a much larger population.

CONCLUSIONS

Anti-alpha-actinin antibody determination may be helpful in the diagnosis of SLE to improve anti-dsDNA specificity. High titers of anti-alpha-actinin/anti-dsDNA Abs were indeed present in sera of SLE patients with active nephritis. Nevertheless, some patients possess anti-alpha-actinin/anti-dsDNA Abs without nephritis, at the lowest levels, suggesting associations with other tissue injury.

ACKNOWLEDGMENTS

Many thanks are due to Cindy Séné and Simone Forest for secretarial assistance.

REFERENCES

1. RENAUDINEAU, Y. *et al.* 2004. Dysfunctional B cells in systemic lupus erythematosus. Autoimmun. Rev. **3:** 516–523.
2. FAABER, P. *et al.* 1986. Cross-reactivity of human and murine anti-DNA antibodies with heparan sulfate: the major glycosaminoglycan in glomerular basement membranes. J. Clin. Invest. **77:** 1824–1830.
3. SHARMA, A., D.A. ISENBERG & B. DIAMOND. 2001. Cross-reactivity of human anti-dsDNA antibodies to phosphorylcholine: clues to their origin. J. Autoimmun. **16:** 479–484.
4. TAKEDA, I., K. RAYNO, M. WOLFSON-REICHLIN & M. REICHLIN. 1999. Heterogeneity of anti-dsDNA antibodies in their cross-reaction with ribosomal P protein. J. Autoimmun. **13:** 423–428.
5. ALBERDI, F. *et al.* 2001. Cross-reaction of lupus anti-dsDNA antibodies with protein translation factor EF-2. Clin. Immunol. **98:** 293–300.
6. MADAIO, M.P. *et al.* 1987. Murine monoclonal anti-DNA antibodies bind directly to glomerular antigens and form immune deposits. J. Immunol. **138:** 2883–2889.
7. DEOCHARAN, B., X. QING, J. LICHAUCO & C. PUTTERMAN. 2002. α-Actinin is a cross-reactive renal target for pathogenic anti-DNA antibodies. J. Immunol. **168:** 3072–3078.
8. MOSTOSLAVSKY, G. *et al.* 2001. Lupus anti-DNA autoantibodies cross-react with a glomerular structural protein: a case for tissue injury by molecular mimicry. Eur. J. Immunol. **31:** 1221–1227.
9. KAPLAN, J.M. *et al.* 2000. Mutations in ACTN4, encoding alpha-actinin 4, cause familial focal segmental glomerulosclerosis. Nat. Genet. **24:** 251–256.
10. KOS, C.H. *et al.* 2003. Mice deficient in α-actinin-4 have severe glomerular disease. J. Clin. Invest. **111:** 1683–1690.
11. GAYNOR, B. *et al.* 1997. Peptide inhibition of glomerular deposition of an anti-DNA antibody. Proc. Natl. Acad. Sci. USA **94:** 1955–1960.
12. MASON, L.J. *et al.* 2004. Is α-actinin a target for pathogenic anti-DNA antibodies in lupus nephritis? Arthritis Rheum. **50:** 866–877.

The Relevance of Autoantigen Source and Cutoff Definition in Antichromatin (Nucleosome) Antibody Immunoassays

DANILO VILLALTA,[a] RENATO TOZZOLI,[b] NICOLA BIZZARO,[c] ELIO TONUTTI,[d] ANNA GHIRARDELLO,[e] AND ANDREA DORIA[e]

[a]Immunologia Clinica e Virologia, Azienda Ospedaliera "S. Maria degli Angeli", Pordenone, Italy

[b]Laboratorio di Chimica Clinica e Microbiologia, Ospedale di Latisana, Latisana, Italy

[c]Laboratorio di Patologia Clinica, Ospedale di Tolmezzo, Tolmezzo, Italy

[d]Immunopatologia e Allergologia, Azienda Ospedaliera "S. Maria della Misericordia", Udine, Italy

[e]Istituto di Reumatologia, Università di Padova, Padova, Italy

ABSTRACT: In the last few years, several reports have shown that chromatin (nucleosome) represents the main autoantigen-immunogen in systemic lupus erythematosus (SLE) and that specific antibodies are an important marker of the disease. To verify the clinical sensitivity and specificity of antinucleosome autoantibodies (Anuas), we evaluated three ELISA immunoassay methods using different autoantigen preparations: Quanta Lite Chromatin, Medizym Anti-nucleo, and Nucleosome IgG Elisa. We compared the results with those obtained using two ELISA assays for determining anti-native DNA (anti-ndNA) antibodies: Axis-Shield and EliA dsDNA. We tested sera from 321 patients: 101 with SLE and 220 controls—48 with infectious diseases; 73 with autoimmune rheumatic disease (20 with rheumatoid arthritis, 30 with systemic sclerosis, and 23 with primary Sjögren's syndrome), and 99 healthy subjects. Using the manufacturer-recommended cutoff, the sensitivity for the three kits was 69%, 78%, and 74%, and specificity was 100%, 94.6%, and 95.0%, respectively. Using the cutoff corresponding to 95% specificity, the sensitivity of the methods for the AnuA assay was 86%, 77%, and 74%—higher than obtained with the two ELISA methods for anti-ndNA (65% and 64%). This study demonstrates that (1) the commercial reagents employed in clinical laboratories for AnuA detection show good sensitivity and high specificity; (2) AnuAs are more sensitive than anti-ndNA antibodies for diagnosing SLE; and (3) different solid-phase antigen preparations and methods used to define cutoff levels may affect a test's clinical performance.

KEYWORDS: antichromatin antibodies; antinucleosome antibodies; autoantigen source; cutoff; anti-native DNA antibodies; receiver operating characteristic (ROC) curves; systemic lupus erythematosus (SLE)

Address for correspondence: Danilo Villalta, Immunologia Clinica e Virologia, Azienda Ospedaliera "S. Maria degli Angeli", Via Montereale 24, 33170 Pordenone, Italy. Voice: +39-0434-399281; fax: +39-0434-399344.
danilo.villalta@aopn.fvg.it

Ann. N.Y. Acad. Sci. 1050: 176–184 (2005). © 2005 New York Academy of Sciences.
doi: 10.1196/annals.1313.018

INTRODUCTION

Patients suffering from systemic lupus erythematosus (SLE) present numerous serum autoantibodies, some of which (e.g., anti-native DNA [ndNA], anti-Sm, anti-ribosomal P proteins) are highly specific.[1–3] In recent years, interest in antichromatin/antinucleosome antibodies (ANuAs) has revived as a result of the development and marketing of enzyme-linked immunosorbent assays (ELISAs), and of the demonstration of ANuAs' pathogenic role in SLE.[4–6] These autoantibodies were the first to be described in SLE, with the demonstration of the LE cell phenomenon by Hargraves in 1948[7] (although the antibody specificity responsible for the phenomenon was not yet known at the time). Later studies proved that LE correlates with the presence of ANuA,[8] especially those that demonstrated that nucleosomes (but not free ndNA or histones) were able to inhibit the LE phenomenon.[9]

Nucleosomes, which are the basic elements of chromatin, are formed by approximately 146 base pairs of DNA wrapped around the $(H2A-H2B-H3-H4)_2$ histone octamer. The full nucleosome also contains a molecule of histone H1 located outside each core particle, where DNA enters and exits the nucleosome. The nucleosome sequence, joined by the length of DNA linker and closely packed by H1 histones, forms chromatin. In addition to ndNA (40%) and histones (40%), in its complex form, it contains nonhistone proteins, RNA, and other macromolecules (20%). Any autoantibodies directed toward these latter molecular structures are not considered to be antichromatin antibodies. Rather, antichromatin antibodies comprise antibodies directed toward histone epitopes exposed in chromatin, toward ndNA (B form), and toward conformational epitopes created by the interactions between ndNA and the various core histones (nucleosome-specific autoantibodies). Consequently, ANuAs and antichromatin antibodies can be considered synonymous for all practical purposes.

In the last decade, numerous studies have been conducted to evaluate the accuracy of ANuAs in the diagnosis of SLE. They have done so nearly always by comparing ANuAs with anti-ndNA antibodies, which are still considered to be the "golden marker" for SLE. In the different studies, the diagnostic sensitivity of ANuAs varied considerably (31–100%) and was generally greater than that of anti-ndNA antibodies (21–82%).[10–21] ANuAs' specificity for SLE was high, though some researchers reported a high percentage of positivity in patients with scleroderma (SSc) and mixed connective tissue disease (MCTD).[11,13,22] ANuAs' different levels of reported diagnostic accuracy can be explained partly by the different characteristics of the populations selected, and partly by the different diagnostic systems and procedures used, by which the cutoff values were obtained.

The purpose of our study was to evaluate the performance of three different commercial ELISA methods for determining ANuAs using three different antigen preparations. We sought to evaluate whether these preparations, associated with the cutoff definition procedure, can significantly influence the diagnostic accuracy of the test.

MATERIALS AND METHODS

Patients

We prospectively investigated 101 consecutive SLE patients who met at least four of the criteria of the American College of Rheumatology (ACR).[23,24] Their male/female ratio was 1/9, mean age 29.8 ± 9.0 years, and mean disease duration 80.2 ± 69.6 months. As controls (N = 220), sera were collected from 99 healthy subjects (HS); 73 patients with other rheumatic diseases (30 with SSc, 23 with primary Sjögren's syndrome [pSS], and 20 with rheumatoid arthritis [RA]); and 48 patients with infectious disease (ID). All the sera were stored at −80°C and assayed in the same laboratory for ANuAs and anti-nDNA antibodies.

ANuA Assay Methods

We used three different commercial ELISAs for the quantitative measurement of ANuA. All the assays were performed in accordance with the manufacturers' instructions.

(a) Quanta Lite Chromatin ELISA (Inova Diagnostics Inc., San Diego, CA). In this method, a highly purified calf thymus chromatin was used as the autoantigen; histone H1 and nonhistone proteins were removed from the chromatin during the purification process, according to the Burlingame and Rubin method.[25]

(b) Medizym Anti-nucleo (Medipan Diagnostika, Selchow, Germany). In this method, the nucleosomes were prepared from chicken erythrocytes according to the procedure of Bruns and colleagues.[26] The absence of histone H1 was verified by electrophoresis; however, the manufacturer supplied no information as to the presence of nonhistone proteins in the preparation.

(c) Nucleosome IgG Elisa kit (D-Tek, Wavre, Belgium). The autoantigen used is prepared from calf thymus chromatin by removing the nonhistone proteins. No nuclease or DNAse is used during the process, so histone H1 is not removed, and the polynucleosome backbone of the chromatin is not enzymatically stripped into mononucleosomes. Agarose gel electrophoresis revealed that the antigen is composed of DNA fragments ranging from 1000 to 4180 bp. SDS-polyacrylamide gel electrophoresis (SDS-PAGE) analysis showed only protein bands corresponding to the core histone subcomponents (H2A, H2B, H3, H4) and histone H1.

Anti-nDNA Antibodies

Immunoglobulin G (IgG) anti-nDNA antibodies were assayed by indirect immunofluorescence (IIF) on *Crithidia luciliae* (cutoff titer = 1:20) (Euroimmun, Lübeck, Germany) and by two ELISA methods: Axis-Shield (Dundee, UK) and EliA (Pharmacia Diagnostics, Freiburg, Germany). For both ELISA methods, the cutoff value was determined by means of receiver operating characteristic (ROC) curves corresponding to a specificity of 95%; the cutoffs proved to be 30 IU/mL and 15 IU/mL, respectively.

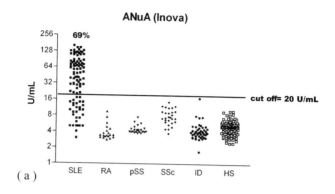

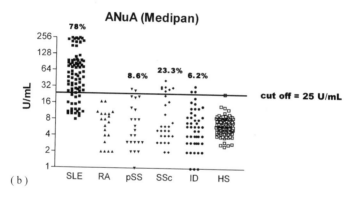

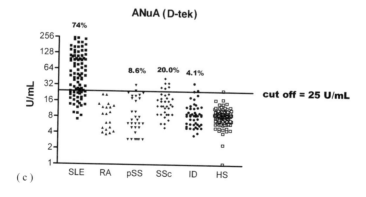

FIGURE 1. Distribution of antinucleosome antibody (ANuA) levels in U/mL, obtained with the Inova (**a**), Medipan (**b**), and D-Tek (**c**) methods, in 101 SLE patients and 220 controls (RA, rheumatoid arthritis; pSS, primary Sjögren's syndrome; SSc, systemic sclerosis; HS, healthy subject; ID, infectious diseases), using the cutoff levels recommended by the manufacturers. The values shown indicate the percentage of positive samples in each group.

TABLE 1. Diagnostic sensitivity (SE) and specificity (SP) of methods employed to measure antinucleosome antibodies

Method	Manufacturer's cutoff (U/mL)	SE (%)	SP (%)	Cutoff value (SP = 95%)	SE (%)	Cutoff value (SP = 98%)	SE (%)	Cutoff value (SP = 99%)	SE (%)
Inova	20	69	100	9.5	86	12.0	81	13.5	77
Medipan	25	78	94.6	26.5	77	33.1	72	35.5	67
D-Tek	25	74	95.0	24.1	74	29.5	67	32.5	64

NOTE: Manufacturer-recommended cutoffs were used. The diagnostic sensitivity of the three methods with cutoff levels corresponding to a specificity of 95%, 98%, and 99% were obtained with ROC curves.

Statistical Analysis

For all three methods relating to the ANuA assay, sensitivity and specificity were first calculated using the cutoff recommended by the manufacturer. We subsequently performed ROC curves and recalculated the sensitivity values for each method, fixing the specificity levels at 95%, 98%, and 99%. The correlations between the nonparametric, unpaired data were calculated with the Mann-Whitney U-test. P values below 0.05 were considered statistically significant.

RESULTS

Using the cutoff value recommended by each manufacturer, the sensitivity was 69%, 78%, and 74%, and the specificity was 100%, 94.6% and 95.0%, for the Inova, Medipan, and D-Tek methods, respectively (TABLE 1). None of the patients in the control population presented an ANuA value exceeding the cutoff value (20 U/mL) with the Inova method (FIG. 1a), whereas 8.6% of pSS patients, 23.3% of SSc patients, and 6.2% of ID patients presented values exceeding the cutoff value (25 U/mL) with the Medipan method (FIG. 1b). Also, 8.6% of pSS patients, 20% of SSc patients, and 4.1% of ID patients presented values exceeding the cutoff (25 U/mL) with the D-Tek method (FIG. 1c).

These data, taken together, reveal that the positivity rate in the control population was always just above the cutoff value. As the graphs clearly show, the section of the control population that presented the greatest number of positives represents the SSc patients. Although none of the SSc patients tested positive with the Inova method, their mean ANuA value was significantly higher (8.1 ± 2.7; $P < .0001$) than in the other control groups (RA, 4.1 ± 1.7; pSS, 4.4 ± 0.9; ID, 4.4 ± 2.2; HS, 5.1 ± 1.6).

To better compare diagnostic accuracy using the data obtained from the ROC curves, cutoff levels corresponding to a specificity of 95%, 98%, and 99% were established for each method, respectively. The new values, expressed in U/mL, and their corresponding diagnostic sensitivity are reported in TABLE 1. Although the Inova method was the least sensitive when the cutoff value recommended by the manufacturer was used, it proved to be more sensitive (86%) than the other two methods at a cutoff corresponding to a specificity of 95%, as well as maintaining

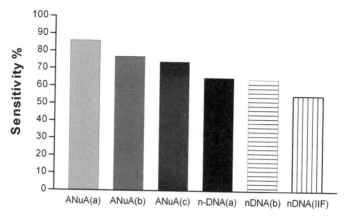

FIGURE 2. Diagnostic sensitivity of the three methods used to assay ANuAs—Inova (a), Medipan (b), and D-Tek (c)—compared with two ELISA methods for anti-nDNA antibody measurement: Axis-Shield (a), EliA (b), and the indirect immunofluorescence (IIF) method on *Crithidia luciliae.*

higher sensitivity at specificity values of 98% and 99%. Overall, when the specificity was set at 95%, the sensitivity of all three ANuA assay methods exceeded that obtained with the two ELISA methods for the anti-nDNA assay (FIG. 2); it was even greater compared with the data obtained using the IIF method on *Crithidia luciliae* (55%).

DISCUSSION

According to recent clinical evidence, nucleosomes play a central role in SLE pathogenesis, at both the immunizing and effector stages. Further, antinucleosome immune response seems likely to be one of the earliest signs of humoral auto-immunity in lupus-prone mice.[27,28] Based on results from observations of murine models, human studies have been conducted in which ANuAs were detected in a high percentage of patients with SLE, both at the initial stages of the disease and in the absence of anti-nDNA antibodies.[10]

After these initial observations in humans, researchers conducted numerous studies to evaluate the diagnostic efficacy of ANuAs in SLE, using ELISA techniques that often differed in terms of the antigen preparation used. The most commonly used antigen preparations were (*a*) reconstituted nucleosomal particles obtained by adding nDNA to the histone core or to histone dimers, and (*b*) purified chromatin, generally obtained by digestion with micrococcal nuclease and subsequent removal of histone H1 and other proteins with 0.5 M NaCl extraction at a neutral pH. An analysis of the main articles that have recently appeared in the literature indicates a diagnostic sensi-tivity of between 70% and 100%,[10,13–16,20,21] although some authors have reported sensitivity below 50%.[11,12] In most cases, specificity exceeded 90%,[20,26,30,31] whereas Wallace and colleagues[11] reported specificity of 45%, Schlumberger and colleagues[22] reported 71%, and Amoura and colleagues[13] reported 90%.

In terms of diagnostic accuracy, these differences can be explained by two main factors: (1) the various antigen substrates used—especially their degree of purification compared with nonhistone proteins, such as transcription factors or other regulatory proteins bound to DNA; and (2) the procedures used to select the cutoff value to distinguish between positive and negative results. In particular, in the three studies reported above,[11,13,22] in which specificity ranged from 45% to 90%, positivity for ANuAs in patients who were not suffering from SLE was found mainly in the group of scleroderma patients.

As other authors have already reported,[6,29] this positivity may have various explanations. The study by Wallace and colleagues[11] used DNA reconstituted with denatured H2A and H2B as antigen, and this may have allowed for the binding of serum autoantibodies present in scleroderma, which are directed towards histone epitopes not usually exposed in native chromatin. Also, in the study by Schlumberger and colleagues,[22] a low-purity-antigen preparation containing residues of Scl70 was used, as the authors themselves later demonstrated.[30] In fact, by using a new antigen preparation, the authors showed that none of the SSc patients tested positive. (They treated the antigen preparation with a high-salt solution and discontinuous sucrose density-gradient centrifugation to eliminate nonhistone proteins that are able to bind strongly to chromatin.) Finally, in the study by Amoura et al.,[13] which used a home-made H1-stripped mononucleosome as the antigen, the definition of the cutoff (2 SDs above the mean value in 406 healthy controls) seems to have been the main factor associated with positivity at a low titer among the scleroderma patients.

IMPLICATIONS

The results of our study confirm the importance of defining the cutoff value in order to determine the diagnostic accuracy of the various ANuA assay methods. If the cutoff recommended by the manufacturer is used, the Inova method is the least sensitive (though demonstrating absolute specificity), whereas the other two methods show greater sensitivity but lower specificity.

To compare the diagnostic accuracy of the three methods more objectively, ROC curves were performed; the specificity levels for each method were set at 95%, 98%, and 99%; and the corresponding sensitivity values were evaluated.

As clearly emerged from analyzing the results obtained, the Inova method was the one that presented the best diagnostic efficiency overall, along with presenting the greatest antigen purity (removal of histone H1 and nonhistone proteins). The other two methods used different antigen substrates and a lower level of purification: the Medipan substrate contained no H1 histones, but no tests for the presence of nonhistone proteins were conducted; the D-Tek substrate did not contain nonhistone proteins, but possessed histone H1. However, patients not suffering from SLE always tested positive for ANuA at a low titer and, consequently, medium or high ANuA values proved highly specific for detecting SLE with all three methods, as already described.[20] Even using the Inova method, which uses a highly purified chromatin preparation, the mean ANuA value in the SSc patients was significantly higher than in the other control groups, though below the cutoff value.

Although autoantibody reactivity to nonhistone proteins such as Scl70 and centromere proteins can therefore be excluded with a high degree of probability in this case, this finding implies the presence of ANuA at low titers in SSc patients, as some authors have already described.[31] In addition, centromere protein A (CENP-A, one of three immunologically related centromere antigens that are important targets of the SSc autoantibody repertoire) has been shown to be a centromere-specific histone H3 variant.[32] SSc sera, by virtue of their polyclonality, may exhibit cross-reactive detection of nucleosomes mediated by homologies in selective regions of core histone H3 and CENP-A.

Finally, our study clearly demonstrates that if the specificity level is set at 95% for all the ELISA methods, the diagnostic sensitivity of all the AnuA assay methods will be greater than that of the anti-ndNA assay methods. This fact establishes the existence of a group of SLE patients (10–15%) who present with ANuAs on diagnosis, but not anti-ndNA antibodies.

In conclusion, ANuAs seem to possess greater diagnostic efficiency than anti-ndNA. Differences in diagnostic accuracy among the ANuA assay methods appear to be caused by the method the manufacturer selected to define the cutoff value, and by the degree of purity of the antigen preparation used. The reasons that low ANuA values are present in SSc patients have not yet been established with certainty.

REFERENCES

1. STOLLAR, B.D. 1975. The specificity and applications of antibodies to helical nucleic acids. CRC Crit. Rev. Biochem. **3:** 45–69.
2. TAN, E.M. 1989. Antinuclear antibodies: diagnostic markers for autoimmune diseases and probes for cell biology. Adv. Immunol. **44:** 93–151.
3. ELKON, K.B., E. BONFA & N. BROT. 1992. Antiribosomal antibodies in systemic lupus erythematosus. Rheum. Dis. Clin. N. Am. **18:** 377–390.
4. TAX, W.J., C. KRAMERS, M.C. VAN BRUGGEN & J.H. BERDEN. 1995. Apoptosis, nucleosomes, and nephritis in systemic lupus erythematosus. Kidney Int. **48:** 666–673.
5. AMOURA, Z., J.C. PIETTE, J.F. BACH & S. KOUTOUZOV. 1999. The key role of nucleosomes in lupus. Arthritis Rheum. **42:** 833–843.
6. KOUTOUZOV, S., A.L. JERONIMO, H. CAMPOS & Z. AMOURA. 2004. Nucleosomes in the pathogenesis of systemic lupus erythematosus. Rheum. Dis. Clin. North Am. **30:** 529–558.
7. HARGRAVES, M.M., H. RICHMOND & R. MORTON. 1948. Presentation of two bone marrow elements: the "tart" cell and the "LE" cell. Mayo Clin. Proc. **23:** 25–28.
8. HOLMAN, H.R. & H.G. KUNKEL. 1957. Affinity between serum factor and cell nuclei and nucleoprotein. Science **126:** 162–163.
9. REKVIG, O.P. & K. HANNESTAD. 1981. Lupus erythematosus (LE) factors recognize both nucleosomes and viable human leukocytes. Scand. J. Immunol. **13:** 597–604.
10. BURLINGAME, R.W., M.L. BOEY, G. STARKEBAUM & R.L. RUBIN. 1994. The central role of chromatin in autoimmune responses to histones and DNA in systemic lupus erythematosus. J. Clin. Invest. **94:** 184–192.
11. WALLACE, D.J., H.C. LIN, G.Q. SHEN & J.B. PETER. 1994. Antibodies to histone (H2A-H2B)-DNA complexes in the absence of antibodies to double-stranded DNA or to (H2A-H2B) complexes are more sensitive and specific for scleroderma-related disorders than for lupus. Arthritis Rheum. **37:** 1795–1797.
12. CHABRE, H., Z. AMOURA, J.C. PIETTE, *et al.* 1995. Presence of nucleosome-restricted antibodies in patients with systemic lupus erythematosus. Arthritis Rheum. **38:** 1485–1491.
13. AMOURA, Z., S. KOUTOUZOV, H. CHABRE, *et al.* 2000. Presence of anti-nucleosome autoantibodies in a restricted set of connective tissue diseases: antinucleosome antibodies of the IgG3 subclass are markers of renal pathogenicity in systemic lupus erythematosus. Arthritis Rheum. **43:** 76–84.

14. MOHAN, C., F. LIU, C. XIE & R.C. WILLIAMS JR. 2001. Anti-subnucleosome reactivities in systemic lupus erythematosus (SLE) patients and their first-degree relatives. Clin. Exp. Immunol. **123:** 119–126.
15. MIN, D.J., S.J. KIM, S.H. PARK, et al. 2002. Anti-nucleosome antibody: significance in lupus patients lacking anti-double-stranded DNA antibody. Clin. Exp. Rheumatol. **20:** 13–18.
16. GHILLANI-DALBIN, P., Z. AMOURA, P. CACOUB, et al. 2003. Testing for anti-nucleosome antibodies in daily practice; a monocentric evaluation in 1696 patients. Lupus **12:** 833–837.
17. CAIRNS, A.P., S.A. MCMILLAN, A.D. CROCKARD, et al. 2003. Antinucleosome antibodies in the diagnosis of systemic lupus erythematosus. Ann. Rheum. Dis. **62:** 272–273.
18. CERVERA, R., O. VINAS, M. RAMOS-CASALS, et al. 2003. Anti-chromatin antibodies in systemic lupus erythematosus: a useful marker for lupus nephropathy. Ann. Rheum. Dis. **62:** 431–434.
19. GONZALEZ, C., B. GARCIA-BERROCAL, O. HERRAEZ, et al. 2004. Anti-nucleosome, anti-chromatin, anti-dsDNA and anti-histone antibody reactivity in systemic lupus erythematosus. Clin. Chem. Lab. Med. **42:** 266–272.
20. GHIRARDELLO, A., A. DORIA, S. ZAMPIERI, et al. 2004. Antinucleosome antibodies in SLE: a two-year follow-up study of 101 patients. J. Autoimmun. **22:** 235–240.
21. SIMON, J.A., J. CABIEDES, E. ORTIZ, et al. 2004. Anti-nucleosome antibodies in patients with systemic lupus erythematosus of recent onset. Potential utility as a diagnostic tool and disease activity marker. Rheumatology (Oxford) **43:** 220–224.
22. SCHLUMBERGER, W. et al. 2002. Diagnostic relevance of autoantibodies against nucleosomes. Autoimmun. Rev. **1:** 32.
23. TAN, E.M., A.S. COHEN, J.F. FRIES, et al. 1982. The revised criteria for the classification of systemic lupus erythematosus. Arthritis Rheum. **25:** 1271–1277.
24. HOCHBERG, M.C. 1997. Updating the American College of Rheumatology revised criteria for the classification of systemic lupus erythematosus. Arthritis Rheum. **40:** 1725.
25. BURLINGAME, R.W. & R.L. RUBIN. 1990. Subnucleosome structures as substrates in enzyme-linked immunosorbent assays. J. Immunol. Methods **134:** 187–199.
26. BRUNS, A., S. BLASS, G. HAUSDORF, et al. 2000. Nucleosomes are major T and B cell autoantigens in systemic lupus erythematosus. Arthritis Rheum. **43:** 2307–2315.
27. AMOURA, Z., H. CHABRE, S. KOUTOUZOV, et al. 1994. Nucleosome-restricted antibodies are detected before anti-dsDNA and/or antihistone antibodies in serum of MRL-Mp lpr/lpr and +/+ mice, and are present in kidney eluates of lupus mice with proteinuria. Arthritis Rheum. **37:** 1684–1688.
28. LADERACH, D., S. KOUTOUZOV, J.F. BACH & A.M. YAMAMOTO. 2003. Concomitant early appearance of anti-ribonucleoprotein and anti-nucleosome antibodies in lupus prone mice. J. Autoimmun. **20:** 161–170.
29. BURLINGAME, R.W. & R. CERVERA. 2002. Anti-chromatin (anti-nucleosome) antibodies. Autoimmun. Rev. **1:** 321–328.
30. SUER, W., C. DAHNRICH, W. SCHLUMBERGER & W. STOCKER. 2004. Autoantibodies in SLE but not in scleroderma react with protein-stripped nucleosomes. J. Autoimmun. **22:** 325–334.
31. HMIDA, Y., P. SCHMIT, G. GILSON & R.L. HUMBEL. 2002. Failure to detect antinucleosome antibodies in scleroderma: comment on the article by Amoura et al. Arthritis Rheum. **46:** 280–282.
32. PALMER, D.K., K. O'DAY, H.L. TRONG, et al. 1991. Purification of the centromere-specific protein CENP-A and demonstration that it is a distinctive histone. Proc. Natl. Acad. Sci. USA **88:** 3734–3738.

Value of a New Automated Fluorescence Immunoassay (Elia) for PR3 and MPO-ANCA in Monitoring Disease Activity in ANCA-Associated Systemic Vasculitis

RENATO ALBERTO SINICO, ANTONELLA RADICE, CATERINA CORACE, LUCAFRANCESCO DI TOMA, AND ETTORE SABADINI

Dipartimento di Nefrologia e Immunologia, Azienda Ospedaliera, Ospedale San Carlo Borromeo, Milano, Italy

ABSTRACT: The value of anti-neutrophil cytoplasmic antibody (ANCA) detection for monitoring disease activity in ANCA-associated systemic vasculitis (AASV) remains controversial. The aim of our work was to rate the performance of a new automated fluorescence PR3 and MPO-ANCA immunoassay (Elia) for monitoring disease activity in AASV. We evaluated 100 serum samples from 71 AASV patients (with Wegener's granulomatosis, microscopic polyangiitis, and Churg-Strauss syndrome) as well as sera from 58 pathological and 35 normal controls. In addition to PR3 and MPO-ANCA Elia, we performed indirect immunofluorescence and "homemade" PR3 and MPO-ANCA ELISA tests. In AASV patients, ANCA levels were correlated with disease activity, according to the Birmingham Vasculitis Activity Score (BVAS). We derived cutoff limits from receiver operating characteristic (ROC) curve analysis comparing AASV with pathological controls. Our results showed that Elia and ELISA had comparable sensitivity (76%) and specificity (95%). The analysis of active versus inactive status and correlation with ANCA levels showed a clear difference between BVAS Group I (score ≤ 4) and BVAS Group II (scores > 4) (AUC = 0.86 vs. 0.72; relative risk [RR] = 2.4; $P < 0.0001$) for PR3-ANCA, but not for MPO-ANCA (AUC = 0.94 vs. 0.87; RR = 1.48; $P = 0.46$). Serial serum samples from 16 patients were examined in detail. For the majority of patients, for both PR3 and MPO-ANCA, change in titer was strongly associated with change in BVAS score. Our data showed a good correlation between ANCA titer (especially for PR3) and AASV disease activity. We recommend that ANCA titer be used to monitor AASV disease activity with the caveat that a few exceptions, in particular with MPO-ANCA, are possible.

KEYWORDS: anti-neutrophil cytoplasmic antibodies (ANCAs); ANCA-associated systemic vasculitis; Wegener's granulomatosis; microscopic polyangiitis; Churg-Strauss syndrome; disease activity; Birmingham Vasculitis Activity Score (BVAS)

Address for correspondence: Dr. R. A. Sinico, Dipartimento di Nefrologia e Immunologia, Azienda Ospedaliera, Ospedale San Carlo Borromeo, Via Pio Secondo, 3, 20153 Milano, Italy. Voice: +39-02-4022-2489/2344; fax: +39-02-4022-2222.
renato.sinico@oscb.sined.net

Ann. N.Y. Acad. Sci. 1050: 185–192 (2005). © 2005 New York Academy of Sciences.
doi: 10.1196/annals.1313.019

INTRODUCTION

Anti-neutrophil cytoplasmic antibodies (ANCAs) are autoantibodies that react with antigens in the cytoplasm of neutrophils and monocytes.[1] They were first described in 1982 by Davies and colleagues in a few patients with necrotizing glomerulonephritis and symptoms of systemic vasculitis.[2] By means of an indirect immunofluorescence (IIF) test on ethanol-fixed neutrophils, two main staining patterns can be identified: a cytoplasmic staining pattern (C-ANCA) and a perinuclear one (P-ANCA).

In 1985, van der Woude and colleagues showed that ANCAs that produced a diffuse granular cytoplasmic staining pattern on ethanol-fixed neutrophils (C-ANCAs) were a sensitive marker for Wegener's granulomatosis.[3] Subsequently, ANCAs producing a perinuclear staining pattern on ethanol-fixed neutrophils (P-ANCAs) were described in patients with idiopathic necrotizing crescentic glomerulonephritis (iNCGN) and microscopic polyangiitis.[4] In these patient categories, myeloperoxidase (MPO) and proteinase 3 (PR3) were identified as the main target antigens of P-ANCA and C-ANCA, respectively.[4,5] Later, it became apparent that ANCA (mainly P-ANCA) could also be found in patients with a wide range of nonvasculitic disorders such as inflammatory bowel disease, primary sclerosing cholangitis, autoimmune liver diseases, rheumatoid arthritis, malignancies, and infections.[6–10] In these disorders, ANCAs are almost always directed against neutrophil constituents other than PR3 and MPO or against unknown antigens.[11–16]

Whereas several studies using meta-analyses[17–21] have confirmed the diagnostic value of ANCAs in ANCA-associated systemic vasculitis (AASV), the role of ANCAs in monitoring disease activity in patients with vasculitis is still controversial. For example, Boomsma and colleagues concluded that taking serial measurements of ANCA levels (detected by enzyme-linked immunosorbent assay [ELISA] or immunofluorescence) is valuable for the early prediction of relapses in patients with Wegener's granulomatosis.[22] However, Kerr and coworkers found that changes in serial C-ANCA titers temporally correlate with changes in disease activity in only 24% of patients.[23] More recently, the predictive value of ANCA testing was investigated in 55 patients with Wegener's granulomatosis enrolled in a randomized prospective trial comparing corticosteroids with oral or pulse cyclophosphamide.[24] Although relapses were more frequent when ANCA remained positive or reappeared, discordance between ANCA titers and disease activity was not unusual. The authors concluded that, in the absence of clinical manifestations, ANCA titers alone could serve only as a warning signal, but not as a tool for making treatment decisions.

The results of a retrospective study published in 2003 were completely different. Here the authors stated that taking serial measurements of PR3- and MPO-ANCA titers in patients with AASV during remission can help predict relapses, and that preemptive increases in immunosuppression following four-fold rises in titer reduce the risk of relapses.[25] Moreover, they reported, adjusting immunosuppression based on lesser titer changes appeared to result in a favorable outcome.

The aim of our work was to evaluate the performance of a new automated enzyme fluoroimmunoassay, the EliA system (Pharmacia Diagnostics GmbH & Co., KG, Freiburg, Germany), for detecting PR3- and MPO-ANCA and monitoring disease activity in AASV. We compared the results with those obtained using indirect immunofluorescence and with a "homemade" classic ELISA.

PATIENTS AND METHODS

Patients

In total, 193 serum samples were studied retrospectively:

(1) 100 serum samples from 71 patients with AASV (27 with Wegener's granulomatosis, 32 with microscopic polyangiitis, and 12 with Churg-Strauss syndrome);

(2) 58 serum samples from 58 disease controls (with cryoglobulinemia, Henoch-Schonlein purpura, systemic lupus erythematosus, other connective tissue diseases, or inflammatory bowel diseases); and

(3) 35 serum samples from blood donors.

The patients with AASV were classified using the names and definitions adopted by the Chapel Hill Consensus Conference.[26] Wegener's granulomatosis and microscopic polyangiitis were diagnosed according to the European Vasculitis Study Group (EUVAS) criteria,[18] and Churg-Strauss syndrome was diagnosed according to the 1990 American College of Rheumatology (ACR) criteria.[27] Disease activity was measured using the Birmingham Vasculitis Activity Score (BVAS).[28]

Methods

PR3 and MPO-ANCA were detected with the EliA system. This system uses single polystyrene wells coated with purified PR3 or MPO, which are automatically dispensed and processed in the UniCAP 100 instrument. ANCAs were also detected using indirect immunofluorescence on ethanol-fixed granulocytes, and antigen-specific PR3 and MPO traditional ELISA, as previously described.[18,29]

Statistical Analysis

Statistical analysis was carried out using the statistical software Analyse-It (Leeds, UK). Cutoff limits were derived from receiver operating characteristic (ROC) curve analysis comparing AASV with pathological controls. For this purpose, only the first serum sample was considered.

RESULTS

Sensitivity and specificity were found to be comparable for both EliA and ELISA (TABLE 1). Sensitivity varied from 50% to 82.3% for ELISA, and from 58.3% to 84.4% for EliA in Churg-Strauss syndrome and microscopic polyangiitis, respectively. Specificity in normal controls was 100%, whereas specificity in disease controls was 95% for both assays. All blood donors tested negative using both test systems.

For the evaluation of C-ANCA and P-ANCA positivity, immunofluororescence on ethanol-fixed granulocytes demonstrated higher sensitivity than ELISA/EliA; in AASV, C-ANCA and P-ANCA combined totaled 81.7% versus 76.1/76.1%. However, specificity was much lower owing to P-ANCA positivity in some patients in the disease control group (data not shown).

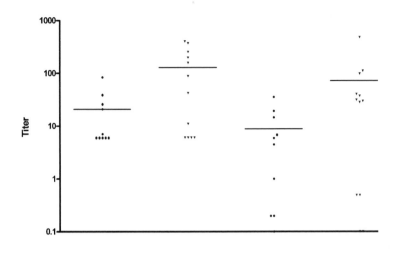

FIGURE 1. Values of PR3-ELISA and PR3-EliA in ANCA-associated systemic vasculitis according to Birmingham Vasculitis Activity Score (BVAS). BVAS Group I: BVAS ≤ 4 (inactive); BVAS Group II: BVAS > 4.

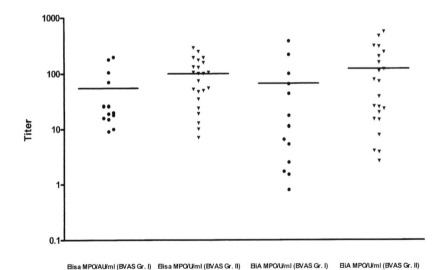

FIGURE 2. Values of MPO-ELISA and MPO-EliA in ANCA-associated systemic vasculitis according to Birmingham Vasculitis Activity Score (BVAS). BVAS Group I: BVAS ≤ 4; BVAS Group II: BVAS > 4.

TABLE 1. Sensitivity and specificity of the various assays

	No.	PR3-ELISA	PR3-EliA	MPO-ELISA	MPO-EliA	PR3 or MPO-ELISA	PR3 or MPO-EliA
		Sensitivity (%)					
Patients							
AASV	71	23.9	25.4	49.3	52.1	76.1	76.1
WG	27	51.9	51.9	25.9	22.2	77.8	74.1
MPA	32	9.4	12.5	68.8	75.0	82.3	84.4
CSS	12	0.0	0.0	50.0	58.3	50.0	58.3
		Specificity (%)					
Controls							
Disease controls	58	98.3	96.6	98.3	98.3	96.6	94.8
Normal controls	35	100.0	100.0	100.0	100.0	100.0	100.0

ABBREVIATIONS: AASV, ANCA-associated systemic vasculitis; WG, Wegener's granulomatosis; MPA, microscopic polyangiitis; CSS, Churg-Strauss syndrome.

A good agreement was found between ELISA and EliA (K = 0.88) and between C-ANCA and PR3-EliA or PR3-ELISA (K = 0.80 and 0.86, respectively), but not between P-ANCA and MPO-EliA or MPO-ELISA (0.55 and 0.52, respectively).

When patients with AASV were arbitrarily subdivided into two groups according to BVAS score (≤ 4 [inactive] or > 4 [active]), there was a good discrimination between the two groups in PR3-ANCA-positive patients ($P < 0.0001$ by F-test for both assays) (FIG. 1) but not in MPO-positive patients ($P = 0.51$ for MPO-ELISA; $P = 0.62$ for MPO-EliA by F-test) (FIG. 2).

To evaluate the ability of ANCA-EliA and ANCA-ELISA to monitor disease activity, 16 AASV patients were studied sequentially, and their ANCA values correlated with BVAS scores. For the majority of patients, a good association in change of titer and change in BVAS score was seen (data not shown). However, a few exceptions were observed with increasing ANCA titer but no change in disease activity.

DISCUSSION

Our study has shown that both systems (ELISA and EliA) have a good diagnostic sensitivity and specificity for AASV. Their overall sensitivity was ~75%, which, taking into account that some patients were studied during a remission phase and 12 patients had Churg-Strauss syndrome (known to be less strongly associated with ANCA), is quite high and compared well with sensitivity reported in previous studies.[18,19] As already known, the sensitivity of immunofluorescence was slightly better.[18,19] Specificity was at least 95% for EliA and ELISA, which was higher than that of immunofluorescence, where the specificity is lower owing both to the presence of P-ANCA not directed against MPO (for example in inflammatory bowel diseases) and to the interference of antinuclear antibodies.[7,8,30,31] For the majority of patients, a good association was found between changes in ANCA titers and changes in disease activity, as measured by BVAS.

Several studies, including large prospective ones, have shown that ANCAs have a high diagnostic value for AASV, provided that the correct methodology is used in the relevant clinical setting.[18–22] Results from these studies have demonstrated that ANCAs, detected by the immunofluorescence test (C-ANCA or P-ANCA), are a sensitive marker for AASV and have 80–90% sensitivity or greater. Unfortunately, immunofluorescence has low specificity (80% or less), which is caused mainly by positive P-ANCA in disease controls, such as ulcerative colitis. In these cases, P-ANCA can also indicate the presence of antinuclear antibodies, especially in systemic lupus erythematosus. The use of ELISA with purified antigens can improve specificity, which can reach 95% or more, but with a slight loss in sensitivity.[18–22]

Even though the value of ANCA for diagnostic purposes has been firmly established, the role of ANCA for monitoring disease activity is more controversial. Some groups have found a close relationship between ANCA titer and disease activity,[22,25] whereas others have not.[23,24]

CONCLUSIONS

In our hands, the new automated fluorescence immunoassay (EliA) performed at least as well as a classic "homemade" ELISA that has been in use in our laboratory for more than 10 years. Our results demonstrate that PR3- and MPO-ANCA EliAs show high sensitivity and very good specificity for AASV. In fact, these EliAs perform as well as a classical "homemade" ELISA. PR3-ANCA EliA (and PR3-ANCA ELISA) correlates with disease activity, although some exceptions are possible. However, MPO-ANCA EliA (and MPO-ANCA ELISA) correlates less strongly with disease activity.

Our data support the practice of measuring ANCA levels to monitor disease activity in AASV. In most instances, we found a significant association between BVAS score and ANCA, as measured by ELISA or EliA. However, exceptions occur regularly. Therefore, we agree with Girard and colleagues[24] that until unequivocal data are available showing that preemptive increases in immunosuppression following ANCA titer rises can reduce the risk of relapses, ANCA levels alone can serve only as a warning signal, but not as a tool for making treatment decisions.

REFERENCES

1. WIIK, A. 1989. Delineation of a standard procedure for indirect immunofluorescence detection of ANCA. APMIS Suppl. **6:** 12–13.
2. DAVIES, D.J., J.E. MORAN, J.F. NIALL & G.B. RYAN. 1982. Segmental necrotizing glomerulonephritis with antineutrophil antibody: possible arbovirus aetiology? Br. Med. J. (Clin. Res. Ed.) **285:** 606.
3. VAN DER WOUDE, F.J., N. RASMUSSEN, S. LOBATTO, et al. 1985. Autoantibodies against neutrophils and monocytes: tool for diagnosis and marker of disease activity in Wegener's granulomatosis. Lancet **1:** 425–429.
4. FALK, R.J. & I.C. JENNETTE. 1988. Anti-neutrophil cytoplasmic autoantibodies with specificity for myeloperoxidase in patients with systemic vasculitis and idiopathic necrotizing and crescentic glomerulonephritis. N. Engl. J. Med. **318:** 1651–1657.

5. GOLDSCHMEDING, R., C.E. VAN DER SCHOOT, D. TEN BOKKEL HUININK, *et al.* 1989. Wegener's granulomatosis autoantibodies identify a novel diisopropylfluorophosphate-binding protein in the lysosomes of normal human neutrophils. J. Clin. Invest. **84:** 1577–1587.

6. CAMBRIDGE, G., D.S. RAMPTON, T.R. STEVENS, *et al.* 1992. Anti-neutrophil cytoplasmic antibodies in inflammatory bowel disease: prevalence and diagnostic role. Gut **33:** 668–674.

7. VECCHI, M., M.B. BIANCHI, R.A. SINICO, *et al.* 1994. Antibodies to neutrophil cytoplasm in Italian patients with ulcerative colitis: sensitivity, specificity and recognition of putative antigens. Digestion. **55:** 34–39.

8. MULDER, A.H., G. HORST, E.B. HAAGSMA, *et al.* 1993. Prevalence and characterization of anti-neutrophil cytoplasmic antibodies in autoimmune liver diseases. Hepatology **17:** 411–417.

9. COREMANS, I.E., E.C. HAGEN, M.R. DAHA, *et al.* 1992. Antilactoferrin antibodies in patients with rheumatoid arthritis are associated with vasculitis. Arthritis Rheum. **35:** 1466–1475.

10. GROSS, W.L., W.H. SCHMITT & E. CSERNOK. 1993. ANCA and associated diseases: immunodiagnostic and pathogenetic aspects. Clin. Exp. Immunol. **91:** 1–12.

11. PEEN, E., S. ALMER, G. BODEMAR, *et al.* 1993. Anti-lactoferrin antibodies and other types of ANCA in ulcerative colitis, primary sclerosing cholangitis, and Crohn's disease. Gut **34:** 56–62.

12. HALBWACHS-MECARELLI, L., P. NUSBAUM, L.H. NOEL, *et al.* 1992. Antineutrophil cytoplasmic antibodies (ANCA) directed against cathepsin G in ulcerative colitis, Crohn's disease and primary sclerosing cholangitis. Clin. Exp. Immunol. **90:** 79–84.

13. KANEKO, K., Y. SUZUKI, Y. YAMASHIRO & K. YABUTA. 1993. Is p-ANCA in ulcerative colitis directed against β-glucuronidase? Lancet. **341:** 320.

14. VECCHI, M., A. SINICO, M.B. BIANCHI, *et al.* 1998. Recognition of bactericidal/permeability-increasing protein by perinuclear anti-neutrophil cytoplasmic antibody-positive sera from ulcerative colitis patients: prevalence and clinical significance. Scand. J. Gastroenterol. **33:** 1284–1288.

15. SINICO, R.A., C. POZZI, A. RADICE, *et al.* 1993. Clinical significance of antineutrophil cytoplasmic autoantibodies with specificity for lactoferrin in renal diseases. Am. J. Kidney Dis. **22:** 253–260.

16. MERKEL, P.A., R.P. POLISSON, Y. CHANG, *et al.* 1997. Prevalence of antineutrophil cytoplasmic antibodies in a large inception cohort of patients with connective tissue disease. Ann. Int. Med. **126:** 866–873.

17. SINICO, R.A., A. RADICE, C. POZZI, *et al.* 1994. Diagnostic significance and antigen specificity of antineutrophil cytoplasmic antibodies in renal disease: a prospective multicentre study. Nephrol. Dial. Transplant. **9:** 505–510.

18. HAGEN, E.C., M.R. DAHA, J. HERMANS, *et al.* 1998. Diagnostic value of standardized assays for anti-neutrophil cytoplasmic antibodies in idiopathic systemic vasculitis. EC/BCR Project for ANCA Assay Standardization. Kidney Int. **53:** 743–753.

19. RAO, J.K., M. WEINBERGER, E.Z. ODDONE, *et al.* 1995. The role of antineutrophil cytoplasmic antibody (C-ANCA) testing in the diagnosis of Wegener granulomatosis: a literature review and meta-analysis. Ann. Intern. Med. **123:** 925–932.

20. JENNETTE, J.C., A.S. WILKMAN & R.J. FALK. 1998. Diagnostic predictive value of ANCA serology. Kidney Int. **53:** 796–798.

21. CHOI, H.K., S. LIU, P.A. MERKEL, *et al.* 2001. Diagnostic performance of antineutrophil cytoplasmic antibody tests for idiopathic vasculitides: metaanalysis with focus on antimyeloperoxidase antibodies. J. Rheumatol. **28:** 1584–1590.

22. BOOMSMA, M.M., C.A. STEGEMAN, M.J. VAN DER LEIJ, *et al.* 2000. Prediction of relapses in Wegener's granulomatosis by measurement of antineutrophil cytoplasmic antibody levels: a prospective study. Arthritis Rheum. **43:** 2025–2033.

23. KERR, G.S., T.A. FLEISHER, C.W. HALLAHAN, *et al.* 1993. Limited prognostic value of changes in antineutrophil cytoplasm antibody titer in patients with Wegener's granulomatosis. Arthritis Rheum. **36:** 365–371.

24. GIRARD, T., A. MAHR, L.H. NOEL, *et al.* 2001. Are antineutrophil cytoplasmic antibodies a marker predictive of relapse in Wegener's granulomatosis? A prospective study. Rheumatology **40:** 147–151.

25. HAN, W.K., H.K. CHOI, R.M. ROTH, et al. 2003. Serial ANCA titers: useful tool for prevention of relapses in ANCA-associated vasculitis. Kidney Int. **63:** 1079–1085.
26. JENNETTE, J.C., R.J. FALK, et al. 1994. Nomenclature of systemic vasculitides: proposal of an international consensus conference. Arthritis Rheum. **37:** 187–192.
27. MASI, A.T., G.G. HUNDER, J.T. LIE, et al. 1990. The American College of Rheumatology 1990 criteria for the classification of Churg-Strauss syndrome (allergic granulomatosis and angiitis). Arthritis Rheum. **33:** 1094–1100.
28. LUQMANI, R.A., P.A. BACON, R.J. MOOTS, et al. 1994. Birmingham Vasculitis Activity Score (BVAS) in systemic necrotizing vasculitis. Q.J.M. **87:** 671–678.
29. RADICE, A., M. VECCHI, M.B. BIANCHI & R.A. SINICO. 2000. Contribution of immunofluorescence to the identification and characterization of anti-neutrophil cytoplasmic autoantibodies: the role of different fixatives. Clin. Exp. Rheumatol. **18:** 707–712.
30. SAVIGE, J., D. DAVIES, R.J. FALK, et al. 2000. Antineutrophil cytoplasmic antibodies and associated diseases: a review of the clinical and laboratory features. Kidney Int. **57:** 846–862.
31. SAVIGE, J., W. DIMECH, M. FRITZLER, et al. for the International Group for Consensus Statement on Testing and Reporting of Antineutrophil Cytoplasmic Antibodies (ANCA). 2003. Addendum to the International Consensus Statement on testing and reporting of antineutrophil cytoplasmic antibodies: quality control guidelines, comments, and recommendations for testing in other autoimmune diseases. Am. J. Clin. Pathol. **120:** 312–318.

Anti-C1q Autoantibodies in Lupus Nephritis

Prevalence and Clinical Significance

RENATO ALBERTO SINICO,[a] ANTONELLA RADICE,[a] MASAMI IKEHATA,[a]
GAIA GIAMMARRESI,[b] CATERINA CORACE,[a] GIROLAMO ARRIGO,[a]
BRUNA BOLLINI,[a] AND MAURIZIO LI VECCHI[b]

[a]Dipartimento di Nefrologia e Immunologia, Azienda Ospedaliera,
Ospedale San Carlo Borromeo, Milano, Italy

[b]Dipartimento di Medicina Interna, Malattie Cardiovascolari e Nefrologiche,
Università di Palermo, Palermo, Italy

ABSTRACT: Recently, anti-C1q autoantibodies have been proposed as a useful
marker in systemic lupus erythematosus (SLE) since their occurrence correlates with renal involvement and, possibly, with nephritic activity. We aimed to
evaluate the prevalence of anti-C1q antibodies in patients with SLE, with and
without renal involvement, and to correlate these markers' presence and levels
with the activity of the disease and nephropathy. We studied 61 patients with
SLE, 40 of whom had biopsy-proven lupus nephritis; 35 patients with other
connective tissue diseases; and 54 healthy controls. In addition, 18 lupus
nephritis patients were followed up during the disease time course. Anti-C1q
antibodies were measured using "homemade" ELISA with high salt concentration (1 M sodium chloride). High anti-C1q antibody titers (> 55 AU) were
present in 27 of 61 (44%) SLE patients and in 4% of normal blood
donors and pathologic controls, respectively. Anti-C1q antibodies were found
in 60% of patients with lupus nephritis compared with only 14% of SLE
patients without nephropathy ($P < 0.05$). Moreover, patients who were positive
for anti-C1q antibodies had a higher European Consensus Lupus Activity
Measurement (ECLAM) score (4.35 vs. 2.2); 89% of patients with active lupus
nephritis showed high titers of anti-C1q antibodies compared with 0% of
patients with inactive nephritis. Anti-C1q and anti-dsDNA antibodies agreed
in 79% of cases. Our results confirm that anti-C1q antibodies are present in a
significant percentage of SLE patients, and that their presence and levels
correlate with disease activity—in particular, during renal flare-ups.

KEYWORDS: systemic lupus erythematosus; SLE; glomerulonephritis; renal
flares; anti-C1q antibodies; anti-DNA antibodies; lupus nephritis; autoimmune
disease

Address for correspondence: Dr. R. A. Sinico, Dipartimento di Nefrologia e Immunologia,
Azienda Ospedaliera, Ospedale San Carlo Borromeo, Via Pio Secondo, 3, 20153 Milano, Italy.
Voice: +39-02-4022-2489/2344; fax: +39-02-4022-2222.
renato.sinico@oscb.sined.net

Ann. N.Y. Acad. Sci. 1050: 193–200 (2005). © 2005 New York Academy of Sciences.
doi: 10.1196/annals.1313.020

INTRODUCTION

Since 1971, it has been known that sera from patients with systemic lupus erythematosus (SLE) contain low- (7S) and high-molecular-weight material binding to C1q,[1] but it was more than fifteen years later before this low-molecular-weight type was identified as monomeric IgG with antibody activity against the collagen-like region of C1q.[2] At that time, a solid-phase assay using purified C1q, coated onto plastic tubes, was used for detecting circulating immune complexes. Using density-gradient ultracentrifugation, researchers demonstrated that not only immune complexes, but also monomeric IgG, bound to solid-phase C1q. Subsequently, an enzyme-linked immunosorbent assay (ELISA) method for detecting anti-C1q antibodies was developed. Using high salt concentrations (0.5–1.0 M sodium chloride), it became possible to differentiate between immune complexes and anti-C1q antibodies (since, under these conditions, the binding of the globular heads of C1q to immune complexes was prevented).[3]

Using this test, researchers discovered that, in addition to SLE, anti-C1q antibodies are found in a variety of diseases, and even in some apparently normal individuals (reviewed by Seelen et al.[4]). In particular, anti-C1q antibodies are detected at a high titer in 100% of patients with hypocomplementemic urticarial vasculitis syndrome.[5]

Anti-C1q antibodies are found in the bloodstream of 30–48% of SLE patients, and their presence is associated with renal involvement.[4] More important, anti-C1q antibodies have been correlated with active renal disease with a sensitivity of 44–100% and a specificity of 70–92%.[6,7] Note that this strong association has been found pertaining only to renal involvement in lupus patients.[3,8] Moreover, researchers have suggested that an increase in anti-C1q antibody titer can predict renal flare-ups in lupus nephritis.[9,10]

The prognostic value (as markers of renal disease activity) of other, more widely used, serological tests (such as anti-double-stranded DNA [anti-dsDNA] antibodies and complement levels) is quite controversial.[11] Thus, the aims of our study were as follows:

(1) To evaluate the prevalence of anti-C1q autoantibodies in SLE patients and control groups;
(2) To verify the correlation with renal involvement and renal disease activity; and
(3) To compare the performance of anti-C1q antibodies for predicting renal flare ups with that of other commonly used assays (anti-dsDNA antibodies and complement levels).

PATIENTS AND METHODS

Patients

We studied 99 serum samples from 40 patients with biopsy-proven lupus nephritis (34 with proliferative forms, WHO Class III or IV; and 6 with membranous nephropathy, WHO Class V) and 35 serum samples from 21 lupus patients without renal involvement. Patients were followed at the Department of Nephrology and Immunology of the Ospedale San Carlo Borromeo in Milano, Italy. All patients fulfilled the 1982 revised American College of Rheumatology (ACR) criteria for SLE.[12] The control groups consisted of 89 people: 35 patients with non-SLE connective tissue diseases (i.e., progressive systemic sclerosis, Sjögren's syndrome, mixed connective tissue disease [MCTD], undifferentiated connective tissue disease, antiphospholipid syndrome) and 54 blood donors.

Serum samples were collected during either a quiescent phase or an active phase of renal disease. The quiescent phase was defined as stable creatinine clearance for at least 6 months, proteinuria of less than 0.5 g/day of protein, and inactive urinary sediment (in the absence of extrarenal signs).[6] Renal flare-ups were defined as (*a*) nephritic flare-ups, characterized by an increase in plasma creatinine level of at least 30% greater than the last value, associated with nephritic urinary sediment; and (*b*) proteinuric flare-ups, characterized by either stable plasma creatinine levels with an increase in proteinuria of at least 2 g/day of protein (if basal proteinuria was less than 3.5 g/day), or doubled proteinuria if the patient already had nephrotic proteinuria.[6] Overall SLE disease activity was measured by means of the European Consensus Lupus Activity Measurement (ECLAM).[13]

Methods

Anti-dsDNA antibodies were measured using the Farr assay (Amersham Biosciences, Buckinghamshire, UK [now part of GE Healthcare]); C3 and C4 plasma levels were measured by nephelometry.

Anti-C1q antibodies were detected using the method described by Siegert and colleagues,[14] with minor modifications. Briefly, 96-well microtiter plates (Greiner Bio-One) were coated overnight with a 10 μg/mL of human C1q in phosphate-buffered saline (PBS) at 4°C. After washing with PBS-Tween 20, plates were blocked with PBS containing 2% fetal calf serum (FCS) for 1 hour at 37°C. After washing, the serum samples (diluted 1/200 in PBS-Tween 20 containing FCS 2% and 1.0 molar/L NaCl) were added to the wells and incubated for 2 hours at room temperature. Serum samples had been previously centrifuged at 16,000*g* for 5 minutes to remove aggregates. Bound IgG was detected using an alkaline phosphatase conjugated F(ab)2 goat anti-human IgG (Sigma) followed by the proper substrate. The results were expressed as arbitrary units (AUs) by reading off a standard curve composed of a pool of positive sera. The normal range was calculated using receiver operating characteristic (ROC) curves.

Statistical Analysis

All the analyses were performed using SPSS software (Cary, NC). The differences between anti-C1q-positive and anti-C1q-negative patients in terrms of continuous variables were tested by the Mann-Whitney U-test, and in categorical variables by Fisher's exact test. Spearman rank and Pearson's correlation coefficient were used to test the correlation between continuous variables (or their log transformation, when necessary). All reported *P* values are two-sided. A *P* value of less than 0.05 was regarded as statistically significant.

TABLE 1. Anti-C1q antibodies in SLE patients and control groups: titer and percentage testing positive

	SLE (n = 21)	SLE-GN (n = 40)	CTD (n = 35)	NHC (n = 54)
Mean (SD)	37 (55)	134 (118)[a]	11 (4)	23 (50)
Positive (%)	14	60[a]	0	4

ABBREVIATIONS: CTD, connective tissue disease; GN, glomerulonephritis; NHC, normal healthy control; SD, standard deviation; SLE, systemic lupus erythematosus. Normal values: <55 AU (arbitrary units).
[a]$P < 0.05$.

TABLE 2. Correlations between the presence of anti-C1q antibodies and other clinical and laboratory parameters

	R	P value
Anti-dsDNA	0.68	0.0001
ECLAM	0.57	0.0001
C3 plasma level	−0.44	0.0001
C4 plasma level	−0.43	0.0001
Hematuria	0.38	0.0002
ESR	0.26	0.0002
Proteinuria	0.23	0.0002

ABBREVIATIONS: dsDNA, double-stranded DNA; ECLAM, European Consensus Lupus Activity Measurement; ESR, erythrocyte sedimentation rate.

RESULTS

High anti-C1q antibody titers (>55 AU) were present in 27/61 (44%) of SLE patients and in 4% and 0% of normal blood donors and pathological controls, respectively. TABLE 1 summarizes the results of anti-C1q antibodies both in SLE patients, with and without lupus nephritis, and in control groups. Patients with lupus nephritis had a statistically significant higher titer of anti-C1q antibodies compared with both normal controls, patients with non-SLE connective tissue diseases, and SLE patients without renal involvement. Sixty percent of lupus nephritis patients tested positive for anti-C1q antibodies compared with 14% of SLE patients without nephritis ($P < 0.05$).

Serum levels of anti-C1q antibodies showed a positive correlation with levels of anti-dsDNA antibodies, ECLAM score, magnitude of hematuria and proteinuria, and erythrocyte sedimentation rate (ESR); they showed a negative correlation with plasma levels of C3 and C4 (TABLE 2). Other significant results include the following:

• Patients who tested positive for anti-C1q antibodies had higher ECLAM scores compared with SLE patients without anti-C1q antibodies (4.35 vs. 2.2).

TABLE 3. Correlations between renal flares and immunologic parameters in SLE

	P value
Anti-C1q	0.0001
Anti-dsDNA	0.0003
C3 plasma level	0.0004
C4 plasma level	0.0030

- Of patients with active lupus nephritis, 89% showed high titers of anti-C1q antibodies compared with 0% of patients with inactive nephritis.
- Anti-C1q and anti-dsDNA antibodies agreed in 79% of cases.
- When the presence or absence of renal flare-ups was correlated with immunologic parameters, the best correlation was found with anti-C1q antibodies, followed by anti-dsDNA and complement levels (TABLE 3). The sensitivity/specificity of anti-C1q antibodies for active renal disease were 86% and 95%, respectively, compared with 79% and 84% for anti-dsDNA antibodies. Both assays combined had a sensitivity of 91% and a specificity of 90%.

DISCUSSION

The present study has confirmed the presence of anti-C1q antibodies in a high percentage of SLE patients. Anti-C1q antibodies were found in 44% of our lupus patients, a number comparable with that reported in other studies.[15–18] We found a strong association between anti-C1q antibodies and (active) renal disease. Even though in our patients anti-C1q antibodies were shown to correlate with other immunologic parameters of disease activity (e.g., complement reduction and anti-dsDNA antibodies), renal flare-ups were related to C1q antibodies more strongly than to these assays.

SLE is characterized by the presence of a wide variety of autoantibodies, comprising antinuclear, anti-Sm, antiphospholipid, and anti-dsDNA antibodies, which are included in the ACR classification criteria and are therefore considered helpful for diagnosis.[12] Anti-dsDNA antibodies and complement levels are also useful for monitoring disease activity. However, even though high levels of anti-dsDNA antibodies are related to lupus nephritis, increases in anti-dsDNA antibodies cannot clearly distinguish between extrarenal and renal relapses.[4,6,10] Moreover, these antibodies are also found in a relatively high percentage in both clinically inactive disease and patients without nephritis.

Glomerulonephritis is a frequent and often severe feature of SLE and is one of the major determinants of poor outcome. Reliable markers for diagnosing and monitoring lupus nephritis are therefore critically important.

With few exceptions,[15] anti-C1q antibodies have been clearly associated with active renal disease in SLE, and especially with severe, proliferative forms.[4,6,8–10,16,17]

It has been postulated that no lupus nephritis can occur in the absence of anti-C1q antibodies.[7,18] Indeed, in our series as well, all the patients with severe proliferative glomerulonephritis had high levels of anti-C1q antibodies, which became undetectable during treatment-induced remission. Whereas anti-dsDNA antibody titer does not seem to be able to accurately predict renal exacerbations, in our experience (as in that of others[6,8,10]), the sensitivity/specificity of anti-C1q antibodies for renal disease activity and renal flares were found to be greater than that of anti-dsDNA antibodies or C3/C4 plasma levels.[6,10]

The association of anti-C1q antibodies with lupus nephritis has been demonstrated not only by the clinical correlation of anti-C1q antibody positivity with active nephritis, but also by the discovery of anti-C1q antibodies in lupus nephritis kidneys.[19,20] Although anti-C1q antibodies are found in a number of diseases other than SLE, and in up to 4% of apparently healthy individuals (reviewed in Seelen[4]), most of these diseases (e.g., hypocomplementemic urticarial vasculitis syndrome, Felty's syndrome, rheumatoid arthritis, rheumatoid vasculitis, classic polyarteritis nodosa, MCTD, and Sjögren's syndrome) are not usually characterized by renal involvement and, in particular, by proliferative glomerulonephritis.

However, do anti-C1q antibodies contribute to the pathogenesis of lupus nephritis, or do they represent only a useful serological marker? Recently, new clues have emerged to explain such controversial findings. For example, it has been shown in experimental models that administering a mouse anti-mouse C1q monoclonal antibody to treatment naive mice resulted in glomerular deposition of C1q and anti-C1q autoantibodies but not in overt renal disease. However, administering anti-C1q antibodies to mice pretreated with C1q-fixing antiglomerular basement membrane antibodies (a model for glomerular immune complex disease) resulted in strong synergistic enhancement of renal disease.[21] Thus, it appears that anti-C1q autoantibodies can be pathogenic to the kidney, but only in the context of C1q-containing glomerular immune complexes, as found in SLE.[21] Moreover, these autoantibodies could serve as an acquired mechanism of complement classical pathway amplification.[22]

Not only is C1q important for complement activation, but it can also help to clear away potentially dangerous nuclear autoantigens from apoptotic cells. Thus, the absence of C1q leads to the development of anti-DNA antibodies and to clinical SLE.[22] In the context of multiple roles for C1q, researchers have hypothesized that anti-C1q autoantibodies affect patients with SLE not only by injuring the kidneys, but also by enhancing the development of anti-DNA and other glomerular-targeting nuclear autoantibodies, because there is too little C1q available for effective clearance of these dangerous antigens.[22] Indeed, researchers have demonstrated an inverse correlation between anti-C1q autoantibody titers and plasma C1q levels.[17] Thus, these autoantibodies play a dual role: not only can they amplify local injury, but they can also accelerate the development of antinuclear autoantibodies by interfering with C1q clearance functions.[22]

What causes anti-C1q reactivity to develop is still unknown. Seelen and colleagues have suggested that in SLE, anti-C1q reactivity might be caused by the large-scale exposure of C1q neo-epitopes during massive complement activation throughout the active course of the disease.[4] Alternatively, impaired and aberrant clearance of apoptotic material might give rise to autoantibody formation to antigens present on apoptotic material, such as C1q.[6]

CONCLUSIONS

Anti-C1q autoantibodies are present in a high percentage of patients with lupus nephritis. These antibodies correlate with renal disease activity and with renal flare-ups better than do other immunologic parameters, such as anti-dsDNA and complement levels. Although by themselves anti-C1q antibodies are not pathogenic, they can exacerbate renal disease when C1q-containing immune complexes are present in the glomerulus. Furthermore, they can increase the severity of a person's autoimmune response by interfering with C1q's functions of clearing out apoptotic material. Thus, anti-C1q antibodies can represent a useful tool for monitoring disease course, prognosis, and response to treatment in SLE patients.

REFERENCES

1. AGNELLO, V., D. KOFFLER, J.W. EISENBERG *et al.* 1971. C1q precipitins in the sera of patients with systemic lupus erythematosus and other hypocomplementemic states: characterization of high and low molecular weight types. J. Exp. Med. **134**(suppl.): 228S–241S.
2. UWATOKO, S. & M. MANNIK. 1988. Low-molecular weight C1q-binding immunoglobulin G in patients with systemic lupus erythematosus consists of autoantibodies to the collagen-like region of C1q. J. Clin. Invest. **82**: 816–824.
3. SIEGERT C.E., M.R. DAHA, C. HALMA, *et al.* 1992. IgG and IgA autoantibodies to C1q in systemic and renal diseases. Clin. Exp. Rheumatol. **10**: 19–23.
4. SEELEN, M.A., L.A. TROUW & M.R. DAHA. 2003. Diagnostic and prognostic significance of anti-C1q antibodies in systemic lupus erythematosus. Curr. Opin. Nephrol. Hypertens. **12**: 619–624.
5. WISNIESKI, J.J. & S.M. JONES. 1992. Comparison of autoantibodies to the collagen-like region of C1q in hypocomplementemic urticarial vasculitis syndrome and systemic lupus erythematosus. J. Immunol. **148**: 1396–1403.
6. MORONI, G., M. TRENDELENBURG, N. DEL PAPA, *et al.* 2001. Anti-C1q antibodies may help in diagnosing a renal flare in lupus nephritis. Am. J. Kidney Dis. **37**: 490–498.
7. TRENDELENBURG, M., J. MARFURT, I. GERBER, *et al.* 1999. Lack of occurrence of severe lupus nephritis among anti-C1q autoantibody-negative patients. Arthritis Rheum. **42**: 187–188.
8. HORVATH, L., L. CZIRJAK, B. FEKETE, *et al.* 2001. High levels of antibodies against C1q are associated with disease activity and nephritis but not with other organ manifestations in SLE patients. Clin. Exp. Rheumatol. **19**: 667–672.
9. SIEGERT, C.E., M.R. DAHA, C.M. TSENG, *et al.* 1993. Predictive value of IgG autoantibodies against C1q for nephritis in systemic lupus erythematosus. Ann. Rheum. Dis. **52**: 851–856.
10. COREMANS, I.E., P.E. SPRONK, H. BOOTSMA, *et al.* 1995. Changes in antibodies to C1q predict renal relapses in systemic lupus erythematosus. Am. J. Kidney Dis. **26**: 595–601.
11. SINICO, R.A., B. BOLLINI, E. SABADINI, *et al.* 2002. The use of laboratory tests in diagnosis and monitoring of systemic lupus erythematosus. J. Nephrol. Suppl. **6**: S20–S27.
12. TAN, E.M., A.S. COHEN, J.F. FRIES, *et al.* 1982. The 1982 revised criteria for the classification of systemic lupus erythematosus. Arthritis Rheum. **25**: 1271–1277.
13. VITALI, C., W. BENCIVELLI, D.A. ISENBERG, *et al.* 1992. Disease activity in systemic lupus erythematosus: report of the Consensus Study Group of the European Workshop for Rheumatology Research. II. Identification of the variables indicative of disease activity and their use in the development of an activity score. The European Consensus Study Group for Disease Activity in SLE. Clin. Exp. Rheumatol. **10**: 541–547.
14. SIEGERT, C.E., M.R. DAHA, E.A. VAN DER VOORT & F.C. BREEDVELD. 1990. IgG and IgA antibodies to the collagen-like region of C1q in rheumatoid vasculitis. Arthritis Rheum. **33**: 1646–1654.

15. OELZNER, P., B. DELIYSKA, R. FUNFSTUCK, *et al.* 2003. Anti-C1q antibodies and anti-endothelial cell antibodies in systemic lupus erythematosus—relationship with disease activity and renal involvement. Clin. Rheumatol. **22:** 271–278.
16. MARTO, N., M.L. BERTOLACCINI, E. CALABUIG, *et al.* 2005. Anti-C1q antibodies in nephritis: correlation between titres and renal disease activity and positive predictive value in systemic lupus erythematosus. Ann. Rheum. Dis. **64:** 444–448.
17. SIEGERT, C., M. DAHA, M.L. WESTEDT, *et al.* 1991. IgG autoantibodies against C1q are correlated with nephritis, hypocomplementemia, and dsDNA antibodies in systemic lupus erythematosus. J. Rheumatol. **18:** 230–234.
18. FREMEAUX-BACCHI, V., L.H. NOEL & J.A. SCHIFFERLI. 2002. No lupus nephritis in the absence of antiC1q autoantibodies? Nephrol. Dial. Transplant. **17:** 2041–2043.
19. MANNIK, M. & M.H. WENER. 1997. Deposition of antibodies to the collagen-like region of C1q in renal glomeruli of patients with proliferative lupus glomerulonephritis. Arthritis Rheum. **40:** 1504–1511.
20. MANNIK, M., C.E. MERRILL, L.D. STAMPS & M.H. WENER. 2003. Multiple autoantibodies form the glomerular immune deposits in patients with systemic lupus erythematosus. J. Rheumatol. **30:** 1495–1504.
21. TROUW, L.A., T.W. GROENEVELD, M.A. SEELEN, *et al.* 2004. Anti-C1q autoantibodies deposit in glomeruli but are only pathogenic in combination with glomerular C1q-containing immune complexes. J. Clin. Invest. **114:** 679–688.
22. HOLERS, V.M.. 2004. Anti-C1q autoantibodies amplify pathogenic complement activation in systemic lupus erythematosus. J. Clin. Invest. **114:** 616–619.

Anti-Endothelial Cell Antibodies Determination by Cyto-ELISA

A Comparative Study between Three Cell Types Used as Substrates

NABIL SAKLY,[a,b] PEJMAN MIRSHAHI,[b] JEANNETTE SORIA,[b] IBTISSEM GHEDIRA,[a] AND MASSOUD MIRSHAHI[b]

[a]Faculty of Pharmacy, Research Unit 03/UR/07-2, 5000 Monastir, Tunisia

[b]INSERM U736, Faculty of Medicine, Paris VI, 75006 Paris, France

ABSTRACT: Cyto-ELISA has been widely used to investigate anti-endothelial cell antibodies (AECAs); however, because various types of endothelial cells have been used, the results among studies differ. The aim of our study was to analyze and compare the results when determining AECAs in patients with connective tissue disease (CTD). We did so using a cyto-ELISA with different cells as antigenic substrates: two different endothelial cells, one microvascular (HMEC-1) and one from human bone marrow (HBMEC), and one epithelial cell line from breast adenocarcinoma as negative controls (MDA-MB-231). In this trial, we performed a retrospective study in 60 patients with CTD [46 with systemic lupus erythematosus, 8 with Sjögren's syndrome, and 6 with systemic sclerosis] and 32 healthy volunteers. Using cyto-ELISA, the antibody against a cell was considered positive when the optical density (OD) obtained was higher than the mean OD obtained in the control group + 2 standard deviations (upper normal range). Patients were classified into three groups according to the OD obtained with the different cell lines: group 1: patients without any antibody; group 2: patients with specific AECAs; and group 3: patients with nonspecific AECAs. According to this classification, we found that 43.3% of patients with CTD have specific AECAs, and 28.3% have nonspecific antibodies. Our study delineates the heterogeneity of AECAs in patients with CTD. The use of HBMEC in cyto-ELISA may increase the sensitivity of the test, and the use of nonendothelial cells as negative controls may improve its specificity.

KEYWORDS: anti-endothelial cell antibodies; autoantibodies; connective tissue diseases; cyto-ELISA; systemic lupus erythematosus; Sjögren's syndrome; systemic sclerosis; scleroderma; Tunisia

INTRODUCTION

Anti-endothelial cell antibodies (AECAs) represent a heterogeneous group of antibodies that react with various poorly defined endothelial cell surface antigens.[1,2]

Address for correspondence: Ibtissem Ghedira, Ph.D., Faculty of Pharmacy, Rue Avicenne, Monastir 5000, Tunisia. Voice: +216-22854790; fax: +216-73461830.

i_ghedira@yahoo.fr

Ann. N.Y. Acad. Sci. 1050: 201–209 (2005). © 2005 New York Academy of Sciences.

doi: 10.1196/annals.1313.021

They were originally identified in the sera of patients with rheumatic diseases by their ability to react with rodent endothelial cells.[3,4] AECAs have been reported in patients with various autoimmune diseases, including systemic lupus erythematosus (SLE),[5,6] systemic sclerosis (SSc [scleroderma]),[7] Sjögren's syndrome (SS),[8] mixed connective tissue disease (CTD),[9] rheumatoid arthritis,[10] vasculitis[10–12] and Wegener's granulomatosis.[13]

These autoantibodies represent an extremely heterogeneous family. Furthermore, endothelial cells present a heterogeneity[14] depending on the organ or the nature of the vessel (e.g., large vessels or capillaries). These heterogeneities could be responsible for the inter-laboratory discrepancies in AECA detection and for the absence of correlation between clinical features and AECA positivity.[15,16]

To improve the detection of these antibodies, a cyto-ELISA was performed to detect AECAs in Tunisian patients with CTD using microvascular (HMEC-1) and human bone marrow (HBMEC) endothelial cells. A negative control was performed using a nonendothelial form of breast cancer epithelial cell (MDA-MB-231) as antigenic substrates.

MATERIALS AND METHODS

Patients and Sera

Sixty sera of Tunisian patients with CTD were enrolled in the study. They comprised 55 women and 5 men (female/male ratio 11:1); mean age = 34.9 ± 13.6 (mean ± SD); age range = 14–73 years. They were distributed as follows: 46 with SLE, 8 with SS, and 6 with SSc. They were treated in the Tunisian University Hospital of Sousse from January 1997 through October 2003. Serum samples were collected at the time of patient presentation at the immunology unit. All patients fulfilled the proposed criteria for their respective disease (SLE, SS, or SSc).[17–20] A group of 32 healthy blood donors without evidence of CTD, 27 males and 5 females aged 17–60 (mean = 36.9 ± 15.37) years, was also investigated. All serum samples were stored at −80°C prior to use.

Cell Culture

The HMEC-1 cell line was provided by Dr. E.W. Ades of the Centers for Disease Control and Prevention in Atlanta, GA. He established this cell line by transfecting human dermal endothelial cells with the gene product SV40A and large T-antigen. The HMEC-1 cell line represents the microvasculature and has properties similar to those of the original primary culture.[21] HMEC-1 cells were cultured in MCDB 131 Medium (Sigma, Saint-Quentin Fallavier, France) supplemented with 10% (v/v) fetal calf serum (FCS), 100 IU/mL penicillin, 100 μg/mL streptomycin, 10 ng/mL epidermal growth factor (Euromedex, France), and 1 mg/mL hydrocortisone (Pharmacia-Upjohn, Saint-Quentin-en-Yveslines, France).

HBMEC cells were isolated from adult human bone marrow and were kindly provided by Prof. Kenneth Pienta of the University of Michigan (Ann Arbor). They were grown in M131 medium supplemented with 10% (v/v) FCS; 5% microvascular growth factors (MVGs [Cascade Biologics], which contain 5% FCS, hydrocortisone, human basic fibroblast growth factor [bFGF], heparin, human epidermal growth factor, and dibutyryl cAMP); 1% L-glutamine; 100 IU/mL penicillin; and 100 µg/mL streptomycin.

Human MDA-MB-231 breast adenocarcinoma cells (controls) were grown in DMEM (GIBCO BRL, Cergy-Pontoise, France) supplemented with 10% (v/v) FCS, 1 mM glutamine, and antibiotics. Cultures were maintained at 37°C in a moist atmosphere of 95% air and 5% CO_2 and subcultured every three days. Cells for ELISA were scraped off the confluent flask mechanically.

Anti-Endothelial Cell Antibody Assay (Cyto-ELISA)

Detection of AECAs of the immunoglobulin G (IgG) isotype was performed as previously described,[22] with minor modifications. In brief: 5×10^4 cells per well were placed in each well of a 96-well microtiter plate (Nunc, Denmark). After two days of incubation, the cells were confluent. Then the cells were fixed with 0.1% glutaraldehyde in phosphate-buffered saline (PBS) for 10 min at 4°C. Nonspecific binding sites were blocked by adding 200 µL of 3% bovine serum albumin (BSA) in PBS to each well. After an incubation period of 30 min at 37°C, the wells were washed three times with 0.2% BSA/PBS. The binding of autoantibodies to cells was performed by adding 200 µL of serum to each well to be tested, previously diluted 1:80 in PBS containing 0.5% BSA.

After 2 h of incubation at 37°C, bound antibodies were detected by adding to each well 200 µL of 1:5000 diluted goat antihuman IgG labeled with peroxydase (Dako). After 1 h of incubation at room temperature, the wells were carefully washed, and immunoperoxidase was detected by adding 200 µL of *o*-phenylenediamine reagent (Sigma) to each well (0.2 g/L in 0.05 mol/L citrate-phosphate buffer, pH 5, containing 0.5 mL/L H_2O_2). After an incubation period of 15 min, the reaction was stopped by adding 50 µL of 3 M sulfuric acid. Then the optical density (OD) was read at 492 nm, using an ELISA reader. For each serum, each test was performed in duplicate, using the three types of cells. Sera from healthy blood donors were used as negative controls.

The mean value of OD + 2 standard deviations (SDs) obtained with the sera of normal healthy volunteers was considered to be the upper normal limit value.

Statistical Analysis

All data were expressed as the mean ± SD. Statistical analysis used chi-square or Fisher's exact test for comparison of percentages. Mean quantitative values were compared using the unpaired Student's *t*-test. The correlation between scale variables was studied using the Pearson correlation coefficient (R). Significance was assessed at $P = 0.05$. All calculated P values are two-tailed.

RESULTS

In this study, we investigated IgG-AECAs using cyto-ELISA with three cell types as antigenic substrates. In the healthy volunteers, using HMEC-1, HBMEC, and MDA-MB-231, the mean OD values were 0.171 (± 0.059), 0.154 (± 0.077), and 0.274 (± 0.082), respectively (TABLE 1).

TABLE 1. Mean OD values and specific IgG-AECA positivity rates for healthy controls and patients with connective tissue disease determined by cyto-ELISA using three cell types: MDA-MB-231, HMEC-1, and HBMEC

	Healthy controls ($n = 32$)	SLE ($n = 46$)	SS ($n = 8$)	SSc ($n = 6$)	Total CTD ($n = 60$)
Cyto-ELISA with MDA-MB-231					
Mean OD (±SD)	0.27 ± 0.08	0.35 ± 0.14	0.38 ± 0.13	0.37 ± 0.10	0.36 ± 0.14
P value[a]	—	$P < 0.005$	$P < 0.005$	$P = 0.068$	$P < 0.002$
Total positivity[b]	0	12 (26.1%)	3 (37.5%)	2 (33.3%)	17 (28.3%)
Cyto-ELISA with HMEC-1					
Mean OD (±SD)	0.17 ± 0.06	0.33 ± 0.11	0.30 ± 0.08	0.33 ± 0.09	0.32 ± 0.10
P value[a]	—	$P < 0.0001$	$P < 0.005$	$P < 0.01$	$P < 0.0001$
Total positivity[b]	1 (3.1%)	26 (56.5%)	4 (50.0%)	4 (66.7%)	34 (56.6%)
Specific anti-HMEC1[c]	1 (3.1%)	14 (30.4%)	1 (12.5%)	2 (33.3%)	17 (28.3%)
Cyto-ELISA with HBMEC					
Mean OD (±SD)	0.15 ± 0.08	0.34 ± 0.10	0.32 ± 0.11	0.32 ± 0.13	0.34 ± 0.10
P value[a]	—	$P < 0.0001$	$P < 0.005$	$P < 0.0001$	$P < 0.0001$
Total positivity[b]	1 (3.1%)	33 (71.7%)	3 (37.5%)	3 (50.0%)	39 (65.0%)
Specific anti-HBMEC[c]	1 (3.1%)	21 (45.7%)	1 (12.5%)	2 (33.3%)	24 (40.0%)
Total Specific AECAs[d]					
	2 (6.2%)	23 (50%)	1 (12.5%)	2 (33.3%)	26 (43.3%)

[a]Student's *t*-test carried out between mean OD values of healthy volunteers (controls) and CTD groups.
[b]Number of sera with OD > mean OD value of healthy volunteers + 2 SDs.
[c]Number of positive sera that do not cross-react with MDA-MB-231.
[d]Number of sera positive with at least one endothelial cell.

According to our results, the patients with CTD were classified into three groups, presented in FIGURES 1a and 1b:

(1) Group 1: Patients for whom the OD was less than the upper normal limit as previously defined, whatever the cell line used. These patients had no AECAs.

(2) Group 2: Patients for whom the OD was higher than the upper normal limit using endothelial cells (HBMEC or HMEC-1) and for whom the OD was less than the upper normal limit with epithelial cancer cells. These patients had specific AECAs. The sensitivity of detection of these AECAs seemed higher when using HBMEC ($n = 24/60$) than when using HMEC-1 as a substrate ($n = 17/60$), especially for patients with SLE ($P < 0.05$).

(3) Group 3: Patients for whom the OD was higher than the upper normal limit, whatever the cells used. These patients were considered to have nonspecific AECAs.

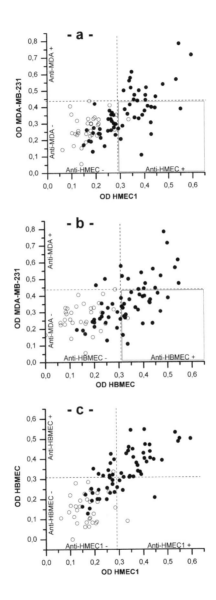

FIGURE 1. Correlation between OD values given by cyto-ELISA using endothelial cells and MDA-MB-231. **(a)** HMEC-1 vs. MDA-MB-231; $R = 0.684$ ($P < 0.001$). **(b)** HBMEC vs. MDA-MB-231; $R = 0.617$ ($P < 0.001$). **(c)** HMEC-1 vs. HBMEC; $R = 0.742$ ($P < 0.001$). *Open circles* are used for healthy volunteer group ($n = 32$), and *black circles* for patient group ($n = 60$). The *vertical* and *horizontal dashed lines* represent the mean OD values + 2 SD of healthy volunteers (for each cell type). The *square* at the right bottom of panels (a) and (b) delimits sera having specific IgG-AECAs.

TABLE 2. Frequency of antibodies against different cell types: MDA-MB-231 epithelial cells, HMEC-1, and HBMEC

		Frequency of antibodies against:		
		Endothelial cells (EC)		
	Epithelial cells	HMEC-1	HBMEC	Both EC
Healthy volunteers ($n = 32$)	0	1/32 (3%)	1/32 (3%)	0
Patients with CTD ($n = 60$)				
Group 1: Patients without any antibody ($n = 17$)	0	0	0	0
Group 2: Patients with specific AECAs ($n = 26$)	0	2/60 (3%)	9/60 (15%)	15/60 (25%)
Group 3: Patients with non-specific AECAs ($n = 17$)	17/60 (28%)	2/60 (3%)	0	15/60 (25%)

None of the studied sera had specific anti–MDA-MB-231 epithelial cell antibodies (i.e., those that recognize exclusively epithelial cells). Also, as seen in FIGURE 1, 26 patients presented high levels of specific AECAs whatever the endothelial cell used. However, 11 patients presented specific AECAs using only one cell line (2 with HMEC-1, 9 with HBMEC). Our results are summarized in TABLE 2.

DISCUSSION

In this study, we investigated IgG AECAs in patients with CTD. We did so using a cyto-ELISA with human microvasculature (HMEC-1) or bone marrow (HBMEC) endothelial cells as antigenic substrates. This investigation was carried out under the same conditions using a cyto-ELISA with a nonendothelial breast cancer epithelial cell line (MDA-MB-231). Note that the cyto-ELISA method remains the most widely used for detecting AECAs.[6]

In our trial, 26 out of the 60 patients with CTD had high specific IgG-AECA (43%) titers, that is, Ig present in their sera bound specifically to at least one endothelial cell but not to MDA-MB-231 cells. The 26 were distributed as follows: 23/46 SLE (50%), 1/8 SS (12%) and 2/6 SSc (33%). Two out of 32 healthy volunteers (6%) were also found to have a slight increase in AECA titer.

Depending on the endothelial cell used as antigenic substrate in cyto-ELISA, we found that the antibodies of 11 of the 26 patients with CTD reacted with only one type of microvascular endothelial cells (2 with HMEC-1 and 9 with HBMEC). AECAs' great heterogeneity has been shown in the literature, according to the endo-thelial cell used as antigen. Shan and colleagues[23] showed that AECAs comprise a highly heterogeneous population of antibodies with respect to the antigens they recognize, as well as VH-gene usage. Lidington and colleagues[24] mentioned that some differences among endothelial cell lines may simply reflect the heterogeneity of endothelial cells derived from different vascular beds. Subsequently, Shoenfeld[25] reported that differences between endothelial cells from large or small vessels may lead to different AECA reactivity in from patients with macro- or microangiopathies.

The parallel investigation of IgG-AECAs by cyto-ELISA with different endothelial cells and the epithelial cell MDA-MB-231 as a negative control permitted us to detect AECAs of various specificities in patients with CTD: 26 sera (43%) were reactive against at least one endothelial cell, and 17 sera (28%) cross-reacted with endothelial cells and MDA-MB-231. We consider the positive rate for specific IgG-AECAs within the patient group to be 43%. Our study made it clear that determining AECAs by cyto-ELISA using individual endothelial cells may lead to nonspecific and overestimated positivity rates. The parallel use of nonendothelial cells (such as the MDA-MB-231 epithelial cells) as negative controls may give more realistic values for antibodies specific to endothelial cells.

Furthermore, because none of the 60 sera studied had antibodies that reacted exclusively with MDA-MB-231 cells, their reactivity against MDA-MB-231 cells was the result of cross-reactive antibodies rather than antibodies specific for this epithelial cell. Hill and colleagues[26] reported that AECAs from patients with SLE presented cross-reactivity against human dermal fibroblasts and the T-cell lymphoma cell line HUT78. In the present study, we showed that a subset of AECAs (nonspecific) are cross-reactive with epithelial MDA-MB-231 cells. Further investigations with advanced techniques such as western blotting are needed to identify specific endothelial cell antigens targeted by AECAs and common cross-reactive antigens.

This study provided the first reported AECA rates in Tunisian SLE patients. The specific IgG-AECA positivity rate in SLE patients was 30.4% (14/46) when determined by cyto-ELISA with HMEC-1 as antigenic substrate and 45.7% (21/46) with HBMEC. These rates concur with the values reported by Vismara and colleagues[27] and Horvathova and colleagues[2] (39.2% and 53%, respectively) but not with those reported by Rosenbaum and colleagues[28] and Hill and colleagues[26] (74% and 78%, respectively). The determination of AECA rates in Tunisian patients with SS and SSc is preliminary and needs a larger study population. Our results showed that the highest specific IgG-AECA positivity rate for the group of patients with CTD (40%) was obtained when using HBMEC as the antigenic substrate. This result agrees with the findings of Renaudineau and colleagues,[29] who showed that cyto-ELISA using HBMEC yielded the highest AECA positivity rate in patients with SSc.

CONCLUSION

The results reported herein delineate the heterogeneity of AECAs as detected by cyto-ELISA with different endothelial cells used as antigenic substrates. We found that some AECAs are specific for endothelial cells, whereas others presented cross-reactivity with epithelial cells. The use of HBMEC in cyto-ELISA may result in increased sensitivity of the test, and the use of nonendothelial cells as negative controls may improve its specificity.

REFERENCES

1. BORDRON, A., R. REVELEN, F. D'ARBONNEAU, *et al.* 2001. Functional heterogeneity of anti-endothelial cell antibodies. Clin. Exp. Immunol. **124:** 492–501.
2. HORVATHOVA, M., E. JAHNOVA & S. NYULASSY. 2002. Detection of anti-endothelial cell antibodies in patients with connective tissue diseases by flow cytometry and their relation to endothelial cell activation. Physiol. Res. **51:** 613–617.

3. TAN, E.M. & C.M. PEARSON. 1972. Rheumatic disease sera reactive with capillaries in the mouse kidney. Arthritis Rheum. **15:** 23–28.
4. LINDQVIST, K.J. & C.K. OSTERLAND. 1971. Human antibodies to vascular endothelium. Clin. Exp. Immunol. **9:** 753–760.
5. SONG, J., Y.B. PARK, W.K. LEE, *et al.* 2000. Clinical associations of anti-endothelial cell antibodies in patients with systemic lupus erythematosus. Rheumatol. Int. **20:** 1–7.
6. RENAUDINEAU, Y., C. DUGUE, M. DUEYMES & P. YOUINOU. 2002. Anti-endothelial cell antibodies in systemic lupus erythematosus. Autoimmun. Rev. **1:** 365–372.
7. RENAUDINEAU, Y., R. REVELEN, Y. LEVY, *et al.* 1999. Anti-endothelial cell antibodies in systemic sclerosis. Clin. Diagn. Lab. Immunol. **6:** 156–160.
8. HEBBAR, M., P. LASSALLE, Y. DELNESTE, *et al.* 1997. Assessment of anti-endothelial cell antibodies in systemic sclerosis and Sjögren's syndrome. Ann. Rheum. Dis. **56:** 230–234.
9. BODOLAY, E., I. CSIPO, I. GAL, *et al.* 2004. Anti-endothelial cell antibodies in mixed connective tissue disease: frequency and association with clinical symptoms. Clin. Exp. Rheumatol. **22:** 409–415.
10. HEURKENS, A.H., P.S. HIEMSTRA, G.J. LAFEBER, *et al.* 1989. Anti-endothelial cell antibodies in patients with rheumatoid arthritis complicated by vasculitis. Clin. Exp. Immunol. **78:** 7–12.
11. CID, M.C., M. SEGARRA, A. GARCIA-MARTINEZ, *et al.* 2004. Endothelial cells, antineutrophil cytoplasmic antibodies, and cytokines in the pathogenesis of systemic vasculitis. Curr. Rheumatol. Rep. **6:** 184–194.
12. BRASILE, L., J.M. KREMER, J.L. CLARKE & J. CERILLI. 1989. Identification of an autoantibody to vascular endothelial cell-specific antigens in patients with systemic vasculitis. Am. J. Med. **87:** 74–80.
13. FERRARO, G., P.L. MERONI, A. TINCANI, *et al.* 1990. Anti-endothelial cell antibodies in patients with Wegener's granulomatosis and micropolyarteritis. Clin. Exp. Immunol. **79:** 47–53.
14. ROOD, P.M., J. CALAFAT, A.E. VON DEM BORNE, *et al.* 2000. Immortalisation of human bone marrow endothelial cells: characterisation of new cell lines. Eur. J. Clin. Invest. **30:** 618–629.
15. YOUINOU, P., P.L. MERONI, M.A. KHAMASHTA & Y. SHOENFELD. 1995. A need for standardization of the anti-endothelial-cell antibody test. Immunol. Today **16:** 363–364.
16. REVELEN, R., A. BORDRON, M. DUEYMES, *et al.* 2000. False positivity in a cyto-ELISA for anti-endothelial cell antibodies caused by heterophile antibodies to bovine serum proteins. Clin. Chem. **46:** 273–278.
17. HOCHBERG, M.C. 1997. Updating the American College of Rheumatology revised criteria for the classification of systemic lupus erythematosus. Arthritis Rheum. **40:** 1725.
18. TAN, E.M., A.S. COHEN, J.S. FRIES, *et al.* 1982. The 1982 revised criteria for the classification of systemic lupus erythematosus. Arthritis Rheum. **25:** 1274–**1277.**
19. VITALI, C., S. BOMBARDIERI, H.M. MOUTSOPOULOS, *et al.* 1993. Preliminary criteria for the classification of Sjögren's syndrome. Results of a prospective concreted action supported by the European Community. Arthritis Rheum. **36:** 340–347.
20. SUBCOMMITTEE FOR SCLERODERMA CRITERIA OF THE AMERICAN RHEUMATISM ASSOCIATION DIAGNOSTIC AND THERAPEUTIC CRITERIA COMMITTEE. 1980. Preliminary criteria for the classification of systemic sclerosis (scleroderma). Arthritis Rheum. **23:** 581-590.
21. ADES, E.W., F.J. CANDAL, R.A. SWERLICK, *et al.* 1992. HMEC-1: establishment of an immortalized human microvascular endothelial cell line. J. Invest. Dermatol. **99:** 683–690.
22. CACOUB, P., P. GHILLANI, R. REVELEN, *et al.* 1999. Anti-endothelial cell auto-antibodies in hepatitis C virus mixed cryoglobulinemia. J. Hepatol. **31:** 598–603.
23. SHAN, H., J. GOLDMAN, G. CUNTO, *et al.* 1998. Heterogeneity of anti-phospholipid and anti-endothelial cell antibodies. J. Autoimmun. **11:** 651–660.
24. LIDINGTON, E.A., D.L. MOYES, A.M. MCCORMACK & M.L. ROSE. 1999. A comparison of primary endothelial cells and endothelial cell lines for studies of immune interactions. Transpl. Immunol. **7:** 239–246.
25. SHOENFELD, Y. 2002. Classification of anti-endothelial cell antibodies into antibodies against microvascular and macrovascular endothelial cells: the pathogenic and diagnostic implications. Cleve. Clin. J. Med. **69**(suppl. 2): SII65–SII67.

26. HILL, M.B., J.L. PHIPPS, A. MILFORD-WARD, *et al.* 1996. Further characterization of anti-endothelial cell antibodies in systemic lupus erythematosus by controlled immunoblotting. Br. J. Rheumatol. **35:** 1231–1238.
27. VISMARA, A., P.L. MERONI, A. TINCANI, *et al.* 1988. Relationship between anti-cardiolipin and anti-endothelial cell antibodies in systemic lupus erythematosus. Clin. Exp. Immunol. **74:** 247–253.
28. ROSENBAUM, J., B.E. POTTINGER, P. WOO, *et al.* 1988. Measurement and characterisation of circulating anti-endothelial cell IgG in connective tissue diseases. Clin. Exp. Immunol. **72:** 450–456.
29. RENAUDINEAU, Y., E. GRUNEBAUM, I. KRAUSE, *et al.* 2001. Anti-endothelial cell antibodies (AECA) in systemic sclerosis—increased sensitivity using different endothelial cell substrates and association with other autoantibodies. Autoimmunity **33:** 171–179.

Prevalence of IgG Anti-α-Fodrin Antibodies in Sjögren's Syndrome

J. L. RUIZ-TÍSCAR,[a] F. J. LÓPEZ-LONGO,[b] S. SÁNCHEZ-RAMÓN,[a]
B. SANTAMARÍA,[a] R. URREA,[a] L. CARREÑO,[b] A. ESTECHA,[b] D. VIGIL,[c]
E. FERNÁNDEZ-CRUZ,[a] AND M. RODRÍGUEZ-MAHOU[a]

*Departments of [a]Clinical Immunology, [b]Rheumatology, and [c]Preventive Medicine,
Gregorio Marañón Hospital, Madrid, Spain*

ABSTRACT: The objective of this study was to determine the prevalence of
antibodies against alpha-fodrin (α-fodrin) of the immunoglobulin G (IgG) isotype in Sjögren's syndrome (SS), as defined by European Community Study
Group (ESG) and ESG-modified criteria. We arrived at the prevalence and
mean concentrations of IgG anti-α-fodrin antibodies using enzyme-linked
immunosorbent assay (ELISA) in 507 patients with SS, primary SS (pSS), and
secondary SS (sSS), classified according to either the ESG or the ESG-modified
criteria. IgG anti-α-fodrin antibodies were detected in 6/507 (1.2%) and 4/228
(1.7%) of the SS group, according to the ESG or ESG-modified criteria, respectively. Similar prevalence was found for patients with pSS or sSS. Anti-Ro/SSA
antibodies were present in 151/409 (36.9%) vs. 149/213 (70.0%) of the SS
group, 85/195 (43.6%) vs. 83/101 (82.2%) of the pSS group, and 66/214 (30.8%)
vs. 66/112 (58.9%) of the sSS group. Anti-La/SSB antibodies were detected in
77/403 (19.1%) vs. 73/212 (34.4%) of the SS group, 47/194 (24.2%) vs. 45/101
(44.5%) of the pSS group, and 30/209 (14.3%) vs. 28/111 (25.2%) of the sSS
group. No clinical associations were found. Only two IgG anti-α-fodrin-positive
sera were anti-Ro/SSA-negative. We conclude that IgG antibodies against α-
fodrin are present in a small percentage of people with SS, pSS, and sSS. The
lower prevalence in patients classified according to the ESG criteria reflects the
lower specificity of these criteria. IgG anti-α-fodrin antibodies can be detected
in some SS patients whose sera do not contain anti-Ro/SSA antibodies.

KEYWORDS: IgG antibodies; α-fodrin; Sjögren's syndrome; immunoglobulin G;
European Community Study Group criteria

BACKGROUND

Sjögren's syndrome (SS) is a frequent chronic autoimmune exocrinopathy of
unknown origin affecting up to 0.1% to 1% of Caucasians.[1,2] It is characterized by
keratoconjunctivitis sicca (dry eyes) and xerostomia (dry mouth) due to lymphocytic
infiltration of the lacrimal and salivary glands.[3] Various sets of classification criteria
have been developed to diagnose this disease. The ESG-modified criteria are highly

Address for correspondence: J. L. Ruiz-Tíscar, Department of Clinical Immunology, Gregorio
Marañón Hospital, 28009 Madrid, Spain.

Ann. N.Y. Acad. Sci. 1050: 210–216 (2005). © 2005 New York Academy of Sciences.
doi: 10.1196/annals.1313.022

stringent, but may lack sensitivity, and require a salivary gland biopsy.[4] The criteria of the European Community Study Group (ESG) are sensitive with less specificity.[5–7]
Sensitive and specific laboratory markers have not been available for the diagnosis of the disease.[8,9] Anti-Ro/SSA antibodies and rheumatoid factor (RF) are sensitive but nonspecific, and anti-La/SSB antibodies lack sensitivity.[10–15] Since 1997, an increasing number of publications have reported that IgA and IgG antibodies against α-fodrin are both sensitive and specific markers for SS.[16–19] These results suggest that anti-α-fodrin antibodies might be able to replace anti-Ro and anti-La antibodies as a more objective serological marker and thereby improve the diagnostic value of classification criteria.[18] Subsequent publications have shown that these antibodies have a lower sensitivity and specificity in patients with SS[20,21] classified according to the ESG criteria.
In this study, we compared the prevalence of IgG antibodies against α-fodrin, anti-Ro/SSA, and anti-La/SSB antibodies in patients with SS, primary SS (pSS), and secondary SS (sSS), classified according to either the ESG[7] or the ESG-modified[22] criteria. In addition, we compared positivity for IgG antibodies against α-fodrin with positivity for anti-Ro/SSA and anti-La/SSB antibodies and clinical manifestations of SS.

MATERIALS AND METHODS

Patients

Sera from 507 patients with SS were recruited from the outpatient rheumatology clinic of the Gregorio Marañón Hospital in Madrid, Spain. All patients provided signed informed consent. All 507 patients were diagnosed with SS according to the ESG criteria: 216 with pSS and 291 with sSS. Of the 507 patients, 228 fulfilled the ESG-modified criteria: 102 for pSS and 126 for sSS (TABLE 1). Sera from 50 healthy blood donors were recruited from the Blood Donor Unit of the Gregorio Marañón Hospital as controls.
The most relevant clinical data from SS patients that were analyzed for correlations were as follows:

- Age at disease onset, current age, and disease evolution time;
- Presence of arthritis;
- Renal, cutaneous, pulmonary, central nervous system, gastrointestinal, liver, thyroid, splenic, and cardiac involvement;
- Leukopenia, thrombocytopenia, and anemia;
- Weight loss;
- Presence of amyloidosis, vasculitis, purpura, peripheral neuropathy, arterial hypertension, diabetes mellitus, and calcinosis;
- Autonomic affectation;
- Immunosuppressive treatment;
- Fetal loss; and
- Infectious disease.

TABLE 1. Anti-Ro, anti-La, and IgG anti-α-fodrin autoantibodies in subjects with SS, pSS, and sSS

Diagnostic category	IgG anti-α-fodrin/N	ELISA (Ro+)	ELISA (Ro−)	ELISA (anti-Ro not performed)	ELISA (La+)	ELISA (La−)	ELISA (anti-La not performed)
SS (ESG criteria)	6/507 (1.2%)	4/151 (2.6%)	2/258 (0.8%)	0/98	0/77	6/326 (1.8%)	0/104
SS (ESG-modified criteria)	4/228 (1.7%)	4/149 (2.7%)	0/64	0/15	0/73	4/139 (2.9%)	0/16
pSS (ESG criteria)	3/216 (1.4%)	1/85 (1.2%)	2/110 (1.8%)	0/21	0/47	3/147 (2%)	0/22
pSS (ESG-modified criteria)	1/102 (1%)	1/83 (1.2%)	0/18	0/1	0/45	1/56 (1.8%)	0/1
sSS (ESG criteria)	3/291 (1%)	3/66 (4.5%)	0/148	0/77	0/30	0/179	0/82
sSS (ESG-modified criteria)	3/126 (2.4%)	3/66 (4.5%)	0/46	0/14	0/28	3/83 (3.6%)	0/15

NOTE: Number of IgG anti-α-fodrin ELISA+/total number of sera tested.

Detection of IgG Antibodies against α-Fodrin by ELISA

IgG antibodies against α-fodrin were tested using a commercial ELISA kit (Aesku.Lab Diagnostika, Wendelsheim, Germany) following the manufacturer's instructions. For the 100 more recent patient samples, another commercial ELISA kit (Orgentec Diagnostika GmbH, Mainz, Germany) was performed.

Detection of Anti-Ro and Anti-La Antibodies by ELISA

Anti-Ro/SSA and anti-La/SSB antibodies were tested using a commercial ELISA kit (Orgentec Diagnostika GmbH, Mainz, Germany) according to the manufacturer's instructions. Not all sera were analyzed with the anti-Ro/anti-La ELISA kit.

Statistical Evaluation

Sera from patients with SS classified according to either the ESG or the ESG-modified criteria were segregated into two categories: with or without IgG antibodies against α-fodrin. The presence of anti-Ro and anti-La antibodies was compared among groups. Associations of both anti-Ro, anti-La antibodies and IgG antibodies against α-fodrin were calculated using cross-tabs. Associations of IgG antibodies against α-fodrin and clinical manifestations were calculated using Fisher's exact test. Probabilities of association (P values) of less than 0.05 were regarded as statistically significant.

RESULTS

IgG Antibodies in the Sera of Healthy Blood Donors

All sera from the 100 healthy blood donors were negative for IgG anti-α-fodrin, anti-Ro/SSA, and anti-La/SSB.

IgG Antibodies in SS Patients: ESG versus ESG-Modified Criteria

IgG antibodies against α-fodrin were detected in 6/507 (1.2%) vs. 4/228 (1.7%) of serum samples, according to ESG and ESG-modified criteria, respectively (TABLE 1). Anti-Ro/SSA antibodies were detected in 151/409 (36.9%) vs. 149/213 (70.0%). Anti-La/SSB antibodies were detected in 77/403 (19.1%) vs. 73/212 (34.4%). In the ESG criteria group, 4/6 IgG anti-α-fodrin positive sera were anti-Ro/SSA positive and 2/6 were anti-Ro/SSA negative. In the ESG-modified criteria group, all IgG anti-α-fodrin positive sera were anti-Ro/SSA positive. In both groups, all IgG anti-α-fodrin positive sera were anti-La/SSB negative. All healthy blood donors were negative for IgG anti-α-fodrin antibodies (TABLE 1).

IgG Antibodies in pSS Patients: ESG versus ESG-Modified Criteria

IgG antibodies against α-fodrin were detected in 3/216 (1.4%) vs. 1/102 (0.9%) pSS patients using ESG and ESG-modified criteria, respectively; anti-Ro/SSA antibodies were detected in 85/195 (43.6%) vs. 83/101 (82.2%). In the ESG criteria group, 1/3 IgG anti-α-fodrin positive sera was anti-Ro/SSA positive, and 2/3 were anti-Ro/SSA negative. In the ESG-modified criteria group, the unique IgG anti-α-fodrin positive sera was anti-Ro/SSA positive. In both groups, all IgG anti-α-fodrin positive sera were anti-La/SSB negative (TABLE 1).

IgG Antibodies in sSS Patients: ESG versus ESG-Modified Criteria

IgG antibodies against α-fodrin were detected in 3/291 (1%) vs. 3/126 (2.4%) sSS patients using ESG and ESG-modified criteria, respectively. Anti-Ro/SSA antibodies were detected in 66/214 (30.8%) vs. 66/112 (58.9%). In both groups, IgG anti-α-fodrin positive sera were anti-Ro/SSA positive and anti-La/SSB negative (TABLES 1 and 2).

The percentages of positive anti-α-fodrin antibodies detected in sera were similar using the two different commercial kits in this study. No significant association between IgG anti-α-fodrin antibodies and clinical data, antinuclear antibodies, RF, anti-Ro/SSA, or anti-La/SSB antibodies was found.

DISCUSSION

The presence of anti-Ro/SSA and anti-La/SSB antibodies is one of the diagnostic criteria for SS, included in the recently established American-European Consensus Group criteria, in which they play a more important role than before.[22] According to these classification criteria, the presence of either anti-Ro/SSA or anti-La/SSB autoantibodies or a positive salivary gland biopsy (lymphocytic focus score [LFS] =

TABLE 2. Main demographic features of the subjects included in the study and distribution of connective tissue diseases associated with Sjögren's syndrome

Diagnostic category	IgG anti-α-fodrin-positive sera	Sex ratio (M/F)	Mean age (years), typical desv.	SLE	RA	SSc	PM/DM	MCTD	Others
SS (ESG criteria)	6/507 (1.2%)	40/467	58.2 13.9	—	—	—	—	—	—
SS (ESG-modified criteria)	4/228 (1.7%)	20/208	57.5 13.8	—	—	—	—	—	—
pSS (ESG criteria)	3/216 (1.4%)	15/201	56.1 13.4	—	—	—	—	—	—
pSS (ESG-modified criteria)	1/102 (1%)	9/93	57.4 14.4	—	—	—	—	—	—
sSS (ESG criteria)	3/291 (1%)	25/266	59.7 14.2	1/41 (2.4%)	2/198 (1%)	0/12	0/3	0/2	0/35
sSS (ESG-modified criteria)	3/126 (2.4%)	11/115	57.5 13.3	1/26 (3.8%)	2/69 (2.9%)	0/3	0/2	0/1	0/25

1.0) is mandatory to establish SS. The disease sensitivities of anti-Ro and anti-La antibodies have been reported to be 60–75% and 30–50%, respectively,[10,11,13–15] while the specificity of particularly anti-La antibodies is generally considered to be reasonably high. Nevertheless, the need remains for an SS-specific marker with a better disease sensitivity and specificity profile.

Haneji and colleagues initially reported that anti-α-fodrin antibodies are highly specific and sensitive markers for SS (with sensitivity of 96% for sera from pSS patients).[16] In follow-up studies, this group and others have detected these auto-antibodies in systemic lupus erythematosus (SLE) patients.[17] In contrast, Witte and collaborators showed much lower disease sensitivities (64% and 47% in pSS and sSS, respectively) when focusing on IgA antibodies against α-fodrin rather than IgG antibodies.[18] Their data suggest a similar sensitivity to that of anti-Ro/SSA antibodies. They also detected two positive sera in rheumatoid arthritis (RA) patients who had no symptoms of SS, possibly indicating lower specificity for anti-α-fodrin antibodies than previously reported. In two recent studies, Ruffatti and colleagues[20,21] found lower prevalence of IgG anti-α-fodrin antibodies in pSS (21.3%) than previously reported. This group also detected these antibodies at a higher prevalence in other chronic connective tissue diseases.

In our cohort of patients with SS, the ELISA test showed the lowest sensitivity for IgG anti-α-fodrin among the literature's data, with a similar sensitivity for anti-Ro/SSA and anti-La/SSB antibodies. IgG anti-α-fodrin antibodies were rarely detected in SS according to the ESG criteria or to the ESG-modified criteria. Therefore, in our study population, the IgG anti-α-fodrin antibodies have not proven useful for the diagnosis of SS, except in some SS patients whose sera lacked anti-Ro/SSA and anti-La/SSB antibodies. Further, statistical analysis revealed no significant association between IgG anti-α-fodrin antibodies and clinical data, antinuclear antibodies (ANAs), RF, anti-Ro/SSA, and anti-La/SSB antibodies. The presence of IgG anti-α-fodrin antibodies in 100% of children with pSS (according to all pediatric reports[23–25]) along with experimental data on the role of α-fodrin as an autoantigen in the pathogenesis of SS[26,27] combined with the low detection in our study indicate that these should be considered early portents rather than diagnostic markers of the disease. To wit, Kobayashi and colleagues detected these antibodies in the sera of childhood patients with SS before anti-Ro/SSA and anti-La/SSB antibodies became positive.[25] Clinical follow-up studies in patients with early signs and symptoms of SS may be able to verify whether anti-α-fodrin antibodies are a predictive marker of SS.

We detected IgG antibodies against α-fodrin more frequently in patients with SS, pSS, and sSS diagnosed according to the ESG-modified criteria. This effect could reflect the higher specificity of these criteria for SS. It is also possible than IgA antibodies against α-fodrin could increase diagnostic sensitivity in Sjögren's disease, but the search for more sensitive and specific diagnostic markers needs to continue. Finally, we cannot rule out racial and geographic differences in the prevalence of IgG anti-α-fodrin antibodies as a cause of our study's atypical findings.

ACKNOWLEDGMENTS

We would like to thank Angela Puché-Torres and Julia Parra for their excellent technical support.

REFERENCES

1. BJERRUM, K.B. 1997. Keratoconjunctivitis sicca and primary Sjögren's syndrome in a Danish population aged 30–60 years. Acta Ophthalmol. Scand. **75:** 281–286.
2. DAFNI, U.G., A.G. TZIOUFAS, P. STAIKOS, *et al.* 1997. Prevalence of Sjögren's syndrome in a closed rural community. Ann. Rheum. Dis. **56:** 521–525.
3. DANIELS, T.E. 1989. Clinical assessment and diagnosis of immunologically mediated salivary gland disease in Sjögren's syndrome. J. Autoimmun. **2:** 529–541.
4. FOX, R.I., C.A. ROBINSON, J. CURD, *et al.* 1986. Sjögren's syndrome: proposed criteria for classification. Arthritis Rheum. **29:** 577–585.
5. VITALI, C. & S. BOMBARDIERI. 1990. Diagnostic criteria for Sjögren's syndrome: the state of the art. Clin. Exp. Rheumatol. **8**(suppl. 5)**:** 13–16.
6. VITALI, C., S. BOMBARDIERI, H.M. MOUTSOPOULOS, *et al.* 1993. Preliminary criteria for the classification of Sjögren's syndrome: results of a prospective concerted action supported by the European Community. Arthritis Rheum. **36:** 340–347.
7. VITALI, C., S. BOMBARDIERI, H.M. MOUTSOPOULOS, *et al.* 1996. Assessment of the European classification criteria for Sjögren's syndrome in a series of clinically defined cases: results of a prospective multicentre study. The European Study Group on Diagnostic Criteria for Sjögren's Syndrome. Ann. Rheum. Dis. **55:** 116–121.
8. HAY, E.M., E. THOMAS, B. PAL, *et al.* 1998. Weak association between subjective symptoms of and objective testing for dry eyes and dry mouth: results from a population based study. Ann. Rheum. Dis. **57:** 20–24.
9. HAGA, H.J., B. HULTEN, A.I. BOLSTAD, *et al.* 1999. Reliability and sensitivity of diagnostic tests for primary Sjögren's syndrome. J. Rheumatol. **26:** 604–608.
10. ALEXANDER, E.L., T.J. HIRSCH, F.C. ARNETT, *et al.* 1982. Ro(SSA) and La(SSB) antibodies in the clinical spectrum of Sjögren's syndrome. J. Rheumatol. **9:** 239–246.

11. HANSEN, B. & R. MANTHORPE. 1986. Antibodies against SS-B/La and SS-A/Ro antigens in patients with primary Sjögren's syndrome. Scand. J. Rheumatol. Suppl. **61:** 93–97.

12. DROSOS, A.A., A.P. ANDONOPOULOS, J.S. COSTOPOULOS, et al. 1988. Prevalence of primary Sjögren's syndrome in an elderly population. Br. J. Rheumatol. **27:** 123–127.

13. REICHLIN, M. 1998. Antibodies to Ro and La. Ann. Med. Interne (Paris) **149:** 34–41.

14. BEER, R.G., M. RISCHMUELLER, T. COATES, et al. 1996. Nonprecipitating anti-La(SS-B) autoantibodies in primary Sjögren's syndrome. Clin. Immunol. Immunopathol. **79:** 314–318.

15. VENABLES, P.J., W. SHATTLES, C.T. PEASE, et al. 1989. Anti-La (SS-B): a diagnostic criterion for Sjögren's syndrome? Clin. Exp. Rheumatol. **7:** 181–184.

16. HANEJI, N., T. NAKAMURA, K. TAKIO, et al. 1997. Identification of alpha-fodrin as a candidate autoantigen in primary Sjögren's syndrome. Science **276:** 604–607.

17. WATANABE, T., T. TSUCHIDA, N. KANDA, et al. 1999. Anti-alpha-fodrin antibodies in Sjögren's syndrome and lupus erythematosus. Arch. Dermatol. **135:** 535–539.

18. WITTE, T., T. MATTHIAS, F.C. ARNETT, et al. 2000. IgA and IgG autoantibodies against alpha-fodrin as markers for Sjögren's syndrome: systemic lupus erythematosus. J. Rheumatol. **27:** 2617–2620.

19. WITTE, T., T. MATTHIAS, M. OPPERMANN, et al. 2003. Prevalence of antibodies against alpha-fodrin in Sjögren's syndrome: comparison of 2 sets of classification criteria. J. Rheumatol. **30:** 2157–2159.

20. RUFFATTI, A., P. OSTUNI, P. GRYPIOTIS, et al. 2004. Sensitivity and specificity for primary Sjögren's syndrome of IgA and IgG anti-alpha-fodrin antibodies detected by ELISA. J. Rheumatol. **31:** 504–507.

21. RUFFATTI, A., P. GRYPIOTIS & P. OSTUNI. 2005. Sensitivity and specificity of anti-α-fodrin antibodies in primary Sjögren's syndrome: Dr. Ruffatti, et al. reply. J. Rheumatol. **32:** 197–198.

22. VITALI, C., S. BOMBARDIERI, R. JONSSON, et al. 2002. Classification criteria for Sjögren's syndrome: a revised version of the European criteria proposed by the American-European Consensus Group. Ann. Rheum. Dis. **61:** 554–558.

23. TAKAHASHI, K., O. TATSUZAWA, K. YANAGI, et al. 2001. Alpha-fodrin auto-antibody in Sjögren's syndrome and other auto-immune diseases in childhood. Eur. J. Pediatr. **160:** 520–521.

24. MAENO, N., S. TAKEI, H. IMANAKA, et al. 2001. Anti-alpha-fodrin antibodies in Sjögren's syndrome in children. J. Rheumatol. **28:** 860–864.

25. KOBAYASHI, I., N. KAWAMURA, M. OKANO, et al. 2001. Anti-alpha-fodrin autoantibody is an early diagnostic marker for childhood primary Sjögren's syndrome. J. Rheumatol. **28:** 363–365.

26. INOUE, H., K. TSUBOTA, M. ONO, et al. 2001. Possible involvement of EBV-mediated alpha-fodrin cleavage for organ-specific autoantigen in Sjögren's syndrome. J. Immunol. **166:** 5801–5809.

27. TODA, I. 2002. Autoantigens and Sjögren syndrome. Cornea **21:** S13–S16.

Effective Use of Autoantibody Tests in the Diagnosis of Systemic Autoimmune Disease

ROBERT LYONS, SONALI NARAIN, CODY NICHOLS, MINORU SATOH, AND WESTLEY H. REEVES

Division of Rheumatology and Clinical Immunology, Center for Autoimmune Disease, University of Florida, Gainesville, Florida 32610, USA

ABSTRACT: Screening for disease-specific autoantibodies may be useful in asymptomatic ANA-positive individuals as a means of evaluating the risk of developing a systemic autoimmune disease such as systemic lupus erythematosus (SLE), polymyositis/dermatomyositis (PM/DM), scleroderma (SSc), Sjögren's syndrome (SS), rheumatoid arthritis (RA), or primary biliary cirrhosis (PBC) in the future. In patients with known or suspected systemic autoimmune disease, a panel of disease-specific markers may help to establish a diagnosis and to assess the prognosis. The great strides in autoantibody testing over the last 20 years make it feasible to use specific autoantibody markers to improve diagnostic accuracy in systemic autoimmune disease. New technology enabling screening for multiple autoantibodies may further enhance the clinical usefulness of autoantibody testing, making it possible to diagnose autoimmune disease in its earliest stages and to intervene before serious end organ damage occurs.

KEYWORDS: antinuclear antibodies (ANA); asymptomatic; autoantibodies; scleroderma; Sjögren's syndrome; SLE; systemic autoimmune disease; test

INTRODUCTION

Disease-Specific Autoantibodies

Systemic autoimmune diseases are generally characterized by the production of autoantibodies that recognize a diverse array of cytoplasmic and nuclear antigens. It is important to distinguish between the terms "autoimmunity" and "autoimmune disease". Autoimmunity is an adaptive immune response (T- or B-cell mediated) against self-antigens either with or without concomitant clinical manifestations, whereas autoimmune disease implies the existence of clinical manifestations (e.g., kidney disease, arthritis, rashes, pleuritis) arising as a consequence of a T- or B-cell-mediated response to self. Thus, the production of antinuclear antibodies (ANA) in the absence of clinical manifestations constitutes autoimmunity, whereas the same antibodies accompanied by arthritis or glomerulonephritis would constitute an autoimmune disease.

Address for correspondence: Westley H. Reeves, Division of Rheumatology and Clinical Immunology, University of Florida, P. O. Box 100221, Gainesville, FL 32610-0221. Voice: 352-392-8600; fax: 352-846-1858.
whreeves@ufl.edu

Ann. N.Y. Acad. Sci. 1050: 217–228 (2005). © 2005 New York Academy of Sciences.
doi: 10.1196/annals.1313.023

TABLE 1. Autoantibody associations with systemic autoimmune disease

Disease	Autoantibody to:	Sensitivity[a] London	Sensitivity[a] Florida	Specificity[b] London	Specificity[b] Florida	Onset prior to disease?
SLE	dsDNA	N/A		N/A		{10272, 12621}[7,8]
	Sm	7	10	100	100	{12621}[7]
	Ribosomal P	3	2	100	100	N/A
	PCNA	3	0.3	100	100	N/A
PM/DM	Jo-1 (tRNA^{his})	25	24	100	100	{12659}[53]
	PL-7 (tRNA^{thr})	3	N/A	100	N/A	N/A
	PL-12 (tRNA^{ala})	N/A	6	N/A	100	N/A
	EJ (tRNA^{gly})	N/A	N/A	N/A	N/A	{4788}[10]
	OJ (tRNA^{ile})	N/A	3	N/A	100	N/A
SSc	Scl-70	16	N/A	100	N/A	{3803}[9]
	Fibrillarin	N/A	2	N/A	100	N/A
	RNAP I/III	N/A	21	N/A	100	N/A
	Th (7–2 RNP)	N/A	N/A	N/A	N/A	{1444}[52]
SS	Ro (SSA)	75	54	87	82	{12621}[7]
	La (SSB)	42	26	96	94	{12621}[7]
RA	CCP^c	N/A	65	N/A	N/A	{12657, 12658}[13,14]
PBC	Pyruvate dehy-drogenase	88	N/A	100	N/A	{7367, 7370}[3,4]

[a]Prevalence of the autoantibody in patients with the associated disease (number positive/number with disease × 100%) from reference 54 {2684} and our own data.
[b]Estimated specificity for the disease.
[c]CCP: Cyclic citrullinated peptide.

Autoantibodies can be used as adjuncts to diagnose autoimmune disease, to monitor disease activity and severity, and to predict the outcome of autoimmune disease. The fluorescent ANA assay using HEp-2 cells is a good initial screening test, but is not specific for a particular diagnosis. It provides information on the presence of serum autoantibodies as well as the subcellular localization(s) of the antigens they recognize.[1] In one population-based study of ANA-positive Caucasians, 18.8% had systemic lupus erythematosus (SLE), 10.9% had drug-induced lupus, 21.7% had other systemic autoimmune diseases (e.g., Sjögren's syndrome, myositis, scleroderma), 10.1% had autoimmune thyroiditis, 5.8% had other organ-specific autoimmune diseases, 8.3% had infections, 2.9% had neoplasms, and 24.3% had other conditions or "idiopathic" autoantibodies.[2] In view of this lack of specificity, attention has focused on tests for disease-specific autoantibodies that can be used to assess diagnosis or prognosis (TABLE 1).

AUTOANTIBODIES APPEAR YEARS BEFORE THE
ONSET OF AUTOIMMUNE DISEASE

Autoantibody production can be the harbinger of autoimmune disease, especially in the case of disease-specific autoantibodies, which may appear months, years, or even decades before the onset of clinical symptoms. Detection of disease-specific autoantibodies in asymptomatic individuals may permit earlier diagnosis and preventative treatment. A striking example is antimitochondrial antibodies in primary biliary cirrhosis (PBC).

Antibodies against the mitochondrial antigen dihydrolipoamide acetyltransferase (E2), a component of pyruvate dehydrogenase, can appear in asymptomatic individuals decades prior to the onset of PBC.[3,4] In one study of 29 asymptomatic individ-

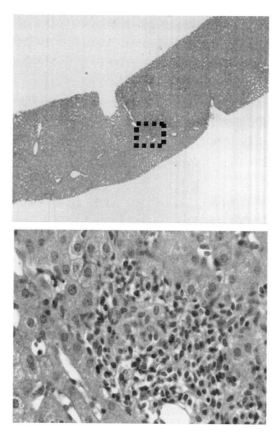

FIGURE 1. Liver biopsy from an SLE patient who developed new onset antimitochondrial antibodies. **(Top)** Low-power view of hematoxylin and eosin staining. An area of inflammatory cell infiltration is apparent within the box. **(Bottom)** High-power view of the area within the box showing mild periportal lymphocytic infiltration.

uals with antimitochondrial antibodies, 22 (76%) developed symptoms of PBC over an 11- to 24-year follow-up period.[3] Antimitochondrial antibodies also may appear before the onset of PBC in the context of another systemic autoimmune disease. For example, we evaluated a 32-year-old woman with SLE with photosensitive malar rash, polyarthritis, Raynaud's phenomenon, a positive ANA, and anti-dsDNA antibodies by *Crithidia luciliae* kinetoplast staining who subsequently developed anti-cytoplasmic autoantibodies. She complained of mild right upper quadrant pain and had a mildly elevated alkaline phosphatase 187, normal AST and ALT, and an elevated serum IgM level of 323 mg/dL (normal range 25–210 mg/dL). IgG and IgA values were normal. Antimitochondrial antibodies were positive at a titer of 1:80. A liver biopsy (FIG. 1) revealed periportal lymphocytic infiltrates, suggesting that she had asymptomatic early PBC. She was treated with ursodeoxycholate, and her alkaline phosphatase and serum IgM levels normalized.

A variety of autoantibodies have been reported to precede the onset of SLE.[5,6] ANA, anti-Ro, anti-La, and antiphospholipid antibodies may be present for extended periods before the onset of autoimmune disease, whereas anti-Sm and anti-nRNP are thought to appear much closer to the onset of disease.[7] Anti-dsDNA antibodies are intermediate. In one study using stored serum samples from military recruits, 55% of individuals who subsequently developed SLE had positive anti-dsDNA antibodies. Anti-dsDNA antibodies were detected as long as 9.3 years before diagnosis, with a mean of 2.7 years.[8] In the same cohort, at least one lupus autoantibody was present before diagnosis in 88% of patients, and ANA were present in 78%.[7] Thus, many or most cases of lupus are preceded by serological abnormalities. Much less is known, however, regarding the likelihood that asymptomatic individuals with lupus autoantibodies will ultimately develop SLE.

Scleroderma-associated autoantibodies also predate disease onset. Anticentromere antibodies, a marker for limited scleroderma, can develop years before the onset of scleroderma or CREST syndrome (calcinosis, Raynaud's phenomenon, esophageal dysfunction, sclerodactyly, telangiectasias), and their presence in individuals with Raynaud's phenomenon is associated with the development of telangiectasias over a period of 1–11 years.[9] In the same study, anti-Scl70 (topoisomerase I) autoantibodies, a marker for diffuse scleroderma, were strongly associated with the subsequent development of skin tightening. Patients who had either of these autoantibodies were 63-fold more likely to develop signs of connective tissue disease by the end of the 11-year observation period.[9]

The production of autoantibodies against tRNA synthetases also may be seen years before the onset of myositis[10] or may shift with alterations in disease manifestations. Autoantibodies also frequently precede the onset of rheumatoid arthritis (RA). Rheumatoid factor (RF) has been detected in RA patients months to years before the onset of clinical symptoms of RA,[11,12] and the presence of RF is associated with a 20- to 40-fold greater risk of developing RA. Although the risk is relatively low (~10–15%),[12] it is highest in those with high RF titers.[11] Autoantibodies to citrulline-modified peptides precede the development of RA by several years.[13] In one study, 93% of patients with these antibodies who were diagnosed with undifferentiated arthritis developed RA within 3 years.[14]

As in the case of systemic autoimmune disease, the onset of organ-specific autoimmune diseases, such as type I diabetes and autoimmune thyroiditis, is frequently preceded by the appearance of specific autoantibodies. Type I diabetes is associated with autoantibodies against insulin, glutamate decarboxylase, and islet cells, which appear before the onset of clinical manifestations. The numbers of autoantibodies against these three antigens, not their specificities, best predict the risk of developing type I diabetes.[15] Among first-degree relatives of patients with type 1 diabetes, the 5-year risk of developing diabetes is 0% if no antibody is present, 15% if 1 antibody is present, 44% if 2 antibodies are present, and 100% if all 3 antibodies are present.[15] About 30–60% of family members of patients with type I diabetes with one of the diabetes-related antibodies develop the disease within 5–10 years.[15–18] Likewise, the presence of thyroid peroxidase antibodies is predictive of the development of elevated TSH or hypothyroidism.[19,20]

These data indicate that disease-specific autoantibodies are useful predictors of the future development of autoimmune disease. However, information about their frequency in at-risk subsets or in the general population is incomplete, and the risk factors determining whether an individual who produces one of these autoantibodies will remain asymptomatic or evolve an autoimmune disease have not been defined.

EVALUATION OF AN ASYMPTOMATIC POSITIVE ANA TEST

A positive ANA test in an asymptomatic individual prompts many referrals to autoimmune disease specialists.[21] In many cases, this is not a cause for concern because some healthy individuals have low-titer ANA.[22,23] The prevalence of a positive ANA is 3–5% in randomly selected healthy Caucasians,[23] but prevalence is strongly age dependent. It is estimated that 10–15% of healthy people over the age of 65 years are ANA positive, although the titers are usually $\leq$ 1:160.[22] Approximately 3% of normal individuals are ANA positive at a 1:320 serum dilution, and 32% are ANA positive at 1:40 serum dilution.[24,25] Nevertheless, in view of the evidence summarized here that disease-specific autoantibodies are highly predictive of the future development of systemic autoimmune disease, an algorithm such as the one shown in FIGURE 2 may be useful for the differential diagnosis of an asymptomatic positive ANA test. This algorithm is based on the immunofluorescence pattern: nucleoplasmic, nucleolar, or cytoplasmic. Nucleoplasmic fluorescence is further categorized as homogeneous, speckled, peripheral, or centromere.

A diverse group of autoantibodies produce homogeneous-, speckled-, peripheral-, or centromere-specific nucleoplasmic staining. Because of the common occurrence of more than one pattern, it is best to consider all nucleoplasmic staining, with the exception of anticentromere staining, under a single differential diagnosis.

Homogeneous Nucleoplasmic Pattern

The differential diagnosis of homogeneous nucleoplasmic staining includes anti-dsDNA, antichromatin, antihistone, and anti-Scl70 (topoisomerase) antibodies. Two of these specificities are disease specific: anti-dsDNA for SLE and anti-Scl70 (topoisomerase I) for scleroderma (see below). Antichromatin and antihistone antibodies are found in a variety of autoimmune disorders and may be helpful for evaluating drug-induced lupus. Like anti-dsDNA, they frequently increase with lupus activity and decrease in remission, but they are poor predictors of disease outcome.

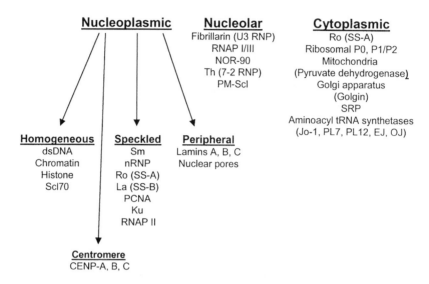

FIGURE 2. Algorithm for the assessment of a positive fluorescent "ANA" test in asymptomatic individuals. Immunofluorescence staining is classified as nucleoplasmic (homogeneous, speckled, peripheral, or centromere), nucleolar, or cytoplasmic, and the specificities of major types of autoantibodies producing these patterns are indicated.

Speckled Nucleoplasmic Pattern

The differential diagnosis of speckled nucleoplasmic staining includes anti-Sm and anti-nRNP (autoantibodies recognizing the U1, U2, U4–6, and U5 small nuclear ribonucleoproteins), anti-Ro60 (autoantibodies recognizing the Y1–5 small ribonucleoproteins), and anti-La (autoantibodies recognizing a 45 kDa protein associated with small RNAs synthesized by RNA polymerase III). The Ro60 antigen is mainly cytoplasmic, although speckled nucleoplasmic staining has been described in some cases. Autoantibodies against proliferating cell nuclear antigen (PCNA), Ku (p70/p80) antigen, and RNA polymerase II (RNAP II) also produce speckled nucleoplasmic staining. Anti-Sm antibodies are pathognomonic of SLE,[1] and when detected in asymptomatic individuals, the onset of SLE generally follows within a year.[7] Anti-PCNA autoantibodies are uncommon but relatively specific for SLE. Their predictive value in asymptomatic individuals is not known. Anti-Ro60 and anti-La are frequently, but not invariably, associated with the development of sicca manifestations regardless of the underlying autoimmune disease. Autoantibodies to RNAP II and Ku are strongly associated with systemic autoimmune disease, but are not specific for a particular subset. There is some evidence that anti-Ku antibodies identify a clinical subset at risk for myositis. Anti-RNAP II autoantibodies are seen in both lupus and scleroderma and may have prognostic significance in the latter (see below).

Peripheral Nucleoplasmic Pattern

Peripheral nucleoplasmic staining results from autoantibodies against components of the nuclear envelope: nuclear lamins A, B, and C and nuclear pore complexes. Autoantibodies to the lamins are associated with SLE, antiphospholipid antibodies, and autoimmune hepatitis,[26–28] whereas autoantibodies to nuclear pore complexes are seen in PBC.[29]

Centromere Pattern

Centromere staining is associated with scleroderma or CREST. The fluorescence pattern consists of discrete nucleoplasmic dots in interphase cells that remain associated with the condensed chromosomes of mitotic cells, making this a distinctive pattern that does not usually require further evaluation.[1]

Nucleolar Pattern

Nucleolar staining is associated with scleroderma.[30] Autoantibodies associated with a nucleolar staining pattern include antifibrillarin (U3 RNP), anti-RNA polymerase I/III (RNAP I/III), anti-NOR-90, and anti-Th (7–2 RNP). With the exception of anti-NOR-90, which may be less disease specific than once thought,[31,32] all of these autoantibodies are highly specific for scleroderma[30] and have both diagnostic and prognostic significance (see below). Autoantibodies against the PM-Scl antigen, which are associated with polymyositis-scleroderma overlap syndrome, also give nucleolar staining. Although most frequent in the overlap syndrome, they are seen in patients with either polymyositis or scleroderma alone but have been reported in patients with neither myositis nor scleroderma, as well.[33]

Cytoplasmic Pattern

The differential diagnosis of cytoplasmic staining includes anti-Ro (SS-A); the ribosomal P0, P1, and P2 antigens; signal recognition peptide (SRP); antimitochondrial antibodies (generally specific for pyruvate dehydrogenase); and an assortment of myositis-associated autoantibodies specific for various aminoacyl tRNA synthetases, including the enzymes specific for tRNA^{his} (Jo-1), tRNA^{thr} (PL-7), tRNA^{ala} (PL-12), tRNA^{gly} (EJ), tRNA^{ile} (OJ), and others.[34] Antiribosomal P autoantibodies, which recognize the P0, P1, and P2 antigens, are highly specific for SLE, and antimitochondrial autoantibodies are a diagnostic marker for PBC (TABLE 1).

USE OF AUTOANTIBODIES FOR DIAGNOSIS AND PROGNOSIS

For individuals with known or suspected systemic autoimmune disease, the detection of specific autoantibodies may be valuable both for confirming the clinical diagnosis and for assessing the prognosis.

SLE

Although the sensitivity of a positive fluorescent ANA test for lupus ranges from 90% to 95% or more,[35,36] the specificity is low[2,37] and the positive predictive value is only 11–13%.[36,38] By contrast, autoantibodies against Sm, dsDNA, the ribosomal P antigens (P0, P1, and P2), and PCNA are highly specific for SLE (TABLE 1). Increasing anti-dsDNA antibody levels may herald exacerbations of lupus nephritis or other organ involvement, and it has been suggested that corticosteroid therapy may be warranted to prevent flares in patients with an increasing anti-dsDNA antibody titer, even in the absence of other clinical evidence.[39]

Anti-Sm antibodies are virtually pathognomonic for SLE and are detected in approximately 7–25% of lupus patients, depending on ethnic origin.[1] Unlike anti-dsDNA, the levels of anti-Sm antibodies do not correlate with disease activity. Anti-nRNP antibodies are associated with anti-Sm (virtually all anti-Sm sera are anti-nRNP positive), but are not disease specific (TABLE 1). Their prevalence in SLE is 20–40%. Antiribosomal P antibodies are reportedly associated with neuropsychiatric manifestations of lupus,[40] although this is somewhat controversial.[41] They are, however, highly specific for the diagnosis of SLE (TABLE 1).

Sjögren's Syndrome

Anti-Ro (SS-A) and La (SS-B) autoantibodies are seen in Sjögren's syndrome and other systemic autoimmune diseases, such as SLE, myositis, and scleroderma, when they are accompanied by sicca symptoms. Anti-Ro60 (SS-A) antibodies are found in 10–50% of SLE and 60–80% of primary Sjögren's syndrome sera.[42] Approximately 10–20% of SLE patients and a somewhat higher percentage of Sjögren's syndrome patients are anti-La (SS-B) positive. Anti-La is virtually always associated with anti-Ro, whereas anti-Ro60 antibodies frequently are detected without anti-La. The 52-kDa Ro52 antigen is recognized by autoantibodies in many sera from patients with Sjögren's syndrome and is associated with anti-Ro60. Anti-Ro52 is seen in the absence of anti-Ro60 in patients with polymyositis[43,44] and less frequently in other disorders. In addition to being associated with sicca syndrome, autoantibodies to Ro52 and La (SS-B) are associated with cardiac conduction abnormalities in neonates.[45] Pregnant women with systemic autoimmune disease and asymptomatic mothers of children with congenital cardiac conduction abnormalities should be screened for these antibodies.

Polymyositis and Dermatomyositis

Polymyositis (PM) and dermatomyositis (DM) are associated with autoantibodies against a group of aminoacyl tRNA synthetases, the most common of which is anti-Jo-1 (histidyl tRNA synthetase), which is produced by approximately 20–25% of adult myositis patients. Other autoantibodies in this group are found in 1–4% of myositis patients. However, because only one antisynthetase autoantibody is usually detected in an individual patient, they are, in aggregate, relatively common. All are highly specific for myositis (TABLE 1) and are associated with a constellation of symptoms (myositis ± skin involvement, interstitial lung disease, Raynaud's phenomenon, inflammatory arthritis, fever, and mechanic's hands) known as antisynthetase autoantibody syndrome.[46] Anti-SRP autoantibodies also are highly specific for polymyositis and are associated with severe disease but not with antisynthetase autoantibody syndrome. Anti-Mi-2 autoantibodies are a dermatomyositis marker generally associated with a relatively more favorable long-term prognosis.

Scleroderma

Anti-Scl70 antibodies are virtually pathognomonic of scleroderma and predict internal organ involvement, proximal scleroderma, and a poor outcome.[30,47,48] Patients who develop both anti-Scl70 and anti-RNA polymerase II autoantibodies have an even worse prognosis.[49] Interestingly, anti-Scl70 autoantibodies are lost by a subset of patients, portending a more favorable outcome.[50] Like anti-Scl-70, anti-RNAP I/III autoantibodies are associated with severe disease and poor outcome.[51] This is the most common disease-specific marker for scleroderma, with a sensitivity of 21% and 100% specificity (TABLE 1).

Antifibrillarin autoantibodies, specific for the nucleolar U3 small ribonucleoprotein, are nearly 100% specific for scleroderma and are found in 2–8% of scleroderma sera (see ref. 30 and TABLE 1). The frequency of anti-Th (7–2 ribonucleoprotein) antibodies, another disease-specific marker for scleroderma, is approximately 4%.[52] Interestingly, 3 of 244 controls were positive for anti-Th, all of whom had primary Raynaud's phenomenon of less than 2 years duration, raising the possibility that these individuals may go on to develop additional manifestations of scleroderma in the future. The PM-Scl antigen is a nucleolar/cytoplasmic complex of 11 proteins reported to be recognized by autoantibodies in approximately 3% of scleroderma, 8% of polymyositis, and 50% of polymyositis-scleroderma overlap syndrome sera.[30]

Patients with limited symptoms and positive centromere staining have a high likelihood of developing additional manifestations of CREST syndrome. The centromere autoantigens recognized most commonly by these sera are CENP-A, -B, and -C.[30] Of these, CENP-B is the most important for predicting the subsequent onset of additional manifestations of CREST syndrome, especially telangiectasias.[9]

CONCLUSIONS

Screening for disease-specific autoantibodies may be useful in asymptomatic ANA-positive individuals as a means of evaluating the risk of developing a systemic autoimmune disease such as SLE, PM/DM, scleroderma, Sjögren's syndrome, RA, or PBC in the future. In this situation, a diagnostic algorithm such as that illustrated in FIGURE 2 may be employed. In patients with known or suspected systemic autoimmune disease, a panel of disease-specific markers may help to establish a diagnosis and to assess the prognosis. A panel for SLE should include assays for anti-dsDNA, anti-Sm, anti-nRNP, anti-ribosomal P, and anti-PCNA. A Sjögren's syndrome panel might include anti-Ro60 (SS-A), anti-Ro52, and anti-La (SS-B). A scleroderma panel would include anti-Scl70, anti-RNA polymerase I/III, antifibrillarin, anti-Th (7–2) ribonucleoprotein, and anticentromere. A myositis panel would include anti-Jo-1, anti-PL-7, anti-PL-12, anti-EJ, anti-OJ, and anti-SRP as well as possibly anti-Mi-2 (specific for dermatomyositis) and anti-Ro52. The great strides in autoantibody testing over the last 20 years make it feasible to use specific autoantibody markers to improve diagnostic accuracy in systemic autoimmune disease. New technology enabling screening for multiple autoantibodies may further enhance the clinical usefulness of autoantibody testing, making it possible to diagnose autoimmune disease in its earliest stages and to intervene before serious end organ damage occurs.

ACKNOWLEDGMENTS

This work was supported by research grants (R01-AR40391 and M01-R00082) from the United States Public Health Service, State of Florida funds to the Center for Autoimmune Diseases, and generous gifts from Lupus Link (Daytona Beach, FL) and Lewis M. Schott.

REFERENCES

1. REEVES, W.H., S. NARAIN & M. SATOH. 2004. Autoantibodies in systemic lupus erythematosus. *In* Arthritis and Allied Conditions, pp. 1497–1521. Lippincott/Williams & Wilkins. Philadelphia.
2. SHIEL, W.C. & M. JASON. 1989. The diagnostic associations of patients with antinuclear antibodies referred to a community rheumatologist. J. Rheumatol. **16:** 782–785.
3. METCALF, J.V., H.C. MITCHISON, J.M. PALMER, *et al.* 1996. Natural history of early primary biliary cirrhosis. Lancet **348:** 1399–1402.
4. MITCHISON, H.C., M.R. LUCEY, P.J. KELLY, *et al.* 1990. Symptom development and prognosis in primary biliary cirrhosis: a study in two centers. Gastroenterology **99:** 778–784.
5. VLACHOYIANNOPOULOS, P.G., V. TZAVARA, U. DAFNI, *et al.* 1998. Clinical features and evolution of antinuclear antibody positive individuals in a rheumatology outpatient clinic. J. Rheumatol. **25:** 886–891.
6. SATOH, M., H. YAMAGATA, F. WATANABE, *et al.* 1995. Development of anti-Sm and anti-DNA antibodies followed by clinical manifestation of systemic lupus erythematosus in an elderly woman with long-standing Sjögren's syndrome. Lupus **4:** 63–65.
7. ARBUCKLE, M.R., M.T. MCCLAIN, M.V. RUBERTONE, *et al.* 2003. Development of autoantibodies before the clinical onset of systemic lupus erythematosus. N. Engl. J. Med. **349:** 1526–1533.
8. ARBUCKLE, M.R., J.A. JAMES, K.F. KOHLHASE, *et al.* 2001. Development of anti-dsDNA autoantibodies prior to clinical diagnosis of systemic lupus erythematosus. Scand. J. Immunol. **54:** 211–219.
9. WEINER, E.S., S. HILDEBRANDT, J.L. SENECAL, *et al.* 1991. Prognostic significance of anticentromere antibodies and anti-topoisomerase I antibodies in Raynaud's disease. Arthritis Rheum. **34:** 68–77.
10. STOJANOV, L., M. SATOH, M. HIRAKATA & W.H. REEVES. 1996. Correlation of anti-synthetase antibody levels with disease course in a patient with interstitial lung disease and elevated muscle enzymes: quantitation of anti-glycyl tRNA synthetase antibodies by immunoprecipitation. J. Clin. Rheumatol. **2:** 89–94.
11. DEL PUENTE, A., W.C. KNOWLER, D.J. PETTITT & P.H. BENNETT. 1988. The incidence of rheumatoid arthritis is predicted by rheumatoid factor titer in a longitudinal population study. Arthritis Rheum. **31:** 1239–1244.
12. AHO, K., M. HELIOVAARA, J. MAATELA, *et al.* 1991. Rheumatoid factors antedating clinical rheumatoid arthritis J. Rheumatol. **18:** 1282–1284.
13. RANTAPAA-DAHLQVIST, S., B.A. DE JONG, E. BERGLIN, *et al.* 2003. Antibodies against cyclic citrullinated peptide and IgA rheumatoid factor predict the development of rheumatoid arthritis. Arthritis Rheum. **48:** 2741–2749.
14. VAN GAALEN, F.A., S.P. LINN-RASKER, W.J. VAN VENROOIJ, *et al.* 2004. Autoantibodies to cyclic citrullinated peptides predict progression to rheumatoid arthritis in patients with undifferentiated arthritis: a prospective cohort study. Arthritis Rheum. **50:** 709–715.
15. VERGE, C.F., R. GIANANI, E. KAWASAKI, *et al.* 1996. Number of autoantibodies (against insulin, GAD or ICA512/IA2) rather than particular autoantibody specificities determines risk of type I diabetes. J. Autoimmun. **9:** 379–383.
16. BONIFACIO, E., P.J. BINGLEY, M. SHATTOCK, *et al.* 1990. Quantification of islet-cell antibodies and prediction of insulin-dependent diabetes. Lancet **335:** 147–149.

17. SCHATZ, D., J. KRISCHER, G. HORNE, *et al.* 1994. Islet cell antibodies predict insulin-dependent diabetes in United States school age children as powerfully as in unaffected relatives. J. Clin. Invest. **93:** 2403–2407.
18. ATKINSON, M.A. & G.S. EISENBARTH. 2001. Type 1 diabetes: new perspectives on disease pathogenesis and treatment. Lancet **358:** 221–229.
19. VANDERPUMP, M.P., W.M. TUNBRIDGE, J.M. FRENCH, *et al.* 1995. The incidence of thyroid disorders in the community: a twenty-year follow-up of the Whickham Survey. Clin. Endocrinol. (Oxf.) **43:** 55–68.
20. HAWKINS, B.R., P.S. CHEAH, R.L. DAWKINS, *et al.* 1980. Diagnostic significance of thyroid microsomal antibodies in randomly selected population. Lancet **2:** 1057–1059.
21. NARAIN, S., H.B. RICHARDS, M. SATOH, *et al.* 2004. Diagnostic accuracy for lupus and other systemic autoimmune diseases in the primary care setting. Arch. Intern. Med. **164:** 2435–2441.
22. HOOPER, B., S. WHITTINGHAM, J.D. MATHEWS, *et al.* 1972. Autoimmunity in a rural community. Clin. Exp. Immunol. **12:** 79–87.
23. HAWKINS, B.R., K.J. O'CONNOR, R.L. DAWKINS, *et al.* 1979. Autoantibodies in an Australian population. I. Prevalence and persistence. J. Clin. Lab. Immunol. **2:** 211–215.
24. TAN, E.M., T.E. FELTKAMP, J.S. SMOLEN, *et al.* 1997. Range of antinuclear antibodies in "healthy" individuals. Arthritis Rheum. **40:** 1601–1611.
25. ROSENBERG, A.M., K.M. SEMCHUK, H.H. MCDUFFIE, *et al.* 1999. Prevalence of antinuclear antibodies in a rural population. J. Toxicol. Environ. Health **A57:** 225–236.
26. REEVES, W.H., N. CHAUDHARY, A. SALERNO & G. BLOBEL. 1987. Lamin B autoantibodies in sera of certain patients with systemic lupus erythematosus. J. Exp. Med. **165:** 750–762.
27. LASSOUED, K., M.N. GUILLY, F. DANON, *et al.* 1988. Antinuclear antibodies specific for lamins: characterization and clinical significance. Ann. Intern. Med. **108:** 829–833.
28. SENECAL, J.L., J. RAUCH, T. GRODZICKY, *et al.* 1999. Strong association of autoantibodies to human nuclear lamin B1 with lupus anticoagulant antibodies in systemic lupus erythematosus. Arthritis Rheum. **42:** 1347–1353.
29. COURVALIN, J.C., K. LASSOUED, E. BARTNIK, *et al.* 1990. The 210-kD nuclear envelope polypeptide recognized by human autoantibodies in primary biliary cirrhosis. J. Clin. Invest. **86:** 279–285.
30. ROTHFIELD, N.F. 1992. Autoantibodies in scleroderma. Rheum. Dis. Clin. North Am. **18:** 483–498.
31. RODRIGUEZ-SANCHEZ, J., C. GELPI, C. JUAREZ & J.A. HARDIN. 1987. A new autoantibody in scleroderma that recognizes a 90-kDa component of the nucleolus organizing region of chromatin. J. Immunol. **139:** 2579–2584.
32. FUJII, T., T. MIMORI, N. HAMA, *et al.* 1996. Detection of anti-NOR-90 in patient sera with anti-nucleolar antibodies using a cDNA that encodes for the NOR-90 autoantigen: correlation of anti-NOR-90 with Sjögren's syndrome. Arthritis Rheum. **39:** 1313–1318.
33. SCHNITZ, W., E. TAYLOR-ALBERT, I. N.TARGOFF, *et al.* 1996. Anti-PM/Scl autoantibodies in patients without clinical poymyositis or scleroderma. J. Rheumatol. **23:** 1729–1733.
34. TARGOFF, I.N. 1992. Autoantibodies in polymyositis. Rheum. Dis. Clin. North Am. **18:** 455–482.
35. TAN, E.M., A.S. COHEN, J.F. FRIES, *et al.* 1982. The 1982 revised criteria for the classification of systemic lupus erythematosus. Arthritis Rheum. **25:** 1271–1277.
36. EMLEN, W. & L. O'NEILL. 1997. Clinical significance of antinuclear antibodies: comparison of detection with immunofluorescence and enzyme-linked immunosorbent assays. Arthritis Rheum. **40:** 1612–1618.
37. EDWORTHY, S.M., E. ZATARAIN, D.J. MCSHANE & D.A. BLOCH. 1988. Analysis of the 1982 ARA lupus criteria data set by recursive partitioning methodology: new insights into the relative merit of individual criteria. J. Rheumatol. **15:** 1493–1498.
38. SLATER, C.A., R.B. DAVIS & R.H. SCHMERLING. 1996. Antinuclear antibody testing. Arch. Intern. Med. **156:** 1421–1425.
39. BOOTSMA, H., P. SPRONK, R. DERKSEN, *et al.* 1995. Prevention of relapses in systemic lupus erythematosus. Lancet **345:** 1595–1599.
40. BONFA, E., S.J. GOLOMBEK, L.D. KAUFMAN, *et al.* 1987. Association between lupus psychosis and anti-ribosomal P protein antibodies. N. Engl. J. Med. **317:** 265–271.

41. TEH, L.S. & D.A. ISENBERG. 1994. Antiribosomal P protein antibodies in systemic lupus eythematosus. Arthritis Rheum. **37:** 307–315.
42. WASICEK, C.A. & M. REICHLIN. 1982. Clinical and serological differences between systemic lupus erythematosus patients with autoantibodies to Ro versus patients with antibodies to Ro and La. J. Clin. Invest. **69:** 835–843.
43. ROZMAN, B., B. BOZIC, M. KOS-GOLJA, *et al.* 2000. Immunoserological aspects of idiopathic inflammatory muscle disease. Wien. Klin. Wochenschr. **112:** 722–727.
44. KUBO, M., H. IHN, Y. ASANO, *et al.* 2002. Prevalence of 52-kd and 60-kd Ro/SS-A autoantibodies in Japanese patients with polymyositis/dermatomyositis. J. Am. Acad. Dermatol. **47:** 148–151.
45. BUYON, J.P. 1993. Congenital complete heart block. Lupus **2:** 291–295.
46. PLOTZ, P.H., M. DALAKAS, R.L. LEFF, *et al.* 1989. Current concepts in the idiopathic inflammatory myopathies: polymyositis, dermatomyositis, and related disorders. Ann. Intern. Med. **111:** 143–157.
47. STEEN, V.D., D.L. POWELL & T.A. MEDSGER. 1988. Clinical correlations and prognosis based on serum autoantibodies in patients with systemic sclerosis. Arthritis Rheum. **31:** 196–203.
48. WEINER, E.S., W.C. EARNSHAW, J-L. SENECAL, *et al.* 1988. Clinical associations of anti-centromere antibodies and antibodies to topoisomerase I: a study of 355 patients. Arthritis Rheum. **31:** 378–385.
49. SATOH, M., M. KUWANA, T. OGASAWARA, *et al.* 1994. Association of autoantibodies to topoisomerase I and the phosphorylated (IIO) form of RNA polymerase II in Japanese scleroderma patients. J. Immunol. **153:** 5838–5848.
50. KUWANA, M., J. KABURAKI, T. MIMORI, *et al.* 2000. Longitudinal analysis of autoantibody response to topoisomerase I in systemic sclerosis. Arthritis Rheum. **43:** 1074–1084.
51. KUWANA, M., Y. OKANO, J. KABURAKI, *et al.* 1994. Racial differences in the distribution of systemic sclerosis-related serum antinuclear antibodies. Arthritis Rheum. **37:** 902–906.
52. OKANO, Y. & T.A. MEDSGER. 1990. Autoantibody to Th ribonucleoprotein (nucleolar 7–2 RNA protein particle) in patients with systemic sclerosis. Arthritis Rheum. **33:** 1822–1828.
53. MILLER, F.W., S.A. TWITTY, T. BISWAS & P.H. PLOTZ. 1990. Origin and regulation of a disease-specific autoantibody response: antigenic epitopes, spectrotype stability, and isotype restriction of anti-Jo-1 autoantibodies. J. Clin. Invest **85:** 468–475.
54. BERNSTEIN, R.M., C.C. BUNN, G.R.V. HUGHES, *et al.* 1984. Cellular protein and RNA antigens in autoimmune disease. Mol. Biol. Med. **2:** 105–120.

Human Antiganglioside Autoantibodies

Validation of ELISA

MEPUR H. RAVINDRANATH, SAKUNTHALA MUTHUGOUNDER,
THIRUVERKADU S. SARAVANAN, NAFTALI PRESSER,
AND DONALD L. MORTON

*Laboratory of Glycoimmunotherapy, John Wayne Cancer Institute,
Santa Monica, California, USA*

ABSTRACT: Gangliosides have a hydrophilic sugar chain that contains antigenic
determinants and a hydrophobic ceramide. In humans, gangliosides elicit a T-
cell independent IgM response; antiganglioside IgM autoantibodies may be
pentameric or polymeric. A correlation between specific neuropathies and antiganglioside autoantibodies has been confirmed. Although many neurologists
attempt to lower titers of antiganglioside autoantibodies, oncologists are developing strategies to augment production of IgM antibodies that will remove
immunosuppressive gangliosides from the circulation of patients and target
gangliosides and kill tumor cells. Antiganglioside IgM antibodies can cause leakage of the blood–nerve barrier in a concentration-dependent and complement-
independent manner, bind to neuronal gangliosides to create a neuromuscular
block and serve as a marker of axonal damage in neuropathies such as multiple
sclerosis. They are also a promising biomarker of early prostate cancer. There
is a need to validate the protocol for enzyme-linked immunosorbent assay
(ELISA) of antiganglioside IgM autoantibodies. This validation must consider
the purity of gangliosides from different commercial sources, the coating of
gangliosides onto a solid matrix in a manner that maximizes exposure of
oligosaccharide epitopes to IgM paratopes, techniques to minimize background noise and eliminate nonspecific antibody binding, and carefully defined
positive and negative controls. The validated protocol also must include a
simple formula to estimate titers for several replicas. Finally, antibody titers
must be converted to natural logs for statistical appraisal.

KEYWORDS: antiganglioside; autoantibodies; ELISA; gangliosides; human;
titer; validate; tumor; antigen

Gangliosides are amphophilic molecules with atomic mass units (AMU) ranging
from 1300 to 3000. They have a hydrophilic sugar chain with one or more sialic acids
and a hydrophobic ceramide with sphingosine and a long-chain fatty acid.[1,2] Diversity in the gangliosides is created by the number and nature of their sugars, the number and length of glycosidic linkages of sialic acids, the number of double bonds, and
the extent of fatty-acid hydroxylation. Gangliosides are expressed on the outer layer

Address for correspondence: Mepur H. Ravindranath, Laboratory of Glycoimmunotherapy,
John Wayne Cancer Institute, 2200 Santa Monica Boulevard, Santa Monica, CA 90404–2302.
Voice: 310-449–5263.
    ravindranathm@jwci.org

Ann. N.Y. Acad. Sci. 1050: 229–242 (2005). © 2005 New York Academy of Sciences.
doi: 10.1196/annals.1313.024

TABLE 1. Structure of gangliosides found in normal and malignant human tissues

Glycolipid	Structure	AMU
GM_3	NeuAcα2,3Galβ1,4Glcβ1Cer	1236
GM_2	GalNAcβ1,4(NeuAcα2,3)Galβ1,4Glcβ1Cer	1385
GD_3	NeuAcα2,8NeuAcα2,3Galβ1,4Glcβ1Cer	1545
GD_2	GalNAcβ1,4(NeuAcα2,8NeuAcα2,3)Galβ1,4Glcβ1Cer	1694
GM_{1a}	Galβ1,3GalNAcβ1,4(α2,3NeuAc)Galβ1,4Glcβ1Cer	1547
GM_{1b}	NeuAcαGalβ1,3GalNAcβ1,4Galβ1,4Glcβ1Cer	1547
GD_{1a}	NeuAcαGalβ1,3GalNAcβ1,4(α2,3NeuAc)Galβ1,4Glcβ1Cer	1838
GD_{1b}	Galβ1,3GalNAcβ1,4(NeuAcα2,8NeuAcα2,3)Galβ1,4Glcβ1Cer	1838
GD_{1c}	NeuAcα2,8NeuAcα2,3Galβ1,3GalNAcβ1,4Galβ1,4Glcβ1Cer	1838
GT_{1b}	NeuAcα2,3Galβ1,3GalNAcβ1,4(NeuAcα2,8NeuAcα2,3)Galβ1,4Glcβ1Cer	2144

of the bilayered lipid membrane of every human cell. Neural tissues and malignant cells overexpress gangliosides. In aqueous media, the molecules aggregate and form irregular micelles. In ethanol, micelle formation requires a higher critical micellar concentration (CMC). Therefore, ethanol suspension is employed to coat polystyrene plates in an enzyme-linked immunosorbent assay (ELISA) to measure antiganglioside antibodies.[3] During drying *in vacuo*, CMC increases, causing attachment of the tail group to the polystyrene plates.

The antigenic determinants of common gangliosides are the sugar chains on the lactosylceramide backbone. TABLE 1 illustrates some of the most common antigenic determinants of gangliosides in neural, extraneural, and malignant human cells. The epitope is the antigenic determinant that binds to the paratope, that is, the complementary combining site (CCS) of an antibody. The upper limit of epitope size is determined by the variable region of the CCS; it is 6 sugar residues for antiganglioside antibodies. The contact areas involve 25.5 nm of sugar residues and 30.4 nm of paratope. Fifteen amino acids of the antibody establish 90 van der Waals forces and 9 hydrogen bonds.[4] Antigen–antibody interactions also may involve salt linkages.

Gangliosides elicit consistent and specific humoral responses without T-cell help.[5–8] They do not elicit specific or consistent cellular immune responses. Although protein or peptide antigens are processed by intracellular enzymes and major histocompatibility complex (MHC) molecules, which transport antigen fragments to the cell surface and present them to T cells as well as to B cells to generate primary and secondary antibody responses, gangliosides are not presented in the context of MHC molecules, and they do not require T-cell help.[8] Oligosaccharide residues of gangliosides are unable to bind into the groove of MHC molecules, which prevents direct and specific recognition by conventional specific T cells.[5–7] Because ganglioside antigens fail to induce a memory response in humans, antiganglioside antibodies are invariably IgM, although antiganglioside IgG (commonly IgG2a or IgG3) antibodies are found in mice and rabbits. In our ELISA system, we rarely encounter IgG antibodies to gangliosides in the sera of patients who have been immunized with ganglioside-based vaccines. To our knowledge, there is no evidence for isotype switching of antiganglioside IgM or any atypical memory responses mediated by T cells. Any IgG antiganglioside antibodies reported in humans could be anti-anti-idiotypic antibodies or antibodies directed against peptides that mimic ganglioside epitopes.

Antiganglioside IgM antibodies may be pentamers, hexamers, heptamers, or other polymers. Unlike conventional pentameric IgM, polymeric IgM may not have a J chain.[9] The polymeric IgM is potentially useful in cancer patients who develop high titers of antiganglioside antibodies, because antibodies without a J-chain fix complement 20-fold more efficiently than do conventional pentamers.[10] Accruing evidence suggests that antiganglioside IgM may be secreted by a separate class of B cells that express the CD5 T-cell marker.[11] Although earlier studies suggested that exogenous adjuvants were necessary to induce an antibody response to ganglioside antigens,[12] our recent study of antiganglioside responses to cryosurgical ablation of liver metastases indicates otherwise: exogenous adjuvants are not required to elicit an antiganglioside IgM response.[13] In this study of patients with advanced colon cancer, we found that cryoablation of metastatic lesions caused tumor necrosis; necrotic cells released tumor gangliosides into circulation, provoking a specific anti-ganglioside antibody response. The increase in antibody levels was followed by a decrease in serum gangliosides, suggesting that gangliosides released during necrosis induced antiganglioside IgM without any exogenous adjuvants. It is possible that necrosis would have acted as a natural adjuvant or would release endogenous adjuvants such as heat shock proteins to stimulate the ganglioside-specific antibody response.

A disease-specific correlation between specific neuropathies and antiganglioside antibodies has been confirmed.[14,15] Although many neurologists attempt to lower the titer of the antiganglioside antibodies in neuropathies, oncologists are developing strategies to boost antiganglioside IgM responses to tumor-associated gangliosides. Some antiganglioside IgM antibodies can increase the permeability of the blood–nerve barrier in a concentration-dependent and complement-independent manner,[16] and some may bind to neuronal gangliosides to create a neuromuscular block.[17–20] While antiganglioside IgM can serve as a marker of axonal damage in neuropathies, including multiple sclerosis, it is far from clear whether the antibodies cause axonal damage or are a result of axonal damage.[21] However, the possible pathogenesis induced by some of the antiganglioside IgM antibodies should caution oncologists against indiscriminate boosting of the antiganglioside IgM response. The development of clinically effective ganglioside vaccines against specific cancers requires biochemical and immunochemical definition of gangliosides associated with specific tumor types. Researchers also must monitor changes in the profile of antiganglioside IgM antibodies during different stages of cancer. This is important to understand and to identify the homeostatic mechanism by which the host eliminates gangliosides that are recognized by the immune system as danger signals.

We recently identified a significant antiganglioside antibody response to early-stage (organ-confined) prostate cancer,[22] and our unpublished observations revealed antiganglioside IgM antibodies in serum and ascites of patients with epithelial ovarian cancer. These findings suggest that glyco-immunomic studies may lead to the development of specific antiganglioside IgM as early biomarkers of human cancer. Many laboratories carry out antiganglioside IgM assays without analyzing the rationale and suitability of each step of the assay system. There is a need to validate the assay protocol for antiganglioside IgM antibodies. Without proper validation of the assay to monitor the antiganglioside IgM, antiganglioside IgM biomarkers may not be identified or introduced into clinical laboratories. No biomarker assay can be proposed for clinical use unless it is properly and rigorously validated. Our first publication in this direction appeared a decade ago.[3] Since then, we have developed a standard operating procedure and validated the ELISA for antiganglioside IgM antibodies.

This ELISA for antiganglioside IgM antibodies has a wide range of clinical and investigative applications in neoplastic and nonneoplastic disease. In cancer patients, it can be used to monitor endogenous immune responses to early or localized disease, evaluate danger signals corresponding to very early stages of disease and ascertain their correlation with prognosis, assess spontaneous and therapeutically induced regression, and check the level of tumor necrosis *in situ*. In neuropathic disease, it may detect autoimmune neuropathies associated with peripheral neuropathies, celiac disease, Guillain-Barré syndrome, amyotrophic lateral sclerosis, Miller-Fischer/Bickerstaff's encephalitis, or multiple sclerosis. Further, it can be a tool for monitoring rheumatoid arthritis, diabetes mellitus I and II, epilepsy, atherosclerosis, Chaga's disease, abortion, and stroke. In infectious disease, the ELISA can be used to check sequelae associated with *Campylobacter jejuni*, *Helicobacter pylori*, cytomegalovirus, HIV, amoebiasis, vaccinia, rotavirus, *Mycoplasma pneumoniae*, and neuroborreliosis. Finally, the ELISA can be used to determine the specificity of antiganglioside monoclonal antibodies and to develop microchip arrays of antiganglioside IgM for human diseases.

VALIDATION OF PROTOCOL FOR ANTIGANGLIOSIDE ANTIBODY ELISA

Since our previous report,[3] we repeatedly validated our standard operating procedures to obtain high-resolution titers of 1 or more antiganglioside IgM antibodies in sera from patients with cancer or other diseases and in sera from healthy controls. Our standard operating procedure entails the following:

(1) Characterizing the purity of ganglioside antigens in different batches and from different commercial sources.
(2) Coating of gangliosides onto microtiter plates.
(3) Blocking to eliminate background noise.
(4) Maximizing epitope–paratope interaction.
(5) Eliminating nonspecific binding of antibodies.
(6) Taking precautions at the final steps.
(7) Establishing positive and negative controls.
(8) Applying a formula to estimate titers for several replicas.
(9) Converting antibody titers to natural logs.

Characterizing the Purity of Ganglioside Antigens in Different Batches and from Different Commercial Sources

We routinely use high-performance thin-layer chromatography (HPTLC) to examine the purity of gangliosides stained with resorcinol or with ganglioside-specific murine monoclonal antibodies. HPTLC is critical because there is no standard definition of purity for gangliosides from different commercial sources. We screened

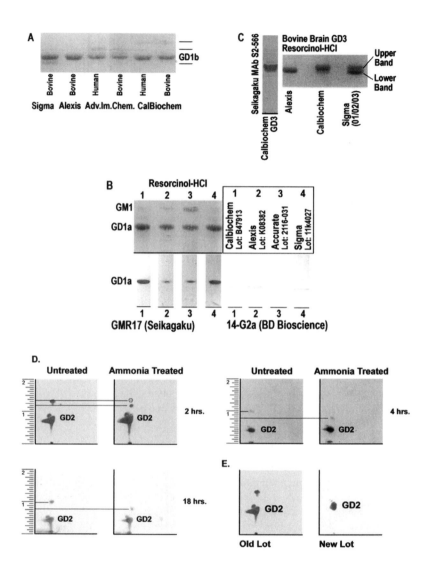

FIGURE 1. Ganglioside purity was assessed by high-performance thin-layer chromatography (HPTLC). Chromatograms were stained by resorcinol-HCl and immunostained with ganglioside-specific murine monoclonal antibodies (MAbs). **(A)** Staining of human and bovine brain GD1b (3 nmol) from 4 different commercial sources (Sigma, Alexis, Advanced Immunochemical, and Calbiochem). Contaminating glycolipids are indicated by the thin lines on the right. The GD1b from Alexis was free of contamination and hence used for ELISA. **(B)** Staining of GD1a (2 nmol) from 4 different commercial sources (Calbiochem, Alexis, Accurate, and Sigma) by resorcinol and antiganglioside monoclonal antibodies against GD1a (GMR17) and GD2 (14.G2a). Resorcinol staining identified a GM1-like contaminant that was distinct for GD1a from Accurate, less apparent for GD1a from Calbiochem and Alexis, and not detectable for GD1a from Sigma. Interestingly, the anti-GD2 monoclonal antibody 14.G2a identified a contaminant in GD1a from Calbiochem, Alexis,

murine monoclonal antibodies for their monospecificity using our ELISA protocol, and we selected a few of these monoclonal antibodies to test the purity of gangliosides on HPTLC.[22]

FIGURE 1A shows our experience with GD1b purified from human and bovine brain by Sigma (St. Louis, MO), Alexis USA (San Diego, CA), Advanced Immunochemical (Long Beach, CA), and Calbiochem (San Diego, CA). In the resorcinol-stained chromatograms, positions of the contaminating glycolipids are indicated by the thin lines on the right. Our preferred source for GD1b is Alexis because its GD1b shows no evidence of contamination.

FIGURE 1B shows contamination in purified GD1a obtained from Calbiochem, Alexis, Accurate Chemical and Scientific (Westbury, NY), and Sigma. Chromatograms were stained by resorcinol and by monoclonal antibodies for all gangliosides including GD1a (GMR17). Resorcinol staining showed a distinct GM1-like contaminant in the preparation from Accurate. This contaminant was less apparent in GD1a from Calbiochem and Alexis and was not detectable in GD1a from Sigma. Staining with MAb 14.G2a, the monoclonal antibody for GD2, identified a contaminant at the position of GD2 in the preparations from Calbiochem, Alexis, and Sigma. Because the contaminant level was very low in Sigma GD1a and because this GD1a did not contain the GM1-like contaminant, we chose GD1a from Sigma. Our second choice was Calbiochem.

FIGURE 1C shows that GD3 from Alexis, Calbiochem, and Sigma was free of contaminants stainable by either resorcinol or anti-GD3 monoclonal antibodies. We selected GD3 from Calbiochem because Sigma stopped its supply.

Unfortunately, no commercially obtained GD2 is free of contamination of other ganglioside fractions. GD2 from Advanced Immunochemical (which is reasonably priced) contains alkali-susceptible GD2, which could be GD2-lactone or O-acetylated GD2. If it is O-acetylated GD2, 1 or both sialic acids in the GD2 can be O-acetylated. Base treatment with ammonia (3N) may remove both lactone and O-acetylated derivatives.

FIGURE 1D shows the result of exposing GD2 to ammonium hydroxide. The scale in the figure shows the position of the O-acetylated GD2 in the untreated preparation. Base treatment for 2 h or 4 h removed the top fraction, which would correspond to lactones or O-acetyl groups in the terminal sialic acid of GD2. However, base treatment also introduced a new fraction midway between GD2 and the top O-acetyl GD2 band, which by its position could be GD2 with an O-acetyl group in the inner sialic acid (FIG. 1D). Additional base treatment with 7 N ammonium hydroxide for

---

and Sigma. However, because this contaminant level was very low in Sigma GD1a and because this GD1a did not contain GM1-like contaminant, we selected GD1a from Sigma for ELISA. (**C**) GD3 from Alexis, Calbiochem, and Sigma was free of contaminants by staining with resorcinol and monoclonal antibodies. We selected GD3 from Calbiochem for ELISA; Sigma no longer produces GD3. (**D**) Two-dimensional chromatogram of GD2 from Advanced Immunochemical shows 2 forms of O-acetyl GD2 before and after treatment with ammonium hydroxide at different time intervals. Treatment of GD2 with 2.5 N ammonium hydroxide de-O-acetylated the terminal sialic, but the O-acetyl group of the internal sialic acid was deacetylated only by treatment with 7 N ammonium hydroxide overnight. (**E**) Two different lots of GD2 from Advanced Immunochemical. The old lot shows base-labile contaminants, including O-AcGD2; the new lot is totally devoid of the contaminants after strong base treatment.

TABLE 2. Anti-GD2 IgM values (expressed in absorbency of sera diluted 1/500) in 40 patients with regional (stage III) metastatic melanoma

Treatment	Background correction	Minimum	Maximum	Median	Mean	STD	P value[a]
None (old lot)	No	0.045	1.609	0.228	0.341	0.318	
	Yes	0.030	1.595	0.195	0.310	0.316	
NH$_4$OH (2.5 N for 4 h)	No	0.038	1.642	0.168	0.294	0.322	**.016**
	Yes	0.031	1.632	0.154	0.278	0.315	.081 (NS)
New lot	No	0.035	2.330	0.285	0.489	0.487	**.0019**
	Yes	0.021	2.310	0.261	0.466	0.484	**.0011**

NOTE: All three batches of GD2 were from Advanced Immunochemical (Long Beach, CA).
[a]Paired-sample test between untreated and other treatment group or new lot.

2 h failed to remove the fraction, but the fraction is eliminated entirely after overnight treatment in 7 N ammonium hydroxide. The new lot provided by Advanced Immunochemical represents the final product (FIG. 1E, new lot).

The importance of base treatment before assessing anti-GD2 titers is shown in FIGURE 1E, which compares 2 lots of GD2 from Advanced Immunochemical. In the first (early) lot, a major fraction of GD2 had both sialic acids *O*-acetylated. The second (new) lot is free of the contamination and is used for routine analyses of sera for anti-GD2 IgM.

TABLE 2 shows the reactivity of sera from 40 patients with stage III melanoma against (1) GD2 (Advanced Immunochemical) treated in the laboratory with 2.5 N ammonium hydroxide for 4 h (FIG. 1D) and (2) new lot of GD2 (FIG. 1E). Base treatment abolished the upper band but not the lower band, which may contain *O*-acetyl group in the inner sialic acid. Base-treated gangliosides show significantly ($P < .02$) lower values than untreated, suggesting that the sera may contain IgM antibodies to *O*-acetyl GD2. The new lot showed significantly ($P < .002$) higher values because 100% of 3 nmol of new lot is GD2. The lower values obtained with the base-treated old lot are due to the presence of 80% or less of GD2/well.

In summary, it is critical to obtain pure ganglioside and to use a precise concentration (3 nmol) of ganglioside per well before measuring the titers of antiganglioside IgM antibodies in ELISA.

Coating of Gangliosides onto Microtiter Plates

The way in which the solid matrix of a microtiter plate is coated with ganglioside will determine how efficiently the ganglioside's sugar domains (epitopes) are exposed for immune recognition. In a previous report,[3] we coated ganglioside antigens onto different polystyrene microtiter plates. Optimal plates were those that had a low reactivity to antibody without gangliosides in the presence of excipient used for gangliosides. Absorbency higher than 0.100 at a serum dilution of 1/200 is not suitable.

Gamma irradiation at 40 kRad (Mark 1-30 irradiator, JL Shepherd and Associates) can lower background reactivity. Although microtiter plates are treated with gamma irradiation during manufacture, the dose and duration of treatment are not available. We selected Falcon 3915 as the best plate for antiganglioside IgM studies; in recent months, we found that some of the lots of Falcon 3915 have differed markedly in their background values, possibly because of differential irradiation or lack of quality control by the manufacturers. Because lot numbers for Falcon 3915 constantly change, there is a need to test background noise for each lot before analysis of antiganglioside IgM antibodies. In countries where these plates are not available, investigators should irradiate the plates in a gamma irradiator and ascertain that the absorbency of the background noise (at dual wavelength, *vide infra*) is less than 0.1.

The major problems encountered are ganglioside differences in the length of fatty acids, the number of double bonds, and the degree of hydroxylation. These characteristics depend, in part, on whether the cell is normal or neoplastic; they also depend on the commercial source (FIG. 1C). We selected 3 nmol as the optimal concentration per well. We use 200-proof ethanol as an excipient, rather than methanol or chloroform or buffer, as cited in the literature.[3] In contrast to other prevailing methods (U.S. patent 6,599,756; 20030049692), we attach the fatty acid residues of the ganglioside to the plate by 24-h vacuum desiccation. Desiccation can be extended up to 1 month if undisturbed; however, after 1 week, the surface of the wells should be checked under a dissection microscope for any evidence of peeling. The oligosaccharide residues should cluster on the plate in a fashion that simulates their appearance on the cell surface and facilitates maximal attachment of IgM. Empirically, we determined that 3 nmol of ganglioside is the optimal concentration per well and upon coating *in vacuo*.

Blocking to Eliminate Background Noise

Intermolecular spaces and ganglioside-free zones of the polystyrene plate are blocked with a buffer that contains 4% human serum albumin (HSA). We strongly discourage using gelatin, milk protein, bovine serum albumin, or other xenogenic proteins for blocking or washing, because they introduce various anomalies. Coating the plates with 4% HSA in phosphate-buffered saline (pH 7.4) for 90 min will block nonspecific binding of the serum proteins, IgM, and other antibodies.

Clinical-grade HSA is available from Baxter Healthcare Corporation (Glendale, CA) and Instituto Grifols (Barcelona, Spain). Known concentrations of this HSA should be subjected to polyacrylamide gel electrophoresis under reducing or native conditions to determine the nature and number of contaminating proteins. The contaminants in some preparations can significantly lower purity. After several such investigations, we selected 20% HSA manufactured by Instituto Grifols (stored at room temperature). This HSA is superior in performance and electrophoretic albumin/nonalbumin ratio to other preparations.

Blocking with HSA yields a baseline or background value (primary negative control) that should not exceed an absorbency of 0.100 at titer dilution or 4 dilutions below titer dilution. For example, if the titer is determined to be 6400, the background noise should be <<<0.100 at 1/3200, 1/1600, 1/800, and 1/400.

Maximizing Epitope–Paratope Interaction

Serum, plasma, or body fluids obtained during clinical investigations are usually stored in liquid nitrogen or in subzero (−35°C) freezers. Because immunoglobulins, particularly IgM cryoglobulins, precipitate during thawing of frozen fluid specimens, measurements based on fluid from the top of the tube will underestimate true antibody titers. Cryopreserved sera should be extensively vortexed immediately upon thawing to resuspend IgM cryoglobulins. Most IgM antibodies against major gangliosides (GM2, GD3, GD1a and GD1b) are not affected by 5 freeze-thaw cycles (unpublished data).

Sera can be aliquoted for analyses soon after vortexing. The aliquoted sera can be refrozen or lyophilized using an accelerated freeze-drying procedure. The lyophilized sera are reconstituted using blocking buffer that contains 4% HSA (Grifols). The volume of blocking buffer will be the same as the volume of the original serum used for lyophilizing. Although we do not use lyophilized serum, others have used it to obtain accurate measurements of antiganglioside titers (personal communication, N. Yuki).

The most critical step required after reconstitution is incubation of aliquoted sera diluted 1/100 [with 4% HSA (Grifols) in phosphate-buffered saline (PBS) pH 7.4] at 37°C for 30 min, before further dilution and addition to microtiter wells. Empirically, we determined that this step is critical to recover IgM precipitated in frozen sera. Serum is further diluted to 1/200, 1/400, 1/800, 1/1600, 1/3200, 1/6400, and 1/12,800 using detergent-free blocking buffer with 4% HSA in PBS. Depending on the nature of the disease, the serum can be diluted up to 1/204,800.

Diluted sera (100 µL) are overlaid onto antigen-coated (or noncoated) microtiter plates either vertically (from rows A to H; i.e., up to 8 dilutions) or horizontally (from rows 1 to 12; i.e., up to 12 dilutions). For maximal resolution, the plates are incubated at 37°C for 2 h.

Eliminating Nonspecific Binding of Antibodies

We previously published a table to show the nature and concentration of detergents that have been used to eliminate nonspecific binding of serum antibodies.[3] We studied varying concentrations of Tween-20 to optimize the concentration required to minimize background noise (optical density below 0.100). Wells overlaid with serum antibody were washed with a buffer containing 0.1% HSA (Grifols) in PBS (pH 7.4) with 0.1% of Tween-20. If Tween-20 is stored for a long time, it becomes ineffective for lowering background noise. We do not store Tween-20 longer than 1 month after opening.

Wells are washed manually with a multichannel pipette that is also used to remove the sera. The washing step is repeated five times, either manually or by an automated washer (BioRad Model 1575 Immunowasher, BioRad, Hercules, CA).

Taking Precautions at the Final Steps

Precautions at the final steps involve conditions to optimize the oxidation of substrates on the solid matrix and the use of a dual wavelength to correct for noise from the solid matrix. The secondary antibody that is conjugated to serum IgM is a peroxidase-conjugated rabbit antihuman $Fc_{5\mu}$ IgM suspended in 4% HSA (Grifols) in PBS (pH 7.4). This antibody is diluted 1/5000 in 4% HSA (Grifols) in PBS (pH 7.4). The incubation time for maximal resolution is 1 h.

Wells overlaid with serum antibody are washed with a freshly prepared buffer comprising 0.1% HSA (Grifols) in PBS (pH 7.4) containing 0.1% of Tween-20 (not stored for more than 1 month). Serum is removed from wells with a multichannel pipette, and wash buffer is manually added to wells (using 150 µL/well). The BioRad washer removes the buffer and automatically adds and removes the wash buffer five times. Then, 100 µL of substrate [50 mL of *ortho*-phenylenediamine dihydrochloride (2 × 25 mg tablets; Sigma) in citrate-phosphate buffer (pH 5.00) with 21 µL of 30% hydrogen peroxide (Sigma, used within 1 month after opening the bottle)] is added to wells. After exactly 45 min of incubation in the dark, enzymatic oxidation of substrate is arrested by 120 µL of 6 N H_2SO_4. Absorbency is measured after 10 min in an ELISA microtiter plate reader at dual wavelength [$A_{490} - A_{650}$] to correct for anomalies in the background and titer plates. The absorption maximum after adding 6 N H_2SO_4 is A_{492}; without 6 N H_2SO_4, it is A_{405}. It is not correct to measure absorbency at A_{490} without adding 6 N H_2SO_4 or at A_{400} after adding 6 N H_2SO_4.

Establishing Positive and Negative Controls

Positive or reference controls for antiganglioside IgM vary with the type of disease or cancer. Serum aliquots are obtained on different days from 1 or more patients who have high antibody titers; cryopreserved specimens are thawed, pooled, and vortexed to obtain 10 to 15 mL of sera, which is further split into 10-µL aliquots in 500-µL Eppendorf (color) vials.

Negative controls are obtained by pooling sera from adult males older than 50 years; age is important because the titers of most antiganglioside antibodies are low in younger patients.[14] Again, about 10 to 15 mL of pooled sera is divided into 10-µL aliquots in 500-µL Eppendorf (colorless) vials.

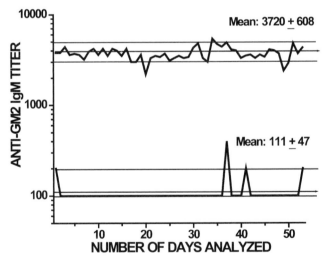

FIGURE 2. Consistency of antiganglioside ELISA. During validation studies, ELISA is repeated on different days with the same positive and negative control sera. The figure illustrates anti-GM2 IgM values in positive control sera pooled from different specimens of a patient with AJCC stage III melanoma (*top*) and negative control sera pooled from healthy volunteers older than 50 years (*bottom*). When control values peaked, ELISA failed. For a valid assay, the coefficient of variation for positive and negative controls must be less than 15%.

One vial each of positive and negative control is analyzed simultaneously with each study specimen. FIGURE 2 shows the values obtained by a single investigator (SM) who repeated the ELISA daily for 50 days.

Applying a Formula to Estimate Titers for Several Replicas

With Microsoft Excel software, the absorbency values of the microtiter plates can be calculated by the following procedure (developed by D. Soh with M. H. Ravindranath, unpublished):

- After reading a plate, use the "copy window (Ctrl + C)" command in Softmax to copy the data in "Window". After opening "Excel" program, paste the data (Ctrl + V). This procedure is repeated for every plate.

- Correct experimental values against background noise by using the subtraction command [e.g., "= (A1 − A2)"]. To find the titer at 0.1 absorbency $(A_{490nm} - A_{650nm})$, only 2 readings are assessed. For example, in the chart below, cell column 1 has a dilution (X) of 1600 and absorbency (Y) of 0.171; cell column 2 has a dilution of 3200 and an absorbency of 0.082. Cell column B and row 3 in Excel (slope value) is used (clicked) to determine slope (change in Y, change in X). After clicking B3, type in the cell "= slope (", and highlight cells B1 and B2 (Y values), insert a comma, highlight cells A1 and A2 (X values), and close parenthesis. The slope should always be negative, and there should always be a comma between the X and Y values:

Cell column	X	Y
1	1600	0.171
2	3200	0.082
3	Slope	−0.000055625
4	Titer	

- The titer at 0.1 is calculated by the following formula: (0.1 − lowest absorbency value)/slope) + highest dilution factor (which corresponds to the lowest absorbency value). Click on B4 cell; type "= ((0.1 − "; highlight B2 (lowest absorbency value) and close parenthesis; type "/" and highlight B3 (slope); Type ") +" and then highlight A2 (highest dilution factor); likewise in the chart: = ((0.1 − B2)/B3) + A2. Round up the titer value by changing the number of decimals to 0. Highlight the B4 cell and right click. In the menu, choose "format cells" and click on "number"; then change the decimal value to 0:

Cell column	A	B
1	1600	0.1710
2	3200	0.082
3	Slope	−0.000055625
4	Titer	2876.404494

- If the copy-and-paste function is used to find slope and titer values, the 2 dilution values must be above and below 0.1. The same procedure also can be used to find titers at a different absorbency such as 0.2, but the titer equation must be changed to 0.2 and all other dilution and absorbency values must be above and below 0.2.

Converting Antibody Titers to Natural Logs

Comparison of the antiganglioside IgM antibody titers for different gangliosides and in relation to treatment or stages of disease cannot use mean or median values because of the large standard deviation. To overcome this problem, we convert values to natural log titers. TABLES 3A and 3B summarize the log titers of different gangliosides obtained from healthy volunteers and patients with benign prostate hyperplasia, organ-confined prostate cancer (stage T1/T2), and unconfined prostate cancer (stage T3/T4). Further elaboration of the same data with an expanded sample size is shown elsewhere.[23]

TABLE 3A. ANOVA assessment of P values showing significant differences in log titers of anti-GD3, anti-GD2, and anti-GD1a IgM antibodies in sera from healthy controls and patients with benign prostatic hyperplasia (BPH) or prostate cancer (CaP)

IgM target	Healthy ($n = 11$) Mean ± SD	Median	BPH ($n = 10$) Mean ± SD	Median	T1/2 CaP ($n = 20$) Mean ± SD	Median	T3/4 CaP ($n = 7$) Mean ± SD	Median	ANOVA P value
GM_1	4.48 ± 1.26	4.61	4.61 ± 0.00	4.61	5.28 ± 0.99	4.61	5.46 ± 1.17	5.70	
GM_2	5.93 ± 0.65	5.97	5.16 ± 0.99	4.61	5.16 ± 0.98	4.61	6.07 ± 1.55	5.99	.073
GM_3	4.43 ± 0.22	4.61	4.68 ± 0.22	4.61	5.19 ± 1.19	4.61	5.15 ± 1.25	4.61	.181
GD_3	5.45 ± 0.91	5.19	4.61 ± 0.00	4.61	4.78 ± 0.86	4.61	4.51 ± 0.27	4.61	**.022**
GD_2	4.18 ± 1.01	4.61	5.06 ± 0.77	4.61	5.62 ± 1.19	5.70	5.74 ± 1.37	6.21	**<.007**
GD_{1a}	4.90 ± 1.09	4.61	4.90 ± 0.63	4.61	5.74 ± 1.18	5.70	4.76 ± 0.58	4.61	**.020**
GD_{1b}	5.19 ± 1.09	5.60	4.88 ± 0.58	4.61	5.04 ± 1.07	4.61	5.74 ± 1.04	5.30	.638
GT_{1b}	5.91 ± 1.04	6.27	5.07 ± 0.83	4.61	5.75 ± 1.29	5.65	6.20 ± 1.24	6.55	.181

TABLE 3B. Pairwise comparison by least significant differences method revealing that anti-GD1a IgM log titers distinguish between T1/2 and T3/4 CaP

Pairwise comparisons	P values		
	Anti-GD$_3$	Anti-GD$_2$	Anti-GD$_{1a}$
Healthy *vs.* BPH	.010^a	.076	.992
Healthy *vs.* T1/2 CaP	.016^a	.001	.018
Healthy *vs.* T3/4 CaP	.009^a	.006	.756
BPH *vs.* T1/2 CaP	.546	.205	.021
BPH *vs.* T3/4 CaP	.757	.224	.767
T1/2 CaP *vs.* T3/4 CaP	.398	.804	.019

^{a}Lower than healthy volunteers.

REFERENCES

1. ANDO, S. 1983. Gangliosides in the nervous system. Neurochem. Int. **5:** 507–537.
2. WIGAND, H. 1985. Gangliosides. New Compr. Biochem. **10:** 199–260.
3. RAVINDRANATH, M.H., R.M. RAVINDRANATH, D.L. MORTON & M.C. GRAVES. 1994. Factors affecting the fine specificity and sensitivity of serum antiganglioside antibodies in ELISA. J. Immunol. Methods **169:** 257–272.
4. RICH, R., R. FLEISHER, T. A. SCHWARTZ, *et al.* 1996. *In* Clinical Immunology: Principles and Practice. Mosby. St. Louis.
5. HARDING, C.V., J. KIHLBERG, M. ELOFSSON, *et al.* 1993. Glycopeptides bind MHC molecules and elicit specific T cell responses. J. Immunol. **151:** 2419–2425.
6. HARDING, C.V., R.W. ROOF, P.M. ALLEN & E.R. UNANUE. 1991. Effects of pH and polysaccharides on peptide binding to class II major histocompatibility complex molecules. Proc. Natl. Acad. Sci. USA **88:** 2740–2744.
7. ISHIOKA, G.Y., A.G. LAMONT, D. THOMSON, *et al.* MHC interaction and T cell recognition of carbohydrates and glycopeptides. J. Immunol. **148:** 2446–2451.
8. FREIMER, M.L., K. MCINTOSH, R.A. ADAMS, *et al.* 1993. Gangliosides elicit a T-cell independent antibody response. J. Autoimmun. **6:** 281–289.
9. RANDALL, T.D., L.B. KING & R.B. CORLEY. 1990. The biological effects of IgM hexamer formation. Eur. J. Immunol. **20:** 1971–1979.
10. DAVIS, A.C., K.H. ROUX & M.J. SHULMAN. 1988. On the structure of polymeric IgM. Eur. J. Immunol. **18:** 1001–1008.
11. RAVINDRANATH, R.M., M.H. RAVINDRANATH & M.C. GRAVES. 1997. Augmentation of natural antiganglioside IgM antibodies in lower motor neuron disease (LMND) and role of CD5+ B cells. Cell Mol. Life Sci. **53:** 750–758.
12. LIVINGSTON, P.O. 1995. Approaches to augmenting the immunogenicity of melanoma gangliosides: from whole melanoma cells to ganglioside-KLH conjugate vaccines. Immunol. Rev. **145:** 147–166.
13. RAVINDRANATH, M.H., T.F. WOOD, D. SOH, *et al.* 2002. Cryosurgical ablation of liver tumors in colon cancer patients increases the serum total ganglioside level and then selectively augments antiganglioside IgM. Cryobiology **45:** 10–21.
14. RAVINDRANATH, M.H., A.M. GONZALES, K. NISHIMOTO, *et al.* 2000. Immunology of gangliosides. Indian J. Exp. Biol. **38:** 301–312.
15. GALLARDO, E., R. ROJAS-GARCIA, R. BELVIS, *et al.* 2001. Antiganglioside antibodies: when, which and for what? Neurologia **16:** 293–297.
16. KANDA, T., T. IWASAKI, M. YAMAWAKI, *et al.* 2000. Anti-GM1 antibody facilitates leakage in an *in vitro* blood-nerve barrier model. Neurology **55:** 585–587.
17. WINER, J.B. 2001. Guillain Barre syndrome. Mol. Pathol. **54:** 381–385.

18. KUWABARA, S., K. OGAWARA, K. MIZOBUCHI, *et al.* 2000. Isolated absence of F waves and proximal axonal dysfunction in Guillain-Barre syndrome with antiganglioside antibodies. J. Neurol. Neurosurg. Psychiatry **68:** 191–195.
19. OBI, T., T. MURAKAMI, M. TAKATSU, *et al.* 1999. Clinicopathological study of an autopsy case with sensory-dominant polyradiculoneuropathy with antiganglioside antibodies. Muscle Nerve **22:** 1426–1431.
20. ARASAKI, K., S. KUSUNOKI, N. KUDO & M. TAMAKI. 1998. The pattern of antiganglioside antibody reactivities producing myelinated nerve conduction block *in vitro*. J. Neurol. Sci. **161:** 163–168.
21. SADATIPOUR, B.T., J.M. GREER & M.P. PENDER. Increased circulating antiganglioside antibodies in primary and secondary progressive multiple sclerosis. Ann. Neurol. **44:** 980–983.
22. RAVINDRANATH, M.H., S. MUTHUGOUNDER, N. PRESSER, *et al.* 2004. Gangliosides of organ-confined versus metastatic androgen-receptor-negative prostate cancer. Biochem. Biophys. Res. Commun. **324:** 154–165.
23. RAVINDRANATH, M.H., S. MUTHUGOUNDER, N. PRESSER, *et al.* 2005. Endogenous immune response to gangliosides in patients with confined prostate cancer. Int. J. Cancer **116:** in press.

A Deiminated Viral Peptide to Detect Antibodies in Rheumatoid Arthritis

GIUSEPPINA MERLINI, CONSUELO ANZILOTTI, DANIELE CHIMENTI, CRISTINA TOMMASI, STEFANO BOMBARDIERI, AND PAOLA MIGLIORINI

Clinical Immunology Unit, Department of Internal Medicine, University of Pisa, Pisa, Italy

ABSTRACT: The data presented suggest that a deiminated viral peptide is specifically recognized by antibodies contained in rheumatoid arthritis (RA) sera. Antipeptide antibodies are not associated with the presence or severity of specific manifestations of RA, but are more frequent in subjects with erosive arthritis. Taking into account the association with rheumatoid factor and with erosive arthritis, we can conclude that antipeptide antibodies are markers of severe forms of RA. Our data also show familial aggregation of anticitrullinated peptide antibodies.

KEYWORDS: rheumatoid arthritis (RA); antipeptide antibodies; deiminated viral peptide

Rheumatoid arthritis (RA) is the most common autoimmune disease in humans. It is characterized by the inflammation of synovial membranes, which can lead to the destruction of synovial joints. RA is diagnosed primarily on clinical manifestations. Serological supporting evidence has long been restricted to the determination of IgM rheumatoid factor; this antibody, however, occurs frequently in many inflammatory diseases and in healthy elderly individuals. In 1964, two Dutch scientists first discovered autoantibodies (antiperinuclear factor, APF) that label a component of the keratohyalin granules surrounding the nucleus of differentiating human buccal mucosa cells. These autoantibodies can be found with a frequency of 49–91% in RA patients' sera, and their specificity for the disease is 73–79%.[1]

In 1979, it was shown that sera from many RA patients bound the stratum corneum of rat esophagus (antikeratin antibodies, AKA). AKA are detected in 36–59% of RA sera and are present almost exclusively in this disease (specificity: 88–99%).[2]

APF and AKA are detected by indirect immunofluorescence. Despite their good sensitivity and high specificity, they have never been routinely used: standardization, in fact, is difficult, and the reproducibility is scarce. In addition, not every normal healthy donor has buccal mucosa cells suitable for APF detection.

The targets of AKA in rat esophagus epithelium are proteins of heterogeneous charge and different molecular weight.[3] In human epidermis, AKA recognize a 40-kDa protein that has been identified as a neutral/acidic isoform of filaggrin.[4] Filaggrin

Address for correspondence: Paola Migliorini, M.D., Clinical Immunology Unit, Department of Internal Medicine, Via Roma 67, 56126 Pisa, Italy. Voice: +39-50-558609; fax: +39-50-558630.
p.migliorini@med.unipi.it

Ann. N.Y. Acad. Sci. 1050: 243–249 (2005). © 2005 New York Academy of Sciences.
doi: 10.1196/annals.1313.025

is a cytokeratin filament–aggregating protein synthesized as a high molecular weight precursor named profilaggrin and stored in keratohyalin granules. During epidermal differentiation, profilaggrin is cleaved, dephosphorylated, and deiminated: the enzyme peptidylarginine deiminase (PAD) transforms, in fact, a variable number of arginine residues into citrulline, thus generating proteins of heterogeneous and more acidic charge. Both APF and AKA recognize the neutral/acidic forms of filaggrin in buccal and esophageal mucosa cells. Thus, two RA-associated autoantibodies previously considered different actually recognize the same target,[5] and both can be labeled antifilaggrin antibodies (AFA).

The posttranslational modification of arginine residues is necessary to generate epitopes recognized by AFA. In fact, recombinant filaggrin is not bound by RA sera before *in vitro* treatment with PAD,[6] and only filaggrin sequences containing citrulline instead of arginine detect RA-associated antibodies.[7]

Immunoenzymatic assays (enzyme-linked immunosorbent assay, ELISA) based on such sequences have been developed[7] and used to screen patient sera. A more sensitive assay is obtained, with a modified peptide that optimally exposes the citrulline moiety and thus allows the detection of antibodies in up to 70% RA patients.[8]

A comparative evaluation of sequences recognized by AFA shows that their critical feature is the presence of citrulline flanked by neutral amino acids such as glycine, serine, or threonine.[6] Similar amino acid repeats are commonly found in viral proteins.[7]

One of the nuclear proteins encoded by Epstein-Barr virus, EBNA I, contains a sequence (35–58) in its N-terminal region that bears a strong sequence homology to the C-terminal protein of SmD, the spliceosome protein recognized by autoantibodies in lupus sera.[9,10] We synthesized this sequence by substituting arginine with citrulline and used it to test sera from patients with connective tissue disorders. The results we obtained indicate that only sera from RA patients react with a citrulline-containing viral peptide.

PATIENTS AND METHODS

Patients

Sera were obtained from 170 RA patients and 147 control subjects, including 20 mixed cryoglobulinemia (MC) patients, 20 systemic lupus erythematosus (SLE) patients, 30 systemic sclerosis (SSc) patients, and 77 normal healthy subjects (NHS). A diagnosis of RA, SLE, and SSc was based on the ACR criteria;[11–13] MC was diagnosed in the presence of Meltzer's triad (purpura, weakness, and arthritis/arthralgia) and of cryoglobulins in the sera.

Anticitrullinated Peptide Antibodies Detection

We developed an ELISA to detect anticitrullinated peptide antibodies. Briefly, ELISA plates (Nunc) were coated with a synthetic peptide (corresponding to the amino acid sequence 35–58 of the EBNA I protein) in which all the arginine residues are substituted with citrulline diluted at 5 µg/mL in phosphate buffer solution (PBS).

After blocking with PBS 3% bovine serum albumin (BSA), sera diluted 1/200 in PBS, 1% BSA, and 0.05% Tween were incubated for 3 h at room temperature. After repeated washings, anti-human IgG F(ab')$_2$ fragment labeled with alkaline phosphatase (Sigma Chemical Co., St. Louis, MO) diluted 1:3000 in PBS, 1% BSA, and 0.05% Tween-20 was added to the wells and incubated for 3 h at room temperature. After washings, the bound enzyme activity was measured using *para*-nitrophenylphosphate as substrate (Sigma Chemical Co.).

Results are expressed as the percentage of an internal positive sample; positivity threshold of the test is 27% (higher than the 97.5th percentile found in a group of healthy control subjects).

Statistical Analysis

All the variables were analyzed independently using the Fisher's exact test for contingency tables. A *P* value of <.05 was considered significant.

RESULTS

We studied 170 serum samples from RA patients (121 women and 49 men; mean age: 60 years; range: 20–88 years; mean disease duration: 8 years; range: 6 months to 41 years) and from 147 control subjects (77 blood donors, 20 MC, 20 SLE, 30 SSc).

Among RA patients, 78/170 (44%) were positive for antipeptide antibodies. In these patients, we evaluated the presence of xerostomia, xerophthalmia, peripheral vasculitis, rheumatoid nodules, morning stiffness, symmetric arthritis, active arthritis, erosive arthritis, rheumatoid factor, and levels of C reactive protein.

The presence of antipeptide antibodies was associated with positivity for rheumatoid factor (*P* < .0001) and erosive arthritis (*P* < .05).

We also analyzed antipeptide antibodies in familial cases of RA. Sera from 16 families in which 2 or more siblings were affected by the disease were studied. In 12/16 families, the levels of antipeptide antibodies were similar in affected siblings; they were discordant in only 4 families.

DISCUSSION

The data presented in this paper suggest that a deiminated viral peptide is specifically recognized by antibodies contained in RA sera.[14] In fact, IgG antibodies that bind the deiminated EBNA I 35–58 sequence are detectable in 44% of RA sera. On the contrary, antibodies with such a specificity are not present in normal subjects or in other connective tissue disorders[15] (FIG. 1). These antibodies are more frequently detected in rheumatoid factor–positive patients, but this association is not due to the interference of rheumatoid factor with their detection. In fact, MC sera that contain rheumatoid factor at high titers do not react with the viral peptide.

Antipeptide antibodies are not associated with the presence or severity of specific manifestations of RA, but are more frequent in subjects with erosive arthritis. Thus, taking into account the association with rheumatoid factor and with erosive arthritis, we can conclude that antipeptide antibodies are markers of severe forms of RA.

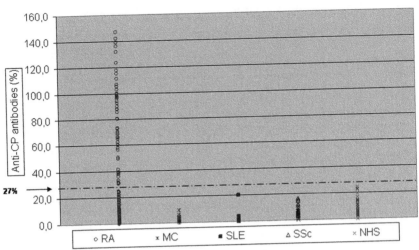

FIGURE 1. Anticitrullinated viral peptide antibodies in connective tissue diseases. The graph shows the reactivity with citrullinated peptide measured in sera from patients with RA and control subjects (other connective tissue diseases and healthy donors). The reactivity is expressed as a percentage of a reference serum. The *dashed line* represents the cutoff value. RA, rheumatoid arthritis; MC, mixed cryoglobulinemia; SLE, systemic lupus erythematosus; SSc, systemic sclerosis; NHS, normal healthy subjects.

Our data also show familial aggregation of anticitrullinated peptide antibodies (FIG. 2). In familial cases of RA, the affected siblings are in most cases both positive or both negative for antipeptide antibodies. Unfortunately, in only one family, a non-affected sibling also was tested; thus, we cannot discriminate between shared genes and shared environment. Familial aggregation has been demonstrated for different families of autoantibodies, such as antinuclear, antiphospholipid,[16] antigoblet,[17] and antithyroid.[18]

In most cases, autoantibodies have been analyzed in relatives and spouses of subjects with autoimmune disorders.[16,17] In the case of antithyroid antibodies, the prevalence of antiperoxidase, antithyroglobulin, and anti–thyroid-stimulating hormone receptor antibodies has been analyzed in twin siblings affected by autoimmune thyroid diseases and healthy twins matched for age, sex, and zygosity.

Significantly more monozygotic twin siblings were positive for two or more auto-antibodies than dizygotic twin siblings, strongly supporting the hypothesis that the familial aggregation of thyroid autoantibodies is genetically determined. The genetic control of the production of anticitrullinated peptide antibodies may be exerted at multiple levels: T and B receptor repertoire, antigen processing, and presentation. In this respect, it is of interest that citrullinated peptides can be bound by the RA-associated DR4 alleles more efficiently than the corresponding noncitrullinated peptides. The *in vivo* relevance of this observation is indicated by the specific T-cell response elicited by citrullinated peptides in HLA-DR4 transgenic mice.[19]

Citrullination is a posttranslational modification operated by PAD and deeply influenced by tissue expression and activity of these enzymes. Genetic factors regulating

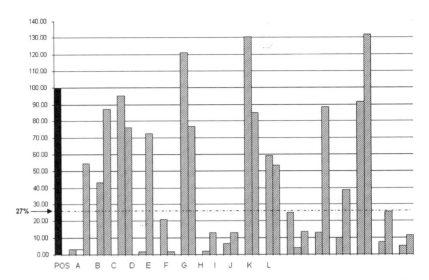

FIGURE 2. Anticitrullinated viral peptide antibodies in familial cases of RA. Histogram bars indicate the levels of anticitrullinated peptides antibodies; groups B to L represent families in which 2 or more siblings are affected by RA. In group A, a healthy sibling is also tested (*white bar*). The affected siblings are, in most cases, both positive or both negative for antipeptide antibodies.

PAD activity have been analyzed recently in subjects affected by RA. In a Japanese population, it has been shown that a PADI4 haplotype is associated with higher mRNA stability and with susceptibility to RA.[20] These data have not been confirmed in Caucasian populations,[21,22] suggesting that further studies are needed to unravel the complex relationship between PAD genes, deimination, and RA.

In conclusion, the anticitrullinated peptide antibodies we described are detectable exclusively in RA and are associated with severe forms of the disease. Both features are typical of AFA, suggesting the overlap of the two antibody populations. However, filaggrin is not the only deiminated protein presently known, and it is not expressed in synovia. Other deiminated proteins have been detected in synovial tissue and one, fibrin, is also a target of RA-specific antibodies.[23]

Therefore, AFA should be more comprehensively labeled as anticitrullinated peptide antibodies (ACPA).[24,25] Because any protein containing several arginine residues in the right amino acidic context can be deiminated by PAD becoming a potential target of ACPA, our deiminated viral peptide might be considered one of the substrates to detect ACPA.

REFERENCES

1. NIENHUIS, R.L.F. & E.A. MANDEMA. 1964. A new serum factor in patients with rheumatoid arthritis: the antiperinuclear factor. Ann. Rheum. Dis. **23:** 302–305.
2. YOUNG, B.J.J., R.K. MALLAYA, R.D.J LESLIE, *et al.* 1979. Anti-keratin antibodies in rheumatoid arthritis. Br. Med. J. **2:** 97–99.

3. GIRBAL, E., M. SEBBAG, V. GOMES-DAUDRIX, *et al.* 1993. Characterisation of the rat oesophagus epithelium antigens defined by the so-called "antikeratin antibodies", specific for rheumatoid arthritis. Ann. Rheum. Dis. **52:** 749–757.

4. SIMON, M., E. GIRBAL, M. SEBBAG, *et al.* 1993. The cytokeratin filament-aggregating protein filaggrin is the target of so-called "antikeratin antibodies", autoantibodies specific for rheumatoid arthritis. J. Clin. Invest. **92:** 1387–1393.

5. SEBBAG, M., M. SIMON, C. VINCENT, *et al.* 1995. The antiperinuclear factor and the so-called antikeratin antibodies are the same rheumatoid arthritis–specific autoantibodies. J. Clin. Invest. **95:** 2672–2679.

6. GIRBAL-NEUHAUSER, E., J.J. DURIEUX, M. ARNAUD, *et al.* 1999. The epitopes targeted by the rheumatoid arthritis-associated antifilaggrin autoantibodies are posttranslationally generated on various sites of (pro)filaggrin by deimination of arginine residues. J. Immunol. **162:** 585–594.

7. SCHELLEKENS, G.A., B.A.W. DE JONG, F.H.J. VAN DEN HOOGEN, *et al.* 1998. Citrulline is an essential constituent of antigenic determinants recognized by rheumatoid arthritis–specific autoantibodies. J. Clin. Invest. **101:** 273–281.

8. SCHELLEKENS, G.A., H. VISSER, B.A.W. DE JONG, *et al.* 2000. The diagnostic properties of rheumatoid arthritis antibodies recognizing a cyclic citrullinated peptide. Arthritis Rheum. **43:** 155–163.

9. SABBATINI, A., S. BOMBARDIERI, P. MIGLIORINI. 1993. Autoantibodies from patients with systemic lupus erythematosus bind a shared sequence of SmD and Epstein-Barr virus-encoded nuclear antigen EBNA I. Eur. J. Immunol. **23:** 1146–1152.

10. MARCHINI, B., M.P. DOLCHER, A. SABBATINI, *et al.* 1994. Immune response to different sequences of the EBNA I molecule in Epstein-Barr virus-related disorders and in autoimmune diseases. J. Autoimmun. **7:** 179–191.

11. ARNETT, F.C., S.M. EDWORTHY, D.A. BLOCH, *et al.* 1988. The American Rheumatism Association 1987 revised criteria for the classification of rheumatoid arthritis. Arthritis Rheum. **31:** 315–322

12. TAN, E.M., A.S. COHEN, J.P. FRIES, *et al.* 1982. The 1982 revised criteria for the classification of systemic lupus erythematosus. Arthritis Rheum. **25:** 1271–1277.

13. SUBCOMMITTEE FOR SCLERODERMA CRITERIA OF THE AMERICAN RHEUMATISM ASSOCIATION DIAGNOSTIC AND THERAPEUTIC CRITERIA COMMITTEE. 1980. Preliminary criteria for the classification of systemic sclerosis (scleroderma). Arthritis Rheum. **23:** 581–590.

14. PRATESI, R. *et al.* 2005. Forthcoming.

15. ANZILOTTI, C. *et al.* 2005. Forthcoming.

16. RADWAY-BRIGHT, E.L., C.T. RAVIRAJAN & D.A. ISENBERG. 2000. The prevalence of antibodies to anionic phospholipids in patients with the primary antiphospholipid syndrome, systemic lupus erythematosus and their relatives and spouses. Rheumatology **39:** 427–431.

17. FOLWACZNY, C., N. NOEHL, K. TSCHOP, *et al.* 1997. Goblet cell autoantibodies in patients with inflammatory bowel disease and their first-degree relatives. Gastroenterology **113:** 101–106.

18. BRIX, T.H., P.S. HANSEN, K.O. KYVIK, *et al.* 2004. Aggregation of thyroid autoantibodies in first-degree relatives of patients with autoimmune thyroid disease is mainly due to genes: a twin study. Clin. Endocrinol. (Oxf.) **60:** 329–334.

19. HILL, J.A., S. SOUTHWOOD, A. SETTE, *et al.* 2003. Cutting edge: the conversion of arginine to citrulline allows for a high-affinity peptide interaction with the rheumatoid arthritis–associated HLA-DRB1*0401 MCH class II molecule. J. Immunol. **171:** 538–541.

20. SUZUKI, A., R. YAMADA, X. CHANG, *et al.* 2003. Functional haplotypes of PADI4, encoding citrullinating enzyme peptidylarginine deiminase 4, are associated with rheumatoid arthritis. Nat. Genet. **34:** 395–402.

21. BARTON, A., J. BOWES, S. EYRE, *et al.* 2004. Functional haplotype of the PADI4 gene associated with rheumatoid arthritis in a Japanese population is not associated in a United Kingdom population. Arthritis Rheum. **50:** 1117–1121.

22. CAPONI, L., E. PETIT-TEIXEIRA, M. SEBBAG, *et al.* 2005. A family-based study shows no association between rheumatoid arthritis and the PADI4 gene in a French Caucasian population. Ann. Rheum. Dis. **64:** 587–593.

23. MASSON-BESSIER, C., M. SEBBAG, E. GIRBAL-NEUHAUSER, *et al.* 2001. The major synovial target of the rheumatoid arthritis–specific antifilaggrin autoantibodies are deiminated forms of the alpha- and beta-chains of fibrin. J. Immunol. **166:** 4177–4184.
24. VAN VENROOIJ, W.J. & G.J. PRUIJN. 2000. Citrullination: a small change for a protein with great consequences for rheumatoid arthritis. Arthritis Res. **2:** 249–251.
25. SEBBAG, M., S. CHAPUY-REGAUD, I. AUGER, *et al.* 2004. Clinical and pathophysiological significance of the autoimmune response to citrullinated proteins in rheumatoid arthritis. Joint Bone Spine **71:** 493–502.

Identification of Thrombin Antibodies in Patients with Antiphospholipid Syndrome

WOLFGANG MIESBACH,[a] TORSTEN MATTHIAS,[b] AND INGE SCHARRER[a]

[a]Medical Clinic III, Johann Wolfgang Goethe University Hospital, Frankfurt/Main, Germany

[b]Aesku.Diagnostics, Wendelsheim, Germany

ABSTRACT: Venous or arterial thrombosis, abortion, and the presence of anti-phospholipid antibodies (aPL) define the criteria for the antiphospholipid syndrome (APS). A heterogeneous group of antibodies against phospholipids and plasma proteins may influence several coagulation pathways and lead to thrombophilia. We investigated the presence of antibodies to thrombin (Thr) in patients with aPL and reviewed their clinical manifestations. IgG and IgM titers of aPL were measured by ELISA (Aesku.Diagnostics, Wendelsheim, Germany). Lupus anticoagulants (LA) were measured according to the criteria of the Scientific and Standardization Committee of the International Society on Thrombosis and Haemostasis. One hundred twenty patients were identified with LA or anticardiolipin (aCL). Of the 120 patients, 98 (82%) had primary APS and 22 (18%) had secondary APS. Further, 76/120 (63%) were suffering from thromboembolic manifestations, mostly venous thrombosis. Anti-thrombin-IgG was detected in 20%, and anti-thrombin-IgM was detected in 23% of the patients. The presence of anti-thrombin antibodies was closely related to the presence of anti-β_2-glycoprotein-I (β_2-GP-I) (96%), aCL (97%), and LA (87%), and less well to the presence of anti-phosphatidylserine/prothrombin (Ser/Pro) antibodies (71%) or anti-prothrombin antibodies (Pro) (50%). Sixty-seven percent of the patients with anti-Thr-IgG suffered from thromboembolic complications, mostly arterial thrombosis. The rate of thrombosis was higher for these patients than for patients with anti-β_2-GP-I antibodies (37/60, 62%), LA (50/79, 63%), or anti-Ser/Pro antibodies (18/28, 64%). Anti-thrombin antibodies were found in 20% of patients with aPL; 67% of these patients were admitted with thrombotic manifestations of APS. The presence of anti-thrombin antibodies was closely associated with the presence of aCL and anti-β_2-GP-I antibodies. The sensitivity of the test for anti-thrombin antibodies for the diagnosis of APS was higher than the sensitivity of the anti-prothrombin assay and similar to the sensitivity of the anti-Ser/Pro assay.

KEYWORDS: antiphospholipid syndrome (APS); antiphospholipid antibodies; thrombin antibodies; thrombotic manifestation; anticardiolipin antibodies

Address for correspondence: Wolfgang Miesbach, M.D., Johann Wolfgang Goethe University, Frankfurt/Main Medical Clinic III, Theodor-Stern-Kai 7, 60590 Frankfurt/Main, Germany. Voice: +49-69-6301-5051; fax: +49-69-6301-6738.
miesbach@em.uni-frankfurt.de

Ann. N.Y. Acad. Sci. 1050: 250–256 (2005). © 2005 New York Academy of Sciences.
doi: 10.1196/annals.1313.026

INTRODUCTION

Antiphospholipid syndrome (APS) is considered to be an autoimmune disease, in which unpredictable episodes of thromboembolism occur.[1] Venous or arterial thrombosis, fetal loss in women, and the laboratory evidence of antibodies against phospholipid-binding proteins are essential criteria for diagnosing APS.[2] Deep vein thrombosis and pulmonary embolism are the most common venous events, whereas the arteries are affected most commonly in the cerebral system.[3] Antiphospholipid antibodies (aPL) consist of a heterogeneous group of antibodies that target phospholipid-binding plasma proteins. In particular, β_2-glycoprotein-I (β_2-GP-I)[4,5] and prothrombin (Pro)[6] are targets of aPL.

More than 20 aPL have been identified. The clinical significance of most of these antibodies has yet to be fully elucidated.

Laboratory criteria for defining the APS include only the most well-established tests for lupus anticoagulants (LA) and anticardiolipin (aCL) antibodies.[3]

Thrombin (Thr) is the key enzyme involved in coagulation and is activated by the prothrombinase complex, which converts Pro to Thr. Thr triggers fibrinogen polymerization into fibrin. Important sites on the surface bind to fibrinogen, thrombomodulin, and anti-thrombin. Numerous effects on platelets and endothelial cells also are described.[7]

It can be presumed that antibodies against Thr play a major role in patients with APS. The aim of this study was to evaluate the presence of anti-thrombin antibodies in these patients and to analyze the relationship of sensitivity and specificity in diagnosis of APS to other aPL.

PATIENTS AND METHODS

Patients

Between 2002 and 2003, we identified 120 patients with LA or aCL present in blood samples and measured the levels of antibodies to Thr, serine/prothrombin (Ser/Pro), and Pro. Most patients were found to be aPL positive on two occasions at least six weeks apart. This finding fulfills the international consensus criteria (Sapporo criteria).[2]

Fifty-two patients (43%) had elevated IgG-aCL antibodies (median 110.5 GPL, range 16–375 GPL). Forty-two patients (35%) had elevated IgM-aCL antibodies (median 42.2 MPL, range 16–393 MPL). In 79 patients (66%), positive LA were detected.

The median age was 53 years (15–85 years), and 25% of the patients were male. Twenty-two patients (18%) suffered from systemic lupus erythematosus, and 98 patients (82%) had a primary APS.

Seventy-one patients (59%) had a history of thrombosis. Of these 71 patients, 52 patients (43%) suffered from venous thrombosis, mostly deep vein thrombosis, and 38 patients (32%) suffered from arterial thrombosis, mostly stroke (17%) and myocardial infarction (13%). Eight patients (7%) reported miscarriages. In 41 patients (34%), no manifestation of APS was found.

Blood samples were obtained by clean venipuncture and were collected into plastic tubes containing sodium citrate in a ratio of 9 parts blood to 1 part anticoagulant. The samples were centrifuged at 4000g for 40 min to obtain platelet-poor plasma, which was either assayed immediately or stored at $-70°C$ until analysis.

Measurement of Anti-Thrombin Antibodies, Anti-Prothrombin Antibodies, and Anti-Ser/Pro Antibodies

Sera were tested for IgG and IgM reactivity against Thr, Pro, and Ser/Pro using commercially available enzyme-linked immunosorbent assays (ELISA) (Aesku. Diagnostics, Wendelsheim, Germany). Human-purified Thr, human-purified Pro, or human-purified Pro with bovine phosphatidylserine was coated on irradiated microtiter plates. ELISA tests were performed according to the manufacturer's instructions. Results are expressed in units/mL in a range from 0 to 300 U/mL; the cutoff value for all tests is <15 U/mL.

Measurement of aCL Antibodies and Anti-β_2-GP-I Antibodies

The IgG-aCL and IgM-aCL antibodies were determined using a solid-phase, β_2-GP-dependent standardized ELISA and were performed according to the method of Harris and Pierangeli.[8] The results for IgG-aCL and IgM-aCL are presented in GPL or MPL units, with values up to 15 considered normal. An Aesku.Diagnostics ELISA method also was used to measure anti-IgG-β_2-GP-I antibodies.

Measurement of LA

LA were measured in platelet-depleted plasma, and the results were positive following the guidelines proposed by the Subcommittee for Standardization of Lupus Anticoagulants of the Scientific and Standardization Committee of the International Society on Thrombosis and Haemostasis.[9] The presence of LA was measured at our institution by the Kaolin-clotting time,[10] the Textarin/Ecarin time,[11] and a modified dilute Russell viper venom time[12] and was confirmed by the Staclot LA test.[10]

Statistical analysis was carried out using Fisher's exact test to compare the frequency of APS-related symptoms for patients with and without Thr antibodies.

RESULTS

Elevated levels of IgG-anti-thrombin antibodies were present in 24 of the 120 patients included in the study (20%, median 34.9 U/mL, range 15.7–100 U/mL). Elevated levels of IgM-anti-thrombin antibodies were present in 28 patients (23%, median 56.2 U/mL, range 15.4–415 U/mL).

Cumulative findings for other aPL in patients with anti-thrombin antibodies are shown in TABLE 1. Most patients with IgG-anti-thrombin antibodies also had elevated levels of IgG -β_2-GP-I (96%), IgG-aCL (92%), or LA (87 %). Elevated levels of IgG-Ser/Pro antibodies or IgG-Pro antibodies were detected much less frequently (71% and 50%, respectively). Similar results were observed for patients with elevated levels of IgM-anti-thrombin antibodies.

TABLE 1. Patients with IgG- and IgM-thrombin antibodies in which various aPL were present

Patients with IgG-anti-thrombin antibodies (n = 24)	
IgG-β_2-GP-I	23/24 (96%)
IgM-aCL	22/24 (92%)
LA	21/24 (88%)
IgM-Ser/Pro	17/24 (71%)
IgM-Pro	12/24 (50%)
Patients with IgM-anti-thrombin antibodies (n = 27)	
IgM-aCL	24/27 (89%)
IgM-Ser/Pro	22/27 (81%)
LA	16/27 (59%)
IgM-Pro	6/27 (22%)

TABLE 2. Presence of aPL in patients with and without clinical manifestations of APS

Manifestation	None	Venous	Arterial
IgG-Thr	8/24 (33%)	9/24 (38%)	11/24 (46%)
IgM-Thr	10/27 (37%)	12/27 (44%)	10/27 (37%)
IgG-aCL	15/52 (29%)	21/52 (40%)	22/52 (42%)
IgM-aCL	15/42 (36%)	18/42 (43%)	13/42 (31%)
IgG-β_2-GP-I	23/60 (38%)	25/60 (42%)	19/60 (32%)
LA	29/79 (37%)	32/79 (41%)	24/79 (30%)
IgG-Ser/Pro	10/28 (36%)	9/28 (32%)	9/28 (32%)
IgM-Ser/Pro	12/37 (32%)	16/37 (43%)	13/37 (35%)
IgG-Pro	7/23 (30%)	10/23 (43%)	8/23 (35%)
IgM-Pro	3/10 (30%)	5/10 (50%)	3/10 (30%)

NOTE: In some patients, both venous and arterial thromboses occurred.

Most patients with elevated levels of IgM-anti-thrombin antibodies also had elevated levels of IgM-aCL antibodies (89%). Elevated IgM-Ser/Pro levels were found in 81% of the patients, and positive tests for LA were found in 59% of the patients, whereas elevated levels of IgM-Pro antibodies were detected in only 22% of the patients.

Cases were analyzed with respect to the type of manifestation of APS and the occurrence of arterial or venous type of thrombosis. Sixty-six percent of patients had clinical features consistent with the Sapporo criteria. The prevalence of anti-thrombin antibodies and other aPL in these patients is shown in TABLE 2.

There were no statistically significant differences between the type of aPL in these 3 groups of patients: (1) patients without APS manifestation; (2) patients with venous thrombosis; (3) patients with arterial thrombosis. Anti-thrombin antibodies were found more frequently in patients with APS than in those without APS [odds ratio (OR) = 1.31; 95% confidence interval (CI) = 0.6–3.4]. The sensitivity of this assay for diagnosing APS was 22.5% (95% CI = 13.4–34), with a specificity of 79% (95% CI = 63–91).

The sensitivity of anti-prothrombin and anti-Ser/Pro antibodies for the diagnosis of APS was 9.86 (95% CI = 4.1–19.3) and 23.3 (95% CI = 15.8–37.1), with a specificity of 92.3 (95%CI = 79.1–98.3) and 74.4 (95% CI = 57.8–86.9), respectively. These data were obtained for the IgG type of these antibodies.

No statistically significant relationship between the presence of anti-thrombin antibodies and the age of the patients was found.

DISCUSSION

The APS is considered to be the most frequently acquired thrombotic disorder. Recently, several reports have provided evidence that anti-prothrombin antibodies are a marker for APS.[13] A number of authors have reported a significant association between anti-prothrombin antibodies and thrombosis and therefore considered these antibodies to be a risk factor for thrombosis.[14,15] Anti-prothrombin antibodies are frequently found in patients with APS, and they are more efficiently recognized when bound to phosphatidylserine-coated ELISA plates.[16] Another group demonstrated that the anti-prothrombin antibodies strongly correlate with the presence of LAC.[17] The clinical relevance of these antibodies, however, has not been established.

Recently, it was demonstrated that some anti-prothrombin antibodies contain anti-thrombin activity.[18] Thr, as the major regulator of the blood coagulation cascade, has various effects. The earliest identified function of Thr is the cleavage of fibrinogen into fibrin monomers and the activation of the fibrin-stabilizing factor XIII and protein C. Thr also has numerous effects on various cells. It alters the synthesis, expression, and release of proteins from endothelial cells[19] and stimulates the aggregation of platelets.[20] Stimulation of platelets and endothelial activation are also the main pathologic effects of aPL.[21]

At present, few data are in the literature, and these are mostly case reports analyzing anti-thrombin antibodies in patients with APS. The first report of anti-thrombin antibodies is from 1953 and involves anti-thrombin antibodies being found in a patient after repeated injections of Thr.[22]

Antibodies that recognize the secondary binding site of Thr were found in a patient with an 18-year history of recurrent arterial thromboses and with no evidence of atherosclerosis or embolism of cardiac origin.[23] It was suggested that Thr antibody production might have resulted from the abnormal generation of Thr.

A 65-year-old patient who had been exposed to topical bovine Thr during cardiac surgery developed markedly prolonged clotting times and a severe bleeding diathesis. The patient's factor V activity was 1% of normal and could not be corrected by mixing with normal plasma. This demonstrated the presence of an inhibitor to factor V. Antibodies to Thr also were found. The authors suggested that detectable amounts of factor V that were found in commercial bovine preparations may have been the cause of the patient developing antibodies to Thr and factor V.[24]

In 1990, a comparative analysis of Thr and anti-thrombin antibody levels in donors and myocardial infarction patients showed increased Thr levels and a decrease of anti-thrombin antibodies in patients with myocardial infarction.[25] In addition, a linear correlation between levels of Thr and its antibodies was demonstrated.[26] Antibodies against thrombomodulin, an inhibitor of Thr, also were found to be related to thrombosis in 83 unselected patients.[27] Recently, it was suggested that Thr inhibition may be a new therapeutic target for cerebral ischemia, because the intracerebral injection of a Thr inhibitor, hirudin, reduced neurological deficits after cerebral ischemia.[28]

In our study, all individuals had been admitted with apL, as either aCL antibodies or LA. It can be presumed that antibodies to Thr play a major role in the APS because the fact that Thr is the key enzyme of coagulation also influences endothelial activity. Thr antibodies were found in more than 20% of the cohort. The prevalence of elevated anti-thrombin antibodies in patients with thrombosis was clearly increased in comparison with those without thrombosis. This finding leads us to suspect a possible role of anti-thrombin antibodies that results in thrombophilic diathesis. No differences were found by distinguishing between the venous and arterial types of thrombosis in patients with APS.

Surprisingly, we could not confirm the close relation between the presence of Thr antibodies and Pro antibodies as demonstrated in an earlier study.[18] The presence of anti-thrombin antibodies is certainly not an epiphenomenon of the presence of anti-prothrombin antibodies. By contrast, the presence of Thr antibodies was closely related to the presence of aCL or anti-β_2-GP-I antibodies. Most patients with Thr antibodies also had elevated levels of aCL or anti-β_2-GP-I antibodies. Further investigations are needed to determine whether there is any benefit in additional measurements of anti-thrombin antibodies.

The sensitivity of the test for anti-thrombin antibodies for the diagnosis of APS was higher than the sensitivity of the anti-prothrombin assay and was similar to the sensitivity of the anti-Ser/Pro assay. It must be considered, however, that the criteria for inclusion in this study were elevated apL, such as aCL antibodies and LA, and as a result all patients had elevated levels of apL.

In conclusion, our investigation suggests that the determination of anti-thrombin antibodies may contribute to a better diagnosis of APS. The role of apL in the pathogenesis of thrombosis requires further and more intensive investigations. As has been shown, the established apL tests cannot be replaced by measurements of apL such as anti-thrombin antibodies. More studies are needed to confirm the pathologic role of Thr antibodies in patients with APS.

REFERENCES

1. SHOENFELD, Y. & M. BLANK. 2004. The infectious etiology of the antiphospholipid syndrome. Autoimmun Rev. **3**(suppl. 1): 32–34.
2. WILSON, W.A., A.E. GHARAVI, T. KOIKE, *et al.* 1999. International consensus statement on preliminary classification criteria for definite antiphospholipid syndrome: report of an international workshop. Arthritis Rheum. **42**: 1309–1311.
3. SHORTELL, C.K., K. OURIEL, R.M. GREEN, *et al.* 1992. Vascular disease in the antiphospholipid syndrome: a comparison with the patient population with atherosclerosis. J. Vasc. Surg. **15**: 158–165.
4. GALLI, M., P. COMFURIUS, C. MAASEN, *et al.* 1990. Anticardiolipin antibodies directed not to cardiolipin but to a plasma protein cofactor. Lancet **335**: 1544–1547.
5. MCNEIL, H.P., R.J. SIMPSON, C.N. CHESTERMAN & S.A. KRILIS. 1990. Anti-phospholipid antibodies are directed against a complex antigen that includes a lipid-binding inhibitor of coagulation: $\beta2$-glycoprotein I (apolipoprotein H). Proc. Natl. Acad. Sci. USA **87**: 4120–4124.

6. GALLI, M. & T. BARBUI. 1999. Antiprothrombin antibodies: detection and clinical significance in the antiphospholipid syndrome. Blood **93**: 2149–2157.

7. SIESS, W. 1989. Molecular mechanisms of platelet activation. Physiol Rev. **69**: 58–178

8. HARRIS, E.N. & S.S. PIERANGELI. 2002. Revisiting the anticardiolipin test and its standardization. Lupus **11**: 269–275.

9. BRANDT, J.T., D.A. TRIPLETT, B. ALVING & I. SCHARRER [on behalf of the Subcommittee on Lupus Anticoagulant/Antiphospholipid Antibody of the Scientific and Standardisation Committee of the ISTH]. 1995. Criteria for the diagnosis of lupus anticoagulants: an update. Thromb. Haemost. **74**: 1185–1190.

10. MACKIE, I.J., S. DONOHOE & S.J. MACHIN. 2000. Lupus anticoagulant measurement. *In* Hughes Syndrome: Antiphospholipid Syndrome, pp. 214–225. Springer. London.

11. TRIPLETT, D.A., K.F. STOCKER & G.A. UNGER. 1993. The Textarin/Ecarin ratio: a confirmatory test for lupus anticoagulants. Thromb. Haemost. **70**: 925–931.

12. THIAGARAJAN, P., V. PENGO & S.S. SHAPIRO. 1986. The use of the dilute Russel viper venom time for the diagnosis of lupus anticoagulants. Blood **68**: 869–874.

13. AMENGUAL, O., T. ATSUMI & T. KOIKE. 2004. Antiprothrombin antibodies and the diagnosis of the antiphospholipid syndrome. Clin. Immunol. **112**: 144–149.

14. DE GROOT, P.G., D.A. HORBACH, M.J. SIMMELINK, *et al.* 1998. Anti-prothrombin antibodies and their relation with thrombosis and lupus anticoagulants. Lupus **7**: S32–S36.

15. VON LANDENBERG, P., T. MATTHIAS, J. ZAECH, *et al.* 2003. Antiprothrombin antibodies are associated with pregnancy loss in patients with the antiphospholipid syndrome. Am. J. Reprod. Immunol. **49**: 51–56.

16. GALLI, M., G. BERETTA, M. DALDOSSI, *et al.* 1997. Different anticoagulant and immunological properties of anti-prothrombin antibodies in patients with antiphospholipid antibodies. Thromb. Haemost. **77**: 486–491.

17. ATSUMI, T., M. IEKO, M.L. BERTOLACCINI, *et al.* 2000. Association of autoantibodies against the phosphatidylserine-prothrombin complex with manifestations of the antiphospholipid syndrome and with the presence of lupus anticoagulant. Arthritis Rheum. **43**: 1982–1993.

18. HWANG, K.K., J.M. GROSSMANN, S. VISVANATHAN, *et al.* 2001. Identification of anti-thrombin antibodies in the antiphospholipid syndrome that interfere with the inactivation of thrombin by antithrombin. J. Immunol. **167**: 7192–7198.

19. DEMICHELE, M.A. & F.L. MINNEAR. 1992. Modulation of vascular endothelial permeability by thrombin. Semin. Thromb. Hemost. **18**: 287–295.

20. VENTURINI, C.M. & J.E. KAPLAN. 1992. Thrombin induces platelet adhesion to endothelial cells. Semin. Thromb. Hemost. **18**: 275–273.

21. MERONI, P.L., E. RASCHI, C. TESTONI & M.O. BORGHI. 2004. Endothelial cell activation by antiphospholipid antibodies. Clin. Immunol. **112**: 169–174.

22. VERWILGHEN, R., M. VERSTRAETE & J. VANDENBROUCKE. 1953. Anti-thrombin specific antibodies of equine origin; description of a case where such antibodies developed following repeated injections of thrombin. Rev. Hematol. **8**: 273–275.

23. COSTA, J.M., J.N. FIESSINGER, L. CAPRON & M. AIACH. 1992. Partial characterization of an autoantibody recognizing the secondary binding site(s) of thrombin in a patient with recurrent spontaneous arterial thrombosis. Thromb. Haemost. **67**: 193–199.

24. ZEHNDER, J.L. & L.L. LEUNG. 1990. Development of antibodies to thrombin and factor V with recurrent bleeding in a patient exposed to topical bovine thrombin. Blood **76**: 2011–2016.

25. POLEVAIA, O., M.A. MIAGKOVA, I.A. BERBITSKAIA, *et al.* 1990. Comparative analysis of thrombin and anti-thrombin antibody levels in donors and myocardial infarction patients. Germatol. Transfuziol. **35**: 8–10.

26. KOROCHKIN, I.M., I.A. VERBITSKAIA, A.N. TUGUTOV, *et al.* 1990. Thrombin and anti-thrombin antibody levels in blood of patients with acute myocardial infarction. Kardiologiia **30**: 45–48.

27. GUERMAZI, S., F. MELLOULI, S. TRABELSI, *et al.* 2004. Anti-thrombomodulin antibodies and venous thrombosis. Blood Coagul. Fibrinolysis **15**: 553–558.

28. HUA, Y., R.F. KEEP, T. SCHALLERT, *et al.* 2003. A thrombin inhibitor reduces brain edema, glioma mass and neurological deficits in a rat glioma model. Acta Neurochir. Suppl. **86**: 503–506.

Antibodies against Erythropoietin and Other Protein-Based Therapeutics

An Overview

ARNO KROMMINGA[a] AND HUUB SCHELLEKENS[b]

[a]Institute for Immunology, Clinical Pathology, Molecular Medicine (IPM), Hamburg, Germany

[b]Central Laboratory Animal Institute and Department of Innovation Studies, Utrecht University, Utrecht, the Netherlands

ABSTRACT: Many factors influence the immunogenicity of protein-based therapeutics. At present, it is inconceivable to manufacture a biopharmaceutical without the risk of this adverse effect. Thus, the detection and characterization of antibodies against protein-based therapeutics is a significant task. Only clinical studies and careful monitoring of the market can be used to conclusively demonstrate rates of immunogenicity in humans for protein therapeutics. Fully validated, reliable, and robust *in vitro* assays, in combination with sensitive bioassays, should be used to address these topics.

KEYWORDS: antibodies; assay; erythropoietin (EPO); immunogenicity; protein; therapeutics

INTRODUCTION

In the past 25 years, an increasing number of biopharmaceuticals produced by genetically modified cells have entered clinical practice. This first generation of products mainly consisted of copies of naturally occurring growth factors, cytokines, or hormones, sometimes with minor modifications to enhance stability or enable expression in bacterial hosts. Powerful new techniques are now available, such as pegylation and hyperglycosylation, which allow the development of second-generation biopharmaceuticals with enhanced therapeutic index, increased bioavailability, or other improvements. These variants of natural products may be immunogenic, which may limit their clinical usefulness.

Immunogenicity has always been associated with the medical use of proteins from both animal and human origin (TABLE 1). In the case of proteins of animal origin, such as bovine and porcine insulin and equine antisera, the foreign nature was considered the main cause of immunogenicity. However, products of human origin, such as growth hormone and clotting factors, also induced an immunological response.

Address for correspondence: Arno Kromminga, Institute for Immunology, Clinical Pathology, Molecular Medicine (IPM), Lademannbogen 61, 22339 Hamburg, Germany. Voice: +49-40-53805514; fax: +49-40-53805854.

arno.kromminga@gmx.de

Ann. N.Y. Acad. Sci. 1050: 257–265 (2005). © 2005 New York Academy of Sciences.
doi: 10.1196/annals.1313.027

TABLE 1. Prevalence of antibodies against biopharmaceuticals

Class	Substance	Indication	Reactivity (%)
Antibodies	Anti-CD3 (OKT3)	Immunosuppressant	<1%
	Anti-Her2	Mamma-tumor	<1%
	Anti-IgE	Allergic asthma	<1%
	Anti-Il-2R	Immunosuppressant	18%
	Anti-TNF-α	RA, M. Crohn	10%
Receptors	CD4	HIV	<1–12%
	TNF receptor	Multiple sclerosis	16%
	Il-1 receptor	Leukemia	<1%
Cytokines	Il-2	Tumor	52%
	Il-3	Tumor	>80%
	Il-12	HCV	<1%
Interferons	IFN-α2a	HCV	27–60%
	IFN-β	Multiple sclerosis	45%
Enzymes	Factor VIII	Hemophilia	10–30%
	DNase	Cystic fibrosis	9%
	Plasm.-activator	Ischemia	<1%
Hormones	Insulin	Diabetes	44–60%
	HGH	Growth	16%
	G-CSF	Neutropenia	4%
	GM-CSF	Tumor	25–80%
	EPO	Anemia	<1%

These products, however, were used to treat innate deficiencies with a supposed lack of development of immune tolerance.

The introduction of recombinant technology made it possible to develop products that could be considered homologues of human proteins. However, in cases in which the protein of animal origin was replaced with a humanized product, the problem of immunogenicity was reduced, but still persisted.[1] In addition, an increasing number of products appeared to be immunogenic in patients who were normally immune tolerant to the natural counterpart.

Many factors influence the immunogenicity of therapeutic proteins (TABLE 2).[2,3] Impurities and contaminants were identified as the main cause of immunogenicity of human growth hormone and insulin. The presence of aggregates by suboptimal production or formulation also has been associated with the induction of antibodies. In addition, patients' characteristics are important. In cancer patients with an impaired immune system, the incidence of antibodies is lower than in patients with viral infection. Route of administration is also a factor. In studies in which the routes of administration were compared, the intravenous and local routes showed a lower incidence of antibodies than the groups treated subcutaneously or intramuscularly.

TABLE 2. Factors that may cause immunogenicity

Product-specific causes

   Structural differences between exogenous and endogenous protein

   Aggregation

   Degradation—oxidation, deamidation, glycosylation differences

   Impurities

   Formulation

Host-specific causes

   Dose and frequency of therapy

   Route of administration

   Host immune competence

   Con-meds

   Genetic predisposition

These antibodies are induced by two mechanisms.[4] First is the classical reaction to foreign proteins such as those caused by the biopharmaceuticals of bacterial or plant origins such as streptokinase and asparaginase. The reaction can be explained easily as a normal reaction to a foreign protein. The other mechanism by which antibodies are induced is based on breaking the normally existing immune tolerance to self-antigens seen in many autoimmune phenomena.[5] This is the mechanism that leads to the antibodies to human homologues, such as the interferons (IFNs), granulocyte-macrophage colony-stimulating factor (GM-CSF), and erythropoietin (EPO). The mechanisms by which tolerance is induced or broken are not completely understood. The presence of impurities such as endotoxins or microbial DNA may act as danger signals and activate autoreactive B cells to self-antigens. An important way to break tolerance is to present the self-antigens in a repetitive way.[6] A periodicity of these antigens as present in aggregates of proteins is apparently very efficient in activating ignorant or anergic B cells that are responsible for tolerance.

In many cases, the antibodies have no or little biological consequences. The main consequence of antibodies is the loss of efficacy of the therapeutic protein. The most dramatic effect of antibodies occurs if a natural protein with an essential biological activity is neutralized. Such a consequence was described for megakaryocyte differentiation and growth factor (MDGF) some years ago. This thrombopoietin-like protein induced antibodies that neutralize endogenous TPO, which leads to severe thrombocytopenia in volunteers and cancer patients. As discussed later, we have seen an upsurge of pure red cell aplasia (PRCA) associated with the use of EPO α in patients with chronic renal failure in Europe, Canada, and Australia between 1998 and 2003 caused by a formulation change.[7,8]

ASSAY METHODOLOGIES

Assays for the detection of antibodies should provide accurate and precise information about the nature of the antibodies.[9] Immunochemical methods, such as binding assays or immunoblotting, and biophysical assays, such as surface plasmon resonance, mainly assess the binding characteristics of the antibodies. Distinguishing between the neutralizing and nonneutralizing potential of those antibodies is done by cell-based assays. The validation of all must consider a number of problems, including the nature of the samples, matrix effects, natural antibodies, immune complexes, and conformational epitopes.[10]

Binding Antibodies

In principle, several assay formats can be used for the analysis of antibodies against protein-based therapeutics. The radioimmunoprecipitation assay (RIPA), which makes use of the radiolabeled antigen, is a direct liquid phase assay and detects linear as well as conformational epitopes with high sensitivity. Because the antigen is not immobilized, the conformation is not altered, and all epitopes are accessible. In addition, its easy use and robustness makes this assay format a "gold standard" for screening purposes.[11,12]

However, standard sandwich enzyme-linked immunosorbent assays (ELISAs) are commonly used as screening assays, although they are hampered by misleading results mainly caused by matrix effects. Nonspecific binding may lead to false-positive results and epitopes that are not accessible because the immobilization of the antigen may lead to false-negative results. In addition, low-affinity antibodies may fail to be detected. Novel bridging types of ELISAs may circumvent the disadvantage of standard ELISAs. In this assay format, antibodies in the serum samples cross-link nonlabeled antigen immobilized on microtiter plates and labeled (biotinylated) antigen in the liquid phase. Antibody–enzyme conjugate, which recognizes the labeled antigen, is used as a secondary antibody for detection. In comparison with standard sandwich ELISAs, this assay format increases the specificity with acceptable sensitivity.

Immunoblotting is the method of choice when other protein components must be separated from the antigen. The electrophoretic separation can be performed under denaturing [in the presence of sodium dodecyl sulfate (SDS)] or nondenaturing conditions, as well as under reducing or nonreducing conditions. Immunoblotting must be carefully controlled to assess the validity of the data generated, and it must be remembered that some antibodies will fail to recognize conformational epitopes after SDS–polyacrylamide gel electrophoresis.

Surface plasmon resonance (SPR) may be used to identify and characterize antibodies without labeling. In addition to the mere detection, SPR can be used to study molecular interaction in real time by determining the relative affinity of the antibodies by the measurement of the dissociation of the antibody from the immobilized antigen. It should be noted that the sensitivity of SPR may be lower than RIPA.

Neutralizing Antibodies

Antibodies whose binding capacity has been identified by immunochemical or biophysical methods must be further characterized by cell-based assays to determine their neutralizing activity. The standardization of bioassays is difficult, and the lab-to-lab variation is high because all bioassays are associated with multiple problems such as matrix effects or interference with nonantibody inhibitory factors.

The detection of antibodies against EPO is based on the proliferative effect of EPO on erythroid progenitor cells from cultured bone marrow cells.[7] Alternatively, the strictly EPO-dependent cell line UT-7 can be used.[13] The growth of those cells can be inhibited in the presence of anti-EPO antibodies. This inhibitory effects on erythroid colony formation can be reversed by the addition of EPO to the cell culture.

Various cell lines are established to measure antibodies against cytokines, including the murine thymoma cell line NOB-1 for Il-1, CTLL2 for Il-2, B9 for Il-6, or the rhabdosarcoma cell line KD4 for tumor necrosis factor-α (TNF-α).[14] In all of those assays, the effect of antibodies is assessed by performing dilution series of antibody preparations and preincubating these with a fixed amount of the appropriate cytokine. Dose–response curves in the presence or absence of the appropriate positive control should be included. The biological activity of anti-GM-CSF can be assessed by using the human cell lines TF-1 and MO7e, which both proliferate in response to GM-CSF.

The measurement of the neutralizing activity of antibodies against IFNs is usually assessed by antiviral assays. In those assays, the cytopathic effect on human lung carcinoma cell lines A549 or MC-5 is detected after challenge by encephalomyocarditis virus (EMCV) in the presence or absence of anti-IFN antibodies.[14,15] This assay measures the interaction of neutralizing antibodies with IFN-β and cultures cells capable of producing MxA. In the presence of neutralizing antibodies, the Mx levels in this model will be reduced.[16,17]

EXAMPLES FOR IMMUNOGENICITY

EPO

EPO is an endogenous growth factor required for erythropoiesis. Since 1998, we have seen an upsurge of PRCA associated with the use of EPO in patients with chronic renal failure in Europe, Canada, and Australia.[7,8] As of September 2004, the number of antibody-mediated cases reported has increased to more than 225. The number of new cases in 2003 dropped dramatically after the s.c. administration of EPO α was banned. The most likely explanation for this serious side effect is a subtle change in the EPO formulation that occurred when human serum albumin was replaced by sorbitol 80.

The development and validation of an assay to detect human anti-EPO antibodies in serum or plasma has been hampered for a long time by the lack of purified antibodies to fully characterize and validate the assay. The preparation of an affinity-purified human antibody to EPO enabled the establishment of a fully validated radio-immunoprecipitation (RIP) assay that can be used for the measurement of anti-EPO antibodies in serum or plasma samples with high sensitivity and reproducibility.[12] The lower limit of detection of this assay is 1 ng/mL; the precision ranges from 5.8% to 15.3%. The mean coefficient of variation ranged from 6.1% to 16.6% for antibody concentrations between 7.8 and 500 ng/mL. Both the sensitivity and specificity of this assay are greater than 98%. Because of its proven practicability in terms of specificity, sensitivity, variability, and robustness, the RIPA format also may be the method of choice for determining the presence of antibodies against other biopharmaceutical therapeutics.

IFN-α2

The immunogenicity of human IFN-α2 (Hu IFN-α2) has been studied most extensively.[18,19] The most striking feature of the immunogenicity of these products is the high variation in incidence reported, which ranges from 0 to more than 60%. As discussed, a number of factors may explain this variation, such as route of administration, length of treatment, and total amount of biopharmaceutical administered. The most important reason for the variation is the assay system used. These assay systems are either immunoassays, which identify binding antibodies, or bioassays, which identify neutralizing antibodies. Because international standards are lacking and materials and methods differ between laboratories, it is impossible to compare results. The World Health Organization has recommended a way to express the neutralizing activity of sera. However, blind panel testing has shown that, even between experienced laboratories employing these calculation methods, results may differ more than 200-fold.[20] Therefore, results on relative immunogenicity of different biopharmaceuticals should be interpreted with caution and are valid only if the preparations are compared in the same trials and the sera are analyzed in a single laboratory.

The type of product also influences immunogenicity. There have been many reports that IFN-α2a is more antigenic than Hu IFN-α2b. These IFNs differ in a single amino acid. Moreover, the gene for IFN-α2a is not present in the population, opening the possibility that this type of IFN carries a neoantigen. However, extensive studies have shown that the structural difference between the two products may not be the reason for the difference in immunogenicity. After analyzing the cause of the differences in immunogenicity between different batches of IFN-α2a, its manufacturer concluded that oxygenation and aggregate formation after prolonged storage at room temperature of an HSA containing freeze-dried preparation were the reason for enhanced immunogenicity. Changing to a liquid HSA-free formulation and storage at 4°C reduced this problem. In the case of IFN-α, the evidence is convincing that antibodies may reduce efficacy, emphasizing the need for reduction of the immunogenicity as much as possible.

IFN-β

Three different IFN-β preparations are being used to treat multiple sclerosis. Because of differences in treatment schedules, dosage, and route of administration, as well as the lack of assay standardization, it is difficult to compare the immunogenicity of the E. coli–derived product (Betaseron) and the two CHO cell-derived products (Avonex and Rebif). It is, however, clear that the bacterial product is more immunogenic than the two products derived from mammalian cells.[21] The E. coli product induces neutralizing antibodies in more than 50% of patients after 6–12 months of treatment. The incidence of antibodies is lower after treatment with CHO products. The relative high immunogenicity of the bacterial product has been linked to the lack of glycosylation, which hides hydrophobic sites of the molecule.[22] The solubility of the protein is reduced, which leads to aggregate formation. Compared with the CHO products, the bacterial-derived IFN-β show a low specific activity, which confirms the presence of inactive material. There is some evidence indicating a difference in immunogenicity between the two CHO preparations, showing that factors other than the host cell also influence the induction of antibodies. There is clear evidence showing that patients with high levels of antibodies lose the response to IFN-β.[15] Large prospective clinical studies are needed to define the level of antibody that can be correlated with the lack of efficacy in individual cases.

Factor VIII

Hemophilia A is a bleeding disorder caused by a deficiency of factor VIII. Replacement therapy with factor VIII has been proven to be successful over the years. The initial factor VIII preparations were natural preparations derived from donated blood. Currently, a number of recombinant DNA-derived products are available. The current plasma-derived factor VIII preparations induce antibodies in 25% of patients, 5–10% of whom show neutralizing activity. In addition, recombinant-derived factor VIII preparations induce antibodies.[23] Hemophilia A is an X-linked genetic disease that results from mutations or deletions that alter the expression and secretion of blood coagulation factor VIII. Factor VIII is completely absent in patients with severe hemophilia A; these patients have never developed immune tolerance, so infused factor VIII represents a foreign antigen to the patient's immune system. This explains why most factor VIII inhibitors develop in severe hemophilia A patients or those whose baseline factor VIII is less than 1%. These patients do not benefit from administration of factor VIII concentrates because their immune systems produce antibodies that inactivate the infused factor VIII. Generally, patients who develop this IgG immune response have factor VIII genes with large deletions, a common inversion, or nonsense mutations that lead to premature termination. Antibody formation rarely occurs in patients with only frameshift or missense mutations. This correlation between type of genetic defect and the development of antibodies is not absolute. It is likely that other genetic and environmental factors contribute to the generation of inhibitors.

Monoclonal Antibodies

Since the introduction of the hybridoma technology in 1975, the development was mainly directed to the use of monoclonal antibodies (mAbs) as therapeutic agents. However, it took a decade before the first monoclonal antibody, OKT-3, was available for the prevention of allograft rejection, followed in 1992 by the marketing authorization of ReoPro to assist percutaneous coronary surgery. The main reason for this slow development as therapeutic agents has been the high immunogenicity of the first generation of murine-derived mAbs.[24]

Recombinant DNA technology has made it possible to exchange the murine constant parts of the immunoglobulin chains with the human counterparts (chimeric mAb) and later to graft murine complementary regions that determine specificity into a human immunoglobulin backbone, creating humanized mAbs. At present, transgenic animals, phage display technologies, and other developments allow the production of completely human mAbs. These technological advances have led to the introduction of an increasing number of therapeutic mAbs, some of which have provided major breakthroughs in the treatment of major chronic diseases. At least 400 others are in development, and some of these will certainly reach the market in the near future. However, the expectation that human mAbs would be devoid of immunogenicity proved to be false. Although humanization has reduced the immunogenicity of mAbs, completely human mAbs have been shown to induce antibodies as has been predicted.[25] Because the antibodies induced by mAbs may interfere with efficacy and may enhance immune-mediated side effects, the issue of immunogenicity should be considered for every new therapeutic mAb.[26]

CONCLUSIONS

Many factors influence the immunogenicity of protein-based therapeutics. At present, it is inconceivable to manufacture a biopharmaceutical without the risk of this adverse effect. Therefore, the detection and characterization of antibodies against protein-based therapeutics is a significant task. Only clinical studies and careful monitoring of the market can be used to conclusively demonstrate rates of immunogenicity in humans for protein therapeutics. Fully validated, reliable, and robust *in vitro* assays, in combination with sensitive bioassays, should be used to address these questions. All assays should be validated according to international guidelines and recommendations.[27] Because of the lack of standardization, the assays must be carefully selected and validated. The validation procedure should include the determination of different factors, including specificity and sensitivity, recovery, and robustness/ruggedness. In addition, other factors, such as sample stability and system suitability, should be considered during assay development. However, one of the most difficult issues associated with assays for antibody detection is the interpretation and evaluation of the results. The results and the analysis are dependent on the type of assay, the assay design, and the issue being considered. It is very important to include adequate control samples. If possible, for positive controls, human sera should be used instead of hyperimmune sera from animals. Reference standards should be provided as is available for antibody preparation against GM-CSF, IFN-α, or IFN-β (NIH in the United States and NIBSC in the United Kingdom). Only antibodies that neutralize the biological activity of the biologicals compromise clinical response. The use of bioassays to assess antibody induction in patients, therefore, provides a useful assessment of potential mediated inhibition of therapeutic response.

REFERENCES

1. PORTER, S. 2001. Human immune response to recombinant human proteins. J. Pharm. Sci. **90:** 1–11.
2. SCHELLEKENS, H. 2002. Bioequivalence and the immunogenicity of biopharmaceuticals. Nat. Rev. Drug. Discov. **1:** 457–462.
3. RYFF, J.C. & H. SCHELLEKENS. 2002. Immunogenicity of rDNA-derived pharmaceuticals. Trends Pharmacol. Sci. **23:** 254–258.
4. SCHELLEKENS, H. 2003. Immunogenicity of therapeutic proteins. Nephrol. Dial. Transplant. **18:** 1257–1259.
5. GOODNOW, C.C. 2001. Pathways for self-tolerance and the treatment of autoimmune diseases. Lancet **357:** 2115–2121.
6. CHAKERIAN, B., P. LENZ, D.R. LOWY & J.T. SCHILLER. 2002. Determinants of autoantibody induction by conjugated papillomavirus virus–like particles. J. Immunol. **169:** 6120–6126.

7. CASADEVALL, N., J. NATAF, B. VIRON, *et al.* 2002. Pure red cell aplasia and antierythropoietin antibodies in patients treated with recombinant erythropoietin. N. Engl. J. Med. **346:** 469–475.

8. WEBER, G., J. GROSS, A. KROMMINGA, *et al.* 2002. Allergic skin and systemic reactions in a patient with pure red cell aplasia and anti-erythropoietin antibodies challenged with different epoetins. J. Am. Soc. Nephrol. **13:** 2381–2383.

9. MIRE-SLUIS, A. 2002. Challenges with current technology for the detection, measurement, and characterization of antibodies against biological therapeutics. Biol. Dev. Biol. (Basel) **109:** 59–69.

10. WADHWA, M., C. BIRD, P. DILGER, *et al.* 2003. Strategies for detection, measurement, and characterization of unwanted antibodies induced by therapeutic biologicals. J. Immunol. Methods **278:** 1–17.

11. KAWASAKI, E. & G.S. EISENBARTH. 2000. High-throughput radioassays for autoantibodies to recombinant autoantigens. Front. Biosci. **5:** e181–e190.

12. TACEY, R., A. GREWAY, J. SMIELL, *et al.* 2003. The detection of anti-erythropoietin antibodies in human sera and plasma. Part I. Validation of the protocol for a radioimmunoprecipitation assay. J. Immunol. Methods **283:** 317–329.

13. CASADEVAL, N. 2002. Antibodies against rHuEPO: native and recombinant. Nephrol. Dial. Transplant. **17**(suppl. 5)**:** 42–47.

14. WADHWA, M., A. MEAGER, P. DILGER, *et al.* 2000. Neutralizing antibodies to GM-CSF, Il-1α and IFN-γ but not other cytokines in human immunoglobulin preparations. Immunology **99:** 113–123.

15. SÖRENSEN, P.S., C. ROSS, K.M. CLEMMESEN, *et al.* 2003. Clinical importance of neutralising antibodies against interferon beta in patients with relapsing-remitting multiple sclerosis. Lancet **362:** 1184–1191.

16. KOB, M., J. HARVEY, F. SCHAUTZER, *et al.* 2003. A novel and rapid assay for the detection of neutralizing antibodies against interferon-beta. Mult. Scler. **9:** 32–35.

17. DEISENHAMMER, F., M. REINDL, J. HARVEY, *et al.* 1999. Bioavailability of interferon 1b in MS patients with and without neutralizing antibodies. Neurology **52:** 1239–1243.

18. PALLERONI, A.V., A. AGLIONE, M. LABOW, *et al.* 1997. Interferon immunogenicity: preclinical evaluation of interferon-α2a. J. Interferon Cytokine Res. **17:** S23–S27.

19. RYFF, J.C. 1997. Clinical investigation of the immunogenicity of interferon-α2a. J. Interferon Cytokine Res. **17:** S29–S33.

20. SCHELLEKENS, H., J.C. RYFF & P.H. VAN DER MEIDE. 1997. Assays for antibodies to human interferon-α: the need for standardisation. J. Interferon Cytokine Res. **17:** 5–8.

21. ROSS, C., K.M. CLEMMESEN, M. SVENSON, *et al.* 2000. Immunogenicity of interferon-β in multiple sclerosis patients: influence of preparation, dosage, dose frequency, and route of administration, Ann. Neurol. **48:** 706–712.

22. KARPUSAS, M. *et al.* 1998. The structure of human interferon-β: implications for activity. Cell. Mol. Life Sci. **54:** 1203–1216.

23. JACQUEMIN, M.G. & J.M. SAINT-REMY. 1998. Factor VIII immunogenicity. Haemophilia **4:** 552–557.

24. KUUS-REICHEL, K., L.S. GRAUER, L.M. KARAVODIN, *et al.* 1994. Will immunogenicity limit the use, efficacy, and future development of therapeutic monoclonal antibodies? Clin. Diagn. Lab. Immunol. **1:** 365–372.

25. CLARK, M. 2002. Antibody humanization: a case of the "emperor's new clothes"? Immunol. Today **21:** 397–402.

26. PENDLEY, C., A. SCHANTZ & C. WAGNER. 2003. Immunogenicity of therapeutic monoclonal antibodies. Curr. Opin. Mol. Ther. **5:** 172–179.

27. DESILVA, B., W. SMITH, R. WEINER, *et al.* 2003. Recommendations for the bioanalytical method validation of ligand binding assays to support pharmacokinetic assessments of macromolecules. J. Pharm. Biomed. Anal. **20:** 1885–1900.

Diagnostic Value of Anti-F-Actin Antibodies in a French Multicenter Study

P. CHRETIEN-LEPRINCE,[a] E. BALLOT,[a,b] C. ANDRE,[a] N. O. OLSSON,[a]
N. FABIEN,[a] A. ESCANDE,[a] F. OKSMAN,[a] S. DUBUQUOI,[a] S. JEGO,[a] J. GOETZ,[a]
A. CHEVAILLER,[a] M. SANMARCO,[a] R. L. HUMBEL,[a] AND C. JOHANET[a,b]

[a]Groupe d'Etude de l'AutoImmunité (GEAI), Laboratoire d'Immunologie,
Hôpital Larrey, Angers, France

[b]Laboratoire d'Immunologie, Hôpital Saint-Antoine, AP-HP, Paris, France

ABSTRACT: According to international criteria, autoimmune hepatitis (AIH)
type 1 is characterized by the presence of antinuclear or anti–smooth muscle
antibodies (SMA) with F-actin specificity. SMA have been found in 85% of AIH
patients, but are not specific to this disease, and anti-F-actin specificity is not
always verified when SMA are detected. The objective of this study was to
determine the diagnostic value of anti-F-actin antibodies in a large population.
A multicenter study involving 12 clinical centers was performed. Patients were
selected on the basis of the presence of F-actin SMA detected by indirect
immunofluorescence (IIF) on rat liver–kidney–stomach sections and was confirmed by IIF on Hep2 cells treated with colchicine, or F-actin dot-blot. The
clinical status of patients was determined from their medical records. One hundred sixty-eight patients were included: 76% women, 24% men; mean age of
45 years (range, 2–88 years), with a bimodal age distribution. Sixty percent had
AIH type 1, and 40% had another disease. In the group of women younger than
25 years, 90% had AIH type 1. Other pathologies associated with antiactin
were other liver diseases (19%), including viral hepatitis C (7%), and nonliver
diseases (21%), including connective tissue diseases (12%). Antibody titers
were higher in AIH than in other diseases. Antiactin antibodies are of major
diagnostic value in AIH, especially in young women; they may be found in
other disease settings, but mostly at low levels.

KEYWORDS: anti–smooth-muscle antibodies; anti-F-actin antibodies; autoimmune hepatitis

INTRODUCTION

Anti–smooth muscle antibodies (SMA) were first described by Johnson et al. in
1965,[1] and the association between SMA and antiactin antibodies in autoimmune
hepatitis (AIH) was established in 1973.[2] AIH is a chronic progressive liver disease
characterized by female predominance (gender ratio, 3.6:1), hypergammaglobu-

Address for correspondence: Dr. C. Johanet, Service d'Immunologie et Hématologie
Biologiques, Hôpital Saint-Antoine, 184 rue du Faubourg Saint-Antoine, 75571 Paris Cedex 12,
France. Voice: +33-1-49-28-20-11; fax: +33-1-49-28-30-46.
catherine.johanet@sat.ap-hop-paris.fr

Ann. N.Y. Acad. Sci. 1050: 266–273 (2005). © 2005 New York Academy of Sciences.
doi: 10.1196/annals.1313.028

linemia, autoantibodies, association with HLA DR3 and DR4, and a good response to immunosuppressive therapy.[3–8] The diagnosis of autoimmune hepatitis, a combination of clinical, laboratory, and histologic findings, is based on a provisional scoring system established in 1993 by the International Autoimmune Hepatitis Group[9] and then revised in 1999.[10] According to these criteria, AIH type 1 is characterized by the presence of antinuclear antibodies (ANA) or SMA.[9–11] SMA are present in 85% of patients with AIH, either alone (35%) or in conjunction with ANA (50%).[8] Unfortunately, they are found in a variety of liver and nonliver diseases, and their utility as diagnostic markers depends on their actin or nonactin specificity,[12–14] which is not always verified when SMA are detected.

Moreover, although antisoluble liver antigen, a nonconventional, specific, AIH type 1 marker,[15,16] has been included in the revised scoring system as an additional parameter, the subspecificity of SMA (e.g., antiactin SMA) is still not included.[10] The aim of this study was thus to determine the diagnostic value of anti-F-actin antibodies in a large population of patients. That is the principal reason that 12 hospital laboratories were involved in this study.

MATERIALS AND METHODS

Patient Selection

This multicenter, retrospective study included 12 clinical centers belonging to the study group for autoimmune diseases (GEAI). Patients were selected on the basis of two criteria: (1) the presence of anti-F-actin SMA in sera and (2) knowledge of their diagnosis. The clinical status of all patients was determined from their medical records. The diagnosis of AIH was based on the criteria defined by the International Autoimmune Hepatitis Group,[9] with an aggregate score of more than 15 (definite AIH) or 10–15 (probable AIH).

Autoantibody Detection: SMA Detection

SMA were routinely detected using indirect immunofluorescence (IIF) on rodent rat liver–kidney–stomach sections. The substrates were either home-prepared[17] or commercially available [Kallestadt™ (Bio-Rad, Marne la Coquette, France) and Biomedica Diagnostic (Marne la Vallée, France)], depending on the laboratory. In most cases, the initial serum dilutions were either 1/10 or 1/40 in phosphate-buffered saline. The sections were revealed using a fluorochrome-labeled, antihuman IgG, IgA, IgM antiserum. The cutoff titer for positivity was fixed at 1/80.

The presence of SMA with F-actin specificity was visualized in accordance with its characteristic fluorescence pattern: in the stomach, the muscular layer (muscularis mucosa) and the vascular axis of the lamina propria of the gastric mucosa were stained; in the liver, the submembrane actin of hepatocytes was stained according to the classic "honeycomb" pattern; in the kidney, the blood vessel wall as well as intracellular fibrils of the renal tubules and mesangial cells of the glomerulus were stained.[18] FIGURE 1 presents these different staining patterns. However, the presence of anti-F-actin antibodies could only be suspected and needed to be confirmed.

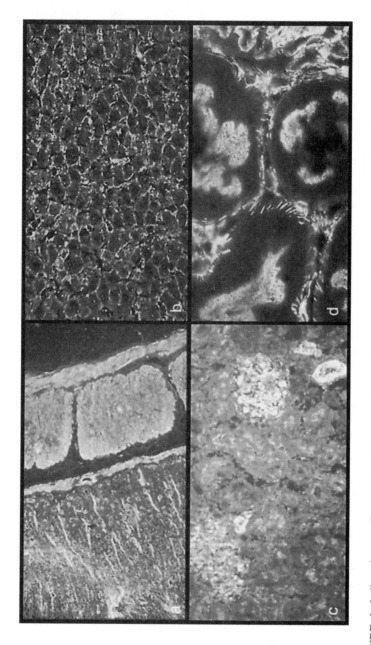

FIGURE 1. Indirect immunofluorescence pattern of anti–smooth muscle antibodies on (**a**) stomach (×100), (**b**) liver (×200), and (**c, d**) kidney (×100 and ×400), respectively.

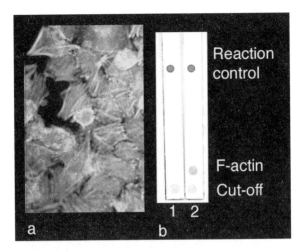

FIGURE 2. Anti-F-actin antibody evaluations: **(a)** using indirect immunofluorescence on colchicine-treated Hep2 cells (×400); **(b)** using immunoDot. Lane 1: negative sera; lane 2: sera with anti-F-actin antibodies.

Autoantibody Detection: Anti-F-Actin Detection

All sera positive for SMA (>1/80) were tested for anti-F-actin antibodies using one of the two following methods:

(1) *Detection of F-actin antibodies on colchicine-treated Hep2 cells*:[13] The standard IIF test was employed, with a 1/80 initial serum dilution in phosphate-buffered saline. Monolayer cells were revealed using a fluorochrome-labeled, antihuman IgG, IgA, IgM antiserum. The presence of anti-F-actin antibodies was assessed according to the typical pattern observed: actin cables were strongly stained, as shown in FIGURE 2a.

(2) *Detection of F-actin antibodies by immunoDot D-TEK® Blue DOT Liver (Mons, Belgium)*: Detection was performed according to the manufacturer's instructions. Briefly, serum diluted 1/151 was incubated for 30 min at room temperature with the coated strip. After three washes, conjugated goat antibodies against human IgG were added for 30 min. After a second washing step, the strip was incubated with the enzyme substrate. The intensity of staining was directly proportional to the amount of antibody present in the sample. The results were interpreted by comparison with the positive control (upper dot corresponding to the control reaction, which must be positive for all patients) and the negative control (last dot corresponding to the cutoff value). A sample was deemed positive for anti-F-actin if the staining intensity was higher than the negative control dot (FIG. 2b).

Statistical Analysis

Data were compared using the Chi-squared test, with Yates' correction applied if necessary. The minimum level of statistical significance was set at $P < .05$.

Number of patients

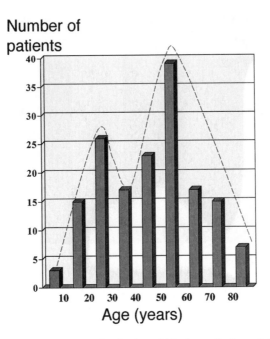

Age (years)

FIGURE 3. Bimodal age distribution within the studied population.

RESULTS

One hundred sixty-eight patients were included in the study. Study of their demographic characteristics revealed a mean age of 45 years (range: 2–88 years). FIGURE 3 shows the bimodal age distribution obtained, with two incidence peaks: at 15–25 years and 50–65 years. The sex ratio was 76%:24% (female:male).

Study of the patients' medical records showed that 60% (101/168) of the 168 patients presented with AIH type 1, 17% had another liver disease, and 23% had a non-liver disease. Moreover, 90% (24/27) of the young females (younger than 25 years) with anti-F-actin antibodies were affected by AIH type 1.

AIH-affected patients included 90 patients with definite AIH and 11 with probable AIH (aggregate score between 10 and 15). Among these patients, 4 were diagnosed as having AIH type 1 associated with primary biliary cirrhosis (1 case), primary sclerosing cholangitis (2 cases), and AIH type 2 (1 case).

With respect to anti-F-actin antibody titers, 58% of patients with levels of 1/640 or higher had AIH, whereas 22% did not ($P < .0001$). Similarly, low titers (1/160 or below) were associated with non-AIH patients (41%), whereas only 11% presented with AIH ($P < .0001$). TABLE 1 shows the other main diseases found to be associated with anti-F-actin autoantibodies.

Twenty-eight patients presented with liver disease such as viral hepatitis C. Other diseases also were associated with these antibodies. Connective tissue diseases (e.g., systemic lupus erythematosus, Sjögren's syndrome, rheumatoid arthritis) were in-

TABLE 1. Pathologies associated with anti-F-actin antibodies

Disease	No.
Liver diseases (*n* = 129)	
AIH type 1	101 (60%)
Viral hepatitis C	12 (7%)
Alcoholic cirrhosis	4
Other types of viral hepatitis (HIV, Hantavirus)	3
Primary biliary cirrhosis	3
Cancer	2
Hepatotoxic drug (statins)	2
Abnormal liver function	2
Nonliver diseases (*n* = 39)	
Connective diseases (SLE, Sjögren's, RA)	20 (12%)
Other autoimmune diseases (celiac, Crohn's, thyroiditis, pernicious anemia, diabetes)	8
Arthritis	6
Other	5

volved in 20 (12%) of cases, as well as autoimmune endocrine diseases (e.g., thyroiditis, pernicious anemia) and inflammatory bowel diseases (e.g., Crohn's disease, celiac diseases).

DISCUSSION

Anti-SMA directed against the actin protein constitute diagnostic criteria for AIH type 1.[9,10] AIH type 1 is a rare disease. To obviate this problem, we initiated a multicenter study to evaluate the diagnostic value of anti-F-actin antibodies. The involvement of 12 laboratories specialized in autoimmune pathologies contributed to circumventing recruitment bias regarding patients. The starting point was biological and aimed at determining the presence of SMA reacting specifically against actin. The determination of anti-F-actin is of paramount importance to improving the characterization of SMA. However, a "gold standard" method is not yet available. Perhaps this is one of the reasons why most centers still use SMA reactivity in the rodent stomach.[19] During our study, specificity was assessed using IIF on rat liver–kidney–stomach sections and confirmed using either immunoDot or IIF on Hep2 treated with colchicine.

The demographic status of our population (bimodal age distribution and female frequency) was fully in line with others involved in studies on AIH type 1.[9,10] It is therefore not surprising that the principal clinical diagnosis in patients was autoimmune hepatitis[9–11] (60%, TABLE 1). This diagnosis was enhanced when young females are considered alone: 90% of the 15- to 25-year-old women studied (with anti-F-actin antibodies) suffered from AIH type 1. If the titer of anti-F-actin antibodies was studied, high levels (≥1/640) were preferentially associated with AIH, whereas low levels (≤1/160) were associated with non-AIH conditions. The study of young females (15–25 years) with high titers of anti-F-actin antibodies concerned 94% of cases of autoimmune hepatitis.

Anti-F-actin antibodies also were found in other liver diseases (17%). Low anti-actin antibody titers previously have been reported in acute viral hepatitis A[20] and in chronic hepatitis C, where Chazouilleres et al. found them at moderate levels.[21] Our findings are in agreement with these data,[21] with 7% of viral hepatitis C. More surprising was the presence of anti-F-actin antibodies associated with connective tissue diseases (12%). During our study, they were found in systemic lupus erythematosus, Sjögren's syndrome, or rheumatoid arthritis. To our knowledge, such findings have not been published elsewhere, except in rheumatoid arthritis, where antiactin antibodies have been described.[22] We also saw antiactin antibodies in patients with inflammatory bowel diseases, such as celiac disease. Our results agree with those published in 2004 by Granito et al.[23] Using both ELISA and IIF on fibroblast cells, 46% of patients with celiac disease presented antimicrofilaments antibodies (IgA). Moreover, in 1997, Corazza et al.[24] described two cases of adults with celiac disease with an atypical antibody pattern: no antiendomysium or antigliadin could be found in their sera, but the authors detected antithyroid antibodies and anti–gastric parietal cells as well as antiactin antibodies. It is well known that hepatitis may be associated with celiac disease, autoimmune thyroiditis, or pernicious anemia. The results of our study are in line with these findings.

In conclusion, anti-F-actin antibodies can be found in numerous disease settings, including both liver and nonliver diseases, although mainly at low levels, but they are of significant interest to the diagnosis of AIH, particularly in young women.

ACKNOWLEDGMENTS

The authors would like to thank all the physicians for their contribution to this study. Members of the Groupe d'Etude de l'AutoImmunité include the following: Dr. Chretien-Leprince, Centre Hospitalier Intercommunal, Créteil; Dr. Andre, CHU Henri Mondor, Créteil; Dr. Olsson, CHU, Dijon; Dr. Fabien, Hôpital Lyon-Sud, Lyon; Dr. Escande, Hôpital Saint-Eloi, Montpellier; Dr. Oksman, Hôpital Rangueil, Toulouse; Dr. Dubuquoi, CHRU, Lille; Drs. Jego and SanMarco, Hôpital de la Conception, Marseille; Dr. Goetz, Hôpital Hautepierre, Strasbourg; Dr. Chevailler, Hôpital Larrey, Angers; Drs. Ballot and Johanet, Hôpital Saint-Antoine, Paris; and Dr. Humbel, Hôpital de Luxembourg, Luxembourg.

REFERENCES

1. JOHNSON, G.D., E.J. HOLBOROW & L.E. GLYNN. 1965. Antibody to smooth muscle in patients with liver disease. Lancet 2: 878–879.
2. GABBIANI, G., B.R. GRAEME, J.P. LAMELIN, et al. 1973. Human smooth muscle autoantibody: its identification as antiactin antibody and a study of its binding to non-muscular cells. Am. J. Pathol. 72: 473–488.
3. MANNS, M.P. & C.P. STRASSBURG. 2001. Autoimmune hepatitis: clinical challenges. Gastroenterology 120: 1502–1517.
4. DIAMANTIS, I. & D.T. BOUMPAS. 2004. Autoimmune hepatitis: evolving concepts. Autoimmun. Rev. 3: 207–214.

5. Czaja, A.J. & D.K. Freese. 2002. Diagnostic and treatment of autoimmune hepatitis. Hepatology **36:** 479–497.
6. Vergani, D. & G. Mieli-Vergani. 2003. Autoimmune hepatitis. Autoimmun. Rev. **2:** 241–247.
7. Donaldson, P.T., D.G. Doherty, K.M. Hayllar, *et al.* 1991. Susceptibility to autoimmune chronic active hepatitis: human leukocytes antigens DR4 and A1-B8-DR3 are independent risk factors. Hepatology **13:** 701–706.
8. Obermayer-Straub, P., C.P. Strassburg & M.P. Manns. 2000. Autoimmune hepatitis. J. Hepatol. **32:** 181–197.
9. Johnson, P.J., I.G. McFarlane, F. Alvarez, *et al.* 1993. Meeting report: International Autoimmune Hepatitis Group. Hepatology **18:** 998–1005.
10. Alvarez, F., P.A. Berg, F.B. Bianchi *et al.* 1999. International Autoimmune Hepatitis Group report: a review of criteria for diagnosis of autoimmune hepatitis. J. Hepatol. **31:** 929–938.
11. Muratori, P., L. Muratori, D. Agostinelli *et al.* 2002. Smooth muscle antibodies and type I autoimmune hepatitis. Autoimmunity **35:** 497–500.
12. Czaja, A.J. & H.A. Homburger. 2001. Autoantibodies in liver disease. Gastroenterology **120:** 239–249.
13. Lindman, K., G. Biberfeld, A. Fagraeus *et al.* 1976. Antiactin specificity of human smooth muscle antibodies in chronic active hepatitis. Clin. Exp. Immunol. **24:** 266–272.
14. Abuaf, N., C. Johanet & J.C. Homberg. 1991. Autoantibodies in autoimmune chronic active hepatitis. *In* Autoimmune Liver Diseases, pp. 93–109. Raven Press. New York.
15. Wies, I., S. Brunner, J. Henninger, *et al.* 2000. Identification of target antigen for SLA/LP autoantibodies in autoimmune hepatitis. Lancet **355:** 1510–1515.
16. Ballot, E., J.C. Homberg & C. Johanet. 2000. Autoantibodies to soluble liver antigen: an additional marker in type 1 auto-immune hepatitis. J. Hepatol. **33:** 208–215.
17. Vergani, D., F. Avarez, F.B. Bianchi, *et al.* 2004. Liver autoimmune serology: a consensus statement from the committee for autoimmune serology of the International Autoimmune Hepatitis Group. J. Hepatol. **41:** 677–683.
18. Bottazzo, G.F., A. Florin-Christensen, A. Fairfax, *et al.* 1976. Classification of smooth muscle autoantibodies detected by immunofluorescence. J. Clin. Pathol. **29:** 403–410.
19. Cançado, E.L., L. Vilas-Boas, C.P. Abrantes-Lemos, *et al.* 1996. Heat serum inactivation as a mandatory procedure for antiactin antibody detection in cell culture. Hepatology **23:** 1098–1104.
20. Lopez, S.I., J. Seia, A. Roy, *et al.* 1998. Anti-actin antibodies in acute viral hepatitis A in children. Acta Gastroenterol. Latinoam. **28:** 261–264.
21. Chazouilleres, O., C. Johanet, L. Serfaty, *et al.* 1996. Anti-actin autoantibodies in patients with chronic hepatitis C. J. Hepatol. **24:** 513.
22. Andresen, I., P. Andersen & H. Graudal. 1980. Smooth-muscle antibodies in rheumatoid arthritis. Acta Pathol. Microbiol. Scand. **88:** 131–135.
23. Granito, A., P. Muratori, F. Cassani, *et al.* 2004. Anti-actin IgA antibodies in severe coeliac disease. Clin. Exp. Immunol. **137:** 386–392.
24. Corazza, G.R., F. Biagi, U. Volta, *et al.* 1997. Autoimmune enteropathy and villous atrophy in adults. Lancet **350:** 106–109.

Paraneoplastic Neurological Antibodies

A Laboratory Experience

ABID R. KARIM,[a] RICHARD G. HUGHES,[b] JOHN B. WINER,[c]
ADRIAN C. WILLIAMS,[c] AND ARTHUR R. BRADWELL[d]

[a]Department of Neuroimmunology, The Medical School, Edgbaston,
Birmingham B15 2TT, United Kingdom

[b]The Binding Site Limited, Birmingham B14 4ZB, United Kingdom

[c]Department of Neurology, Queen Elizabeth Hospital, Edgbaston,
Birmingham B15 2TH, United Kingdom

[d]Department of Immunity and Infection, The Medical School, Edgbaston,
Birmingham B15 2TJ, United Kingdom

ABSTRACT: Antineuronal antibodies are associated with rare paraneoplastic
neurological syndromes, and their identification alerts clinicians to examine
for the presence of a tumor. Presented here is laboratory experience (prevalence, difficulties, and procedures) and several interesting but inconclusive results. A total of 1045 samples were screened over a 2-year period; 91 showed a
degree of binding of antibodies to the cerebellum, and 22 of these 91 were confirmed, by Western blot, to have specific antineuronal antibodies. Thirteen of
22 were Hu-positive, and 6 of these also had antinuclear antibodies. Six were
Yo-positive, 2 had anti-Ma antibodies, and 1 was Tr-positive. An additional 27
of 91 patients had cerebellar antibodies giving recognized staining patterns
(Hu, Yo, and Ma). However, Western blot did not confirm these specificities,
and hence they were reported as atypical. Six of 27 of these patients had neoplasms; 3 of the 6 gave nucleolar patterns (not Ma). Two appeared similar to
Yo, and 1 similar to Hu. Antineuronal antibodies are rare, and in the absence
of a specific etiology patients should be examined further for the possible
presence of an underlying tumor. Methodical classification of the antibodies
must be conducted to avoid incorrect reporting. Further criteria on the typing/
reporting of atypical results may aid diagnosis of paraneoplastic neurological
syndromes.

KEYWORDS: autoantibodies; immunofluorescence; screen; Yo; Hu; Tr; Ma

INTRODUCTION

Paraneoplastic neurological disorders are rare debilitating neurological illnesses
associated with remote effects of malignant neoplasm (predominantly small cell
lung cancer, breast, and gynecological tumors). Very often the symptoms precede the

Address for correspondence: Abid R. Karim, Department of Neuroimmunology, The Medical
School, Edgbaston, Birmingham B15 2TT, United Kingdom.
a.r.karim@bham.ac.uk; <http://www.ii.bham.ac.uk/clinicalimmunology/neuroimmunology>

Ann. N.Y. Acad. Sci. 1050: 274–285 (2005). © 2005 New York Academy of Sciences.
doi: 10.1196/annals.1313.029

TABLE 1. Paraneoplastic antineuronal antibodies[5]

Antibody	MW (kDa)	Staining pattern	PND	Associated tumor(s)
Recoverin	23, 65	Retinal photoreceptor	Retinopathy	SCLC
Yo (PCA-1)	34, 52, 62	Purkinje cell cytoplasm and axons	PCD	Ovary, breast
Zic4 (6)	~37	Nuclei of granular neurons, weaker on Purkinje cell nuclei	PCD	SCLC
Ma (Ma1)	37, 40	Neuronal nucleoli	PCD, BE	Various, lung cancer
Ta (Ma2)	41.5	Neuronal nucleoli, perikaryon	BE, LE	Testicular cancer
Hu (ANNA1)	34–40	Nuclei of both central and peripheral neurons	PCD, PEM, SN	SCLC
Ri (ANNA2)	55, 80	Nuclei of central neurons	OM, PCD, BE	Breast, SCLC, gynecologic
GAD	65, 67	Islet cells and gray matter	SPS	Breast, colon, SCLC
CV2/CRMP5	66	Oligodendrocyte cytoplasm	PEM/SN	SCLS, thymoma
Amphiphysin	128	Central presynaptic terminals	SPS, PEM	Breast cancer, SCLC
GluR1	~140	Purkinje cell cytoplasm, climbing fiber	PCD	Hodgkin's lymphoma
ANNA-3 (8)	170	Purkinje cell cytoplasm and nucleus + glomerular podocytes	PCD, PEM, SN	SCLC
PCA-2 (7)	280	Purkinje cell cytoplasm and other neurons	PEM, PCD, LEMS	SCLC
Tr	[??]	Purkinje cell cytoplasm with "dots" in molecular layer	PCD	Hodgkin's lymphoma

NOTE: PND, paraneoplastic neurological disorder; PCD, paraneoplastic cerebellar degeneration; PEM, paraneoplastic encephalomyelitis; SN, sensory neuropathy; OM, opsoclonus/myoclonus; BE, brain stem encephalomeyelitis; LE, limbic encephalmyelitis; LEMS, Lambert–Eaton myasthenic syndrome; SPS, stiff person syndome; SCLC, small cell lung carcinoma. Question marks [??] indicate that no common band has been identified by Wetern blot analysis.

detection of the paraneoplastic tumors.[1] The ailment is thought to arise from autoimmune response against neuronal antigens. The autoimmune attack is evident in the postmortem brains where there is severe loss of Purkinje cells and inflammatory infiltrates are present.[2] The consequential presence of high titer, specific antineuronal antibodies in the blood and cerebral spinal fluid provides a useful and early diagnostic marker, alerting the clinician to undertake a thorough examination for a possible presence of a tumor.[3,4] Many of the well-defined antineuronal antibodies and associated tumors are listed in TABLE 1.[5–8]

The neuronal antigens, expressed in the cytoplasm and/or nuclei of the neurons (in particular, Purkinje cells), are identical to those expressed in the associated tumor. The antigen–antibody interaction can be visualized by using indirect immuno-fluorescence (IIF) on normal cerebellar cryosections. Although rodent cerebellum sections are considered sufficient and are frequently used, monkey tissues are probably preferable for reasons of antigenic similarity. This is the method of choice when screening for antineuronal antibodies for most laboratories, including ours. The immunofluorescent pattern can be difficult to interpret, partly because of the co-localization of both neuronal-specific and nonspecific antigens. The patterns are only indicative and specificity must always be confirmed by other techniques. To eliminate false-positive results (together with the uncharacterized antibodies), the final confirmation must rest with results from a Western blot, preferably one that includes recombinant proteins.[9]

Neuroimmunology laboratories are faced with an ever-increasing number of requests to screen for antineuronal antibodies and are frequently challenged to characterize antibody-binding patterns in the cerebellum which are negative by Western blot but have a very similar distribution to the antineuronal antibodies of known clinical relevance. In the literature, there is a lack of information dealing with this issue. This study aims to address this by exploring some of the interactions of uncharacterized antineuronal antibodies (presently of undetermined clinical significance), which could lead to confusion, lost time, inefficient use of resources and possibly incorrect reporting of the results.

METHODS

Appropriateness of Test

Requests for screening for paraneoplastic antibodies were received and accepted from referring neurologists at specialist centers regardless of the clinical details being supplied. The information provided on the request form did not influence the selection of the test. Furthermore, tests were repeated at the request of the specialist center.

Subjects

Over a 2-year period from 2002 to 2003, we screened 1045 serum samples on cerebellum for paraneoplastic neurological autoantibodies. These samples originated from neurology centers around the West Midlands region of the United Kingdom.

Screening Procedure

Detection of paraneoplastic antineuronal-specific antibodies is based on and closely follows the guidelines published by Moll *et al.*[10] With this screening procedure, most of the antibodies in TABLE 1 can be detected. The antineuronal antibody screen offered includes the detection of Yo, Hu, and Ri (also known as PCA, ANNA1, and ANNA2, respectively), which are the most commonly detected paraneoplastic neurological autoantibodies. The screen is conducted by indirect immuno-fluorescence. All relevant staining patterns were further investigated. Full details of the methodology are given elsewhere.[11] In brief, frozen sections of monkey cerebellum are incubated with test sera at a dilution of 1:50, allowing specific antibody-antigen binding to take place. Unbound immunoglobulins are removed by a wash step; bound human immunoglobulins (IgG class) are visualized using sheep anti-human IgG (monkey-absorbed) conjugated to fluorescein (all the IIF reagents were sourced from The Binding Site Ltd.). Where considered appropriate, the positive samples also were tested on separate slides containing stomach-liver-kidney composite tissue, Hep-2, and testis cryosections.

All positive sera were subjected to commercial preparation of Western blots as per the manufacturer's recommendation (Euroimmun). These contained separated extract of primate cerebellum with additional recombinant Hu and Yo proteins. We considered samples to be positive when antibodies were shown to bind both the recombinant antigen and a protein band on the cerebellar extract of the relevant molecular weight.

RESULTS

From the initial screen of 1045 samples, 91 (~9%) showed a degree of binding to the cerebellum. The staining patterns of 49 gave what was considered to be characteristic antineuronal patterns. Of these, 22 were typed as typical antineuronal antibodies, with known clinical relevance, and 27 were atypical, that is, antineuronal antibodies with undetermined clinical significance. The remaining 42 samples showed neither characteristic antineuronal staining patterns nor any significant bands on the Western blot; hence they were reported negative for the known paraneoplastic neurological autoantibodies.

Antineuronal Antibodies of Known Clinical Relevance

The 22 sera identified as having antineuronal antibodies of known clinical relevance conformed to the well-publicized criteria.[2,11–13] Antineuronal nuclear auto-antibody type 1 (Hu or ANNA1) was identified in 13 of these sera, five of which showed no other reactivity. Six of these Hu samples also contained antibodies against nuclear antigens (antinuclear antibody [ANA]–positive), with titers ranging from 1:40 to 1:1600. The ANA pattern ranged from fine to coarse-speckled and one was nucleolar. Antimitochondrial antibodies (M2 type) were present in two of the Hu sera. In one case, the antineuronal pattern on the cerebellum was totally masked by the presence of a strong mitochondrial antibody (M2 >100 AU/mL), and the Hu specificity was shown only by Western blot analysis. There was another case of strong antimitochondrial antibodies on cerebellum that proved to be negative by Western blot for the presence of antineuronal antibodies. The serum samples with additional antibody reactivities also recognized additional bands on the Western blots.

Five females and one male patient were seropositive for the Yo antibody. Only one anti-Yo serum had additional antibodies. In this case, the coexisting ANA gave a centromere pattern on Hep-2 cells. Two (2/22) males had the Ma antibody and one (1/22) had Tr antibody.

Atypical Antineuronal Antibodies

The 27 atypical antineuronal antibodies detected can be divided into three groups based on their IIF patterns on cerebellum. The three patterns resemble Hu, Yo, and Ma antibody staining. All these samples were negative for Hu, Yo, and Ma when analyzed by Western blot. Among those seropositive for atypical antineuronal antibodies, six patients had some form of neoplasm (TABLE 2).

Non-Ma Nucleolar Antibodies

Six serum samples had antibodies to the nucleoli of cerebellar neurons, giving a distribution that resembled the anti-Ma pattern. None of these conformed to anti-Ma characterization. Only one of the samples reacted with all the substrates tested (Hep-2, liver, testis, and peripheral neurons), implying a general antinucleolar antibody. Two (2/6) samples in this group were weakly positive on Hep-2 cells with a nucleolar pattern, and the activity of the remaining three was exclusively confined to nucleoli in cells of the cerebellum.

Three of the patients (two males and one female) with antinucleolar antibodies on the cerebellum had concurrent neoplasm (gastric cancer, rectal adenocarcinoma, and myeloma). Only one was nucleolar-positive on the testis. This sample satisfied laboratory IIF criteria for Ma/Ta, but the reactivity was not confirmed by Western blot.

Atypical Yo (PCA)

Six sera had IIF features resembling the distribution of Yo antibody. Unlike Yo, the reactivity was not confined to the central nervous system. Most (4/6) of these were positive on rodent myenteric neurons. Five were positive on Hep-2 cells; the staining was restricted to the cytoplasm. In one case, specificity for ribosomal P protein, which is a cytoplasmic antigen, was identified, and this could be causing the observed cerebellar pattern resembling Yo. In all other cases antibodies against mitochondria, Jo1, and ribosomal P protein were excluded. All six samples were negative for the Yo antibody by Western blot. A 35-kDa protein was detected in one serum sample, which was negative for recombinant Yo. The sixth serum had anti-neuronal antibodies that stained both the nucleoli and the cytoplasm of Purkinje cells, giving an impression of a combination pattern consisting of non-Ma nucleolar and atypical Yo. This antibody also reacted both with peripheral neurons and HEp-2 cell cytoplasm but did not react with testis. On Western blot, bands were detected in the region of Ma and Yo proteins (43 and 62 kDa); however, the recombinant Yo was negative. Two of the patients, one male and one female, with atypical Yo also had neoplasms.

This group of antibodies stained the cytoplasm of the Purkinje cells together with some dendrites, a pattern resembling Yo, but the Western blot was negative for Yo, and in all cases there were no immunohistochemical indications that the antibody reaction observed on the primate cerebellum was an anti–Tr antibody reaction.

Atypical Hu (ANNA1)

The sera of 13 patients gave Hu-like staining on the cerebellum; these sera also reacted with the nucleus of HEp-2 cells, myenteric neurons, and proteins on Western

TABLE 2. Details of patients with atypical PCA and non-Ma nucleolar antibody

Patient ID	Age & sex	Diagnosis	Cerebellum	EN	HEp-2	Western blot	Comments
40367	84 (F)	Gastric cancer, odd sensory disturbance of extremities	Nucleolar	N	WP speckled	46 & 54 kDa	Gangliosides negative
44717	52 (F)	Axonal sensorimotor neuropathy	Nucleolar	N	N	65 kDa	Gangliosides negative
6758	55 (M)	Complex clinical picture with peripheral neuropathy	Nucleolar	N	N	50 kDa	Gangliosides negative
26930	73 (M)	Peripheral neuropathy, rectal adenocarcinoma	Nucleolar (1/400)	N	WP nucleolar	49–52 kDa	Ma/Ta-negative
6941	71 (M)	Myeloma, IgG lambda paraprotein	Nucleolar	N	WP nucleolar	N	Testis nucleoli-positive
14567	64 (F)	Motor neuron disease	Strong nucleolar	P	Strong nucleolar	114 kDa	—
39004	58 (M)	Complex clinical picture, death from pneumonia & polymyositis	Nucleolar with atypical PCA	P	Cytoplasmic staining	43 & 62 kDa	
23745	80 (F)	Motor neuron disease	Atypical PCA	—	Cytoplasmic staining, ribosomal by ELISA	100 kDa	
36939	73 (M)	Lung adenocarcinoma, deceased	Atypical PCA and white matter neurons	P	Cytoplasmic staining	51, 66, & 74.5 kDa	
40303	43 (M)	Polymyositis	Atypical PCA	P	Cytoplasmic staining (not ribosomal)	—	
31047	78 (F)	Peripheral neuropathy	Atypical PCA with granular-layer staining	N	N	35 kDa	Recombinant negative for PCA
29283	71 (F)	Metastatic adenocarcinoma of unknown primary	Atypical PCA	P	Cytoplasmic staining	22.5 kDa	CA-125 elevated

NOTE: Some of the images associated with these antibodies can be viewed at <http://www.ii.bham.ac.uk/clinicalimmunology/neuroimmunology>. Terms: P, positive; N, negative; EN, enteric neurons; M, male; F, female.

blot extract of primate cerebellum. The patterns resembled IIF criteria for Hu (specific for both central and peripheral neurons); however, all the samples in this group were negative for both Hu and Ri by Western blot. A range of antinuclear patterns on HEp-2 cells were observed, consisting of coarse-speckled (32 and 66 kDa), homogeneous (ranging from 53 to 105 kDa), and multinuclear dots (50, 53, and 82 kDa).

There were two samples positive for SS-B/SS-A, which could be mistaken for anti-Hu antibody by IIF and that also recognized protein on the Western blot in the same region as anti-Hu (between 34 and 40 kDa) but did not react with the recombinant Hu.

DISCUSSION

By the end of 2003, the requests for the paraneoplastic screen increased by 165% in comparison with the percentage in 2002. Only a small proportion (2.1%) of samples were positive for paraneoplastic neurological antibodies. In 22 patients (13 Hu, 6 Yo, 2 Ma, and 1 Tr), the antineuronal antibody specificities were confirmed using Western blots with the exception of the Tr antibody. No common bands have been identified for the Tr antigen on Western blots; however, in this case the identification was strictly based on IIF criteria in which Purkinje cell cytoplasmic staining was combined with a characteristic punctuated staining in the molecular layer.

More than 50% of Hu samples also showed specificity for antigens of HEp-2 cells, causing potential difficulties in pattern recognition during the initial screening process. In addition to anti–Hu antibody, ANA was the most commonly occurring antibody encountered in this series of patients. The presence of coexisting auto-antibodies was evident from the observed additional bands on the Western blot of primate cerebellum extract. The presence of ANA may reflect the age of patients in this group because it is well documented that autoantibodies increase in prevalence with age, particularly in women. Elsewhere, the coexistence of anti-Hu and ANA in patient sera has been reported,[14,15] and 29% of Ri coexists with ANA.[16] Other autoantibodies appearing in conjunction with anti-Hu includes anti-DNA[17] and anti-Ro/SS-A and anti-La/SS-B.[14] However, note that some sera from patients with Sjögren's syndrome may recognize proteins of identical molecular weight as Hu antigen on the Western blots of neuronal extract,[17] thus resembling anti-Hu specificity.[9,18] These antibodies do not bind to the recombinant Hu antigen.

The coexistence of anti–Hu and antimitochondrial antibodies is reported here in 15% of Hu-positive sera (2/13). This is similar to the frequency of antimitochondrial antibodies reported in conjunction with Ri.[16] Interestingly, a female aged 71 years with established diagnosis of primary biliary cirrhosis/sclerosing cholangitis with subacute onset of patchy sensory neuropathy and autonomic neuropathy (no tumor found so far) had a strong antimitochondrial antibody masking the anti-Hu antibody to the extent that it could not be visualized on the cerebellum (FIG. 1a) despite titration to the end point. The coexistence of the two antibodies in both cases was resolved by Western blot analysis where, in addition to recombinant Hu and 38-kDa bands, other proteins were recognized by the antibody with molecular weights between 80–83 and 53–54 kDa. The latter is similar in size to the protein recognized by antimitochondrial antibody in cerebellar extract reported by Moll et al.[14] Most

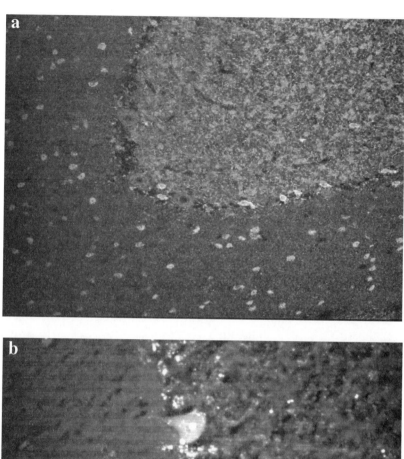

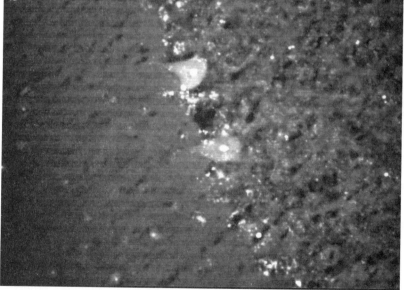

FIGURE 1. Monkey cerebellum showing coexistence of antimitochondrial antibody masking anti-Hu pattern (**a**), and two atypical autoantibodies: atypical Ma (**b**) and a Yo-type antibody that recognizes a 35-kDa protein on Western blot but shows no reaction with the recombinant antigen (**c**).

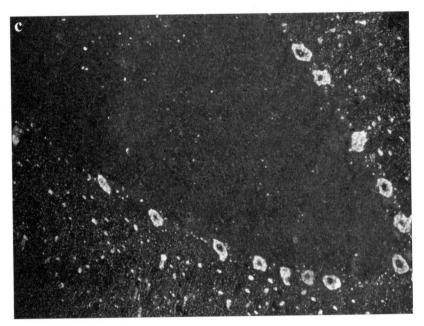

FIGURE 1 — *continued.*

laboratories use IIF as the initial tool to screen out all the negative samples. Our observations emphasize the importance of carrying out Western blot analysis on samples that show significant antibody binding on the initial IIF screen. On occasion, strong mitochondrial antibodies may mask the presence of coexisting antineuronal antibodies and will require additional procedures to ascertain this. Note therefore that, in exceptional cases, primary biliary cirrhosis markers might conceal anti–Hu antibodies.

Atypical Antineuronal Antibodies

In this publication, "atypical antineuronal antibodies" is defined as those antineuronal antibodies that have morphological distribution similar to the established and well-characterized neuronal antibodies (such as Hu, Ri, Ma, etc.) yet display different antigenic specificities. Furthermore, this definition is intended to avoid complicating the existing dual nomenclature, which is based on both the morphological distribution and the first two letters of the patients' surnames.

Three IIF patterns with comparable morphological distribution to Hu (ANNA1), Yo (PCA), and Ma/Ta antibody were detected. In our experience, the frequency of detection of atypical antineuronal antibodies was similar to that of the antineuronal antibodies of known clinical relevance.

Atypical Hu antibodies found in 13 samples reacted with both central and peripheral neurons. Most of these samples reacted with HEp-2 cells producing patterns commonly seen with autoimmune antibodies. It is important for the laboratory to distinguish between antineuronal antibodies and ANAs because the latter are not neuronal specific. There is the possibility that the ANAs observed with the atypical samples were coexisting with neuronal-specific antibodies, as observed with the typical neuronal autoantibody samples. Therefore, where an ANA is observed there could also be a novel neuronal-specific antibody present in the sample. There is also the possibility that on occasion the neuronal-specific antibodies are detected on the tissue sections but not by the Western blots. This is because of the possibility that some epitopes on the native antigens may be lost when presented on the Western blots because of the inevitable denaturing conditions.

In a case of a non-Ma nucleolar pattern, such as Ma, the nucleoli of primate cerebellar neurons (FIG. 1b) and testis were positive. It was unlikely that the 73-year-old male subject was suffering from a testicular germ-cell tumor. However, the patient did have a rectal adenocarcinoma, which may have been coincidental to the serologic findings. In 50% (3/6) of non-Ma nucleolar-positive patients, the sera reacted with primate cerebellar antigens having molecular weights ranging from 45 to 65 kDa. Only one serum sample was strongly positive for antinucleolar antibodies on both neuronal and nonneuronal tissue (cerebellum, Hep-2, testis, and liver). This recognized a protein of molecular weight 114 kDa on Western blot of the cerebellar extract. It is important to be able to correctly identify the anti-Ma specificity because it is so rare that only approximately 40 cases have been identified worldwide.[12]

Two atypical Yo (one recognized a 35-kDa protein [FIG. 1c] and the other a 62-kDa protein on Western blot) had all the hallmarks of anti–Yo antibody but failed to react with the recombinant Yo protein. It is likely to be coincidental that the identified bands on the extract were of similar molecular weights to those reported for Yo. It is important to mention that previous findings concluded that the final interpretation paraneoplastic antibodies should be based on both the presence of appropriate bands on the cerebellar extract and the recombinant antigens.

Patients with neurological disorders other than the paraneoplastic can have antibodies that have a comparable IIF pattern and are negative by Western blot for the known reactivities, including those to recombinant antigens, and often may be coincidentally associated with tumors. Atypical antineuronal antibodies may also be found in various neurological conditions without a specific significance, thus creating the possibility that a paraneoplastic neurological disorder may exist, which on careful clinical evaluation of the patient may lead to identification of a novel autoantibody.

In our experience, specialist laboratories with high turnover are better equipped for dealing with the detection of paraneoplastic autoantibodies. This is in view of the low frequency of paraneoplastic neurological syndromes (<1 case per 200,000 per year) as mentioned by Grant,[19] together with the fact that not all patients with paraneoplastic syndromes have identifiable antibodies in their serum.[2,20] This is further exemplified by the immunology audit conducted in 2002 in which five laboratories from the United Kingdom took part and only three identified the paraneoplastic antibodies correctly (unpublished report).

In conclusion, we have successfully detected antineuronal antibodies (both typical and atypical) using monkey cerebellum cryosections as the substrate and consider that the atypical results are significant enough to be reported. It therefore is important to provide along with the atypical results both any staining patterns observed and the molecular weights of any significant bands on the Western blots. The atypical antineuronal antibodies may not currently be viewed as clinically relevant, but will provide insight into the types of reactivities that can cause difficulties in pattern recognition. Furthermore, recognition of the coexistence of other antibodies may ease the interpretation of the IIF patterns during the initial screening process and provide an addition to the guidelines on the detection of paraneoplastic antineuronal antibodies.[10] Laboratories need to be aware of these types of samples to avoid wasting resources and confusion, lost time, and possible incorrect reporting of the results.

ACKNOWLEDGMENTS

A.R.B. is the chairman and shareholder and R.G.H. is an employee of The Binding Site, UK, which manufacturers and sells immunodiagnostic kits and reagents. We thank Euroimmun UK for conducting the ribosomal P protein ELISA.

REFERENCES

1. GULTEKIN, A.H. *et al.* 2000. Paraneoplastic limbic encephalitis: neurological symptoms, immunological findings and tumour association in 50 patients. Brain **123:** 1481–1494.
2. DARNELL, R.B. & J.B. POSNER. 2003. Paraneoplastic syndromes involving the nervous system. N. Engl. J. Med. **349:** 1543–1554.
3. CHUANG, V.J. *et al.* 1996. Inflammatory infiltrates and complete absence of Purkinje cells in anti-Yo-associated paraneoplastic cerebellar degeneration. Acta Neuropathol. (Berl.) **91:** 519–525.
4. POSNER, J.B. 2004. Paraneoplastic opsoclonus/myoclonus: B cells, T cells, both, or neither? Neurology **62:** 1466–1467.
5. SHAMS'ILI, S.S. *et al.* 2003. Paraneoplastic cerebellar degeneration associated with antineuronal antibodies: analysis of 50 patients. Brain **126:** 1409–1418.
6. BATALLER, L. *et al.* 2004. Antibodies to Zic4 in paraneoplastic neurological disorders and small-cell lung cancer. Neurology **62:** 778–782.
7. VERNINO, S. & V.A. LENNON. 2000. New Purkinje cell antibody (PCA-2): marker of lung cancer-related neurological autoimmunity. Ann. Neurol. **47:** 297–305.
8. CHAN, H.K. *et al.* 2001. ANNA-3 anti-neuronal nuclear antibody: marker of lung cancer-related autoimmunity. Ann. Neurol. **50:** 301–311.
9. SMITT, P.S. *et al.* 1996. Pitfalls in the diagnosis of autoantibodies associated with paraneoplastic neurological disease. Neurology **46:** 1739–1741.
10. MOLL, J.W.B. *et al.* 1995. Guidelines on detection of paraneoplastic anti-neuronal-specific antibodies. Neurology **45:** 1937–1941.
11. BRADWELL, A.R. 2000. Paraneoplastic neurological syndromes associated with Yo, Hu, and Ri autoantibodies. Clin. Rev. Allergy Immunol. **19:** 19–29.
12. VOLTZ, R. 2002. Paraneoplastic neurological syndromes: an update on diagnosis, pathogenesis, and therapy. Lancet Neurol. **1:** 294–305.
13. SUTTON, I. & J.B. WINER. 2002. The immunopathogenesis of paraneoplastic neurological syndromes. Clin. Sci. **102:** 475–486.
14. MOLL, J.W.B. *et al.* 1993. Antineuronal antibodies in patients with neurological complications of primary Sjögren's syndrome. Neurology **43:** 2574–2581.
15. CARPENTIER, A.F. *et al.* 2001. Systemic lupus erythematosus with anti-Hu antibodies and polyradiculoneuropathy. Neurology **57:** 558–559.
16. PITTOCK, S.J. *et al.* 2003. Anti-neuronal nuclear autoantibody type 2: paraneoplastic accompaniments. Ann. Neurol. **53:** 580–587.
17. BENYAHIA, B. *et al.* 2003. Paraneoplastic antineuronal antibodies in patients with systemic autoimmune diseases. J. Neuro-Oncol. **62:** 349–351.

18. VIANELLO, M. *et al.* 2004. The spectrum of antineuronal autoantibodies in a series of neurological patients. J. Neurol. Sci. **220:** 29–36.
19. GRANT, R. 2002. What neurologist needs to know about the paraneoplastic syndromes. Practical Neurol. **2:** 318–327.
20. REES, J.H. 2004. Paraneoplastic syndromes: when to suspect, how to confirm, and how to manage. J. Neurol. Neurosurg. Psychiat. **75**(suppl. II): ii43–ii50.

Determination of ANA Specificity Using the UltraPlex™ Platform

JODIE SMITH, DAVID ONLEY, CAROLINE GAREY, STUART CROWTHER, NICHOLAS CAHIR, ADAM JOHANSON, SIANIE PAINTER, GRANT HARRADENCE, RICARDO DAVIS, AND PETER SWARBRICK

SmartBead Technologies Limited, Babraham, Cambridge CB2 4AT, United Kingdom

ABSTRACT: SmartBead Technologies has developed a multiplexed immunofluorescence assay, the UltraPlex ANA Profile, which determines nine antinuclear antibodies simultaneously. The UltraPlex assay platform uses bar-coded microparticles to track analytes through assays. These bar-coded microparticles were used to tag and track key ANA markers: Jo-1, Scl-70, Sm, SmRNP, SSA, SSB, U1RNP, Centromere B, dsDNA, and a blank control microparticle. The immunofluorescence assays are fully automated and are performed on a Perkin-Elmer multiprobe II liquid handling system that performs all sera dilutions, additions of reagents, washes, and incubation steps. Results were determined by the automated UltraPlex plate reader. This fully automated multiplex antinuclear antibody (ANA) immunoassay was used to screen commercially available ANA-positive sera and negative control samples. The UltraPlex ANA Profile enables the panels of samples to be screened simultaneously for nine ANA antoantibodies, requiring significantly less labor and fewer reagents, with performance equivalent to existing gold-standard methods.

KEYWORDS: UltraPlex ANA Profile; dsDNA antibodies; autoantibodies; antigens; multiplex; bar-code

INTRODUCTION

Measurement of antinuclear antibodies (ANAs) is an important tool in the diagnosis and therapeutic monitoring of systemic rheumatic diseases including systemic lupus erythematosus, Sjögren's syndrome, scleroderma, dermatomyositis and polymyositis, and mixed connective tissue disease.[1] Antinuclear antibodies are autoantibodies directed against a variety of components of the cell nucleus.[2,3]

Indirect Immunofluorescence Assays

This is the most common method to determine ANA and is performed by incubating patient sera with substrate cells such as human epithelial cell line HEp-2. Bound antibodies are detected by incubation with a dye-conjugated anti-human immunoglobulin and visualized by fluorescent microscopy. Highly trained personnel

Address for correspondence: Jodie Smith, SmartBead Technologies Limited, Babraham Hall, Babraham, Cambridge CB2 4AT, United Kingdom.
jsmith@smartbead.com

Ann. N.Y. Acad. Sci. 1050: 286–294 (2005). © 2005 New York Academy of Sciences.
doi: 10.1196/annals.1313.030

usually can identify the pattern of fluorescent staining, which suggests which type of ANAs are present, because different disease states may have different patterns of fluorescence, although pattern recognition is highly subjective.

ELISA

Enzyme immunoassays such as ELISA are gaining popularity for ANA testing. Specific antigens (or mixtures of antigens) are bound to ELISA microtiter plates and incubated with patient sera; semi-quantitative measurement of antibodies is made by subsequent incubation with an enzyme-conjugated anti-human antibody that in the presence of bound ANA antibodies results in a color change when reacted with the substrate. This method has the advantage of sensitivity, quantification, and micro-titer format and is relatively quick but requires one microtiter plate well for each data point generated for each antigen tested.

UltraPlex

SmartBead Technologies has developed an immunofluoresence-based multiplex-ing assay called UltraPlex ANA Profile. Bar-coded microparticles act as supports with antigens attached to the surface, providing a permanent tag for the tracking of analytes through the assay. The UltraPlex ANA Profile allows nine ANAs to be de-termined simultaneously on microparticles that have been coated with specific anti-gens (one antigen per bar-code number). Combined ANA antigens are incubated in wells of microtiter filter plates with one patient serum sample per well. Assay out-comes are determined by incubation with anti-human antibody coupled to a fluoro-phore. Analysis is performed by the UltraPlex Plate Reader system, which identifies each microparticle, reads the bar-code number, and measures the levels of fluorescence.

This approach has the advantage that nine determinations are made per serum sample in a similar time that it takes to perform a standard ELISA. Unlike other multiplex technologies such as fluorescent beads, the bar-coded microparticles pro-vide a robust, permanent, non-bleaching tag. The inert microparticle material does not interfere with the bioassay, and the system provides built-in controls and high levels of redundancy for data confidence.

MATERIALS AND METHODS

Microparticle Design and Manufacture

The microparticles were manufactured using established semi-conductor processes by SMC (Edinburgh, UK). In brief, a quartz plate mask with transparent and opaque regions that defined the shape and the bar-code pattern was manufactured by Compugraphics International Ltd. (Glenrothes, UK). The pattern from the mask was transferred to aluminum by means of photolithography and acid etch techniques using standard semi-conductor equipment. FIGURE 1 shows the microparticles at this stage of manufacture; each particle is $100 \times 10 \times 1$ μm and is sitting on an organic release layer.

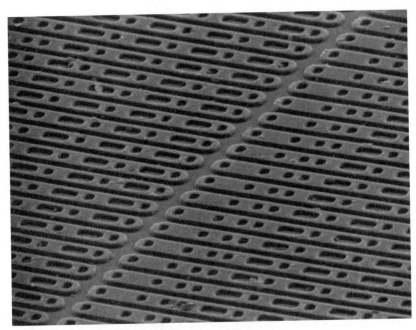

FIGURE 1. Electron micrograph showing aluminum microparticles on wafer before release (original magnification: ×67; figure reduced to 40%).

The three-inch wafer format used allows approximately two million microparticles to be manufactured per wafer. They are released from the wafer by suspension in an organic solvent, which dissolves the organic layer beneath the microparticles.

Reagents

The recombinant antigens Centromere B, dsDNA, Jo-1, Scl-70, SSB (La), and U1RNP were purchased from Diarect (Freiburg, Germany), and purified antigens SSA (Ro), Sm, and SmRNP were from The Binding Site (Birmingham, UK). Detection antibodies were purchased from Rockland Immunochemicals (Gilbertsville, PA). Control serum samples were obtained from The Binding Site (Birmingham, UK) and Immunovision (Springdale, AR) and UKNEQAS Nuclear Antibody scheme (Sheffield, UK). The ANA Human Reference Sera panel for nine antigens (SSA, SSB, Jo-1, Scl-70, U1RNP, Centromere B, dsDNA, Sm, and SmRNP) markers was obtained from the Centers for Disease Control (Atlanta, GA).

Attachment of Antigens to the Microparticles

The released particles were coated with either Amino or BTSE silanes (Sigma, Poole, UK), which increased the hydrophobicity of the microparticle surfaces. Each of the nine antigens was assigned to a specific bar-code-numbered microparticle. Antigens were adsorbed onto the surface of approximately 1.25 million silanized microparticles, by incubation with each antigen (concentration ranges 10–50 μg/mL in PBS or PBS + 0.05% Tween) for 16 h. The coupled microparticles were washed to remove excess antigen and blocked in a buffer containing 0.5% BSA (Sigma, Poole, UK). A tenth bar-coded microparticle was added as an internal control and was treated in the same fashion, but no antigen was absorbed onto the microparticle. These microparticles were used as a control to monitor non-specific binding in every reaction.

Accuspheres

For ease of handling, extended shelf life, and ensuring that the correct number of microparticles per reaction were present, all reagents for the multiplexed assay were combined and lyophilized to form a small solid sphere of approximately 5 mm in diameter. The manufacturing process was performed by Biomerieux (Boxtel, the Netherlands) and included resuspension of the nine antigen-coated and single-control microparticles to a concentration of 15,000 microparticles per mL in lyophilization buffer (Biomerieux). The solution then was dropped in 50-μL volumes into liquid nitrogen, snap-freezing the droplets to form "Accuspheres," each containing approximately 750 of each microparticle type. The Accuspheres then were lyophilized and dispensed into 96-well filter plates (one Accusphere per well) in a dry atmosphere, and the plates were sealed.

ELISA

ELISAs were performed on all samples before testing using UltraPlex ANA Profile. In brief, wells were coated with 2 μg/mL of antigen in PBS overnight at room temperature. After a wash cycle, the wells were blocked with PBS, 0.5% BSA, and 0.01% Tween for 1 h at room temperature. The wells were washed again, and then diluted serum specimens (1:100) were added to the wells for 1 h to allow the antibodies to bind to the antigens immobilized to the surface of the wells. The wells then were washed before addition of the horseradish peroxidase–conjugated anti-human IgG antibody for 1 h. Another wash step was performed before adding the OPD substrate for another 5 min followed by the addition of stop solution (2 M HCl). Absorbances were measured at 490 nm using a microplate reader (Bio-Tek Instruments, Vermont).

Multiplexed ANA Assay

The assay procedure was fully automated and was performed on a Perkin-Elmer Multiprobe II liquid handling system (Seer Green, UK). A 96-well microtiter plate shaking/plate vacuum station was incorporated into the robotic system for automated incubation and liquid removal steps. The system tracked all samples via bar-codes and performed all the liquid handling steps, washes, sample dilutions, and incubations. In brief, bar-code-labeled test serum samples and controls, all reaction buffers, and microtiter plates were loaded onto the liquid handling system, which read the serum sample bar-codes and tracked these through the assay. Samples were diluted 1 in 100 and then dispensed in each well and incubated for 30 min with shaking. After three wash cycles, 100 μL of 1 μg/mL Texas red–conjugated anti-human IgG antibody was added to each well, and the plate was incubated for another 30 min with shaking.

The wells were washed and resuspended in 150 μL of 90% PBS, 0.05% Tween, and 10% glycerol, and 75-μL samples were transferred to a reading plate.

UltraPlex Reader System

SmartBead Technologies has developed an automated 96-well microtiter plate-reader system based an Olympus IX51 (inverted) fluorescent microscope (Tokyo, Japan). Samples are read in clear-bottom 96-well microtiter plates. The system automatically scans each well, identifies and decodes all microparticles, and measures the amount of fluorescence associated with each particle via a CCD camera and image-capture software. Proprietary software (CodeCaller™) controls all aspects of the reader system operation and assigns a positive or negative value to each sample for the nine analytes. In addition, quantitative data (IU/mL) were generated for the dsDNA analyte.

Determination of ANA Specificity

The UltraPlex ANA Profile Assay was tested against the Arthritis Foundation/Centers for Disease Control (AF/CDC) ANA Human Reference Sera panel. Each ANA Human Reference Sera had been evaluated using conventional Ouchterlony immunodiffusion techniques and performed as monospecific reagents in this context (CDC datasheet). The AF/CDC reference sera were also highly reactive in solid-phase assays using purified and/or recombinant antigens, but the AF/CDC literature accompanying the sera states that they may not perform as monospecific reagents in such assays; therefore, the UltraPlex ANA Profile results were compared with ELISA test results for all samples. A cutoff of 0.5 OD units was assigned to discriminate between positive and negative samples (based on the analysis of 50 serum samples from normal healthy blood donors; data not shown).

A panel of commercial control samples comprising 38 ANA-positive and 42 ANA-negative sera was also tested using the UltraPlex ANA Profile. Once again, the samples were first assayed using ELISA to confirm the ANA specificity. The sensitivity and specificity of each test within the UltraPlex ANA Profile Assay was determined by comparison with the ELISA results. Samples were designated positive or negative depending on the ratio of the fluorescent signals of the antigen-coated particles to the control (no antigen coating) particles, which are present in every well and thus every reaction. This allowed the contribution to the fluorescent signal obtained from non-specific binding to be accounted for in each sample. The cutoff ratio for each assay was determined using several samples that previously had been characterized for ANAs.

RESULTS AND DISCUSSION

The UltraPlex ANA Profile was developed at SmartBead Technologies Ltd. for the multiplexed detection of ANA autoantibodies. Initial studies involved identifying suitable antigens, particle manufacturing techniques, immobilization chemistries, establishing suitable capture protein-coating concentrations, serum specimen and detection antibody dilution, as well as suitable buffers, molecular tags, and incubation times (data not shown). Once the parameters for the assays were determined, studies were undertaken in both uniplex and multiplexed format to demonstrate that the individual assays were not affected when performed simultaneously (data not shown). In cross-reactivity studies, only the assays for autoantibodies to Sm, SmRNP, and U1RNP cross-reacted. This was expected as these antigens are all part of the SmRNP polypeptide complex.

The use of the system to determine ANA specificity was tested using various commercial samples. All of the samples were first tested using an in-house ELISA for the detection of ANA antibodies to the recombinant antigens Centromere B, Jo-1, Scl-70, SSB, U1RNP, and the purified antigens Sm, SmRNP, and SSA. For the plas-

TABLE 1. Analysis of AF/CDC Human Reference Sera with the UltraPlex ANA Profile Assay and in-house ELISA

	Test									
Sera	Control	Cent B	SSA	SSB	Scl-70	Jo-1	Sm	SmRNP	U1 RNP	dsDNA (IU/mL)
AF/CDC 1 (dsDNA)										
UP	–	–	–	–	–	–	+	–	–	320
EL	–	–	–	–	–	–	–	–	–	+
AF/CDC 2 (SSB)										
UP	–	–	+	+	–	–	–	–	–	12.3
EL	–	–	+	+	–	–	–	–	–	–
AF/CDC 4 (U1 RNP)										
UP	–	–	–	–	–	–	–	+	+	12.3
EL	–	–	–	–	–	–	–	+	+	–
AF/CDC 5 (Sm)										
UP	–	–	–	–	–	–	+	+	–	12.3
EL	–	–	–	–	–	–	+	+	–	–
AF/CDC 7 (SSA)										
UP	–	–	+	–	–	–	–	–	–	12.3
EL	–	–	+	–	–	–	–	–	–	–
AF/CDC 8 (Cent)										
UP	–	+	–	–	–	–	–	–	–	12.3
EL	–	+	–	–	–	–	–	–	–	–
AF/CDC 9 (Scl-70)										
UP	–	–	–	–	+	–	–	–	–	12.3
EL	–	–	–	–	+	–	–	–	–	–
AF/CDC 10 (Jo-1)										
UP	–	–	–	–	–	+	–	–	–	12.3
EL	–	–	–	–	–	+	–	–	–	–

NOTE: UP, qualitative result from the UltraPlex system; EL, qualitative result from ELISA.

mid dsDNA antigen, the Pharmacia Varelisa assay kit (Uppsala, Sweden) was used to quantify the autoantibody response in IU/mL. The same antigens were used in the ANA Profile Assay described here.

AF/CDC ANA Human Reference Sera

The UltraPlex ANA Profile correctly identified the specificity of each of the nine AF/CDC ANA Human Reference sera (TABLE 1). The assay identified the CDC 1 sera to be positive for Sm autoantibodies in addition to anti–dsDNA antibodies ($n = 8$); this, however, was not observed in the corresponding ELISA. It may be that the ANA Profile is more sensitive than the ELISA and thus detects low levels of these antibodies in CDC 1. CDC 2 was shown to be positive for SSB (La) autoantibodies as indicated and also for SSA (Ro) autoantibodies; this was also observed in the ELISA. As expected, CDC 4 was positive for antibodies to both U1 RNP and SmRNP antigens, both of which contain the U1 polypeptide. Similarly, CDC 5 was positive for antibodies to Sm and SmRNP antigens. The cross-reactivity between these antigens was also observed in the ELISA assay. The results demonstrate that the ANA Profile Assay correctly identified the specificities of all the AF/CDC sera and gave almost identical results to the "gold standard" method.

Commercial Control Samples

The specificity of the ANA Profile was excellent: all nine assays exhibited 100% specificity (TABLE 2). The sensitivity was 100% for all assays except SSA for which the figure was 93.33%. For this assay, one sample was assigned the wrong profile (SSA-negative rather than SSA-positive), most likely caused by a liquid handling error because the signal from the control particle suggests that serum was not added to this well (sample diluent alone produces a lower background fluorescent signal than that from diluted sera).

The sensitivity and specificity of the dsDNA assay was determined on a qualitative basis. The autoantibody content of all dsDNA-positive sera was determined quantitatively using both the ANA Profile Assay and the Pharmacia Varelisa assay kit, both of which are standardized to the international reference preparation Wo/80.[4]

TABLE 2. Sensitivity and specificity of the UltraPlex ANA Profile Assay

	Sensitivity (%)	Specificity (%)	No. of positive samples
Centromere B	100.00	100.00	3
Jo-1	100.00	100.00	2
Scl-70	100.00	100.00	2
Sm	100.00	100.00	1
SmRNP	100.00	100.00	12
SSA	93.33	100.00	15
SSB	100.00	100.00	12
U1 RNP	100.00	100.00	10
dsDNA	100.00	100.00	7

TABLE 3. Intra- and inter-assay variation of the UltraPlex ANA Profile Assay

	Test								
	SSA	SSB	Sm	SmRNP	U1RNP	Scl-70	Jo-1	Cent-B	dsDNA
Intra-assay (*n* = 8)									
Mean	144.43	199.92	160.89	166.93	95.43	175.55	96.13	151.46	320.48
SD	4.67	4.90	4.76	14.15	14.82	2.77	8.34	3.27	27.61
CV%	3.23	2.45	2.96	8.48	15.53	1.58	8.68	2.16	8.62
Inter-assay (*n* = 5)									
Mean	73.45	98.34	47.44	151.43	95.07	101.87	40.32	111.57	1794.54
SD	14.32	15.84	2.69	12.30	31.01	9.07	4.83	10.36	574.84
CV%	19.50	16.11	5.67	8.12	32.61	8.90	11.99	9.28	32.03

NOTE: Values are mean fluorescence except for dsDNA values, which are given in IU/mL.

For five of seven samples, the assigned IU/mL values were within 30 units of each other. The correlation coefficient, r, has a value of 0.97, which indicates a positive correlation when $P = 0.001$.

A selection of samples from this study was used to determine the intra- and inter-assay variation ANA Profile Assay. The intra-assay variation was calculated from replicate determinations on each of eight samples in a single assay ($n = 8$). The inter-assay was calculated from single determinations of nine samples in five separate test runs. The results are shown in TABLE 3. The intra-assay variation was comparable to that generally observed with ELISAs. The inter-assay variation was somewhat higher, particularly for the dsDNA and U1 RNP assays. These were caused by the presence of one anomalous replicate for each of the assays, which may be caused by a sampling problem with the robotics system.

SUMMARY

The UltraPlex ANA Profile system is a multiplexed, microparticle-based fluorescent immunoassay designed to determine ANA specificity of human serum samples in a single reaction. The system is fully automated by means of a front-end liquid handling system and bench-top reader designed to decode each individual microparticle and measure the associated fluorescence. The UltraPlex ANA Profile Assay kit contains the multiplexed antigen-coated microparticles lyophilized in Accuspheres presented in a ready-to-use 96-well format. All other reagents are in liquid format for ease of use. The system provides a simple alternative to either IFA or ELISA and has been shown to correctly profile the well-characterized AF/CDC ANA Human Reference Sera. Studies with both commercially available sera and clinical samples have shown the system to be highly specific while offering high levels of sensitivity for each of the nine multiplexed ANA tests.

UltraPlex™ and CodeCaller™ are trademarks of SmartBead Technologies Ltd.

REFERENCES

1. KAVANAUGH, A., R. TOMAR, J. REVEILLE *et al.* 2000. Guidelines for clinical use of the antinuclear antibody test and tests for specific autoantibodies to nuclear antigens: American College of Pathologists. Arch. Pathol. Lab. Med. **124:** 71–81.
2. MONGEY, A.B. & E.V. HESS. 1991. Antinuclear antibodies and disease specificity. Adv. Intern. Med. **36:** 151.
3. HILLIQUIN, P. 1995. Biological markers in inflammatory rheumatic diseases. Cell. Mol. Biol. **41:** 993–1006.
4. FELTKAMP, T.E.W. *et al.* 1988. The first international standard for antibodies to double stranded DNA. Ann. Rheum. Dis. **47:** 740–746.

Association of Anti–Cyclic Citrullinated Peptide Antibodies, Anti-Citrullin Antibodies, and IgM and IgA Rheumatoid Factors with Serological Parameters of Disease Activity in Rheumatoid Arthritis

ALEXANDER GREINER, HERBERT PLISCHKE, HERBERT KELLNER, AND RUDOLF GRUBER

Rheumazentrum München, Klinikum der Universität, Medizinische Poliklinik, 80336 München, Germany

ABSTRACT: We evaluated the association of anti–cyclic citrullinated peptide (CCP) antibody titers with serological markers of disease activity. We also compared three different anti-CCP antibody ELISAs with an anti-citrullin ELISA and the IgM and the IgA rheumatoid factor (RF) in their performance of discriminating between rheumatoid arthritis (RA) and other rheumatic diseases. Sera from 333 consecutive patients of the Rheumaeinheit der Medizinischen Poliklinik München, an outpatient clinic for rheumatic diseases, were collected and tested. Anti-CCP antibodies were assayed with three different commercially available ELISAs. Antifilaggrin antibodies were tested with a commercially available ELISA using *in vitro* deiminated recombinant rat filaggrin. IgA-RF was analyzed with an ELISA, whereas IgM-RF was measured by latex-enhanced turbidimetry. Rheumatoid arthritis (RA) was diagnosed in 87 patients according to the revised classification criteria of the American College of Rheumatology (ACR), probable RA was diagnosed in 23 patients in an early phase not (yet) fulfilling the ACR criteria, and 223 patients had other rheumatic diseases. Differences in sensitivity and specificity were calculated using McNemar's test. A measure of agreement (kappa statistic) was used to examine whether the tests tended to identify the same patients as positive or negative. Correlations between CCP titers and other tests were analyzed by Spearman nonparametric rank correlation. No significant differences in sensitivity and specificity were found between the tested CCP assays (80.0–80.9% and 97.3–98.1%, respectively). All three CCP tests were slightly but not significantly more sensitive and specific than the anti-citrullin assay (77% and 92%, respectively), comparably sensitive but significantly more specific compared with the IgM-RF (86% and 82%, respectively), and significantly more sensitive but comparably specific compared with the IgA-RF (63% and 94.4%, respectively) in detecting the patients with RA. There was no significant correlation between anti-CCP, anti-citrullin, or IgM-RF or IgA-RF antibody titers and C-reactive protein, erythrocyte sedimentation rate, or white blood cell count. A weak but significant linear correlation was found between anti-CCP titers and IgM-RF

Address for correspondence: Priv. Doz. Dr. med. Rudolf Gruber, Klinikum der Universität München, Medizinische Poliklinik, Innenstadt, Pettenkoferstrasse 8a, 80336 München, Germany. Voice: +089-5160-3347; fax: +089-5160-7680.
rudolf.gruber@med.uni-muenchen.de

Ann. N.Y. Acad. Sci. 1050: 295–303 (2005). © 2005 New York Academy of Sciences.
doi: 10.1196/annals.1313.031

titers ($r = 0.2$, $P = 0.03$). We could not find a significant difference between the three tested anti-CCP assays and the anti-citrullin test in terms of sensitivity and specificity. Compared with the IgM-RF, all the anti-CCP assays were superior in specificity and comparable in sensitivity. Compared with the IgA-RF, they were more sensitive and comparably specific in the discrimination of patients with RA from other rheumatic diseases. No correlation of any tested autoantibody titer with serological parameters of inflammation was found.

KEYWORDS: autoantibodies; filaggrin; peptidyl-arginine deiminase; PADI

INTRODUCTION

Rheumatoid arthritis (RA) is the most common inflammatory joint disease and one of the most common autoimmune diseases, affecting 0.5–1% of the population in Western countries. RA is a systemic, chronic, inflammatory disease characterized by joint inflammation that often leads to joint destruction. Because of the highly variable and unpredictable course of the disease, current therapeutic strategies in RA are increasingly aggressive regimens early in the course of the disease. Therefore, diagnostic tests with high specificity are desirable for choosing the optimal treatment.[1] The rheumatoid factor, usually the IgM rheumatoid factor (RF), is currently used in the diagnosis of RA and constitutes one of the classification criteria proposed by the American College of Rheumatology (ACR).[2] However, IgM-RF positivity shows low diagnostic specificity because IgM-RF is present in patients with other autoimmune and infectious diseases, and even in a considerable percentage of normal healthy subjects, particularly in aging individuals.[3] During recent years, various other circulating antibodies have been reported to be of potential diagnostic value, including antiperinuclear factor antibodies, antikeratin antibodies, and anti-RA33 with adequate specificity but rather low sensitivity for RA.[4–6] These antibodies were later recognized to bind to citrullinated proteins, especially citrullinated filaggrin or fibrin. The use of cyclic synthetic peptides with a high content of citrullin as antigen turned out to improve sensitivity substantially without loss of specificity. These assays for anti–cyclic citrullinated peptide (CCP) antibodies are of great interest in the diagnosis of RA. They are reported to have a high specificity (91–98%) but wide variability in diagnostic sensitivity (41–80%).[7–10] We therefore compared the sensitivities and specificities of three commercially available anti-CCP antibody tests of the second generation (CCP2) with those of an anti-citrullinated fibrin antibody ELISA and IgM-RF and IgA-RF. We evaluated the association of all methods with serological parameters of disease activity (erythrocyte sedimentation rate [ESR], C-reactive protein [CRP], and white blood cell [WBC] count) and disease duration. We also investigated the differences of anti-CCP–negative versus anti-CCP–positive patients with RA within these parameters.

PATIENTS AND METHODS

Patients and Controls

In a cross-sectional study, we recruited 333 patients with suspected rheumatic diseases in the outpatient rheumatology unit of the University Hospital of Munich (median age, 54.8 years; range, 13–90 years); 87 patients had definite RA according to the 1987 revised ACR criteria[2] (median age, 58.6 years; range, 19–84 years); 75% were women; 23 patients had suspected early RA, not (yet) fulfilling the ACR criteria according to the clinical evaluation; and 223 non-RA control patients with other rheumatological diagnoses were included in the study. To analyze the sensitivity and specificity of the tests, we used the definite and early RA groups and for controls pooled data from the other 223 patients with degenerative or other inflammatory joint diseases, including psoriatic arthritis, reactive arthritis, crystal arthropathy, osteoarthritis, and spondylarthropathy. The patients were evaluated by clinical examination and laboratory tests. The final clinical diagnosis according to the ACR criteria served for the diagnosis of definite RA, and clinically suspicious RA patients not (yet) fulfilling the ACR criteria were classified as possible "early RA". The examiner was blinded to the anti-CCP, anti-citrullin, and IgA-RF results at the time of diagnosis. Blood samples were obtained at first clinical presentation and stored at −20°C until assayed. Disease activity of patients with RA was assessed at their first visit according to clinical and serological parameters (ESR, CRP, and WBC count).

Autoantibody Assays

The IgM-RF was measured by turbidimetry on a latex-enhanced agglutination assay (Roche Integra, Penzberg, Germany). Results were expressed in units per mL. The IgM-RF was considered positive at values greater than 10 U/mL. The RF isotypes for IgA were measured by a commercially available ELISA (Orgentec, Heidelberg, Germany) according to the manufacturer's instructions for use. The IgA-RF was considered positive at values greater than 20 U/mL. The anti-CCP antibodies were analyzed by three commercially available second-generation ELISAs (Menarini/ INOVA, Florence, Italy; Euroimmun, Lübeck, Germany; Generic Assays/Euro-Diagnostica, Dahlewitz, Germany) and were conducted according to the manufacturers' instructions for use. Results were expressed in arbitrary units. The samples were considered positive according to the manufacturer's manual if the antibody titer was greater than 5 (Euroimmun), 20 (Menarini), or 25 (Generic Assays/Euro-Diagnostica) arbitrary units. For the purpose of this study, each company was assigned a letter (A–C). The anti-citrullinated fibrin antibody ELISA was provided by BIOZOL/ Genesis (Eching, Germany). For statistical analysis, the results were analyzed as continuous and dichotomous variables. The serological disease activity parameters ESR, CRP, and WBC count were measured according to standard methods and used as continuous values. Statistic correlations between the autoantibody tests used, serological activity parameters, and the disease duration were determined by Spearman's rank correlation. The sensitivity and specificity for each assay was determined with respect to the clinical diagnosis. Differences between the tests were calculated with the McNemar's test. The concordance between the tests were assessed by coefficient kappa. In addition, receiver operating characteristic (ROC) analysis was performed to compare test characteristics independently of predefined cutoff points. Student's *t*-test for continuous variables was used to examine the significance of differences between the different groups. A P value of less than 0.05 was considered statistically significant. All statistical analyses were done with Medcalc statistical software (Version 6.10; Belgium).

TABLE 1. Sensitivity and specificity of the tests, alone or combined, for the diagnosis of rheumatoid arthritis

	Sensitivity	Specificity
CCP (A)	0.80	0.97
CCP (B)	0.81	0.98
CCP (C)	0.81	0.98
Citrullin	0.77	0.92
IgA-RF	0.63^a	0.94
IgM-RF	0.86	0.82^b
CCP + IgM-RF	0.90	0.81^b

[a]Significantly less sensitive compared with all other tests according to McNemar's statistics.
[b]Significantly less specific compared with all other tests according to McNemar's statistics.

RESULTS

Sensitivity and Specificity of the Assays for the Diagnosis of RA

When individual tests were considered, sensitivity for RA was highest for IgM RF (86%), followed by anti-CCP antibodies (81%), anti-citrullin antibodies (77%), and IgA RF (63%). The difference between IgM RF and the three anti-CCP antibodies was not significant. Specificity was significantly greater for anti-CCP antibodies (98%) and IgA RF (94%) and anti-citrullin antibodies (92%) than for IgM RF (82%). Sensitivity for the diagnosis of RA could be further increased by a combination of the anti-CCP and IgM-RF test, which resulted in a respectably high sensitivity of 89.9% (TABLE 1). IgA-RF and anti-citrullin antibodies could not further increase the overall sensitivity. Furthermore, in our study cohort, three of the anti-CCP–positive patients in the "non-RA" group with the diagnosis of SLE, osteoarthritis, and undifferentiated spondylarthropathy presented with articular manifestations. They were positive in all three anti-CCP assays and also for IgM-RF, but negative for IgA-RF, and two of them were also negative for anti-citrullin antibodies. For further comparisons of the diagnostic value of each assay, we did an ROC analysis and calculated the area under the curve. The ROC analysis displays the pairs of sensitivity and specificity for different cutoff points of anti-CCP, anti-citrullin, IgA-RF, and IgM-RF concentrations. The area under the curve was best for the anti-CCP assays, at 0.94–0.95. The values for anti-citrullin, IgM-RF, and IgA-RF were 0.88, 0.88, and 0.89, respectively. It could be clearly shown that CCP ELISA provided the best combination of sensitivity and specificity for detecting RA with no significant difference between the three tested anti-CCP assays. We also analyzed the benefit of single or combined use of all four antibody assays. We found a significant additional diagnostic value of anti-CCP compared with the single use of IgM-RF alone. The combination with anti-citrullin antibodies or IgA-RF could not further increase the sensitivity. In 56.3% of the 87 definite RA patients investigated, all antibody assays were positive. However, in 10 patients (11.5%) with clinically diagnosed RA, the conventionally used RF (IgM-RF) and in 31 patients (35.6%) the IgA-RF were negative. In four (40%) of these IgM-RF–negative patients, all three anti-CCP tests were positive. In 9 (10.3%)

TABLE 2. Agreement between the assay expressed as the concordance coefficients of the kappa test (95% confidence interval)

	CCP (B)	CCP (C)	Citrullin	IgM	IgA
CCP (A)	0.91 (0.86–0.96)	0.93 (0.88–0.97)	0.76 (0.69–0.84)	0.60 (0.51–0.69)	0.58 (0.47–0.69)
CCP (B)		0.94 (0.89–0.98)	0.81 (0.74–0.88)	0.64 (0.56–0.73)	0.62 (0.52–0.73)
CCP (C)			0.80 (0.73–0.88)	0.63 (0.54–0.71)	0.62 (0.52–0.72)
Citrullin				0.57 (0.47–0.66)	0.53 (0.43–0.64)
IgM					0.54 (0.45–0.64)

TABLE 3. Difference in the serological activity parameter in the CCP-negative versus CCP-positive definite RA patients

	Leukocytes (g/L)	ESR (mm/h)	CRP (mg/L)
CCP-negative ($n = 9$)	8.4	26.3	16.9
CCP-positive ($n = 78$)	8.6	28.5	18.6
P value	n.s.	n.s.	n.s.

NOTE: n.s., not significant.

of the 87 patients with definite RA, anti-CCP was negative and in one of these nine patients anti-citrullin was positive, in two patients IgA-RF was positive, and in four patients IgM-RF was positive. For the comparison of the antibody assays, we used the kappa coefficient test, where we could show a very good agreement between the anti-CCP assays (>0.9). There was also a good agreement between the anti-CCP and the anti-citrullin test (>0.8), but only a medium agreement between the mentioned assays and the IgM-RF and IgA-RF (0.5–0.64). [See TABLE 2.]

Specific Antibodies as Markers for Disease Activity

The analysis of serological parameters of disease activity (ESR, CRP, and WBC count) between the anti-CCP–positive and –negative patients with RA showed no significant differences in any parameter (TABLE 3). There was also no correlation between disease duration and the anti-CCP antibody titers. We could find a small, but significant correlation between the IgM-RF titer and the anti-CCP antibody titer ($r = 0.2$, $P = 0.03$). There was no significant correlation between anti-CCP, IgM-RF, IgA-RF, or anti-citrullin antibody titers and ESR, CRP, or WBC count.

DISCUSSION

There is evidence that early intensive therapeutic intervention ("hit hard and early") in patients with RA may stop disease progression and joint damage, resulting in a better prognosis. It therefore is important to differentiate between RA and other forms of arthritis early after the onset of symptoms.[11,12] First reported by Schellekens et al.,[13] there is now growing evidence that the diagnostic properties of the anti-CCP autoantibody in the specific diagnosis of RA outplays other available antibody tests, especially IgM-RF.[14–16]

This study is to our knowledge the first to compare three commercially available second-generation anti-CCP antibody tests (CCP2) and an anti-citrullin antibody assay with the IgM-RF and IgA-RF tests. The patient groups tested in our study were biased, because all patients came into a university outpatient rheumatology unit. These patients all had "rheumatology" problems and most of them had been sent to the unit by an other physician. Therefore, the pretest probability for the diagnosis RA is higher than for other patients with joint problems, and the percentage of patients positive for any test was relatively high compared with other studies.[17,18] On the other hand, the clinical situation of these patients may be less clear and the specificity of any test for the diagnosis of RA is challenged. Therefore, a very important finding from the data of our patient groups was that anti-CCP is a highly specific marker in the diagnosis of RA. Comparable with the results of some other studies using the CCP1 and CCP2 assay, we found a specificity of 98%.[19,20] The somewhat lower specificity and sensitivity of some other studies using anti-CCP assays may reflect different cutoff levels and different patient populations. The sensitivity of anti-CCP has also been increased by the second test generation anti-CCP assays used in this study. Now there is no longer a significant difference in sensitivity to the IgM-RF. We found a high sensitivity of 80% as described by others.[20,21] On the other hand, lower sensitivities of approximately 65% also had been described.[22,23] The lower sensitivity in those study cohorts may reflect the presence of a relatively high percentage of early rheumatoid patients and higher cutoff levels. By combining the use of all antibodies (anti-CCP, anti-citrullin, and IgM/A-RF), only the combination of anti-CCP with IgM-RF could increase the sensitivity (to 90%). Like others,[13,22,23] we could also find an additional diagnostic value of anti-CCP compared with IgM-RF; as in 40% of the sero-negative (IgM-RF–negative) RA patients, anti-CCP antibodies could be detected. Also interesting was the observation that all anti-CCP–positive patients in the control group had an articular disease manifestation. As it was shown that the anti-CCP antibody may precede the clinical manifestation of RA by many years, these patients may not have received false-positive results but may develop RA or have a clinically undiagnosed RA. Rantapaa-Dahlqvist et al. showed that anti-CCP and IgA-RF predict the development of RA, with anti-CCP having the highest predictive value of all tested antibodies (IgG-RF, IgA-RF, and IgM-RF and CCP2).[24] The value of anti-CCP and antifilaggrin antibodies and RF for predicting the outcome of RA, clinical signs of disease activity, and the severity of radiographic joint damage has been investigated recently. Bas et al. showed an association of IgA-RF and anti-CCP with clinical signs of disease activity.[7,25] The high prevalence of anti-CCP in RA patients with extensive disease activity and severe radiological changes, and even more impressively in RA patients who are IgM-RF–negative, suggests that anti-CCP is more useful than the RF alone in the early prediction of disease outcome and disease activity. Vencovsky *et al.* showed that patients with erosive RA were more likely to be anti-CCP–positive and IgM-RF–negative than RF-positive and anti-CCP–negative.[26] Using anti-citrullin antibody tests, some studies failed to predict joint destruction and radiological progression by a positive test result using an assay with purified human filaggrin[27] or citrullinated rat filaggrin but could show a high diagnostic value for an anti-citrullin antibody assay in the diagnosis of RA.[28,29]

A special interest of our study was the correlation of the antibody titers of anti-CCP and anti-citrullin antibodies and IgM-RF and IgA-RF with the serological markers of disease activity, the ESR, CRP, and WBC count. ESR and CRP are, along with the number of swollen and painful joints, one of the major criteria for the "clinical" disease activity score and the ACR scores. First, we could not find an association of disease duration or patient's age with any of the tested antibodies (data not shown). Furthermore, we could find no significant differences between anti-CCP–negative and anti-CCP–positive patients comparing ESR, CRP, and WBC count (TABLE 3). And finally, there was no correlation between anti-CCP antibody titers or any other antibody titer with ESR, CRP, or WBC count.

In conclusion, the IgM-RF is still mostly used as a screening marker in the diagnosis of RA. However, the second-generation anti-CCP antibody assays have a comparable sensitivity in the diagnosis of RA but a much higher specificity. To establish the diagnosis of RA in a preselected patient group, we would suggest the use of the highly specific anti-CCP antibody test in the first line. The use of IgM-RF and IgA-RF could be restricted to a few unclear cases of anti-CCP–negative patients. Especially in ambiguous cases or in RF-negative patients with suspected RA, the anti-CCP assay has proved to be very helpful and seems to now be the diagnostic marker of choice for the diagnosis of RA. In our study, the combined use of IgM-RF and anti-CCP assays reached a sensitivity of 90%, but loses specificity. Therefore, the use of anti-CCP is the best diagnostic tool and also a good prognostic marker and would allow the clinician to choose a more intensive disease-modifying antirheumatic therapy early in the course of the disease, and also in patients for whom the clinical and radiological findings are not conclusive or indicative for such a therapy.

ACKNOWLEDGMENTS

We thank Ms. B. Danne, Ms. J. Partzsch, and Ms. M. Siwy for excellent technical assistance. Part of this work is included in the doctoral thesis of Mr. Alexander Greiner at the Ludwig-Maximilians-University of Munich.

REFERENCES

1. OLSEN, N.J. & C.M. STEIN. New drugs for rheumatoid arthritis. N. Engl. J. Med. **350:** 2167–2179.
2. ARNETT, F.C., S.M. EDWORTHY, D.A. BLOCH, *et al.* 1988. The American Rheumatism Association 1987 revised criteria for the classification of rheumatoid arthritis. Arthritis Rheum. **31:** 315–324.
3. DORNER, T., K. EGERER, E. FEIST & G.R. BURMESTER. 2004. Rheumatoid factor revisited. Curr. Opin. Rheumatol. **16:** 246–253.

4. HASSFELD, W., G. STEINER, K. HARTMUTH, et al. 1989. Demonstration of a new anti-nuclear antibody (anti-RA33) that is highly specific for rheumatoid arthritis. Arthritis Rheum. **32:** 1515–1520.

5. CORDONNIER, C., O. MEYER, E. PALAZZO, et al. 1996. Diagnostic value of anti-RA33 antibody, antikeratin antibody, antiperinuclear factor and antinuclear antibody in early rheumatoid arthritis: comparison with rheumatoid factor. Br. J. Rheumatol. **35:** 620–624.

6. SIMON, M., E. GIRBAL, M. SEBBAG, et al. 1993. The cytokeratin filament-aggregating protein filaggrin is the target of the so-called "antikeratin antibodies," autoantibodies specific for rheumatoid arthritis. J. Clin. Invest. **92:** 1387–1393.

7. BAS, S., T.V. PERNEGER, M. SEITZ, et al. 2002. Diagnostic tests for rheumatoid arthritis: comparison of anti-cyclic citrullinated peptide antibodies, anti-keratin antibodies and IgM rheumatoid factors. Rheumatology **41:** 809–814.

8. NIJENHUIS, S., A.J. ZENDMAN, E.R. VOSSENAAR, et al. 2004. Autoantibodies to citrulli-nated proteins in rheumatoid arthritis: clinical performance and biochemical aspects of an RA-specific marker. Clin. Chim. Acta **350:** 17–34.

9. VAN VENROOIJ, W.J., E.R. VOSSENAAR & A.J. ZENDMAN. 2004. Anti-CCP antibodies: the new rheumatoid factor in the serology of rheumatoid arthritis. Autoimmun. Rev. **3**(suppl. 1): S17–S19.

10. ZENDMAN, A.J., E.R. VOSSENAAR & W.J. VAN VENROOIJ. 2004. Autoantibodies to citrulli-nated (poly)peptides: a key diagnostic and prognostic marker for rheumatoid arthritis. Autoimmunity **37:** 295–299.

11. LINDQVIST, E., K. EBERHARDT, K. BENDTZEN, et al. 2005. Prognostic laboratory markers of joint damage in rheumatoid arthritis. Ann. Rheum. Dis. **64:** 196–201.

12. VISSER, H. 2005. Early diagnosis of rheumatoid arthritis. Best Pract. Res. Clin. Rheumatol. **19:** 55–72.

13. SCHELLEKENS, G.A., B.A. DE JONG, F.H. VAN DEN HOOGEN, et al. 1998. Citrulline is an essential constituent of antigenic determinants recognized by rheumatoid arthritis-specific autoantibodies. J. Clin. Invest. **101:** 273–281.

14. KASTBOM, A., G. STRANDBERG, A. LINDROOS & T. SKOGH. 2004. Anti-CCP antibody test predicts the disease course during 3 years in early rheumatoid arthritis (the Swedish TIRA project). Ann. Rheum. Dis. **63:** 1085–1089.

15. SODERLIN, M.K., A. KASTBOM, H. KAUTIAINEN, et al. 2004. Antibodies against cyclic citrullinated peptide (CCP) and levels of cartilage oligomeric matrix protein (COMP) in very early arthritis: relation to diagnosis and disease activity. Scand. J. Rheumatol. **33:** 185–188.

16. VISSER, H., S. LE CESSIE, K. VOS, et al. 2002. How to diagnose rheumatoid arthritis early: a prediction model for persistent (erosive) arthritis. Arthritis Rheum. **46:** 357–365.

17. VAN JAARSVELD, C.H., E.J. TER BORG, J.W. JACOBS, et al. 1999. The prognostic value of the antiperinuclear factor, anti-citrullinated peptide antibodies and rheumatoid factor in early rheumatoid arthritis. Clin. Exp. Rheumatol. **17:** 689–697.

18. GOLDBACH-MANSKY, R., J. LEE, A. MCCOY, et al. 2000. Rheumatoid arthritis associated autoantibodies in patients with synovitis of recent onset. Arthritis Res. **2:** 236–243.

19. BIZZARO, N., G. MAZZANTI, E. TONUTTI, et al. 2001. Diagnostic accuracy of the anti-citrulline antibody assay for rheumatoid arthritis. Clin. Chem. **47:** 1089–1093.

20. SUZUKI, K., T. SAWADA, A. MURAKAMI, et al. 2003. High diagnostic performance of ELISA detection of antibodies to citrullinated antigens in rheumatoid arthritis. Scand. J. Rheumatol. **32:** 197–204.

21. PALOSUO, T., R. TILVIS, T. STRANDBERG & K. AHO. 2003. Filaggrin related antibodies among the aged. Ann. Rheum. Dis. **62:** 261–263.

22. LEE, D.M. & P.H. SCHUR. 2003. Clinical utility of the anti-CCP assay in patients with rheumatic diseases. Ann. Rheum. Dis. **62:** 870–874.

23. VALLBRACHT, I., J. RIEBER, M. OPPERMANN, et al. 2004. Diagnostic and clinical value of anti-cyclic citrullinated peptide antibodies compared with rheumatoid factor isotypes in rheumatoid arthritis. Ann. Rheum. Dis. **63:** 1079–1084.

24. RANTAPAA-DAHLQVIST, S., B.A. DE JONG, E. BERGLIN, et al. 2003. Antibodies against cyclic citrullinated peptide and IgA rheumatoid factor predict the development of rheumatoid arthritis. Arthritis Rheum. **48:** 2741–2749.

25. BAS, S., S. GENEVAY, O. MEYER & C. GABAY. 2003. Anti-cyclic citrullinated peptide antibodies, IgM and IgA rheumatoid factors in the diagnosis and prognosis of rheumatoid arthritis. Rheumatology **42:** 677–680.
26. VENCOVSKY, J., S. MACHACEK, L. SEDOVA, *et al.* 2003. Autoantibodies can be prognostic markers of an erosive disease in early rheumatoid arthritis. Ann. Rheum. Dis. **62:** 427–430.
27. PAIMELA, L., T. PALOSUO, K. AHO, *et al.* 2001. Association of autoantibodies to filaggrin with an active disease in early rheumatoid arthritis. Ann. Rheum. Dis. **60:** 32–35.
28. VITTECOQ, O., B. INCAURGARAT, F. JOUEN-BEADES, *et al.* 2004. Autoantibodies recognizing citrullinated rat filaggrin in an ELISA using citrullinated and non-citrullinated recombinant proteins as antigens are highly diagnostic for rheumatoid arthritis. Clin. Exp. Immunol. **135:** 173–180.
29. VITTECOQ, O., S. POUPLIN, K. KRZANOWSKA, *et al.* 2003. Rheumatoid factor is the strongest predictor of radiological progression of rheumatoid arthritis in a three-year prospective study in community-recruited patients. Rheumatology **42:** 939–946.

Detection of TT Virus in Patients with Idiopathic Inflammatory Myopathies

PETER GERGELY, JR.,[a,b] ANTAL BLAZSEK,[a] KATALIN DANKÓ,[c] ANDREA PONYI,[c] AND GYULA POÓR[a,b]

[a]National Institute of Rheumatology and Physiotherapy, H-1023 Budapest, Hungary

[b]Musculoskeletal Molecular Biology Research Group at the National Institute of Rheumatology and Physiotherapy, Hungarian Academy of Sciences, H-1023 Budapest, Hungary

[c]Third Department of Internal Medicine, Division of Clinical Immunology, Medical and Health Science Center, University of Debrecen, H-4004 Debrecen, Hungary

ABSTRACT: The TT virus, a recently identified single-stranded DNA virus with unknown pathogenicity, has been shown to commonly infect humans. Viruses have been considered to contribute to disease pathogenesis in autoimmune disorders including idiopathic inflammatory myopathies (IIMs) and rheumatoid arthritis (RA). We assessed the prevalence of TTV infection in IIM compared with that in patients with RA and healthy blood donors. Detection of TTV was conducted by nested PCR and real-time PCR in the sera of 94 patients with IIM, 95 RA patients. and 95 age- and sex-matched healthy blood donors. Identity of the PCR products was confirmed by sequencing. TTV DNA was detected in 61 of 94 (64.9%) patients with IIM, in 64 of 95 (67.4%) patients with RA, and in 62 of 95 (65.3%; $P > 0.05$) healthy individuals. Age, sex, activity, or duration of disease had no influence on TTV positivity in either group. However, patients with severe IIM ($n = 36$) had a significantly higher rate of TTV infection (31/36, 86.1%) than patients with mild disease (30/58, 51.7%, $P < 0.05$, $\chi^2 = 10.0$). Disease was considered severe in IIM when immunosuppressive treatment was necessary because of continuous high activity and/or serious inner-organ involvement despite corticosteroid treatment. In conclusion, although we found the detection rate of TTV similar in patients with idiopathic inflammatory myopathies and rheumatoid arthritis and comparable to that in healthy controls, our data suggest that infection with TT virus may result in a more severe disease in patients with idiopathic inflammatory myopathies.

KEYWORDS: TT virus; idiopathic inflammatory myopathies; myositis; rheumatoid arthritis

Address for correspondence: Dr. Gyula Poór, 1st Department of Rheumatology and Metabolic Osteology, National Institute of Rheumatology and Physiotherapy, Frankel Leó u. 38–40, H-1023 Budapest, Hungary. Voice: +36-1-438-8300; fax: +36-1-355-2779.
orfireum@axelero.hu

Ann. N.Y. Acad. Sci. 1050: 304–313 (2005). © 2005 New York Academy of Sciences.
doi: 10.1196/annals.1313.032

INTRODUCTION

Idiopathic inflammatory myopathies (IIMs), or polymyositis-dermatomyositis (PM/DM) syndrome as traditionally termed, represent a heterogeneous group of conditions characterized by proximal muscle weakness and nonsuppurative inflammation of skeletal muscle. The unknown etiology, the very low (approximately 5–10 cases per million population) incidence rate, and the often inadequate response to therapy all contribute to the difficulties both researchers and clinicians must overcome when studying or treating patients with IIM. Constant inflammation and involvement of various internal organs result in significant worsening of quality of life and decreased survival rates.[1,2] Although the etiopathogenesis is believed to be mediated by autoimmune processes in genetically susceptible individuals, the cause and exact pathomechanisms are still unclear.[3]

Several lines of indirect evidence have been accumulated suggesting that certain strains of viruses belonging to the family of picornaviruses, coxsackieviruses, enteroviruses, or retroviruses may play a role in the etiopathogenesis of IIM.[4] These findings include seasonal variations on the onset of the disease, signs of viral infections preceding or coincident with inflammatory myopathies, sequence homology and molecular mimicry between self and viral antigens, results of cultures from affected muscle tissues, elevated titers of antibodies to viral proteins, identification of viral antigens in muscle biopsies, and development of chronic myositis in animal models after certain viral infections.[4,5] However, currently no virus has been unequivocally identified as a causative agent in IIM.

Clarification of mechanisms by which viruses initially can trigger autoimmunity and differentiation between causative and consequential events upon viral infection in IIM are necessary to understand the exact role of viruses in inflammatory myopathies. Furthermore, in addition to certain known pathogens already suggested to have an etiological role, newly or not yet identified viral agents may also be responsible for triggering IIM. TTV is a recently discovered small DNA virus with a unique unenveloped single-stranded circular DNA genome.[6] TTV is known to cause persistent infection in humans, and various genotypes of the virus have been detected with frequencies ranging from 2 to 90% in serum of healthy blood donors.[7–9] However, there is no clear direct or indirect evidence so far suggesting that the virus has a pathogenic role in any disease.[7,10]

Although several hundreds of published studies on TTV infection are available today, there are very few data regarding the prevalence (or possible role) of the virus in autoimmune disorders. Recent studies were undertaken to determine the prevalence of TTV infection in rheumatic diseases: patients with unselected pathologies had similar rates of infection as patients with systemic lupus erythematosus,[11] and the percentage of TTV DNA positivity was similar in serum samples of patients with rheumatoid arthritis (RA) and systemic sclerosis and was comparable to that of patients with osteoarthritis and normal blood donors.[12] Although these studies did not support the role of TTV in autoimmunity, association of TTV infection with autoimmune diseases cannot be ruled out.

In this article, we describe a sensitive real-time PCR and melting curve analysis using the conservative primer sets described by Leary *et al.* for the detection of TTV DNA in serum samples.[13] We, for the first time, analyzed sera of patients with IIM and compared the TTV infection rate with that of patients with RA and that of healthy blood donors matched for age and sex. We also investigate whether the continuing infection with TTV DNA relates to the clinical and laboratory parameters, disease activity, and severity in patients with idiopathic inflammatory myopathies.

PATIENTS AND METHODS

Patients

Serum samples were obtained from Hungarian patients with IIM (n = 94, mean age 40.5 ± 10.7 years, 25 males), from patients with RA (n = 95, mean age 46.8 ± 9.65 years, 21 males), and from healthy blood donors (n = 95, mean age 43.5 ± 11.2 years, 23 males). IIM was diagnosed according to the criteria of Bohan and Peter,[14] and patients were divided into five subgroups based on clinicopathological findings: polymyositis (PM; n = 51), dermatomyositis (DM; n = 15), overlap myositis (OM; n = 16), malignancy-associated myositis (MAM; n = 6), and juvenile dermatomyositis (JDM; n = 6). All patients with RA met the criteria of the American College of Rheumatology[15] and had no other connective tissue diseases. There were no significant differences in age and sex distribution between the patient and control groups. Disease activity in patients with IIM was assessed by the criteria based on manual muscle strength and activities of creatine kinase and lactate dehydrogenase, as recently suggested by the International Myositis Assessment and Clinical Studies Group.[16] Disease activity in RA was calculated by the 28 joint disease activity score (DAS28).[17] Patients were receiving 0.5–2 mg prednisolone/kg of body weight per day or equivalent in the IIM group and a total of 5–15 mg prednisolone or equivalent per day in the RA group. Immunosuppressive drugs included methotrexate (7.5–20 mg per week), azathioprine (50–150 mg per day), or cyclosporin A (2.5–7.5 mg/kg of body weight per day).

Laboratory Evaluation

Antinuclear antibodies, rheumatoid factor, erythrocyte sedimentation rate, C-reactive protein, and serum levels of creatine kinase and lactate dehydrogenase were routinely evaluated for all patients; anti–Jo-1 antibody was detected in patients with IIM.

Detection of TTV DNA

Serum samples from patients and controls were stored at −80°C and assayed for TTV DNA in parallel. Viral DNA was extracted from 200 μL of serum using the Roche High Pure Viral Nucleic Acid kit (Roche Diagnostics, Mannheim, Germany). TTV DNA (GenBank Accession number AB008394.1) was amplified by PCR as described by Leary et al. using the nested SetB primer sets forward 1 (5'-GTGG-GACTTTCACTTGTCGGTGTC-3' corresponding to nucleotide positions 3087–3110) and reverse 1 (5'-GACAAATGGCAAGAAGATAAAGGCC-3' corresponding to nucleotide positions 3392–3368) followed by forward 2 (5'-GGTCACTAAG-CACTCCGAGCG-3' corresponding to nucleotide positions 3120–3141) and reverse 2 (5'-GCGAAGTCTGGCCCCACTCAC-3' corresponding to nucleotide positions 3362–3342).[14] The thermocycler program included preheating to 95°C for 5 min, followed by 35 cycles consisting of denaturation at 94°C for 45 s, annealing at 55°C for 30 s, and extension at 72°C for 30 s using an Applied Biosystems (ABi) Geneamp 2700 thermocycler (Applera Corporation, Foster City, CA). PCR products were detected by electrophoresis (FIG. 1A) on 2% agarose gels, stained with ethidium bromide, photographed under UV light using an AlphaDigiDoc System 1000 gel documentation system (Alpha Innotech Corporation, San Leandro, CA). The size of the PCR product (243 bp) was estimated according to the migration pattern of a 250-bp DNA ladder. Identity of PCR products was confirmed by automated sequencing

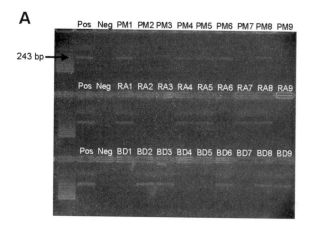

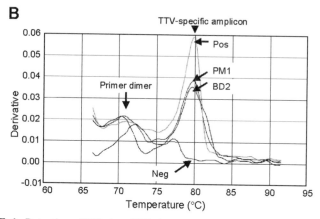

FIGURE 1. Detection of TT virus DNA in sera of healthy blood donors (BD1-9) and patients with RA (RA1-9) and IIM (PM1-9) by two different PCR methods. Viral DNA extracts were specifically amplified by nested PCR. For positive control (Pos), TTV DNA that previously had been identified by sequencing was used. Negative control (Neg) refers to a reaction with serum containing no TTV DNA. (**A**) TTV positivity or negativity was determined by the presence or absence of the 243-bp PCR product. (**B**) After amplification by PCR, SYBR Green I–based real-time PCR and melting curve analysis was performed to detect TTV. TTV-specific amplicon was verified by its melting temperature (Tm = 80°C). Unspecific primer dimers are seen between 70°C and 76°C.

using an ABi 377 sequencer. For positive control, viral DNA extract from serum containing TTV that had been identified previously by the method of Okamoto *et al.*[18] and sequenced by an ABi Prism 310 automatic sequencer was kindly provided by Gyorgyi Szladek, Department of Microbiology, University of Debrecen, Debrecen, Hungary.[9] SYBR Green I real-time PCR and melting curve analysis of TTV DNA (FIG. 1B) was also performed as previously described for the detection of DNA of various origin.[19,20] SYBR Green I–based PCR amplification was performed as the second nested step in the ABi 7300 Sequence Detection PCR system. After optimization of the primer pair, samples were assayed in a 96-well plate with 30 μL reaction mixture volume containing 1 μL of the previous reaction and optimal concentration of each of the primers. Reaction was performed with the AmpliTaq Gold SYBR Mastermix (ABi). The thermal profile for the SYBR Green–based PCR consisted of a 10-min hotstart enzyme activation step at 95°C, followed by 40 cycles of PCR at 95°C for 30 s (denaturation), 55°C for 30 s (annealing), and 72°C for 30 s (extension). After amplification, a melting curve analysis was performed to verify the correct product by its specific melting temperature (Tm = 80°C). Melting curve analysis consisted of a denaturation step at 95°C for 0.5 min, lowered to 55°C for 30 s, and followed by several cycles of incubation in which the temperature was increased to 95°C, with continuous reading of fluorescence. Results were analyzed with the melting curve analysis software of the ABi SDS 7300. For SYBR Green–based PCR amplification, amplification plots and Tm values were routinely analyzed to verify TTV positivity (presence of TTV DNA) and the specificities of the amplicons.

Statistics

Differences in TTV prevalence in the IIM, RA, and control groups were calculated with Yates corrected χ^2 statistics using Prism Version 3.0 software for Windows (GraphPad, San Diego, CA). Nonparametric data were compared with Mann-Whitney *U* test. Differences were considered significant at $P < 0.05$.

RESULTS

TTV DNA was detected in 61 of 94 (64.9%) patients with IIM, in 64 of 95 (67.4%) patients with RA, and in 62 of 95 (65.3%; $P > 0.05$) healthy individuals. Age, sex, and duration of disease had no influence on TTV positivity in either group. Disease activity, treatments with immunosuppressive agents or corticosteroids, and presence of autoantibodies (antinuclear antibodies or rheumatoid factor) were independent of the presence of TTV DNA in the sera of patients with RA (data not shown). We found no association between clinicopathological subsets (PM, DM, JDM, OM, MAM) and TTV positivity in IIM (TABLE 1). Note, however, that all six patients with juvenile dermatomyositis were infected with the virus.

Patients with inner-organ or joint involvement including interstitial lung disease ($n = 10$ of 18, 55.6%), dysphagia ($n = 11$ of 19, 57.9%), cardiac manifestations ($n = 10$ of 18, 55.6%), respiratory muscle involvement ($n = 1$ of 1, 100%), Raynaud's phenomenon ($n = 28$ of 44, 63.6%), or arthritis/arthralgia ($n = 27$ of 42, 64.3%) were more likely to be tested positive for TTV DNA. However, none of these clinical fea-

TABLE 1. Prevalence of TTV infection in different subgroups of patients with IIM

	All patients (%)[a]	TTV-pos (%)[b]	TTV-neg (%)[b]
No. of patients	94	61 (64.9)	33 (35.1)
Age (years ± SD)	40.5 ± 10.7	40.2 ± 11.9	40.9 ± 9.5
Age at onset of IIM (years ± SD)	32.8 ± 13.4	32.3 ± 14.1	33.7 ± 12,2
Male/female patients	25/69	14/47	11/22
Diagnosis			
Polymyositis	51 (54.3)	33 (64.7)	18 (35.3)
Dermatomyositis	15 (16)	8 (53.3)	7 (46.7)
Juvenile dermatomyositis	6 (6.4)	6 (100)	0 (0)
Overlap myositis	16 (19.1)	10 (62.5)	6 (37.5)
Malignancy-associated myositis	6 (6.4)	4 (66.7)	2 (33.3)
Organ involvement			
Interstitial lung disease	18 (19.1)	10 (55.6)	8 (44.4)
Dysphagia	19 (20.2)	11 (57.9)	8 (42.1)
Cardiac involvement	18 (19.1)	10 (55.6)	8 (44.4)
Respiratory muscle involvement	1 (1.1)	1 (100)	0 (0)
Raynaud's phenomenon	44 (46.8)	28 (63.6)	16 (36.4)
Arthritis/arthralgy	42 (44.7)	27 (64.3)	15 (35.7)
Laboratory parameters			
Elevated CK	22 (23.4)	15 (68.2)	7 (31.8)
Elevated LDH	23 (24.5)	17 (73.9)	6 (26.1)
Anti–Jo-1 positivity	13 (13.8)	6 (46.2)	7 (53.8)
Patients with active disease	49 (52.1)	34 (69.4)	15 (30.6)

[a]Percentage of all patients.
[b]Percentage of TTV-positive or -negative patients within the subgroup.

tures correlated significantly with the presence of TTV. Similarly, patients who had elevated creatine kinase ($n = 15$ of 22, 68.2%) or lactate dehydrogenase ($n = 17$ of 23, 73.9%) levels were more often positive for TTV. Of 13 anti–Jo-1 antibody–positive patients, six (46.2%) showed detectable TTV DNA in their sera (TABLE 1). The presence of other autoantibodies such as antinuclear antibody was also unrelated to TTV positivity (not shown). Forty-nine patients had active disease and 34 of these (69.4%) tested positive for TTV DNA.

Although none of these parameters correlated significantly with TTV positivity in IIM, we observed a tendency that patients with active disease, extramuscular manifestations, and elevated levels of muscle-specific enzymes were more likely to carry TTV DNA, indicating that the virus might influence disease course. To further investigate this issue, we also determined disease severity in IIM, which is a more complex parameter than a single clinical or laboratory marker and reflects disease

TABLE 2. Correlation between TTV infection and disease severity in patients with idiopathic inflammatory myopathies

	TTV-positive	TTV-negative	Total
Severe disease (n)	31	5	36
Mild disease (n)	30	28	58
Total (n)	61	33	94

NOTE: Statistical analysis was performed with Yates corrected chi-square test: $\chi^2 = 10.0$; $P = 0.0015$; relative risk (95% confidence interval): 1.67 (1.3–2.2); odds ratio (95% confidence interval): 5.79 (2.0–16.9).

progression rather than a momentary stage of the disease. Thirty-six patients with continuous high activity and/or serious inner-organ involvement despite corticosteroid treatment had required immunosuppressive agents at some point of time since the onset of the disease; these patients were considered "severe" by the physician. "Mild" disease was deemed in cases of 58 patients who had responded adequately to corticosteroids and needed no immunosuppressants. Interestingly, 31 (86.1%) of the 36 severe patients tested positive for TTV DNA, which resulted in a significant correlation and an increased relative risk ($P = 0.0015$, TABLE 2). These data would probably indicate a myositis-specific phenomenon, because immunosuppressive treatment, severity, or activity of the disease was unrelated to TTV infection in RA.

DISCUSSION

TTV is a recently discovered small DNA virus with a unique unenveloped single-stranded circular DNA genome of negative polarity that has been provisionally classified into the Circoviridae family.[6,21,22] The TT virus originally was named after the initials of the first patient (TT) who had hepatitis of unknown origin and then was renamed transfusion-transmitted virus.[6,22] Although several studies have attempted to clarify its pathogenicity since then, TTV has not been causally associated with any disease.[10] Moreover, several open issues (i.e., method of replication, antibody production against TTV-derived proteins, significance of its global presence, and high genomic variability) are to be clarified. TTV has not been transmitted to tissue culture cells or visualized with certainty by electron microscopy; however, TTV has been transmitted to chimpanzees and rhesus monkeys by intravenous inoculation of virus-positive human sera or fecal extracts.[23]

Because of difficulties in the expression of full-length TTV protein in prokaryotic or eukaryotic cells and in the generation of pan-specific TTV antibodies, diagnosis of TTV infection has been dependent on PCR detection of viral DNA using primers specific for the conservative noncoding regions.[23,24] TTV has been documented previously in various types of human samples including peripheral blood mononuclear cells, saliva, bile, and serum.[7] So far, serum has been used most often as the most convenient (but not necessarily the optimal) human sample for the detection of TTV. We have developed a novel SYBR Green–based real-time PCR method using conservative primer sets corresponding to the untranslated regions of TTV described by Leary *et al.* to detect TTV DNA in the serum.[13]

In this study, we used this method to assess the rate of infection in patients with autoimmune rheumatic disorders; specificity was confirmed by sequencing. We for the first time to our knowledge detected TT virus in the sera of patients with IIM and found its prevalence similar (64.9%) to that in patients with RA (67.4%) and healthy blood donors (65.3). These values are higher than those regarding the infection rate of Hungarian blood donors (20%) or patients with hepatitis of unknown origin (50%).[25] Differences may be explained by the extremely high genome heterogeneity of TTV and the use of different primer sets. Szladek *et al.* recently detected TTV in 57% of renal transplant patients and in 20% of healthy blood donors in Hungary using primers specific for genogroup 1, but the prevalence of TTV was above 90% in both groups with a different method capable of detecting most known genotypes.[9]

Although the prevalence of TTV infection in IIM was similar to that in RA or healthy blood donors and no clinical or laboratory parameter correlated significantly with TTV positivity in IIM, we observed a tendency that patients with IIM with active disease, extramuscular manifestations, and elevated levels of muscle-specific enzymes were more likely to carry TTV DNA. Furthermore, we found that patients with more severe IIM had a significantly higher rate of TTV infection. Thus, TTV infection may be a risk factor for developing a progressive and corticosteroid-refractory disease in IIM. Ours is the first evidence that TT virus may play a role in IIM; it might be an additive factor to the pathomechanism of the serious organ manifestations rather than a direct causative agent.

Viruses have long been considered as etiological factors in IIM. The seasonal variation in the onset of disease among different subsets characterized by myositis-specific autoantibodies suggests that viral agents may play a role. Retroviruses have also been hypothesized in IIM. Higuchi and Osame suggested that IIM might be associated with HTLV-I infection because of T-cell–mediated immunological processes triggered by HTLV-I–infected CD4+ lymphocytes.[26] Although cause and effect remain to be proved, there are reports of hepatitis C virus infections preceding or co-incident with IIM.[27] Certain picornaviruses can also serve as a substrate for amino-acyl-tRNA synthetase activity, and homology has been found between amino acid sequences corresponding to muscle proteins and a capsid protein of encephalomyo-carditis virus, a picornavirus that induces myositis in the mouse.[28] Coxsackievirus A9 that has been cultured from muscle can also cause myositis[29] and coxsackievirus-specific antibodies have been found in some children with JDM.[30] Furthermore, mumps virus antigen and enteroviral genomes have been detected in muscle of a few patients with IIM.[31,32] Animal models have provided strong evidence that viruses can trigger autoimmunity and IIM: infecting neonatal Swiss mice with coxsackie-virus B1 or injecting encephalomyocarditis virus 221A into adult BALB/c mice resulted in chronic myositis.[33,34]

The mechanism by which TT virus can contribute to disease pathomechanism, however, remains unclear. In this study, we used a descriptive approach to examine whether TTV has any role in IIM and found that TTV infection may be associated with the severity of the disease. It is important that further studies with detailed functional analyses and examination of cause and effect relationships clarify how TT virus can contribute to the development of serious manifestations in idiopathic inflammatory myopathies.

ACKNOWLEDGMENTS

This work was supported by the Hungarian Scientific Research Fund OTKA T042637.

REFERENCES

1. DANKO, K., A. PONYI, G. SZEGEDI, et al. 2004. Long-term survival of patients with idiopathic inflammatory myopathies according to clinical features: a longitudinal study of 162 cases. Medicine **83:** 35–42.
2. PONYI, A., L. GERGELY, K. DANKO, et al. 2005. Functional outcome and quality of life in adult patients with idiopathic inflammatory myositis. Rheumatology **44:** 83–88.
3. CHRISTOPHER-STINE L. & P.H. PLOTZ. 2004. Myositis: an update on pathogenesis. Curr. Opin. Rheumatol. **16:** 700–706.
4. WORTMAN, R.L. 2001. Inflammatory diseases of muscle and other myopathies. *In* Kelley's Textbook of Rheumatology. Sixth edition, pp. 1281–1282. Saunders. Philadelphia.
5. TAM, P.E., A.M. SCHMIDT, P.P. MESSNER, et al. 1994. Duration of virus persistence and its relationship to inflammation in the chronic phase of coxsackievirus B1-induced murine polymyositis. J. Lab. Clin. Med. **123:** 346–356.
6. NISHIZAWA, T., H. OKAMOTO, M. MAYUMI, et al. 1997. A novel DNA virus (TTV) associated with elevated transaminase levels in posttransfusion hepatitis of unknown etiology. Biochem. Biophys. Res. Commun. **241:** 92–97.
7. BIAGINI, P. Human circoviruses. 2004. Vet. Microbiol. **98:** 95–101.
8. HUANG, L.Y., T. OYSTEIN JONASSEN, B. GRINDE, et al. 2001. High prevalence of TT virus-related DNA (90%) and diverse viral genotypes in Norwegian blood donors. J. Med. Virol. **64:** 381–386.
9. SZLADEK G., A. JUHASZ, L. ASZTALOS, et al. 2003. Persisting TT virus (TTV) genogroup 1 variants in renal transplant recipients. Arch. Virol. **148:** 841–851.
10. SAGIR, A., O. KIRSCHBERG, T. HEINTGES, et al. 2004. SEN virus infection. Rev. Med. Virol. **14:** 141–148.
11. MAGGI, F., C. FORNAI, M. BENDINELLI, et al. 1999. High prevalence of TT virus viremia in Italian patients, regardless of age, clinical diagnosis, and previous interferon treatment. J. Infect. Dis. **180:** 838–842.
12. SEEMAYER, C.A., S. VIAZOV, S. GAY, et al. 2001. Prevalence of TTV DNA and GBV-C RNA in patients with systemic sclerosis, rheumatoid arthritis, and osteoarthritis does not differ from that in healthy blood donors. Ann. Rheum. Dis. **60:** 806–809.
13. LEARY, T.P., J.C. ERKER, I.K. MUSHAHWAR, et al. 1999. Optimized PCR assay for the detection of TT virus. J. Virol. Methods **82:** 109–112.
14. BOHAN, A. & J.B. PETER. 1975. Polymyositis and dermatomyositis. N. Engl. J. Med. **292:** 344–347.
15. ARNETT, F.C., S.M. EDWORTHY, H.S. LUTHRA, et al. 1988. The American Rheumatism Association 1987 revised criteria for the classification of rheumatoid arthritis. Arthritis Rheum. **31:** 315–324.
16. RIDER, L.G., E.H. GIANNINI, F.W. MILLER, et al. 2004. International Myositis Assessment and Clinical Studies Group. International consensus on preliminary definitions of improvement in adult and juvenile myositis. Arthritis Rheum. **50:** 2281–2290.
17. PREVOO, M.L.L., M.A. VAN'T HOF, H.H. KUPER, et al. 1995. Modified disease activity scores that include twenty-eight-joint counts. Arthritis Rheum. **38:** 44–48.
18. OKAMOTO, H., T. NISHIZAWA & M. UKITA. 1999. A novel unenveloped DNA virus (TT virus) associated with acute and chronic non-A to G hepatitis. Intervirology **42:** 196–204.
19. TAN, S.W., A.R. OMAR, I. AINI, et al. 2004. Detection of Newcastle disease virus using a SYBR Green I real time polymerase chain reaction. Acta Virol. **48:** 23–28.
20. RIRIE, K.M., R.P. RASMUSSEN & C.T. WITTWER. 1997. Product differentiation by analysis of DNA melting curves during the polymerase chain reaction. Anal. Biochem. **245:** 154–160.

21. OKAMOTO, H., M. FUKUDA, I. HAYASAKA, *et al.* 2000. Species-specific TT viruses and cross-species infection in nonhuman primates. J. Virol. **74:** 1132–1139.
22. MUSHAHWAR, I.K., J.C. ERKER, S.M. DEXAI, *et al.* 1999. Molecular and biophysical characterization of TT virus: evidence for a new virus family infecting humans. Proc. Natl. Acad. Sci. USA **96:** 3177–3182.
23. OKAMOTO, H., M. TAKAHASHI, T. SAI, *et al.* 2000. Replicative forms of TT virus DNA in bone marrow cells. Biochem. Biophys. Res. Commun. **270:** 657–662.
24. KAKKOLA, L., K. HEDMAN, M. SODERLUND-VENERMO, *et al.* 2003. Cloning and sequencing of TT virus genotype 6 and expression of antigenic open reading frame 2 proteins. J. Gen. Virol. **83:** 979–990.
25. TAKACS, M., K. BALOG, G. BERENCSI, *et al.* 2003. TT virus in Hungary: sequence heterogeneity and mixed infections. FEMS Immunol. Med. Microbiol. **35:** 153–157.
26. HIGUCHI, I. & M. OSAME. 1997. Recent progress of molecular immunology on inflammatory myopathy. Nippon Rinsho **55:** 3331–3335.
27. MCMURRAY, R.W. & K. ELBOURNE. 1997. Hepatitis C virus infection and autoimmunity. Semin. Arthritis Rheum. **26:** 689–701.
28. WALKER, E.J. & P.D. JEFFREY. 1988. Sequence homology between encephalomyocarditis virus protein VPI and histidyl-tRNA synthetase supports a hypothesis of molecular mimicry in polymyositis. Med. Hypotheses **25:** 21–25.
29. GYORKEY, F., G.A. CABRAL, J.L. MELNICK, *et al.* 1978. Coxsackievirus aggregates in muscle cells of a polymyositis patient. Intervirology **10:** 69–77.
30. CHRISTENSEN, M.L., L.M. PACHMAN, J.M. FRIEDMAN, *et al.* 1986. Prevalence of coxsackie B virus antibodies in patients with juvenile dermatomyositis. Arthritis Rheum. **29:** 1365–1370.
31. BOWLES, N.E., T.A. BAYSTON, L.C. ARCHARD, *et al.* 1993. Persistence of enterovirus RNA in muscle biopsy samples suggests that some cases of chronic fatigue syndrome result from a previous, inflammatory viral myopathy. J. Med. **24:** 145–160.
32. CHOU, S.M. 1986. Inclusion body myositis: a chronic persistent mumps myositis? Hum. Pathol. **17:** 765–777.
33. RAY, C.G., L.L. MINNICH & P.C. JOHNSON. 1979. Selective polymyositis inducted by coxsackievirus B1 in mice. J. Infect. Dis. **140:** 239–243.
34. MILLER, F.W., L.A. LOVE, P.H. PLOTZ, *et al.* 1987. Viral and host genetic factors influence encephalomyocarditis virus-induced polymyositis in adult mice. Arthritis Rheum. **30:** 549–556.

Clinical Utility of the Anti-CCP Assay

Experiences with 700 Patients

ULRICH SAUERLAND, HEIDEMARIE BECKER, MATTHIAS SEIDEL,
HEIKO SCHOTTE, PETER WILLEKE, ANNETTE SCHORAT,
BERNHARD SCHLÜTER, WOLFRAM DOMSCHKE, AND MARKUS GAUBITZ

*Medizinische Klinik und Poliklinik B, Universitätsklinikum Münster,
D-48129 Münster, Germany*

ABSTRACT: Our objective was to determine the frequency of antibodies to
cyclic citrullinated peptides (CCPs) in a series of patients with a variety of
rheumatic diseases. Seven hundred consecutive serum samples from patients at
an outpatient clinic were tested for the presence of rheumatoid factor (RF) and
anti-CCP. Clinical diagnosis, radiographic information, and other laboratory
data were taken from patients' charts. The sensitivity and specificity of anti-
CCP reactivity for the diagnosis of rheumatoid arthritis (RA) were 74.0% and
94.5%, respectively; the corresponding results for RF were 69.7% sensitivity
and 81.0% specificity. Highest rates of false-positive RF tests were found in patients with SLE (18.3% vs. 12.7% CCP), Sjögren's syndrome (73.3% vs. 3.3%
CCP), and a control group with chronic hepatitis (24.7% vs. 1.3% CCP). The
detection of anti-CCP is useful for the diagnosis of RA because of its similar
sensitivity but higher specificity compared with RF. Anti-CCP also helps to
diagnose other inflammatory and noninflammatory diseases (especially connective tissue diseases) by reducing the rate of false-positive results in comparison
with RF.

KEYWORDS: cyclic citrullinated peptide (CCP); rheumatoid factor; sensitivity;
specificity; rheumatoid arthritis; rheumatic diseases

Testing for the rheumatoid factor, an immunoglobulin (Ig) that binds to the constant
portion of IgG, is often applied in diagnostic procedures in patients with rheumatic
symptoms. However, approximately 20% of patients with rheumatoid arthritis (RA)
remain RF-negative for the course of their disease. In early RA, the percentage of
rheumatoid factor (RF)–positive patients may be below 50%.[1] In addition, RFs are
not specific for RA. High percentages of RF-positive patients can be found in other
rheumatic diseases, especially connective tissue diseases (in Sjögren's syndrome in
up to 70%), other chronic inflammatory diseases such as hepatitis,[2] and also in elder
people.[3] These shortcomings of the RF assay have provided an impetus for identification of other assays for RA. Recent publications announced antibodies against cyclic
citrullinated peptides (CCPs) to be a promising alternative. Anti-CCP antibodies have

Address for correspondence: Markus Gaubitz, M.D., Department of Medicine B, Münster
University Hospital, Albert-Schweitzer-Strasse 33, D-48129 Münster, Germany. Voice: +49-251-
83-57562; fax: +49-251-83-56429.

gaubitz@uni-muenster.de

Ann. N.Y. Acad. Sci. 1050: 314–318 (2005). © 2005 New York Academy of Sciences.
doi: 10.1196/annals.1313.033

a high specificity, mostly above 95%, for RA combined with a sensitivity comparable to the traditional RF. In addition, anti-CCP antibodies appear early in the disease, often even preceding the symptoms of RA.[4] Finally, anti-CCP is the most reliable predictor of a progressive and erosive course of RA.[5]

With regard to limited experiences with anti-CCP, we examined the ability to distinguish RA from other chronic inflammatory rheumatic and hepatic diseases. In addition, we compared the enzyme-linked immunosorbent assay results with an automated test system.

PATIENTS

We collected blood from 700 consecutive patients from our outpatient department, mostly referred for diagnosis of rheumatic symptoms. Patient data were sampled by reviewing patient charts and medical reports, also taking account of technical tests and laboratory data. Diagnoses were made based on internationally accepted diagnostic criteria—American Rheumatism Association criteria,[6] when possible. In this series, 231 patients had RA; 71 had systemic lupus erythematosus (SLE); 30 had Sjögren's syndrome; 38 had other forms of connective tissue disease such as scleroderma, polymyositis, or overlap syndromes; 50 had different forms of vasculitis such as Wegener's granulomatosis, giant cell arteritis, or polymyalgia rheumatica; 40 had osteoarthritis; 52 had noninflammatory myopathies/myalgias such as local tendomyalgias or fibromyalgia; and the remaining 111 patients suffered from other rheumatic diseases such as infectious arthritis, seronegative spondyloarthropathy, psoriatic arthritis, sarcoidosis, and other rare entities. Seventy-seven patients with chronic hepatitis (C and B) served as controls.

METHODS

Anti-CCP activity was determined by an enzyme-linked immunosorbent assay using a commercial assay (Euroimmun, Lübeck, Germany). The rheumatoid factor was measured by agglutination in the Waaler-Rose test and by Latex-Immuno-nephelometry (BN II, Dade Behring, Marburg, Germany). A positive Waaler-Rose test and/or a concentration of the Latex-RF above 20 IU/mL was considered RF-positive. The first 500 samples were additionally tested in an automated test system (EliA; Pharmacia Diagnostics, Freiburg, Germany).

RESULTS

In this cohort of 700 patients with a variety of rheumatic diseases (herein 231 patients with RA) and hepatitis, 250 samples (35.7%) tested positive for RF, and 197 (28.1%) tested positive for anti-CCP (TABLE 1).

In the subgroup of 231 patients with RA diagnoses according to the American Rheumatism Association criteria, the sensitivity of anti-CCP was 74% compared with 69.7 for RF. From 171 anti-CCP–positive sera, 11 (6.4%) were between 5 and 10 units, 21 (12.3%) were between 10 and 30 units, 56 (32.7%) were between 30 and

TABLE 1. Patients in different diagnosis groups and positive results for RF and anti-CCP, respectively

Diagnosis	n	RF-positive	Anti-CCP–positive
RA	231	161 (69.7%)	171 (74.0%)
SLE	71	13 (18.3%)	9 (12.7%)
Sjögren's syndrome	30	22 (73.3%)	1 (3.3%)
Other connective tissue disease	38	4 (10.5%)	0
Vasculitis	50	7 (14%)	1 (2%)
Osteoarthritis	40	5 (12.5%)	3 (7.5%)
Noninflammatory myalgia	52	10 (19.2%)	4 (7.7%)
Others	111	9 (8.1%)	7 (6.3%)
Hepatitis	77	19 (24.7%)	1 (1.3%)
Total	700	250 (35.7%)	197 (28.1)
Non-RA	469	89 (19.0%)	26 (5.5%)

TABLE 2. Sensitivity and specificity of RF and anti-CCP for presence of rheumatoid arthritis

	Rheumatoid factor	Anti-CCP antibodies
Sensitivity	69.7%	74.0%
Specificity	81.0%	94.5%

100 units, and 83 (48.5%) were above 100 units; the proposed cutoff recommended by the company was 5 units.

Ten sera were found to be RF-positive but anti-CCP–negative; vice versa, 20 sera were anti-CCP–positive but RF-negative.

In the non-RA rheumatic diseases, RF and anti-CCP were rarely found with the expected exception of sera from patients with Sjögren's syndrome, in which the RF could be detected in 73.3%, anti-CCP in 3.3%. In patients with chronic hepatitis, 24.7% were RF-positive, but only 1.3% were anti-CCP–positive.

TABLE 2 summarizes the sensitivity and specificity of RF and anti-CCP.

The first 500 sera were tested in parallel with the EliA CCP (Pharmacia Diagnostics). Controversial results were found in only 8 sera, distributed over several diseases. All controversial results were close to the cutoff of the tests. In 6 of these 8 sera, the EliA-CCP correlated with the diagnosis according to accepted criteria.

DISCUSSION

In our cohort of 700 patients with different rheumatic diseases and a subgroup with chronic hepatitis, testing for anti-CCP was confirmed to be very helpful in diagnosing patients with different rheumatic symptoms. Anti-CCP was moderately more sensitive, but clearly more specific than was testing by traditional RF.

In patients with RA, our results correlate with published data. Lee and Schur[7] found a sensitivity of 66% for anti-CCP and 71.6% for RF, whereas specificity of anti-CCP and RF was 90.4% and 80.3%, respectively. Dubucquoi *et al.*[8] described a sensitivity of 85% for anti-CCP and 94% for RF, whereas specificity was 90.9% for anti-CCP but only 53% for RF. The decision to take either positive Waaler-Rose agglutination test and/or positive testing in Latex-Immunonephelometry as a positive result obviously did not decrease the specificity of RF in our series.

A general problem of testing these diagnostic tools is, of course, the fact that RF is part of the American Rheumatism Association criteria for the classification of RA. It seems not unrealistic that the sensitivity of RF might be slightly overrated when accepting a diagnosis of RA which eventually is made in part by the diagnostic tool we want to evaluate. The presence of RF as a classification criterion will also make it more difficult for anti-CCP testing to substitute for RF testing, although there are some evident advantages that argue for anti-CCP testing.

In our opinion, the high specificity of anti-CCP is especially valuable for the rheumatologist. Patients with arthralgias or arthritis showing a combination of anti-bodies and RF herein are still a frequent diagnostic problem. The differential diag-nosis between early rheumatoid arthritis versus systemic lupus erythematosus versus Sjögren's syndrome versus rheumatoid arthritis with secondary Sjögren's syndrome also has therapeutic impact. In our series, the anti-CCP–positive patients with SLE were less frequent than those with RF; however, especially in patients with Sjögren's syndrome, other connective tissue diseases, and vasculitic disorders, we found posi-tive anti-CCP extremely rare. In a recent article, Gottenberg *et al.*[3] confirmed this observation. Correlating with our results, they found 59% of their patients with Sjögren's syndrome to be RF-positive, but only 7.5% anti-CCP–positive.

In patients with hepatitis who frequently show RF positivity as an immunological epiphenomenon, arthralgias may be explained as an extrahepatic feature of hepatitis; on the other hand, early RA cannot be excluded. Thus, a positive RF is puzzling. In our hepatitis patients, only one was found to be anti-CCP–positive but 24.7% were RF-positive. Werner *et al.*[9] recently described 79 patients with chronic hepatitis C virus infection, of whom 44% were RF-positive, but anti-CCP could not be observed in any patient.

In summary, the detection of anti-CCP is useful for the diagnosis and exclusion of RA. It seems to be advantageous compared with testing for traditional RFs. Automated test systems provide a reliable cost-effective means of testing for anti-CCP antibodies.

REFERENCES

1. STEINER, G. 2003. Autoantibodies in rheumatoid arthritis. *In* Rheumatology, pp. 833–841. Mosby. Edinburgh/London/New York.
2. BOMBARDIERI, M., C. ALESSANDRI, G. LABBADIA, *et al.* 2004. Role of anti-cyclic citrulli-nated peptide antibodies in discriminating patients with rheumatoid arthritis from patients with chronic hepatitis C infection-associated polyarticular involvement. Arthritis Res. Ther. **6:** R137–R141.
3. GOTTENBERG, J-E., S. MIGNOT, P. NICAISE-ROLLAND, *et al.* 2005. Prevalence of anti-cyclic citrullinated peptide and anti-keratin antibodies in patients with primary Sjögren's syndrome. Ann. Rheum. Dis. **64:** 114–117.
4. NIELEN, M.M.J., D. VAN SCHAARDENBURG, H.W. REESINK, *et al.* 2004. Specific autoanti-bodies precede the symptoms of rheumatoid arthritis: a study of serial measurements in blood donors. Arthritis Rheum. **50:** 380–386.

5. KROOT, E-J.J.A., B.A.W. DE JONG, M.A. VAN LEEUWEN, *et al.* 2004. The prognostic value of anti-cyclic citrullinated peptide antibody in patients with recent-onset rheumatoid arthritis. Arthritis Rheum. **43:** 1831–1835.
6. ARNETT, F.C., S.M. EDWORTHY, D.A. BLOCH, *et al.* 1988. The American Rheumatism Association 1987 revised criteria for the classification of rheumatoid arthritis. Arthritis Rheum. **31:** 315–324.
7. LEE, D.M. & P.H. SCHUR. 2003. Clinical utility of the anti-CCP assay in patients with rheumatic diseases. Ann. Rheum. Dis. **62:** 870–874.
8. DUBUCQUOI, S., E. SOLAU-GERVAIS, D. LEFRANC, *et al.* 2004. Evaluation of anti-citrullinated filaggrin antibodies as hallmarks for the diagnosis of rheumatic diseases. Ann. Rheum. Dis. **63:** 415–419.
9. WERNER, M.H., K. HUTCHINSON, C. MORISHIMA, *et al.* 2004. Absence of antibodies to cyclic citrullinated peptide in sera of patients with hepatitis C virus infection and cryoglobulinemia. Arthritis Rheum. **50:** 2305–2308.

Prevalence of Anticentromere F Protein Autoantibodies in 347 Patients with Non-Hodgkin's Lymphoma

CELINE BENCIMON,[a] GILLES SALLES,[b] ANNICK MOREIRA,[a] STEPHANIE GUYOMARD,[a] BERTRAND COIFFIER,[b] JACQUES BIENVENU,[a] AND NICOLE FABIEN[a]

[a]Department of Autoimmunity, [b]Department of Clinical Hematology, Centre Hospitalier Lyon-Sud, HCL, Pierre-Bénite, France

ABSTRACT: An association between autoimmunity and hematological malignancies has been reported including the detection of antinuclear autoantibodies (ANAs) in patients suffering from non-Hodgkin's lymphoma (NHL), with a high prevalence of ANAs directed to components of the mitotic apparatus or the mitosis-associated proteins. Previous studies have demonstrated that one of the targets of such ANAs could be the CENP-F protein, especially in some carcinomas. The prevalence and specificity of anti–CENP-F autoantibodies (aAbs) thus were analyzed in 347 patients with different histological subgroups of NHL before any treatment of NHL, along with 150 controls. The detection of these aAbs was performed using two techniques: a radioimmunological assay (RIA) and an indirect immunofluorescence technique (IIF). Twenty-five (7.2%) NHL patients and 2 (1.3%) control patients displayed anti–CENP-F aAbs using RIA. This difference between the two groups was found to be significant ($P < 0.01$), with a higher prevalence of aAbs in the follicular (13%) and in the marginal zone B and MALT (10.2%) lymphoma subgroups. By IIF, 10 (2.9%) patients with NHL displayed aAbs with a CENP-F or CENP-F–like pattern, whereas none of the control group did. In conclusion, these data demonstrate that a significant incidence of anti–CENP-F aAbs is observed, before any treatment, in some histological subgroups of NHL patients. In addition to the usefulness of anti–CENP-F aAbs as a marker for some NHL subgroups, prospective studies may be important to evaluate the predictive value of anti–CENP-F aAbs for the development of carcinomas.

KEYWORDS: non-Hodgkin's lymphoma; antinuclear autoantibodies; centromeric protein F; radioimmunological technique; indirect immunofluorescence technique

Different clinical and biological autoimmune features have been observed in patients with non-Hodgkin's lymphoma (NHL).[1–5] A significant incidence of antinuclear autoantibodies (ANAs) before any treatment already has been described in NHL. This

Address for correspondence: Nicole Fabien, Laboratoire d'Auto-Immunité, Centre Hospitalier Lyon-Sud (Hospices Civils de Lyon), Chemin du Grand Revoyet, 69495 Pierre-Bénite cedex, France. Voice: +33-4-78-866681; fax: +33-4-78-863344.
nicole.fabien@chu-lyon.fr

Ann. N.Y. Acad. Sci. 1050: 319–326 (2005). © 2005 New York Academy of Sciences.
doi: 10.1196/annals.1313.034

occurrence has been reported to be higher in some histological subgroups with particular ANAs, such as ANAs directed against mitotic proteins or mitosis-associated proteins.[6] One of the targets of such autoantibodies (aAbs) could correspond to centromeric proteins. Indeed, aAbs against the CENP-F have been described previously in breast and lung cancer.[7-9] The CENP-F, also known as p330d and mitosin, is a 367-kDa nuclear protein that depends on both the nuclear matrix and the centromere, and it has already been cloned.[10] Its chromosomal localization is at 1q32–41, and some abnormalities in chromosomes 1q have been reported in several types of carcinomas including head and neck cancer.[7,10,11] CENP-F is expressed in low amounts in GO/G1 cells and accumulates in the nuclear matrix during S-phase, with a maximum expression in G2/M cells. The amount of CENP-F decreases rapidly after the end of mitosis.[10-13]

The aim of our study was to evaluate the prevalence of aAbs directed against this protein in our population of patients with NHL. Indeed, this population has been shown to display a significant incidence of aAbs that could be directed to proteins related to mitosis as the CENP-F protein. Two different techniques were performed to detect the aAbs against CENP-F: a radioimmunological assay (RIA) and an indirect immunofluorescence technique (IIF) on HEp2 cells. For the RIA method, the fragment p-F4 of the CENP-F was selected because it represents the peptide that is the most commonly reactive with human sera from patients with neoplasms.[8]

PATIENTS, MATERIALS, AND METHODS

Patients

Three hundred forty-seven serum samples of patients with NHL were examined for the presence of anti–CENP-F aAbs. These sera were collected from the Department of Clinical Hematology (Centre Hospitalier Lyon-Sud, Hospices Civils de Lyon) in consecutive patients providing informed consent. They were selected at the time of diagnosis before any specific treatment of NHL. The 347 patients consisted in 202 males and 145 females, with a median age of 63 years (range 17–86). All cases were classified according to the criteria of the Revised European-American Classification of Lymphoid Neoplasm,[14,15] and the study population included 43 small lymphocytic, 49 mantle cell, 70 marginal zone, 37 MALT, 54 follicular, 60 diffuse large B cell, and 33 T cell lymphomas. As a control population, 150 serum samples (78 males and 72 females; median age 60 years; range 42–76) were selected from individuals who were undergoing examination in different clinical departments of the same hospital who had no evidence of malignancy or known autoimmune disease. All sera were frozen at −80°C before use. To set up the technique of detection of anti–CENP-F aAbs, we used 100 serum samples from blood donors.

Detection of Anti–CENP-F aAbs

Indirect Immunofluorescence Technique

This detection was performed using HEp2 cells (Biorad, Marnes la Coquette, France) with a technique previously described.[6] The different nuclear immunofluorescence patterns, for example, homogeneous, speckled, nucleolar, and mitotic apparatus, were noted along with the CENP-F pattern previously described.[16,17] A classic titration of each ANA positive at a titer of 1:80 was performed by serial (1 in 2) dilutions. A titer equal to or greater than 1:160 was interpreted as a positive result.

Radioimmunological Technique: In Vitro–*Coupled Transcription/Translation of Human p-F4 Fragment of the CENP-F Protein*

The cDNA of the p-F4 fragment of the CENP-F protein corresponding to nucleotide positions 7538–10,116, inserted in the vector pGex 5X3, was a gift from J. Rattner. According to the manufacturer's instructions, the ^{35}S-labeled p-F4 peptide was obtained by coupled transcription/translation of the cDNA template (Promega, Southampton, U.K.). In brief, 1 µg of circular plasmid DNA was transcribed and translated using T3 RNA polymerase in a 50-µL reaction mix for 30 min at 37°C in presence of 2 µL of ^{35}S-Met (10 mCi/mL; Amersham Pharmacia Biotech, Buckinghamshire, U.K.) and methionine-free rabbit reticulocyte lysate (Promega). The translated products then were purified using NAP5 Sephadex column (Pharmacia Biotech, Uppsala, Sweden).

Immunoprecipitation

The *in vitro*–labeled products (30,000 cpm) were incubated overnight at 4°C with 20 µL of patient sera or 20 µL of diluted (1:500) rabbit polyclonal antibody against the CENP-F (polyclonal 911; gift from J. Rattner) or a goat polyclonal antibody (C19; Santa Cruz Biotechnology, distributed by TEBU, Le Perray en Yvelines, France) in phosphate-buffered saline (PBS; 0.15 M NaCl, 10 mM phosphate, pH 7.4) and Tween 0.1%. Fifty µL of protein A–Sepharose 4 Fast Flow (Pharmacia Biotech) was added and incubated for 1 h at 4°C. The protein A–Sepharose antibody complexes were collected by centrifugation and washed three times with ice-cold PBS. Immunoprecipitated radioactivity was evaluated on a beta-scintillation analyzer in the presence of 2 mL Ultimagold (Tri-Carb, Packard, Rungis, France). The reaction was considered as positive when the result was greater than 1.4 arbitrary units (AU). This cutoff value was determined from the mean value obtained from the control group of blood donors plus 5 standard deviations. The reproducibility of the assay throughout its sensitivity range was determined with the same polyclonal Abs (C19) analyzed five times in a same run and in five separated runs. The intra- and interassay variation coefficients were found to be 3.8% and 7.4%, respectively.

Statistical Analysis

The χ^2 test was used to analyze the statistical significance of the presence of the aAbs in NHL compared with the control group and between the different histological NHL subgroups. A *P* value less than 0.05 was considered statistically significant.

RESULTS

Detection of Anti–CENP-F Autoantibodies by RIA

Twenty-five (17 males and 8 females) of the 347 sera samples from NHL (7.2%) and 2 (2 males) of the 150 control sera (1.3%) displayed anti–CENP-F aAbs (see

TABLE 1. Detection of anti–CENP-F autoantibodies in the NHL population and in the control group using RIA

	Control	NHL	LL	DLCL	MZL + MALT	FL	MCL	TCL
No. of positive sera	2/150	25/347[a]	0/43[b]	3/60[b]	11/108[a]	7/54[c]	2/49[b]	2/33[b]
Percentage	1.33	7.2[a]	0[b]	5[b]	10.2[a]	13[c]	4.1[b]	6.1[b]
Titers (AU)				1.9, 2, 3.5	2, 2.1, 2.3, 2.3, 2.4, 2.4, 2.4, 3.4, 3.8, 4.7, 6.8	1.1, 1.8, 1.8, 2.1, 2.5, 2.8, 2.8	1.9, 1.9	2.2, 2.8
Male	2/78	17/202	0/24	2/32	8/60	4/29	2/36	1/20
Female	0/72	8/145	0/19	1/28	3/48	3/25	0/13	1/12

[a]$P < 0.01$; [b]$P < 0.05$; [c]$P < 0.001$.
ABBREVIATIONS: LL, lymphocytic lymphoma; MCL, mantle cell lymphoma; MZL, marginal zone B lymphoma; FL, follicular lymphoma; TCL, T cell lymphoma; DLCL, diffuse large B cell lymphoma.

TABLE 1). This difference between the two groups was found to be significant ($P < 0.01$). No significant difference is observed between the two sexes in the NHL population. The prevalence of the aAbs was similar for some histological subgroups, for example, 6.1% for T cell lymphomas, 4.1% for mantle cell lymphomas, and 5% for diffuse large B cell lymphomas. The highest prevalence was observed in follicular lymphomas and in marginal zone/MALT lymphomas (13% and 10.2%). Most of the sera with the highest titers belonged to the marginal zone B and MALT lymphoma subgroups (TABLE 1). No positive sera were detected in the small lymphocytic lymphoma subgroup. The polyclonal C19 was positive (titer: 2.89 ± 0.35 AU; $n = 10$), whereas the polyclonal 911 directed to the CENPpF2 fragment gave no reactivity.

Detection of Anti–CENP-F Autoantibodies by IIF

Sixty-six (19%) of the 347 patients had ANAs. Twenty-four of them had aAbs directed against the components of the mitotic apparatus or the mitosis-associated proteins, with 10 (2.8%) giving a CENP-F pattern or a CENP-F–like pattern. The presence of such aAbs can be identified during the progression of the cell cycle into prophase, which is accompanied by the localization of the protein to the entire kinetochore region. At the onset of anaphase, CENP-F is no longer associated with the kinetochore, but is found at the spindle midzone. By telophase, it is concentrated into a narrow band on either side of the midbody.[10,18,19] This pattern has also already been reported as "MSA3" for mitotic spindle apparatus 3.[16] Six of the 10 sera giving a CENP-F pattern or a CENP-F–like pattern were positive by RIA. Twelve of the 42 sera giving a homogeneous, nucleolar, or speckled pattern and 7 of 281 negative sera were also positive by RIA. The sera positive in RIA and IIF with a CENP-F pattern were mostly from patients with marginal zone and follicular lymphoma subgroups. The polyclonal anti–CENP-F antibodies (911 and C19) gave a CENP-F pattern and a CENP-F–like pattern, respectively. (See FIG. 1.)

DISCUSSION

A previous study has reported a high frequency of ANAs directed against mitotic proteins or mitosis-associated proteins in patients with NHL.[6] The antigens recognized by these aAbs could correspond to centromeric proteins as CENP-F, which is one of the targets of aAbs previously described in breast and lung cancer.[7–9] In our study, we found a prevalence of anti–CENP-F aAbs in 7.2% of NHL patients in comparison with 1.3% of the control group using the RIA technique. The difference between the two groups was found to be significantly higher in NHL patients ($P < 0.01$). Using IIF, we found a prevalence of only 2.9% in NHL in comparison with none of the control patients. This result is in accordance with previous data demonstrating that the prevalence of anti–CENP-F aAbs detectable with IIF is very low.[7,9] The difference between the two techniques could be explained by the better sensitivity of the RIA technique. Furthermore, the simultaneous presence of other aAbs can mask the CENP-F pattern of fluorescence; indeed, 29% of the RIA-positive sera gave a homogeneous, speckled, or nucleolar pattern. In contrast, only 60% of the sera positive by RIA showed a CENP-F or CENP-F–like pattern by RIA. The p-F4 fragment was chosen in this study because it represents the peptide the most com-

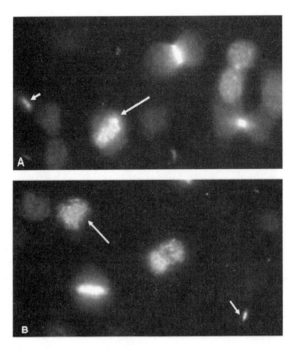

FIGURE 1. Immunofluorescence pattern of antibodies directed to CENP-F protein using HEp2 cells. The fluorescence is observed at the spindle midzone of cells in anaphase (*long arrow*). By telophase, it is concentrated into a narrow band on either side of the midbody (*short arrow*). (**A**) Sera from a patient with NHL; (**B**) polyclonal anti–CENP-F antibody (911).

monly reactive with human sera from patients with neoplasia.[8] Regarding our data, different peptides corresponding to other fragments of the CENP-F protein have to be further tested using the RIA method.

The NHL are categorized in different entities based on histological, immunological, genetic, and major clinical features.[17] The frequency of anti–CENP-F aAbs therefore could depend on the type of the histological subgroup. We found that the frequency of these aAbs was especially high in the follicular (13%) and in the marginal zone B and MALT (10.2%) lymphoma subgroups. Furthermore, titers in aAbs were also different among the histological subgroups, with the highest values in the marginal zone B and MALT subgroups.

The secretion of monoclonal components frequently is observed in follicular lymphoma with an ANA specificity;[20] anti–CENP-F aAbs could be associated with these monoclonal components. Further, the germinal center, from which follicular lymphomas appear to originate, is characterized by a large number of apoptotic cells. Numerous antigens can be modified during the apoptotic process, with these modifications leading to an autoimmune process.[21,22] In parallel, overexpression of CENP-F protein has been described in some neoplasia, especially in head and neck squamous cell carcinomas.[11] Structural alterations in CENP-F associated with its overexpression in tumors might increase the immunogenicity of the protein.

The correlation between the presence of anti–CENP-F aAbs and particular clinical manifestations has to be evaluated along with their prognostic significance; indeed, it was demonstrated that the presence of ANAs in the serum of patients with breast cancer was associated with higher risk of recurrence or metastases in a follow-up of 2 years.[23] Surprisingly, we found that the 2 positive patients in the control group suffered from hepatocarcinoma (1 case) and alcoholic cirrhosis (1 case). Anti–CENP-F aAbs already have been described in patients before the diagnosis of hepatocarcinoma.[24,25] They also have been found in patients with hepatitis B and C, and all these pathologies are characterized by an increased cellular proliferation and by a high risk of developing a cancer.[7]

In conclusion, anti–CENP-F aAbs may be used as markers for some NHL subgroups. In addition, prospective studies may be important to evaluate the predictive value of anti–CENP-F aAbs for carcinomas, especially in hepatic disorders.

ACKNOWLEDGMENTS

We thank Professor J. Rattner (Departments of Anatomy, Medical Biochemistry, and Medicine, University of Calgary, Calgary, Canada) for the gift of the CENP-F4 cDNA and the polyclonal antibody 911; all clinical departments of the Centre Hospitalier Lyon-Sud that contributed to work on the control group population; and Paola Damaso for secretarial help. This work was supported in part by the Hospices Civils de Lyon.

REFERENCES

1. SWISSA, M., Y. COHEN & Y. SCHOENFELD. 1992. Autoantibodies in the sera of patients with lymphoma. Leuk. Lymphoma 7: 117–122.
2. ABU-SHAKRA, M., D. BUSKILA, M. EHRENFELD, *et al.* 2001. Cancer and autoimmunity: autoimmune and rheumatic features in patients with malignancies. Ann. Rheum. Dis. 60: 433–440.
3. EHRENFELD, M., M. ABU-SHAKRA, D. BUSKILA, *et al.* 2001. The dual association between lymphoma and autoimmunity. Blood Cells Mol. Dis. 27: 750–756.
4. TIMURAGAOGLU, A., A. DUMAN, G. ONGUT, *et al.* 2000. The significance of autoantibodies in Non-Hodgkin's lymphoma. Leuk. Lymphoma 40: 119–122.
5. VAROCZY, L., L. GERGELY, M. ZEHER, *et al.* 2002. Malignant lymphoma-associated autoimmune diseases: a descriptive epidemiological study. Rheumatol. Int. 22: 233–237.
6. GUYOMARD, S., G. SALLES, M. COUDURIER, *et al.* 2003. Prevalence and pattern of antinuclear autoantibodies in 347 patients with non-Hodgkin's lymphoma. Br. J. Hematol. 122: 1–10.
7. CASIANO, C.A., R.L. HUMBEL, C. PEEBLES, *et al.* 1995. Autoimmunity to cell-cycle dependent centromere protein p330d/CENP-F in disorders associated with cell proliferation. J. Autoimmun. 8: 575–586.
8. RATTNER, J.B., J. REES, C.M. WHITEHEAD, *et al.* 1997. High frequency of neoplasia in patients with autoantibodies to centromere protein CENP-F. Clin. Invest. Med. 20: 308–319.
9. GOSRAU, G., K. CONRAD & K.H. FRANK. 1998. Non-organ-specific autoantibodies in tumor patients. *In* Pathogenic and Diagnostic Relevance of Autoantibodies, pp. 415–416. Pabst Sci. Pub. Berlin.
10. LIAO, H., R.J. WINKFEIN, G. MACK, *et al.* 1995. CENP-F is a protein of the nuclear matrix that assembles onto kinetochores at late G2 and is rapidly degraded after mitosis. J. Cell Biol. 130: 507–518.

11. DE LA GUARDIA, C., C.A. CASIANO, J. TRINIDAD-PINEDO, *et al.* 2001. CENP F gene amplification and overexpression in head and neck squamous cell carcinomas. Head Neck **23:** 104–112.

12. LANDBERG, G., M. ERLANSON, G. ROOS, *et al.* 1996. Nuclear autoantigen p330d/CENP F: a marker for cell proliferation in human malignancies. Cytometry **25:** 90–98.

13. FLETCHER, L., T.J. YEN & R.J. MUSCHEL. 2003. DNA damage in HeLa cells induced arrest at a discrete point in G2 phase as defined by CENP F localization. Radiat. Res. **159:** 604–611.

14. HARRIS, N.L., E.S. JAFFE, H. STEIN, *et al.* 1994. A revised European-American classification of lymphoid neoplasms: a proposal from the International Lymphoma Study Group. Blood **84:** 1361–1392.

15. CHAN, J.K. 2001. The new world health organization classification of lymphomas: the past, the present and the future. Hematol. Oncol. **19:** 129–150.

16. HUMBEL, R.L. 1986. Autoantibodies to the cellular mitotic apparatus. Immunobiology **173:** 211.

17. RATTNER, J.B., G.J. MACK & M.J. FRITZLER. 1998. Autoantibodies to components of the mitotic apparatus. Mol. Biol. Rep. **25:** 143–155.

18. CASIANO, C.A., G. LANDBERG, R.L. OCHS, *et al.* 1993. Autoantibodies to a novel cell cycle-regulated protein that accumulates in the nuclear matrix during S phase and is localized in the kinetochores and spindle midzone during mitosis. J. Cell. Sci. **106:** 1045–1056.

19. RATTNER, J.B., A. RAO, M.J. FRITZLER, *et al.* 1993. CENP-F is a ca. 400 kDa kinetochore protein that exhibits a cell-cycle dependent localization. Cell Motil. Cytoskeleton **26:** 214–226.

20. DIGHIERO, G., S. HART, A. LIM, *et al.* 1991. Autoantibody activity of immunoglubulins isolated from B cell follicular lymphomas. Blood **78:** 581–585.

21. RODENBURG, R.J.T., J.M.H. RAATS, G.J.M. PRUIJN, *et al.* 2000. Cell death: a trigger of autoimmunity? Bioassays **22:** 627–636.

22. ROVERE, P., M.G. SABBADINI, F. FAZZINI, *et al.* 2000. Remnants of suicidal cells fostering systemic autoaggression. Arthritis Rheum. **43:** 1663–1672.

23. WASSERMAN, J., U. GLAS & H. BLOMGREN. 1975. Autoantibodies in patients with carcinoma of the breast: correlation with prognosis. Clin. Exp. Immunol. **19:** 417–422.

24. REEVES, W.H. 2001. Tumor immunity and autoimmunity: a case of Dr. Jekyll and Mr. Hyde. Clin. Exp. Immunol. **100:** 129–133.

25. ZHANG, J.Y., W. ZHU, H. IMAI, *et al.* 2001. *De-novo* humoral immune responses to cancer-associated autoantigens during transition from chronic liver disease to hepatocellular carcinoma. Clin. Exp. Immunol. **125:** 3–9.

Comparison of Different Test Systems for Simultaneous Autoantibody Detection in Connective Tissue Diseases

PETRA EISSFELLER,[a] MICHAEL STICHERLING,[b] DIETMAR SCHOLZ,[c] KIRSTEN HENNIG,[d] TANJA LÜTTICH,[a] MANFRED MOTZ,[a] AND ARNO KROMMINGA[d]

[a]MIKROGEN GmbH, Martinsried, Germany

[b]Department of Dermatology, University of Leipzig, D-04103 Leipzig, Germany

[c]Dialysis Center Hamburg, D-22391 Hamburg-Poppenbüttel, Germany

[d]Institute for Immunology, Clinical Pathology, and Molecular Medicine (IPM), D-22339 Hamburg, Germany

ABSTRACT: The serological diagnosis of connective tissue diseases (CTDs) is based on the analysis of circulating autoantibodies to cytoplasmic and nuclear proteins (extractable nuclear antigens [ENAs]). The determination of autoantibody specificities supports the clinical diagnosis of the type of CTD and also often the prognosis of the disease. The former indirect immunofluorescence (IIF) technique still provides a useful screening method that currently is supplemented by a range of different techniques allowing the exact determination of single autoantibody specificities. These ENA profiling techniques include ELISA, immunoblotting, line-blot assays, and flow cytometric bead–based multiplex assays. The novel line immunoassay (LIA) from Mikrogen has been introduced in a recent study as a suitable technique for the simultaneous detection of autoantibodies in a routine clinical laboratory, providing comparable results as ELISA and ELiA (both from Pharmacia Diagnostics) (see Damoiseaux et al., this volume). In this study, LIAs from three different manufacturers were performed in 30 serum samples from patients with dermatological manifestations and 27 samples from SLE patients with renal involvement. The line assays from Mikrogen (recomLine ANA/ENA), Innogenetics (Inno-Lia ANA Update), and Imtec (ANA-LIA) were compared for antigen composition, handling, and statistical analysis including sensitivity and concordance. Autoantibody frequencies detected by the Mikrogen, Innogenetics, and Imtec line assays were 14.0%, 19.3%, and 15.8% for RNP; 14.0%, 22.8%, and 14.0% for Sm; 26.3%, 31.6%, and 40.3% for SSA; 3.5%, 12.3%, and 14.0% for SSB; and 3.5%, 14.0%, and 10.5% for histones. Our studies show that the line assay format is an easy-to-use, sensitive, and specific method for ENA antibody detection in human sera.

KEYWORDS: connective tissue diseases; simultaneous autoantibody detection; ENA; recombinant autoantigens; line immunoassay; test comparisons; SLE

Address for correspondence: Petra Eissfeller, Mikrogen GmbH, Fraunhoferstrasse 20, D-82152 Martinsried, Germany. Voice: +49-0-89-8565-2817; fax: +49-0-89-8565-2829. eissfeller@mikrogen.de

Ann. N.Y. Acad. Sci. 1050: 327–339 (2005). © 2005 New York Academy of Sciences.
doi: 10.1196/annals.1313.035

INTRODUCTION

The measurement of autoantibodies against nuclear antigens (ANAs) is commonly used for screening, diagnosis, and monitoring of connective tissue diseases (CTDs) such as systemic lupus erythematosus (SLE), mixed connective tissue disease (MCTD), Sjögren's syndrome (SS), scleroderma, and polymyositis.[1,2] The indirect immunofluorescence (IIF) assay for ANA testing is the standard method used for the initial evaluation of patients with suspected CTD.[3] Although ANA IIF testing on HEp-2 cells is a good screening method for connective tissue diseases,[4] it lacks specificity because of considerable overlap in the clinical features of those diseases, as well as in the presence of the various extractable nuclear antigen (ENA) antibodies.[3–5] Typical immunofluorescence pattern, for example, for proliferating cell nuclear antigen (PCNA), which is specific for SLE, may be overlaid by the homogeneous pattern caused by anti-dsDNA antibodies. Another problem of the IIF may be that certain antigens are not represented in sufficient amount, as known for the SSA.[6] Furthermore, the immunofluorescence is very time-consuming and requires elaborate experience. Follow-up testing of patient sera with ANA IIF-positive results therefore is needed to identify antibodies specific to ENA.

Traditional methods for detecting antibodies to ENA include the Ouchterlony double-diffusion assay,[7] which has now been widely replaced by enzyme-linked immunosorbent assays (ELISAs). ELISAs using purified or recombinant ENA have proved to be highly sensitive and specific while being less subjective and time-consuming than ANA HEp2 IIF.[4,7–9]

More recently, cell-derived or recombinant antigens are also used in line assays. This innovative assay format allows the simultaneous determination of autoantibodies against a broad spectrum of antigens.

In a recent study, the good correlation between the line assay produced by Mikrogen (recomLine ANA/ENA) to ELISA (Pharmacia) and ELiA (Pharmacia) has been proved. RecomLine ANA/ENA contains all antigens important for the diagnosis of SLE, SS, MCTD, myositis, and scleroderma: in detail, the three RNP proteins RNP 68 kDa, RNP A, and RNP C, SmB, SmD, SSA60, SSA52, SSB, ribosomal phosphoprotein P0, PCNA, CENP-B (CENP = centromere-associated protein), DNA topoisomerase I (Scl70), histidyl-tRNA synthetase (Jo-1), and histone (all antigens are recombinant, except for the histone).[10]

Specificities and sensitivities of autoantibodies against those antigens vary, depending on the source of the antigen, assay format, and clinical manifestation of the disease.[4] Antibodies to U1 snRNP typically appear in both SLE and MCTD; however, whereas they are required for the diagnosis of MCTD, they are found in only 30–40% of patients with SLE.[11] The presence of RNP 68 kDa (also described as RNP 70 kDa) alone strongly suggests a diagnosis of MCTD.[12] Antibodies to SSA (Ro) are found in 40–60% of patients with SS[13] and in 25–35% of patients with SLE.[2,14–17] SSB (La) antibodies are found in 50–60% of patients with SS and 5–15% of SLE patients.[16–18] Smith (Sm) antibodies are highly specific for SLE, but show relatively low sensitivity. Because of the high specificity for SLE, their presence constitutes one of the revised American Rheumatism Association criteria.[2] Their overall prevalence ranges from only 10–20% of white SLE patients to 30–40% or more of Asian and black SLE patients.[11,19,20,34] Antibodies against DNA topoisomerase I (Scl-70) are found in 18–30% of patients with systemic sclerosis with high specificity. Anti-CENP-B antibodies are detected in 12–43% of patients with general systemic sclerosis, but in up to 82% in patients with the limited form of the disease (CREST syndrome). In rare cases, anti–CENP-B antibodies are found in SLE and other CTDs and may indicate the potential for the development of scleroderma in these patients.[19]

In this study, we have compared three line assays, produced by Mikrogen (*recom*-Line ANA/ENA), Innogenetics (Inno-Lia ANA Update), and Imtec (ANA-LIA), regarding their performance with clinically defined SLE sera (from 30 with cutaneous manifestations and 27 with renal insufficiencies). The aim of the study was to demonstrate the usefulness of line assays with respect to the detection of ANA and to elucidate possible differences between the line assays produced by different manufacturers.

MATERIALS AND METHODS

Clinical Samples

This study included 57 serum samples from patients with clinically defined SLE. Sera of 30 patients with dermatological manifestations (cutaneous lupus erythematosus [CLE]) were obtained from the Department of Dermatology of the University of Leipzig. The CLE patients presented clinically with characteristic erythematous or erythemato-squamous skin lesions and (partly) UV sensitivity. The clinical diagnosis was supported by histological and immunohistochemical examination of skin biopsies. In addition, internal organ involvement was evaluated by clinical chemistry, serological and hematological testing, and respective imaging techniques. The CLE patients were diagnosed as having either chronic discoid or subacute cutaneous LE. All CLE serum samples were taken at the time of first diagnosis before initiating the relevant therapy.

The remaining 27 sera were provided by the Dialysis Center (Hamburg) and samples from consecutive patients with lupus nephritis were taken.

All samples have undergone IIF testing on ANA HEp2 cells (slides from The Binding Site, U.K.) before the comparative study of the line assays.

Line Assays

Three comparable line assays from different manufacturers were used in this study. The *recom*Line ANA/ENA from Mikrogen, the Inno-Lia ANA Update from Innogenetics, and the ANA-LIA from Imtec. All of the assays are labeled for *in vitro* diagnostic use and are CE-certified.

The line assays from Mikrogen and Innogenetics contain the same antigens, respectively, RNP 68 kDa (70 kDa), RNP A, RNP C, SmB, SmD, SSA60, SSA52, SSB, P0 (Ribosomal P), PCNA, CENPB, DNA-topoisomerase (Scl70), histidyl-tRNA-synthetase (Jo-1), and histones. The Imtec assay presents the complete U1snRNP complex. SmB, PCNA, and P0 are not included in the Imtec assay, but nucleosomes are offered in addition.

Mostly recombinant human antigens are used, except for the native bovine histone used by Mikrogen and the native SSA60 and histone used by Innogenetics. No

TABLE 1. Comparison of the frequencies of antibodies to the ENA in the literature and the three line assays included in the study

	Frequencies (%), $n = 57$ lupus patients			
	Literature	recomLine Mikrogen	INNO-LIA Innogenetics	ANA-LIA Imtec
RNP 68/70 kDa		5.3	8.8	—
RNP A		5.3	10.5	—
RNP C		14.0	17.5	—
RNP[a]	10–30	14.0	19.3	15.8
SmB		14.0	22.8	—
SmD		0	5.3	14.0
Sm	10–30	14.0	22.8	14.0
Sm/RNP[a]	30–45	24.6	26.3	22.8
SSA60		10.5	28.1	38.6
SSA52		26.3	26.3	26.3
SSA[a]	25–35	26.3	31.6	40.3
SSB	5–15[b]	3.5	12.3	14.0
PO/RPP	10–20	7.0	1.8	—
PCNA	0.3–2	0	—	—
CENP-B[c]	—	1.8	3.5	3.5
Scl70[c]	—	0	1.8	1.8
Jo-1[c]	—	0	0	0
Histone		3.5	14.0	10.5
dsDNA	60–90	—	—	—
Nucleosomes		—	—	24.6

[a]Because the subspecification of certain antigens (RNP, Sm, and SSA) is possible only recently by the use of recombinant technique, corresponding numbers in literature are rare and not sufficiently confirmed yet. Therefore, data comparisons have been mainly performed on the level of the better described complexes.

[b]According to a study by Sontheimer and McCauliffe, the prevalence of SSB achieves 25–35% in subacute cutaneous lupus erythematosus.[21]

[c]Antibodies to CENP-B, Scl 70, and Jo-1 are specific for scleroderma, respectively, polymyositis. As they occur in SLE only exceptionally, there are no numbers from the literature available.

information about the antigen source is given in the instruction manual of the Imtec assay.

The test procedure is common to all three line assays with more or less the same duration (Mikrogen: 2 h 25 min; Innogenetics: 2 h 30 min – 2 h 50 min; Imtec: 2 h 50 min). The samples are diluted 1:100 in the Mikrogen assay, 1:200 in the Innogenetics assay, and 1:50 in the Imtec assay. The test procedure includes serum incubation, washing steps, and incubation with an antihuman IgG conjugate coupled with an enzyme, for example, peroxidase. The specifically bound patient IgG is recognized by the antihuman conjugate. The positive bands become visible by the following enzyme-substrate reaction, which must be stopped in time.

The solutions used in the assays from Mikrogen and Imtec are supplied as only three different bottles, that is, washing/diluting buffer, conjugate, and substrate. The line test kit of Innogenetics is more complex, because it comprises eight different bottles (diluent, cutoff control, conjugate buffer, conjugate, substrate buffer, substrate, wash buffer, and stop solution) and therefore increases the risk of error-prone handling.

Each strip of the Mikrogen and Imtec assay possesses a separate cutoff band, which allows an easy comparison of the intensities of the different antigen bands with the cutoff. Innogenetics offers a separate cutoff serum. An additional strip has to be incubated with this serum in each run, which means a higher consumption of strips.

Data Analysis

The visible bands on the strips of the different assays have been assessed in comparison with the strip internal cutoff (Imtec, Mikrogen), respectively, to the cutoff on the extra strip (Innogenetics).

The data have been summarized as frequencies of specificities in each assay, expressed in percentage in relation to the total number of samples ($n = 57$) and compared with numbers from the literature (TABLE 1).

Correspondences between each two of the assays, respectively, have been calculated as the ratio of concordant results to the total of samples ($n = 57$; TABLE 2).

Finally, the method of consensus calculation has been applied: for each autoantibody specificity of each specimen a consensus was established from the three test results as agreement of at least two of three results. The percentage of agreement with the consensus was determined for each assay with regard to each antigen.

RESULTS

The panel of 57 defined SLE sera has been tested by the three line assays, and frequencies of the antibody specificities for each assay, correspondences between each of the assays, and the percentage of agreement with the consensus result have been determined.

Because the autoantibody frequencies between the groups of cutaneous and nephrological lupus did not differ significantly, these sera are considered as one group unless otherwise mentioned.

The differences in antigen grouping between these assays have to be taken into consideration to compare the frequencies of antibodies detected by the three line assays.

Although in the Imtec line assay the whole U1snRNP complex is presented in native form, Innogenetics and Mikrogen line assays present the three major proteins of the U1snRNP complex separately. As shown in this study, the selection of the three proteins RNP 70 kDa (Innogenetics), respectively, RNP 68 kDa (Mikrogen), RNP A, and RNP C does not impair the overall sensitivity, because the addition of antibody frequencies of the separate proteins yields numbers at least as high as in the Imtec assay, with Mikrogen 14%, Innogenetics 19.3%, and Imtec 15.8% (TABLE 1). The correspondences with respect to the RNP reactivities between the Innogenetics and Mikrogen assay, between Imtec and Mikrogen, and between Imtec and Innogenetics were 87.7%, 94.7%, and 86% respectively (TABLE 2).

The best concordance within the RNP comparison appears between Imtec and Mikrogen assay with two discrepant positives in Imtec versus Mikrogen and one discrepant positive in Mikrogen versus Imtec.

Considering the a-RNP reactivities on the level of the proteins RNP 68/70 kDa, RNP A, and RNP C, the highest frequencies are achieved against the RNP C in the Mikrogen assay as well as in Innogenetics assay with 14% and 17.5%, whereas the frequencies are lowest against the RNP 68/70 kDa. In fact, almost the full anti-RNP prevalence is already achieved by the frequency of the anti-RNP C within this panel of SLE patients.

TABLE 2. Correspondence between two line assays

RNP

Mikrogen	Innogenetics −	Innogenetics +	Mikrogen	Imtec −	Imtec +	Innogenetics	Imtec −	Imtec +
−	44	5	−	47	2	−	43	3
+	2	6	+	1	7	+	5	6
correspondence:	87.7%			94.7%			86.00%	

Sm

Mikrogen	Innogenetics −	Innogenetics +	Mikrogen	Imtec −	Imtec +	Innogenetics	Imtec −	Imtec +
−	43	6	−	45	4	−	41	3
+	1	7	+	4	4	+	8	5
correspondence:	87.7%			86.00%			80.7%	

SSA60

Mikrogen	Innogenetics −	Innogenetics +	Mikrogen	Imtec −	Imtec +	Innogenetics	Imtec −	Imtec +
−	41	10	−	35	16	−	35	6
+	0	6	+	0	6	+	0	16
correspondence:	82.5%			71.9%			89.5%	

SSA52

Mikrogen	Innogenetics −	Innogenetics +	Mikrogen	Imtec −	Imtec +	Innogenetics	Imtec −	Imtec +
−	42	0	−	42	0	−	42	0
+	0	15	+	0	15	+	0	5
correspondence:	100%			100%			100%	

SSA

Mikrogen	Innogenetics −	Innogenetics +	Mikrogen	Imtec −	Imtec +	Innogenetics	Imtec −	Imtec +
−	39	3	−	34	8	−	34	5
+	0	15	+	0	15	+	0	18
correspondence:	94.7%			86.00%			91.2%	

SSB

Mikrogen	Innogenetics −	Innogenetics +	Mikrogen	Imtec −	Imtec +	Innogenetics	Imtec −	Imtec +
−	50	5	−	49	6	−	48	2
+	0	2	+	0	2	+	1	6
correspondence:	91.2%			89.5%			94.7%	

Histone

Mikrogen	Innogenetics −	Innogenetics +	Mikrogen	Imtec −	Imtec +	Innogenetics	Imtec −	Imtec +
−	49	6	−	51	4	−	46	3
+	0	2	+	0	2	+	5	3
correspondence:	89.5%			93.00%			86.00%	

The Sm proteins, the core proteins of the snRNP complexes, are represented by the immunodominant components SmB and SmD in the Mikrogen and in the Inno-genetics assay, whereas the SmD1 protein is included in the Imtec assay exclusively. Comparison of frequencies therefore has taken place on the level of all Sm frequencies together determined by one assay, respectively. The resulting frequencies are 14% each for the Imtec and the Mikrogen, but 22.8% for Innogenetics. The correspondences between two of the assays each lay between 80% and 87.7%, with the numbers of discrepants at least as high as the number of positive results. (In detail, the comparison between Innogenetics and Mikrogen shows 87.7% correspondence, with six discrepant positives for Innogenetics and one discrepant positive in Mikrogen, 86% correspondence between Imtec and Mikrogen with four discrepant positives in Mikrogen and four discrepant positives in Imtec, 80.7% correspondence between Imtec and Innogenetics with three more positives in Imtec and eight positives in Innogenetics.)

Antibodies to SSA60 were detected in only 10.5% of cases by the Mikrogen assay, but in 28.1% and 38.6% of cases by the Innogenetics and Imtec LIA. The Innogenetics assay showed 10 more cases positive than the Mikrogen assay, and the Imtec assay showed six more positives compared with the Innogenetics.

In contrast with great differences in detection mode regarding the SSA60, the detection of the a-SSA52 antibodies corresponded overwhelmingly well, with 26.3% in total agreement between all three line assays.

The a-SSB antibodies, which are considered as the serological hallmark for SS, are described to occur also in 5–15% of cases of SLE.[21,22] The frequencies of a-SSB antibodies within the SLE sera tested in this study varied from 3.5% in Mikrogen assay, to 12.3% in Innogenetics, and up to 14% in Imtec. According to the studies by Reichlin[22] and Venables,[23] the occurrence of anti-SSB precipitins are associated with a lower prevalence of renal disease. Although better known for their association with anti-SSA, 25–35% of subacute cutaneous lupus erythematosus (SCLE) patients also have anti-SSB.[21,34] To verify these findings from the literature, we considered the a-SSA/a-SSB positives of our study separately as one group of 30 subacute cutaneous LE and as another group of 27 patients with nephrological SLE. The a-SSA/a-SSB frequencies in the SCLE sera were detected by Mikrogen as 15.8%/3.5%, by Inno-genetics as 19.3%/8.8%, and by Imtec as 26.3%/10.5%; in the nephrological SLE sera, however, the frequencies were detected as 10.5%/0%, 12.3%/3.5%, and 14.0%/3.5% in each of the assays. The tendency described in the literature is confirmed by higher SSA and SSB frequencies in the dermatological versus the nephrological SLE samples for each of the assays included.

The ribosomal phosphoproteins (RPP), which are represented by the phospho-protein 0 (PO) in Mikrogen assay, show lower frequency in Inno-Lia ANA Update than in *recom*Line ANA/ENA with one versus four positive reactions and are not presented on the ANA-LIA (Imtec) at all. PCNA is highly specific, but very rare, with occurrences as few as 2% in SLE. By chance, in this selection of 57 samples tested, none of the SLE sera showed a-PCNA reactivity in either the Mikrogen or the Innogenetics assay. PCNA is not included in the Imtec ANA-LIA.

The scleroderma markers CENP-B and Scl70 are not typical in SLE, but may occur and might be a hint for possible development of scleroderma. Anti–CENP-B antibodies were observed overlapping in two sera of dermatological SLE by the Imtec and Innogenetics assay and in one of these sera by the Mikrogen assay; in the other serum,

TABLE 3. Percentages of agreement with the consensus result

	Mikrogen	Innogenetics	Imtec
RNP	98.2	93	96.5
Sm	96.5	94.7	89.5
SSA60	82.5	100	89.5
SSA52	100	100	100
SSA (60 + 52)	94.7	100	91.2
SSB	93	98.2	96.5
Histone	98.2	91.2	96.5
CENP-B	98.2	100	100
Scl70	100	98.2	98.2
Jo1	100	100	100

CENP-B was borderline, which means below the cutoff intensity, in the Mikrogen assay. Antibodies against Scl70 were detected in one dermatological sample by Imtec and in another dermatological sample by Innogenetics, but none in Mikrogen.

Antibodies to histidyl-tRNA synthetase (Jo-1), which are indicative of myositis, were not detected in this study of SLE sera by any of the assays.

The frequencies of a-histone strongly varied depending on the assay used: from 3.5% in Mikrogen, to 10.5% in Imtec, and 14.0% in the Innogenetics assay. Nucleosomes are detected by Imtec only, in 24.6% of the SLE samples within this study.

According to the method of consensus calculation, for each autoantibody specificity of each specimen a consensus was established from the three test results according to the agreement of at least two of three results. The percentage of agreement with the consensus was determined for each assay with regard to each antigen.

The Mikrogen, Innogenetics, and Imtec LIA provided percentages of agreement with the consensus as follows: RNP 98.2%, 93%, and 96.5%; Sm 96.5%, 94.7%, and 89.5%; SSA60 82.5%, 100%, and 89.5%; SSA52 100% for each assay; SSB 93%, 98.2%, and 96.5%; and histone 98.2%, 91.2%, and 96.5% (TABLE 3).

In summary, the Mikrogen assay shows highest percentages of agreement with the consensus with respect to the RNP, Sm, and histones, whereas Innogenetics displayed the best agreement with the consensus for SSA60 and SSB.

DISCUSSION

ANA specificities in the literature comprise wide-spread ranges of frequencies, depending on factors such as the assay format, source of antigens used, conditions of protein extraction and denaturation, and depending on the type, stage, or organ manifestation of the disease. Accordingly, differences in separate results became obvious by the use of three different line assays. Antigen amounts, antigen sources, especially whether native or recombinant, and the test conditions, including ionic strengths and cutoff determination, are some of the most important features that may account for differences in test results between the three assays.

The overall expected frequencies of ENA antibody specificities have been more or less achieved by all line assays included.

An interesting finding from this study was the good correlation between the reactivities to the U1snRNP on the Imtec strip to the combined reactivities to the three RNP proteins (RNP 68 kDa, RNP A, RNP C) on the Mikrogen strip. This confirms that these proteins are the major targets of the autoantibodies directed to the U1snRNP complexes, and that the antigenic reactivity of the U1snRNP complex is apparently independent of the RNA components. Until recently, the detection of RNP antibodies had to be performed as exclusion diagnosis, as by the hitherto known methods the RNPs could be isolated only in conjunction with the Sm. By the recombinant RNP proteins on the Innogenetics and Mikrogen strip, direct and save identification of the RNP proteins became possible, and, moreover, the frequencies of subspecificities to RNP 68 kDa on the one hand and to RNP A and RNP C on the other may provide additional information for better classifying a patient between MCTD and SLE. High titers of RNP, especially in the absence of Sm or dsDNA antibodies are very specific for MCTD. Nearly all MCTD patients demonstrate anti-RNP 68-kDa activity, whereas in SLE patients the RNP appears isolated only in rare cases and the anti–protein A and anti–protein C antibodies appear to be twice as common as the anti-RNP 68-kDa antibodies.[34]

According to the literature, anti-Sm reactivity ranges from 10% to 30% depending on the autoantibody detection system and the racial background of the SLE population.[11,19,20] The most frequently targeted polypeptides of the Sm autoantigen complex are the B and D polypeptides.[24] Because the SmBB' shares cross-reactive epitopes with U1snRNPs, respective sera that are reacting with U1snRNP and SmB at the same time should not be considered as Sm-positive specific for SLE.[19] SmD, in contrast, is regarded as the more specific autoantigen for SLE because of an auto-epitope within the carboxyl-terminus of the D1 and D3 and also of the BB' poly-peptides containing symmetrically dimethylated arginines by posttranslational modification. In our study, only two of eight SmB-positive sera in the Mikrogen line assay reacted with RNP proteins at the same time, whereas 5 of 13 SmB positives in the Innogenetics line assay reacted with at least one of the three RNP proteins. These overlapping reactivities in the Innogenetics and in the Mikrogen assay could be caused by shared motifs between the SmBB' and the RNPs, whereas the four sera that are positive in the Imtec SmD1 and the Imtec U1snRNP complex might pick up the SmD reactivity within the U1snRNP complex because the RNP proteins are not offered separately. Interestingly, the three sera which were positive in SmD in Innogenetics were also positive in the SmB (and to the RNP proteins) and therefore did not contribute to higher sensitivity. A striking fact is also the nonreactivity of the SmD in the Mikrogen assay within this study. At the time of the study, recombinant SmD expressed in insect cells Sf21 has been used without further modification. As a result of this study, Mikrogen is under way to improve its SmD according to the described necessity of symmetrical dimethylation. Considering the different results with respect to SmB and SmD reactivity obtained from different tests, it is not definitely clear which results are the correct SLE-specific ones. Further studies are necessary for further elucidation.

The reactivities to the SSA52 within this study were identical in all three line assays applied, occurring in 26.3% of the SLE samples tested. This 52-kDa protein was first described by Ben-Chetrit *et al.* in 1988 as an important component of the

SSA particle for the serological confirmation of SS and SLE.[25] The importance of the diagnostic completion of the formerly known SSA complex by the recombinant 52-kDa SSA has been proved in further studies.[26] The strong association of SSA52 in mothers to risk of congenital heart block (CHB) in their children, however, has been disproved in a very recent study from December 2004.[27] According to this study and contrary to previous reports, 52-kDa SSA as detected by Inno-Lia ANA Update is not more specific for or frequent in CHB than 60-kDa SSA. However, the presence of anti-SSB antibodies significantly increases the risk for CHB.

With respect to a-SSA60, the prevalences in this study ranged from 10.5% in Mikrogen, to 28.1% in Innogenetics, and up to 38.6% in Imtec line assay. Because the SSA60 almost always co-occur with SSA52 in the samples tested, the numbers of the reactivity to total SSA (60 + 52) finally does not differ to the same extent between the assays. However, the high detection of anti-SSA60 in Imtec assay is ostentatious, especially because four samples are exclusively positive in SSA60 in Imtec, whereas no other assay confirmed any ANA reactivity, not even the initial IIF. Whether these elevated a-SSB reactivities in the Imtec assay are true-positives or whether they are rather an indication of a lack in specificity remains to be evaluated at assessed negative control sera.

The frequency of SSB with 3.5% in the *recom*Line ANA/ENA (Mikrogen) in this panel of SLE-defined sera was lower than numbers in the competitive assays, respectively, from the literature. The frequencies achieved by *recom*Line ANA/ENA in SLE patients was considerably higher in the company's internal evaluations, with 9% a-SSB reactivity. Also in the comparison with ELISA and ELiA, both Pharmacia, within the Dutch study,[10] the frequency of a-SSB also corresponded very well between the Mikrogen line assay with 13.8% and the ELISA from Pharmacia with 15.5% in 123 SLE sera tested. This shows that frequencies are varying in different studies according to the random selection of SLE patients in diverse activity stages of the disease.

Antibodies to ribosomal phosphoproteins (RPPs) are very specific markers for SLE and comprise the phosphoproteins P0, P1, and P2. In the Mikrogen assay, the RPPs are represented by the recombinant produced P0, which covers the necessary sensitivity because the reactivity of RPP antibodies is mainly directed against the well-preserved C-terminal region of the phosphoproteins which is common to all three of the ribosomal P proteins. According to the insert of the Inno-Lia ANA Update (Innogenetics), synthetic ribosomal P is indicated. In this study, the Mikrogen assay was even more sensitive with four positive results (7%) than the Innogenetics, with only one positive result (1.8%) from the 57 SLE samples tested. The Imtec assay does not contain the RPP at all. According to the literature, the frequency of anti-P antibodies in randomly selected SLE populations is 10–20%.[28] A strong association of anti-P antibodies with neuropsychiatric manifestations of SLE, particularly psychosis and severe depression, were found in several studies[29–31] and have also been recently confirmed in a mouse model by the induction of depression by intrathecal instillation of a-RPP.[20] It should be emphasized that this antibody may be present in lupus sera even when other "ANA-positive" antibodies are not detected; therefore, in these circumstances they are a valuable means of confirming the diagnosis of SLE.[32]

The PCNA is also very specific for SLE but rare, with a described frequency of approximately 2%.[33] Anti-PCNA reactivity is visible as a typical pleomorphic nuclear staining in IIF, because of its cell cycle–dependent expression, but can be detected only by immunofluorescence when no other antinuclear antibodies are present in the serum or when the PCNA antibodies are present in much higher titers than the coexisting antibodies. Because other uncharacterized autoantibodies also produce a cell cycle–related staining pattern, the line assay provides a useful tool for the clear identification of the PCNA. The PCNA is included in the Mikrogen and the Innogenetics line assays.

Reactivity to the scleroderma markers, CENP-B and Scl70, was low, as expected, because they occur only exceptionally in SLE patients. Anti-Scl70 antibodies are known as a highly specific marker for scleroderma with a specificity greater than 99%.[19] Accordingly, it has not been detected in the serum panel of diagnosed SLE patients by the Mikrogen line assay. However, there was one a-Scl70 reactivity detected in the Innogenetics and another in the Imtec line assay, which are most likely false-positive test results.

On the other hand, the excellent sensitivity of the Scl70 and CENP-B on the Mikrogen strip has been demonstrated in the comparative study to Pharmacia ELISA and ELiA by Damoiseaux in scleroderma patients.[10] In this study, including 123 diagnosed SLE and 25 scleroderma patients, the Mikrogen *recom*LineANA/ENA showed excellent agreement for CENP-B with 99.5% toward the ELISA and with 98.9% toward the ELiA and for Scl70 98.4% versus ELISA and ELiA. In contrast, the parallel tested in-house counter-immunoelectrophoresis exhibited a great lack of sensitivity, detecting none of the 20 a-CENP-B positives and none of the 4 a-Scl-70–positive sera, which were consistently positive by the *recom*Line ANA/ENA, ELISA, and ELiA.

Considering the correlation between the initial routinely performed IIF and the three line assays included in our study, interestingly, the deficiency in detection of SSA by IIF is confirmed by two negative IIF screening results, which turn out to be positive by a-SSA in the line assays.

In conclusion, the line assay format provides a useful means for the confirmation and discrimination of ENA markers, either as confirmation of ANA-positive IIF results or as confirmation of urgent clinical suspicion of SLE, even without a positive ANA-IIF screening result.

The line assays have the advantage of reporting results for all important ENAs from a single run, resulting in saving of reagents, labor, sample volume, and storage space.

When the *recom*Line ANA/ENA is used in conjunction with an automated system (e.g., Profiblot by Tecan) and an automated scanning software (*recom*Scan by Mikrogen), a highly automated, cost-effective system for the detection of autoantibodies to the most important ENAs was achieved.

REFERENCES

1. OSTERLAND, C.K. 1994. Laboratory diagnosis and monitoring in chronic systemic autoimmune diseases. Clin. Chem. **40:** 2146–2153.
2. TAN, E.M. *et al.* 1982. The 1982 revised criteria for the classification of systemic lupus erythematosus. Arthritis Rheum. **25:** 1271–1277.
3. TAN, E.M. 1982. Autoantibodies to nuclear antigens (ANA): their immunobiology and medicine. Adv. Immunol. **33:** 167–240.

4. PHAN, T.G., R.C. WONG & S. ADELSTEIN. 2002. Autoantibodies to extractable nuclear antigens: making detection and interpretation more meaningful. Clin. Diagn. Lab. Immunol. **9:** 1–7.
5. TAN, E.M. 1989. Antinuclear antibodies: diagnostic markers for autoimmune diseases and probes for cell biology. Adv. Immunol. **44:** 93–151.
6. POLLOCK, W. & B.-H. TOH. 1999. Routine Immunofluorescence detection of Ro/SS-A autoantibody using Hep-2 cells transfected with human 60 kDa Ro/SS-A. J. Clin. Pathol. **52:** 684–687.
7. ORTON, S.M. et al. 2004. Practical evaluation of methods for detection and specificity of autoantibodies to extractable nuclear antigens. Clin. Diagn. Lab. Immunol. **11:** 297–301.
8. JAKOWSKI, T.D. et al. 1996. Screening for antinuclear antibodies by enzyme immunoassay. Am. J. Clin. Pathol. **105:** 468–473.
9. SANCHEZ-GUERRERO, J. et al. 1996. Utility of anti-Sm, anti-RNP, anti-Ro/SS-A, and anti-La/SSB (extractable nuclear antigens) detected by enzyme-linked immunosorbent assay for the diagnosis of systemic lupus erythematosus. Arthritis Rheum. **39:** 1055–1061.
10. DAMOISEAUX, J. et al. 2004. Evaluation of a novel line-blot immunoassay for the detection of antibodies to extractable nuclear antigens. This volume.
11. CRAFT, J. 1992. Antibodies to snRNPs in systemic lupus erythematosus. Rheum. Dis. Clin. N. Am. **18:** 311–335.
12. MARTINS, T.B. et al. 2004. Evaluation of multiplexed fluorescent microsphere immunoassay for detection of autoantibodies to nuclear antigens. Clin. Diagn. Lab. Immunol. **11:** 1054–1059.
13. JONSSON, R., H.J. HAGE & T.P. GORDON. 2000. Current concepts on diagnosis, autoantibodies and therapy in Sjögren's syndrome. Scand. J. Rheumatol. **29:** 341–348.
14. ALEXANDER, E.L. et al. 1982. Ro(SSA) and La(SSB) antibodies in the clinical spectrum of Sjögren's syndrome. J. Rheumatol. **9:** 239–246.
15. KEPHART, D.C., A.F. HOOD & T.T. PROVOST. 1981. Neonatal lupus erythematosus: new serological findings. J. Invest. Dermatol. **77:** 331–333.
16. MADDISON, P.J., T.T. PROVOST & M. REICHLIN. 1981. Serological findings in patients with "ANA-negative" systemic lupus erythematosus. Medicine **60:** 87–94.
17. PROVOST, T.T. et al. 1977. Antibodies to cytoplasmic antigens in lupus erythematosus. Serological marker for systemic disease. Arthritis Rheum. **20:** 1457–1463.
18. SCOPELITIS, E., J.J. BIUNDU & M.A. ALSPAUGH. 1980. Anti-SSA antibody and other antinuclear antibodies in systemic lupus erythematosus. Arthritis Rheum. **23:** 287–293.
19. CONRAD, K., W. SCHÖßLER & F. HIEPE. 2002. Autoantibodies in systemic autoimmune disease. Pabst Science Publishers. Lengerich, Germany.
20. SHOENFELD, Y. 2004 (Nov.). Autoantibodies: predictive, pathogenic and protective. Presented at the 4th International Congress on Autoimmunity. Budapest, Hungary.
21. SONTHEIMER, R.D. & D.P. MCCAULIFFE. 1990. Pathogenesis of anti-Ro/SS-A autoantibody-associated cutaneous lupus erythematosus. Dermatol. Clin. **8:** 751–758.
22. REICHLIN, M. 1986. Significance of the Ro antigen system. J. Clin. Immunol. **6:** 339–348.
23. VENABLES, P.J. et al. 1989. Anti-La (SS-B): a diagnostic criterion for Sjögren's syndrome? Clin. Exp. Rheumatol. **7:** 181–184.
24. MAHLER, M., M.J. FRITZLER & M. BLÜTHNER. 2004. Identification of a SmD3 epitope with a single symmetrical dimethylation of an arginine residue as a specific target of a subpopulation of anti-Sm antibodies. Arthritis Res. Ther. **7:** R19–R29.
25. BEN-CHETRIT, E., E.K. CHAN, K.F. SULLIVAN & E.M. TAN. 1988. A 52-kD protein is a novel component of the SS-A/Ro antigenic particle. J. Exp. Med. **167:** 1560–1571.
26. MCCAULIFFE, D.P. et al. 1997. Recombinant 52 kDa Ro(SSA) ELISA detects autoantibodies in Sjögren's syndrome sera that go undetected by conventional serological assays. J. Rheumatol. **5:** 860–866.
27. GORDON, P. et al. 2004. Anti-52 kDa Ro, anti-60 kDa Ro, and anti-La antibody profiles in neonatal lupus. J. Rheumatol. **12:** 2480–2487.
28. FRANCOUER, A.M. et al. 1985. Identification of ribosomal protein autoantigens. J. Immunol. **135:** 2378–2384.
29. BONFA, E. et al. 1987. Association between lupus psychosis and antiribosomal P protein antibodies. N. Engl. J. Med. **30:** 265–271.

30. SCHNEEBAUM, A.B. *et al.* 1991. Association of psychiatric manifestations with antibodies to ribosomal P proteins in systemic lupus erythematosus. Am. J. Med. **90:** 54–62.
31. NOJIMA, Y. *et al.* 1992. Correlation of antibodies to ribosomal P protein with psychosis in patients with systemic lupus erythematosus. Ann. Rheum. Dis. **51:** 1053–1055.
32. BONFA, E. & K.B. ELKON. 1986. Clinical and serological associations of the antiribosomal P protein antibody. Arthritis Rheum. **29:** 981–985.
33. FRITZLER, M.J. *et al.* 1983. Clinical features of patients with antibodies directed against PCNA. Arthritis Rheum. **26:** 140–145.
34. PETER, J.B. & Y. SHOENFELD. 1996. Autoantibodies. Elsevier. Amsterdam/New York.

Evaluation of a Novel Line-Blot Immunoassay for the Detection of Antibodies to Extractable Nuclear Antigens

J. DAMOISEAUX, K. BOESTEN, J. GIESEN, J. AUSTEN, AND J. W. COHEN TERVAERT

Department of Clinical and Experimental Immunology, University Hospital Maastricht, Maastricht, the Netherlands

ABSTRACT: We have evaluated the performance of a novel line-blot immunoassay (LIA; Mikrogen) and compared results with those obtained by CIE (in-house), ELISA (Pharmacia Diagnostics), and FEIA (Pharmacia Diagnostics). Sera from systemic lupus erythematosus (SLE) patients ($n = 123$), systemic sclerosis patients ($n = 25$), and healthy controls ($n = 40$) were analyzed for the presence of antibodies to RNP, Sm, SSA, SSB, CENP-B, Scl-70, and Jo-1. Reading of LIA results, as compared with a cutoff control, was performed by automatic analysis of the test strips. Because LIA enables recognition of separate subunits of RNP (68, A, and C), Sm (B and D), and SSA (52 and 60), at least two of the RNP antigens and either one of the Sm or SSA antigens should be detected for considering the test RNP, Sm, or SSA-positive, respectively. LIA had the highest sensitivity in patients with autoimmune connective tissue diseases: 131 specificities (not PO, PCNA, or histones), as compared with ELISA (121), FEIA (119), and CIE (80). However, LIA revealed three positive reactions in healthy controls; other assays were completely negative. LIA is better than CIE, but similar to ELISA and FEIA, in terms of detecting systemic sclerosis–associated antibodies (CENP-B and Scl-70). Furthermore, LIA had the highest sensitivity (17.9%) for the SLE-specific anti-Sm antibodies, as compared with ELISA (11.4%), CIE (8.1%), and FEIA (5.7%). Finally, anti-SSA antibodies were far more prevalent by LIA in the systemic sclerosis samples because of anti-SSA52 reactivity. The clinical relevance of the latter finding remains to be determined. In conclusion, LIA is suitable for routine evaluation of autoantibodies to extractable nuclear antigens.

KEYWORDS: connective tissue disease; autoantibodies; extractable nuclear antigens; systemic lupus erythematosus; systemic sclerosis

INTRODUCTION

Antibodies to extractable nuclear antigens (ENAs) are prevalent in patients with autoimmune connective tissue diseases, such as systemic lupus erythematosus

Address for correspondence: Jan Damoiseaux, Ph.D., Department of Clinical and Experimental Immunology, University Hospital Maastricht, P. O. Box 5800, 6202 AZ Maastricht, the Netherlands. Voice: +31-43-3881433; fax: +31-43-3884164.

  jdam@limm.azm.nl

Ann. N.Y. Acad. Sci. 1050: 340–347 (2005). © 2005 New York Academy of Sciences.
doi: 10.1196/annals.1313.036

(SLE), Sjögren's syndrome, systemic sclerosis (SSc), and myositis.[1,2] These ENAs are ribonucleoproteins and nonhistone proteins that can be eluted from cell nuclei by neutral buffer solutions. Most common specificities include RNP, Sm, SSA, SSB, Scl-70 (also referred to as topoisomerase I), CENP-B, and Jo-1, but also additional specificities have been described. These antibodies may be diagnostic and/or prognostic. Although clinical associations originally were determined after detection by counterimmunoelectrophoresis (CIE),[3,4] many different alternative techniques are available for the detection of ENAs in a clinical immunology laboratory.[5-7] Especially the new-generation techniques apply recombinant instead of native antigens, and this may be important because several ENAs consist of distinct subunits. Moreover, distinct ENAs may be attached to the same RNA molecule.[8] For instance, RNP consists of three subunits (68, A, and C) and Sm is composed of six subunits (B, B', D, E, F, and G), whereas both are linked to U1 RNA molecules. Similarly, SSA contains two subunits (52 and 60) and is coupled together with SSB to Y-RNA. Obviously, different epitopes may be available if the subunits are present as separate (recombinant) antigens, or in a native configuration. Replacement of CIE is of interest because this technique is hampered by being laborious and by having a rather subjective read-out system. The new-generation ENA detection systems are less laborious, and some are even fully automated and have an objective read-out system.

In this study, we evaluated a novel line-blot immunoassay (LIA) for the detection of antibodies to ENAs. This LIA presents the most common ENAs as separate, recombinant subunits and combines the two test stages, that is, screening and typing, which is typical for most other ENA detection systems. The performance of the LIA was determined in sera from SLE patients ($n = 123$), SSc patients ($n = 25$), and healthy controls ($n = 40$). Results were compared with those obtained by CIE, enzyme-linked immunosorbent assay (ELISA), and fluorescent-enzyme immunoassay (FEIA).

MATERIALS AND METHODS

Patients

From 123 patients who were assigned the clinical diagnosis SLE in our university hospital, we were able to find at least one sample in our laboratory store. If more than one sample of the same patient was available, we selected for a sample that was clearly positive for antinuclear antibodies (ANAs). Similarly, we selected serum samples from patients with SSc ($n = 25$), that is, diffuse SSc and CREST syndrome. In addition, sera of 40 healthy controls (laboratory personnel) were included in this study.

ENA Detection by CIE, ELISA, and FEIA

In our laboratory, ENAs are regularly detected by an in-house CIE assay and a commercial ELISA (Varelisa; Pharmacia Diagnostics, Freiburg, Germany). These tests are performed upon finding a positive result in testing for ANA by indirect immunofluorescence. The CIE is started as a screening assay for antibody reactivity to thymic extracts of both rabbit and calf origin. In case a positive precipitation line is observed, the test serum is typed in a second step by running it next to well-defined reference sera (RNP, Sm, SSA, SSB, Scl-70, Jo-1, and PCNA; the CIE is not able to detect antibodies to CENP-B). If the precipitation line is confluent with that formed by the reference serum, it involves identical antigen specificity.[9] The presence and confluence of precipitation lines is read by at least two observers.

Also, the ELISA is a two-step assay starting with screening for antibodies to a mixture of antigens: U1-snRNP, RNP-Sm, Sm, SSA, SSB, Scl-70, CENP-B, and Jo-1 (Varelisa ANA 8 Screen; Pharmacia Diagnostics). If a positive reaction is observed, the reactivity of the antibodies is determined for individual antigens: RNP (68, A, C), Sm (B, B', D), SSA (52, 60), SSB, Scl-70, CENP-B, and Jo-1 (Varelisa ReCombi ANA Profile; Pharmacia Diagnostics). Except for the native Sm antigen, all antigens in the profile assay are of recombinant origin. Both ELISAs were performed according to the manufacturer's instructions.

Finally, the automated FEIA (EliA Symphony; Pharmacia Diagnostics) again is a screening assay followed by testing using specific ENA antigens. The antigens used in the FEIA system are recombinant RNP (68, A, C), SSA (52, 60), SSB, CENP-B, Scl-70, and Jo-1 and highly purified SmD. These tests were performed according to the instructions of the manufacturer and were conducted on a UniCAP 100 instrument (Pharmacia Diagnostics).

ENA Detection by LIA

The recomLine immunoblot (Mikrogen, Martinsried, Germany) is a multiplex LIA that combines screening and typing of 14 antigens (RNP68, RNPA, RNPC, SmB, SmD, SSA60, SSA52, SSB, PO, PCNA, CENP-B, Scl70, Jo-1, and histones) in a single procedure. Except for the native histones, all antigens are of recombinant origin. The assay was performed according to the manufacturer's instructions. Test strips were incubated in 2 mL, 1:100 diluted sample for 1 h. After three wash steps in washing buffer, the antihuman IgG peroxidase conjugate was added and incubated for another 45 min. After three further wash steps in washing buffer, staining solution was added for approximately 4 min. Staining was terminated by washing in distilled water. After drying the strips for 2 h, results were read automatically by scanning the strip and applying the recomScan software (Mikrogen). Staining intensities above the cutoff control on the same strip were reported as positive results. For comparison with the other assays, RNP was considered positive if at least two of the three RNP antigens were recognized, whereas Sm and SSA were considered positive if one of the two Sm or SSA antigens were recognized, respectively.

Statistics

Sensitivity is defined as the probability of a positive test result in a patient with the disease under investigation. Sensitivity is calculated as the number of test-positive samples within the disease population (true-positives), divided by the total number of samples from patients with the respective disease (true-positives + false-negatives). Specificity is the probability of a negative test result in a patient without the disease under investigation. Specificity is calculated as the number of test-negative samples within the population without the disease (true-negatives), divided by the total number of samples from patients without the disease (false-negatives + true-negatives).

Concordance between two assays is the percentage of samples that give similar results. Concordance is calculated as the number of samples that are positive in both assays plus the number of samples that are negative in both assays, and this sum is divided by the total number of samples under evaluation.

RESULTS

ENAs in SLE Samples

The overall reactivities to the conventional ENAs (RNP, Sm, SSA, SSB, CENP-B, Scl-70, and Jo-1) detected by the different techniques revealed that ELISA ($n = 95$), FEIA ($n = 91$), and LIA ($n = 100$) gave a similar amount of reactivity, whereas the CIE ($n = 78$) clearly had a reduced sensitivity. In contrast with the other assays, the LIA detected a substantial amount of additional ENAs, like the ribosomal protein PO ($n = 14$) and histones ($n = 25$); the CIE detected only a single PCNA-positive serum.

The sensitivities of antibodies to RNP (11.4–14.6%), SSA (26.8–34.2%), and SSB (13.8–17.1%) were quite similar for the four different techniques, and there was good concordance between results obtained by CIE, ELISA, or FEIA with LIA (TABLE 1). The most discordant results were obtained for Sm: sensitivities ranged from 5.7% (FEIA) to 17.9% (LIA). In case of LIA, this was almost exclusively caused by reactivity to the SmB antigen; only a single SmD-positive serum was discovered by LIA, and this positivity could not be confirmed by any of the other techniques. Because the LIA enabled detection of SSA52 and SSA60 as two separate entities, it became apparent that samples reacting with both antigens in the LIA were also detected by the other techniques (TABLE 2). However, when LIA detected only antibodies to SSA52 ($n = 14$), anti-SSA was found to be negative in approximately half of the samples by CIE (64%) and ELISA (43%).

TABLE 1. Sensitivity and concordance of ENA detection by different techniques

	CIE	ELISA	FEIA	LIA
SLE ($n = 123$)				
RNP	11.4 (94.3)	14.6 (94.3)	13.8 (95.9)	12.2
SSA	26.8 (89.4)	32.5 (88.6)	34.2 (90.2)	32.5
SSB	15.5 (95.1)	15.5 (95.1)	17.1 (91.9)	13.8
Sm	8.1 (85.4)	11.4 (88.6)	5.7 (84.6)	17.9
SSc ($n = 25$)				
CENP-B	0 (36)	68 (96)	72 (92)	64
Scl-70	0 (84)	20 (96)	20 (96)	16
SSA	16 (72)	16 (72)	20 (76)	44

NOTE: Numbers represent sensitivity in percentages; numbers in parentheses represent the concordance in percentages of the respective assay with the LIA (obviously, the concordance is omitted in the last column). CIE, counterimmunoelectrophoresis; ELISA, enzyme-linked immunosorbent assay; ENA, extractable nuclear antigen; FEIA, fluorescent-enzyme immunoassay; LIA, line-blot immunoassay; SLE, systemic lupus erythematosus; SSc, systemic sclerosis.

TABLE 2. Recognition of separate SSA52 and SSA60 by LIA

	LIA		CIE	ELISA	FEIA
	SSA52	SSA60			
SLE (n = 123)					
23	+	+	23	23	21
14	+	−	5	8	12
3	−	+	2	2	2
SSc (n = 25)					
1	+	+	1	1	1
10	+	−	3	3	4
0	−	+	NA	NA	NA

NOTE: Numbers in the first column represent the sera that are positive for SSA52 and/or SSA60 by LIA. Results (last three columns) are presented as the number of sera with the respective SSA subunit profile that are positive by CIE, ELISA, or FEIA. CIE, counterimmunoelectrophoresis; ELISA, enzyme-linked immunosorbent assay; FEIA, fluorescent-enzyme immunoassay; LIA, line-blot immunoassay; NA, not applicable; SLE, systemic lupus erythematosus; SSc, systemic sclerosis.

With respect to the other antigens, the Jo-1 antigen was not recognized in any of the SLE sera. The LIA detected two sera positive for Scl-70, but this reactivity could not be confirmed by any of the other techniques, and the CENP-B antigen was detected by ELISA, FEIA, and LIA in the same four samples.

ENAs in Systemic Sclerosis Samples

As for the SLE samples, the SSc samples (n = 25) also revealed similar overall reactivities to the conventional ENAs by ELISA (n = 26), FEIA (n = 28), and LIA (n = 31). In contrast, the CIE detected hardly any antibodies (n = 4). These reactivities were essentially confined to the SSc-associated antibodies to CENP-B and Scl-70, but also contained antibodies to SSA. No other antibodies were detected by any of the techniques. The sensitivities of the SSc-associated antibodies to CENP-B (64–72%) and Scl-70 (16–20%) were quite similar for the ELISA, FEIA, and LIA (TABLE 1). However, the CIE did not detect any of these two antibody specificities. There was good concordance between results obtained by either ELISA or FEIA, but obviously not CIE, with LIA. Finally, LIA detected SSA reactivity in 11 of 25 samples (44%). As shown in TABLE 2, this predominantly concerned reactivity to SSA52 only, and again these antibodies were poorly recognized by the other techniques.

ENAs in Healthy Control Samples

With regard to the specificity of the four techniques evaluated in this study, we examined reactivity in healthy control samples (n = 40). The CIE, ELISA, and FEIA did not show any positive reaction, whereas the LIA revealed reactivity to Sm(D) (n = 1), SSA (60) (n = 1), SSB (n = 1), and PO (n = 1) in three different samples.

DISCUSSION

In the current study, we evaluated a novel LIA for detection of ENAs in sera of patients with autoimmune connective tissue diseases, that is, SLE and SSc, and healthy controls. Our results reveal that sensitivities for the conventional ENAs, as obtained by LIA, are increased as compared with CIE, but quite similar to ELISA and FEIA. In case of the LIA, but not ELISA and FEIA, this increased sensitivity is associated with a slightly reduced specificity. The LIA detected not only four positive reactions in sera of healthy controls, but also unexpectedly antibodies to Scl-70 in two samples of SLE patients. Although none of these reactivities could be confirmed by any of the other techniques, it seems to have become more difficult to discard these data as false-positive. Indeed, antibodies to ENAs may be present several years before clinical symptoms become apparent or a definite diagnosis can be made.[10]

As compared with ELISA and FEIA, increased sensitivities are observed for Sm(B) and SSA(52). Antibodies to Sm are considered specific for SLE, and it has been suggested that this high specificity holds in particular for antibodies to the SmD, but less the SmB subunit.[6,11] The prevalence in SLE of SmB antibodies has been reported to be higher (28.1%) than of SmD antibodies (13.6%).[12] Our data reveal lower sensitivities, but it should be stressed that our current study was not designed to determine the prevalences of antibodies to the distinct ENAs in sera of SLE and SSc patients. We hardly detected any anti-SmD reactivity and this was not even confined to SLE patients (one SLE and one healthy control). Moreover, the Sm reactivity in these two samples could not be confirmed by any of the other techniques, including the FEIA which is considered highly specific for SmD. Antibodies to SmB, on the other hand, appeared specific for SLE.

The increased sensitivity for antibodies to SSA52 by LIA is also reported by others using another commercial LIA[6] and was apparent in both the sera of SLE patients as well as SSc patients. Although antibodies to SSA are not specific for any of the auto-immune connective tissue diseases, these antibodies may be prognostic for the development of neonatal lupus and/or a congenital heart block.[13,14] Interestingly, it has been reported recently that maternal autoantibodies directed to a specific epitope within the leucine zipper amino acid sequence 200–239 (p200) of the SSA52 protein correlate with prolongation of fetal atrioventricular time and heart block.[15] This indicates that detection of antibodies specific for the SSA52 subunit is clinically relevant in pregnant women.

The multiplex LIA evaluated in this study has the advantage over the other techniques in that it enables the detection of antibodies with additional specificities, like PCNA, PO, and histones. Antibodies to PCNA are considered to be highly specific for SLE, but are extremely infrequently (<3%) found.[16] Indeed, these antibodies were not detected by LIA in this study. Antibodies to ribosomal P proteins (PO, P1, and P2) are detected in 10–20% of SLE patients, but are rarely detected in patients with other autoimmune diseases. In patients with SLE, an association of antibodies to ribosomal P proteins with psychosis has been noted, and although there has been some controversy about this association, ample evidence suggests a meaningful relationship between these antibodies and central nervous system disease.[17] However, more recently it has been suggested that antiribosomal P protein antibodies are a marker of SLE-associated hepatitis to differentiate it from autoimmune hepatitis and other liver dysfunctions in SLE patients without renal dysfunction or central nervous system involvement.[18] Finally, high titer antihistone antibodies are found almost exclusively in patients with SLE and, in particular, with drug-induced lupus.[19] Especially the detection of these antibodies in the absence of SLE marker antibodies is characteristic of drug-induced lupus. Although we observed anti-PO antibodies in 14 (11.4%) and antihistone antibodies in 25 (20.3%) of our SLE patients, clinical studies were not performed to study the clinical relevance of these antibodies.

In conclusion, the novel LIA *recom*Line is a suitable technique for the detection of autoantibodies to ENAs in a clinical immunology laboratory and is comparable to ELISA and FEIA. Obviously, further evaluation in daily practice is recommended. Furthermore, the clinical significance of detection of additional antigens (PCNA, PO, histone) and split-antigens of RNP, Sm, and SSA in terms of diagnosis and prognosis of autoimmune connective tissue diseases remains to be determined.

REFERENCES

1. TAN, E.M. 1989. Antinuclear antibodies: diagnostic markers for autoimmune diseases and probes for cell biology. Adv. Immunol. **44:** 93–151.
2. VON MÜHLEN, C.A. & E.M. TAN. 1995. Autoantibodies in the diagnosis of systemic rheumatic diseases. Semin. Arthritis Rheum. **24:** 323–358.
3. TAN, E.M. & H.G. KUNKEL. 1966. Characteristics of a soluble nuclear antigen precipitating with sera of patients with systemic lupus erythematosus. J. Immunol. **96:** 464–471.
4. CLARK, G., M. REICHLIN & T.B. TOMASI, JR. 1969. Characterization of a soluble cytoplasmic antigen reactive with sera from patients with systemic lupus erythematosus. J. Immunol. **102:** 117–122.
5. BIZZARO, N., R. TOZZOLI, E. TONUTTI, et al. 1998. Variability between methods to determine ANA, anti-dsDNA and anti-ENA autoantibodies: a collaborative study with the biomedical industry. J. Immunol. Methods **219:** 99–107.
6. MEHEUS, L., W.J. VAN VENROOIJ, A. WIIK, et al. 1999. Multicenter validation of recombinant, natural, and synthetic antigens used in a single multiparameter assay for the detection of specific anti-nuclear autoantibodies in connective tissue disorders. Clin. Exp. Rheumatol. **17:** 205–214.
7. ROUQUETTE, A.M., C. DESGRUELLES & P. LAROCHE. 2003. Evaluation of the new multiplexed immunoassay, FIDIS, for simultaneous quantitative determination of antinuclear antibodies and comparison with conventional methods. Am. J. Clin. Pathol. **120:** 676–681.
8. LERNER, M.R., J.A. BOYLE, J.A. HARDIN, et al. 1981. Two novel classes of small ribonucleoproteins detected by antibodies associated with lupus erythematosus. Science **211:** 400–402
9. KURATA, N. & E.M. TAN. 1976. Identification of antibodies to nuclear acidic antigens by counterimmunoelectrophoresis. Arthritis Rheum. **19:** 574–580.
10. ARBUCKLE, M.R., M.T. MCCLAIN, M.V. RUBERTONE, et al. 2003. Development of autoantibodies before the clinical onset of systemic lupus erythematosus. N. Engl. J. Med. **349:** 1526–1533.
11. VAN VENROOIJ, W.J., P. CHARLES & R.N. MAINI. 1991. The consensus workshops for the detection of autoantibodies to intracellular antigens in rheumatic diseases. J. Immunol. Methods **140:** 181–189.
12. HOFFMAN, I.E., I. PEENE, L. MEHEUS, et al. 2004. Specific antinuclear antibodies are associated with clinical features in systemic lupus erythematosus. Ann. Rheum. Dis. **63:** 1155–1158.
13. WATSON, R.M., A.T. LANE, N.K. BARNETT, et al. 1984. Neonatal lupus erythematosus: a clinical, serological and immunogenetic study with review of the literature. Medicine **63:** 362–378.
14. SINGSEN, B.H., J.E. AKHTER, M.M. WEINSTEIN, et al. 1985. Congenital complete heart block and SSA antibodies: obstetric implications. Am. J. Obstet. Gynecol. **152:** 655–658.

15. SALOMONSSON, S., S.E. SONESSON, L. OTTOSSON, *et al.* 2005. Ro/SSA autoantibodies directly bind cardiomyocytes, disturb calcium homeostasis, and mediate congenital heart block. J. Exp. Med. **201:** 11–17.
16. ASERO, R., L. ORIGGI, S. CRESPI, *et al.* 1987. Autoantibody to proliferating cell nuclear antigen (PCNA) in SLE: a clinical and serological study. Clin. Exp. Rheumatol. **5:** 241–246.
17. REICHLIN, M. 2003. Ribosomal P antibodies and CNS lupus. Lupus **12:** 916–918.
18. OHIRA, H., J. TAKIGUCHI, T. RAI, *et al.* 2004. High frequency of anti-ribosomal P antibody in patients with systemic lupus erythematosus–associated hepatitis. Hepatol. Res. **28:** 137–139.
19. MONESTIER, M. & B.L. KOTZIN. 1992. Antibodies to histones in systemic lupus erythematosus and drug-induced lupus syndromes. Rheum. Dis. Clin. N. Am. **18:** 415–436.

A Prospective Study of 1038 Pregnancies on the Predictive Value of Anti–Annexin V Antibodies for Fetal Loss

N. BIZZARO,[a] A. ANTICO,[b] M. MUSSO,[c] S. PLATZGUMMER,[d] L. CAMOGLIANO,[e] R. TOZZOLI,[f] AND D. VILLALTA[g]

[a]Laboratorio di Patologia Clinica, Ospedale di Tolmezzo-Gemona, Tolmezzo, Italy

[b]Laboratorio Analisi, Ospedale di Cittadella, Cittadella, Italy

[c]Laboratorio Analisi, Ospedale di Cuneo, Cuneo, Italy

[d]Laboratorio Analisi, Ospedale di Merano, Merano, Italy

[e]Laboratorio Analisi, Ospedale di Novi Ligure, Novi Ligure, Italy

[f]Laboratorio di Chimica-Clinica e Microbiologia, Ospedale di Latisana, Latisana, Italy

[g]Servizio di Immunologia Clinica e Virologia, Az. Osp. S. Maria degli Angeli, Pordenone, Italy

ABSTRACT: Retrospective studies have demonstrated that anti–annexin V (anti-AnxV) antibodies are linked to miscarriage. Their predictive value is, however, unknown. We have carried out a prospective study to evaluate the relationship between anti-AnxV antibodies and the pregnancy outcome. A serum sample was taken from 1038 consecutive healthy women at the beginning of pregnancy. IgG and IgM anti-AnxV antibodies were measured by an ELISA method. The cutoff value was set at 5 units for both IgG and IgM. Out of 1038 women, 116 (11.4%) had a miscarriage by the 22nd week; 10 were lost to follow-up, 10 had an induced abortion, 6 had a preterm delivery, and 896 carried their pregnancy through to term. An adverse outcome of the pregnancy proved to be directly related to the number of previous miscarriages ($P = .008$) and the age of the woman ($P = .002$). IgG and IgM anti-AnxV were present in 25% and 27% of the women who miscarried, and in 23% and 28% of those who gave birth (mean antibody concentration IgG, 4.2 vs. 4.4 U/mL; IgM, 3.7 vs. 3.5 U/mL). IgG and IgM anticardiolipin and anti-β_2GPI, together with antinuclear, antithyroperoxidase, and antithyroglobulin antibodies, were also measured in the 116 sera of the women with miscarriage and in an equal number of women who gave birth. Their positivity or level proved not to be useful in discriminating between the risk of miscarriage and term delivery. This large-scale prospective study demonstrates that the presence of IgG and IgM anti-AnxV antibodies, when measured in healthy women, does not give a positive predictive lead towards the possibility of a miscarriage, and it is not useful in evaluating the risk of miscarriage at the beginning of pregnancy.

Address for correspondence: Nicola Bizzaro, M.D., Laboratorio di Patologia Clinica, Ospedale Civile, via Morgagni, 18, 33028 Tolmezzo (UD), Italy. Voice: +39-0433-488261; fax: +39-0433-488264.

nbizzaro@ass3.sanita.fvg.it

Ann. N.Y. Acad. Sci. 1050: 348–356 (2005). © 2005 New York Academy of Sciences.
doi: 10.1196/annals.1313.037

KEYWORDS: annexin V; pregnancy outcome; miscarriage; prospective study

INTRODUCTION

Miscarriage is the most frequent complication of pregnancy, with an incidence ranging between 8% and 25%, depending on the population studied and the data collection method.[1]

Many factors are considered potentially liable to cause miscarriage: chromosomal abnormalities, uterine abnormalities, hormonal imbalances, coagulation defects, and infectious and immunological causes. In general, however, it is considered that chromosomal abnormalities are strongly prevalent before the 8th week of gestation[2,3] and that a high percentage of the miscarriages occurring after the 8th week of gestation may have immunological causes.[4,5] It has been extensively demonstrated that the presence of a medium–high level of β_2-glycoprotein I (β_2GPI)–dependent anti-cardiolipin antibodies (aCL) or lupus anticoagulant (LAC) plays a specific role in the genesis of placental thrombosis and miscarriage.[6-11] Both antibodies constitute one of the fundamental criteria for the diagnosis of the antiphospholipid syndrome (APS), a disorder characterized by arterial or venous thromboembolism and miscarriage.[12] However, in addition to aCL and LAC, other antiphospholipid antibodies or antiphospholipid-binding proteins are probably involved, including anti–annexin V (AnxV) antibodies, which numerous retrospective studies have found to be associated with a higher frequency of occasional and recurrent miscarriages.[13-15] Annexin V is a glycoprotein with natural anticoagulant activity and a high affinity for anionic phospholipids; it is expressed by trophoblasts and endothelial cells, and its anticoagulant activity is associated with its ability to act competitively with coagulation factors for the phospholipid-binding sites, preventing their activation. Anti-AnxV monoclonal antibodies have proved able to divert annexin V from the surface of the trophoblast cells, thus promoting a procoagulant effect.[16] In an earlier retrospective study, we observed that, among the various antiphospholipid antibodies and anti-phospholipid-binding proteins, anti-AnxV antibodies were the only ones significantly associated with recurrent miscarriage.[17] However, the correlation between a clinical event and the subsequent detection of antibodies may simply represent an epiphenomenon resulting from the event. To establish whether anti-AnxV antibodies are not only associated with miscarriage, but also have a predictive value, we performed a prospective study on healthy women without any history of thromboembolism or autoimmune disease, evaluating the correlation between the presence and concentration of anti-AnxV antibodies at the start of pregnancy and the outcome of the pregnancy.

MATERIALS AND METHODS

Patients

One thousand thirty-eight healthy women (mean age, 31.5 years; range, 16–45 years) at the start of pregnancy with a documented positive β-hCG test or the presence of a gestational sac on ultrasound were recruited consecutively from 6 general hospitals in northern Italy in the period of September 2001 to June 2002. Age, ethnic origin, week of gestation at the blood draw (between 5 and 8 weeks), parity, and use of medicines were recorded for each patient. The exclusion criteria were pregnancy over the 8th week, the presence of autoimmune diseases (systemic or organ-specific) or any other chronic disease, and a history of thromboembolic events. None of the patients refused to enroll in the study, and all of them signed an informed consent form stating that they were healthy and agreed to the performance of the tests and a follow-up until the end of the pregnancy.

Anti-AnxV Antibodies

IgG and IgM anti-AnxV antibodies were assayed in serum samples drawn at the beginning of pregnancy. The tests were conducted with a commercially available enzyme-linked immunosorbent assay (ELISA) (Orgentec Diagnostika GmbH, Mainz, Germany), according to the manufacturer's instructions. The assays were performed on microtiter plates coated with purified human annexin V. A polyclonal rabbit anti-human IgG (or IgM) conjugate, labeled with horseradish peroxidase, and a 3,3',5,5'-tetramethyl-benzidine enzymatic substrate were used. The anti-AnxV antibody concentrations were calculated with a six-point calibration curve and expressed in units (U)/mL. Tests were performed in one laboratory by a single operator. All assays were validated by the inclusion of one positive and one negative control, as an internal quality control. Calibrators and controls were run in duplicate, and the patient samples in single determinations.

The optimal cutoff levels were determined in a previous study[17] by receiver operating characteristic (ROC) curves and set at 5 U/mL for both IgG and IgM anti-AnxV.

Other Autoantibodies

At the end of the study, the following tests were conducted on the same serum samples, stored frozen at $-80°C$, in the women who miscarried and an equivalent number of women of the same age and parity, selected at random, whose pregnancy had reached full term: IgG and IgM aCL and anti-β_2GPI antibodies were determined with an ELISA method (Orgentec); antinuclear antibodies (ANA) were determined with the indirect immunofluorescence method (Inova Diagnostics, San Diego, CA) at the starting dilution of 1:40 in phosphate buffer solution; and antithyroperoxidase (TPO) and antithyroglobulin (Tg) antibodies were detected with an ELISA method (Varelisa Pharmacia, Freiburg, Germany). The assay procedures and calculation of the results were conducted in one laboratory by personnel unaware of the outcome of the pregnancy, according to the instructions given by the various manufacturers; the calibrators and controls were run in duplicate, and the patient samples in single determinations.

The optimal cutoff levels for IgG and IgM aCL and anti-β_2GPI antibodies were determined by ROC curves in a previous study,[17] and set at 13.3 GPL and 10.6 MPL for aCL, and 13.6 U/mL for IgG and 11.9 U/mL for IgM anti-β_2GPI antibodies. The cutoffs for the anti-TPO (56 U/mL) and anti-Tg (62 U/mL) antibodies were those provided by the manufacturer.

Approval of the study protocol was obtained from the Ethics Committee of the S. Donà di Piave Hospital.

Statistical Analysis

The association between the dichotomic variables (prior miscarriage and antibody positivity) and the outcome of pregnancy was evaluated with the χ^2 test. The association between age and outcome was evaluated with the t test. The correlation between antibody concentration and the outcome was verified by means of the Mann-Whitney U-test. The variables that, on bivariate analysis, were associated with the outcome with $P \le 0.1$ were inserted in a multiple binomial logistic regression model. The statistical analyses were performed with the Stata IF Package for Windows 8.2 (StataCorp, College Station, TX). Two-sided P values <.05 were considered to have statistical significance.

RESULTS

Of the 1038 women enrolled in the study, 1028 completed the follow-up and 10 dropped out because they moved to another town during the study. Of the 1028 women, 1018 were Caucasian and 10 were black Africans. None of them were taking any medicines or suffered from any infectious disease at the time of blood draw. One hundred twenty-six had a miscarriage or abortion as the outcome of the pregnancy: 10 had an induced abortion (1 due to trisomy 21 established by cytogenetic test and 9 for personal reasons) and 116 (11.4%) miscarried. Anatomical abnormalities of the uterus were not found in any case. The cause was established in 5 cases: 2 due to fetal malformations, 2 to cervical incontinence, and 1 to hormonal insufficiency. Of the remaining 111, 16 had a miscarriage by the end of the 8th week, 76 between the 9th and 12th weeks, and 19 after the 12th week.

Of the 902 (87.7%) women who gave birth, 6 had a premature birth between the 22nd and 33rd week of gestation (1 baby died at 3 weeks after the birth), while 896 pregnancies went to term. In 1 case, the baby died after 8 months due to cardiac malformations.

Two patients diagnosed with Hashimoto's thyroiditis during the pregnancy gave birth at term.

Incidence of Miscarriage in Relation to Age and Parity

The mean age of the women who miscarried was 32.8 ± 5.1 years, while the mean age of those who gave birth was 31.4 ± 4.6 years ($P = .002$). Of the 1018 women evaluated (excluding the 10 women who had an induced abortion and the 10 lost to follow-up), 499 were pregnant for the first time, 336 had had earlier full-term pregnancies (1–5), 93 had had both miscarriages and births, and 90 had had only miscarriages (1–5 earlier miscarriages). The percentages of miscarriages recorded in this study in the four groups were 7.4%, 13.1%, 18.2%, and 20%, respectively. Moreover, the 30.1% (35/116) of women with miscarriage had a history of miscarriages vs. 19.5% of the women with full-term pregnancy (175/896) (odds ratio [OR], 1.78; 95% CI, 1.16–2.72; $P = .008$). Thus, an adverse outcome of pregnancy proved to be directly related to the number of previous miscarriages and the age of the woman. The stratification of the outcome of pregnancy in relation to parity is set out in TABLE 1.

TABLE 1. Distribution of pregnancy outcome and frequency of anti-AnxV antibodies in relation to parity

Obstetric history	No. of women	Mean age	Outcome of pregnancy		% of positive anti-AnxV	
			Birth	Miscarriage	IgG	IgM
Primigravidae	499	30.0	462	37 (7.40%)	20.6	26.8
Births only	336	32.9	292	44 (13.1%)	26.8	29.2
Both births and miscarriages	93	34.9	75	17 (18.2%)	27.9	29.0
Miscarriages only	90	31.7	73	18 (20.0%)	23.3	26.7
Total	1018	31.5	902	116 (11.4%)	23.6	27.8

NOTE: Ten women with an induced abortion and 10 who were lost to follow-up were excluded.

Anti-AnxV Antibodies

IgG anti-AnxV antibodies were present in 29 of the women who miscarried (25%) and 211 (23.5%) of those who gave birth at full term (OR, 1.08; 95% CI, 0.69–1.69; $P = .71$). IgM anti-AnxV antibodies were present in 32 (27.5%) of the women who miscarried and 251 (28%) of those who gave birth at full term (OR, 0.97; 95% CI, 0.63–1.50; $P = .51$). None of the 6 women who gave birth prematurely tested positive for IgG anti-AnxV, and only 2 tested positive for IgM at low levels.

The mean antibody concentration did not differ significantly between the two groups—for anti-Anx IgG: 4.2 U/mL in the group that miscarried and 4.4 U/mL in the group that gave birth ($P = .56$); for anti-Anx IgM: 3.7 U/mL in the group that miscarried and 3.5 U/mL in the group that gave birth ($P = .27$). The risk of miscarriage is thus not correlated with the presence of anti-Anx antibodies or antibody level.

If the four different groups of patients are divided on the basis of obstetric history (TABLE 1), the percentages of antibody positivity in each group are not significantly different.

aCL and Anti-β_2GPI Antibodies

aCL and anti-β_2GPI antibodies were measured in the 116 women who miscarried and in an equivalent number of women who gave birth. aCL antibodies were present, always at low level and without statistical significance, in 6 women who miscarried (5 IgG, $P = .09$; 1 IgM, $P = .31$) and 1 woman who gave birth. Anti-β_2GPI antibodies were also positive, again at low level, in 2 women who gave birth (1 IgG; 1 IgM) and in none of the patients who miscarried.

ANA and Antithyroid Antibodies

ANA and antithyroid antibodies were also measured in the 116 women who miscarried and in an equivalent number of women who gave birth. Three positives (titer 1:40 – 1:80) for ANA were observed among the patients who miscarried and 2 (titer 1:40 and 1:160) in the group who gave birth, with no statistical significance ($P = .65$). In 1 patient with ANA titer 1:160, the subsequent test for antinuclear specific antigens and anti-dsDNA antibodies gave a negative result.

Anti-TPO and anti-Tg antibodies proved to be present in exactly the same number of patients: in 21 (18.1%) of the women who miscarried and 19 (16.3%) of the women who gave birth (anti-TPO, $P = .72$; anti-Tg, $P = .72$). The two antibodies were simultaneously present in 13 women in both the miscarriage group and the birth group.

DISCUSSION

In unselected pregnant women, the most common cause of miscarriage in the pre-embryonic or embryonic period (from conception to the 8th week of gestation) is chromosomal abnormality.[3] In later periods, the chromosomal cause declines drastically in frequency and other causes prevail, including immunological causes, which seem to have a high incidence.[18] Pregnancy loss, typically in the second trimester, is one of the most consistent features of APS, which is characterized by the presence of aCL antibodies and LAC. Histologic examination of placentas from APS pregnancies often shows infarction and thromboses of the uteroplacental vasculature. However, some women with persistently elevated aCL or LAC levels and a history of thrombosis have no fetal complications at all, and in many cases repeated miscarriages with no recognizable cause occur in women without aCL or LAC. Several autoantibodies other than aCL and LAC are involved in cases of reproductive failure.[5] Among them, a significant role seems to be played by anti-AnxV antibodies. In murine models, annexin V is needed to maintain the integrity of the placental structure, and probably performs a thromboregulatory action at the maternal-fetal interface.[19] In fact, annexin V was found to be markedly reduced in placentas from patients with APS[20,21] and in cultured trophoblasts and endothelial cells exposed to antiphospholipid antibodies.[22] It has been suggested that annexin V forms an antithrombotic shield around procoagulant anionic phospholipids, which blocks their participation in phospholipid-dependent coagulation reactions, and that the binding of specific high-affinity antibodies to annexin V can compromise the antithrombotic shield and contribute to reproductive failure.[23,24] It has recently been demonstrated by atomic force microscopy that annexin V binding to phospholipids or its anticoagulant activity was significantly reduced by plasmas of patients with antiphospholipid antibodies and thrombosis compared with healthy controls and patients with thromboembolism and without antiphospholipid antibodies.[25] In addition, monoclonal antibodies against annexin V block intertrophoblastic fusion, suggesting another possible mechanism whereby these antibodies may induce miscarriage.[26]

The association between miscarriage and anti-AnxV antibodies has already been described in numerous retrospective studies, in women with recurrent miscarriages[14,15,27] and in women with systemic lupus erythematosus.[13,28,29] In an earlier study, we found that anti-AnxV antibodies were present in 17% of subjects with recurrent miscarriage and were the only immunological marker among aCL, anti-β_2GPI, and antiprothrombin, which was correlated with the occurrence of miscarriage, though to a moderate extent ($P = .02$).[17] Conversely, Arnold *et al.* observed the presence of anti-AnxV antibodies in 35% of aCL-positive women with miscarriage and 19% of aCL-negative women, but did not find that anti-AnxV constituted a risk factor for miscarriage;[30] equally, Ogawa *et al.* found no correlation between AnxV and miscarriage in patients with APS.[31] These conflicting observations, all based on retrospective studies, led us to design this prospective study of over 1000 pregnant women.

The results of this study, which confirm those of earlier studies,[32,33] demonstrate that primigravidae and women with earlier favorable obstetric outcomes have a much lower incidence of miscarriage than those whose case history includes only miscarriages or miscarriages alternating with normal pregnancies, and that the risk of recurrence increases cumulatively in relation to the number of earlier miscarriages.

The association between miscarriage and maternal age is well documented in the literature; according to Bulletti et al.,[34] the frequency of miscarriage increases from 12% at the age of 20 to 26% over the age of 40. Although in this study the difference in mean age between the women who miscarried and those who gave birth was statistically significant, there is such an overlap that this finding has no clinical usefulness.

What does emerge clearly from this study is that anti-AnxV antibodies of class IgG or IgM measured at the beginning of pregnancy are not predictive of the outcome of the pregnancy. In fact, we recorded similar percentages of antibody positivity for IgG (25% vs. 23%) and IgM (27% vs. 28%) in the women who miscarried and those who gave birth, and the antibody concentrations did not differ significantly between the two groups.

Equally, we found no significant increase in aCL, anti-β_2GPI, or ANA antibodies in women who miscarried compared with the women in the control group, confirming the results obtained in other studies.[35,36] Although antithyroid antibodies were frequent, their prevalence was the same in both groups, and thus not helpful. Moreover, their frequency is similar to that found in the general female population (12–17%).[37]

In conclusion, although retrospective studies have demonstrated a close correlation between miscarriage and anti-AnxV antibodies, this large-scale prospective study did not confirm that these antibodies have a prognostic significance in predicting miscarriage when measured in healthy women. However, it is possible that anti-AnxV antibodies are predictive of miscarriage in patients with APS or other autoimmune diseases, who were not enrolled in this study. It is also possible that other antibodies against other members of the annexin family of proteins are involved and play a pathogenic role,[38] or that anti-AnxV antibodies appear after one or more miscarriages, thus representing an immunological epiphenomenon of miscarriage. At present, therefore, the determination of this new antibody parameter does not seem useful to evaluate the risk of miscarriage at the beginning of pregnancy in healthy women.

REFERENCES

1. REGAN, L. & R. RAI. 2000. Epidemiology and the medical causes of miscarriage. Bailliere's Clin. Obstet. Gynaecol. **14:** 839–854.
2. SIMPSON, J.L. 1980. Genes, chromosomes, and reproductive failure. Fertil. Steril. **33:** 107–116.
3. BE, C., P. VELASQUEZ & R. YOULTON. 1997. Spontaneous abortion: cytogenetic study of 609 cases. Rev. Med. Chile **125:** 317–322.
4. MAIER, D.B. & A. PARKE. 1989. Subclinical autoimmunity in recurrent aborters. Fertil. Steril. **51:** 280–285.
5. SHOENFELD, Y. & M. BLANK. 2004. Autoantibodies associated with reproductive failure. Lupus **13:** 643–648.

6. LEE, R.M., W. EMLEN, J.R. SCOTT *et al.* 1999. Anti-beta2-glycoprotein-I antibodies in women with recurrent spontaneous abortion, unexplained fetal death, and antiphospholipid syndrome. Am. J. Obstet. Gynecol. **181:** 642–648.
7. OUT, H.J., C.D. KOOIJMAN, H.W. BRUINS *et al.* 1991. Histo-pathological findings from patients with intrauterine fetal death and antiphospholipid antibodies. Eur. J. Obstet. Gynecol. **41:** 179–186.
8. BLANK, M., I. COHEN, V. TODER *et al.* 1991. Induction of anti-phospholipid syndrome in naïve mice with mouse lupus monoclonal and human polyclonal anti-cardiolipin antibodies. Proc. Natl. Acad. Sci. USA **88:** 3069–3073.
9. PIONA, A., L. LA ROSA, A. TINCANI *et al.* 1995. Placental thrombosis and fetal loss after passive transfer of mouse lupus monoclonal or human polyclonal anti-cardiolipin antibodies in pregnant naive BALB/c mice. Scand. J. Immunol. **41:** 427–432.
10. GEORGE, J., M. BLANK, Y. LEVY *et al.* 1998. Differential effects of anti-beta2-glycoprotein I antibodies on endothelial cells and on the manifestations of experimental antiphospholipid syndrome. Circulation **97:** 900–906.
11. LYNCH, A., R. MARLAR, J. MURPHY *et al.* 1994. Antiphospholipid antibodies in predicting adverse pregnancy outcome: a prospective study. Ann. Intern. Med. **120:** 470–475.
12. WILSON, W.A., A.E. GHARAVI, T. KOIKE *et al.* 1999. International consensus statement on preliminary classification criteria for definite antiphospholipid syndrome. Arthritis Rheum. **42:** 1309–1311.
13. NOJIMA, J., H. KURATSUNE, E. SUEHISA *et al.* 2001. Association between the prevalence of antibodies to β_2-glycoprotein I, prothrombin, protein C, protein S, and annexin V in patients with systemic lupus erythematosus and thrombotic and thrombocytopenic complications. Clin. Chem. **47:** 1008–1015.
14. MATSUDA, J., M. GOTOH, N. SAITOH *et al.* 1994. Anti-annexin antibody in the sera of patients with habitual fetal loss or preeclampsia. Thromb. Res. **75:** 105–106.
15. MATSUBAYASHI, H., T. ARAI, S. IZUMI *et al.* 2001. Anti–annexin V antibodies in patients with early pregnancy loss or implantation failure. Fertil. Steril. **76:** 964–969.
16. RAND, J.H. 2002. Effects of antiphospholipid antibodies upon the morphology and anticoagulant function of annexin-V [abstract]. Lupus **11:** 571.
17. BIZZARO, N., E. TONUTTI, D. VILLALTA *et al.* 2005. Prevalence and clinical correlation of antiphospholipid-binding protein antibodies in anticardiolipin-negative patients with systemic lupus erythematosus and women with unexplained recurrent miscarriages. Arch. Pathol. Lab. Med. **129:** 61–68.
18. GOLDSTEIN, S. 1994. Embryonic death in early pregnancy: a new look at the first trimester. Obstet. Gynecol. **84:** 294–297.
19. WANG, X., B. CAMPOS, M.A. KAETZEL *et al.* 1999. Annexin V is critical in the maintenance of murine placental integrity. Am. J. Obstet. Gynecol. **180:** 1008–1016.
20. RAND, J.H., X. WU, S. GULLER *et al.* 1994. Reduction of annexin-V (placental anticoagulant protein I) on placental villi of women with antiphospholipid antibodies and recurrent spontaneous abortion. Am. J. Obstet. Gynecol. **171:** 1566–1572.
21. KRIKUN, G., C.J. LOCKWOOD, X. WU *et al.* 1994. The expression of the placental anticoagulant protein, annexin-V, by villous trophoblasts: immunolocalization and *in vitro* regulation. Placenta **15:** 601–612.
22. RAND, J.H., X. WU, H.A.M. ANDREE *et al.* 1997. Pregnancy loss in the antiphospholipid antibody syndrome—a possible thrombogenic mechanism. N. Engl. J. Med. **337:** 154–160.
23. RAND, J.H., X. WU, S. GULLER *et al.* 1997. Antiphospholipid immunoglobulin G antibodies reduce annexin V levels on syncytiotrophoblast atypical membranes and in culture media of placental villi. Am. J. Obstet. Gynecol. **177:** 918–923.
24. RAND, J.H. 1999. "Annexinopathies": a new class of diseases. N. Engl. J. Med. **340:** 1035–1036.
25. RAND, J.H., X. WU, R. LAPINSKI *et al.* 2004. Detection of antibody-mediated reduction of annexin A5 anticoagulant activity in plasmas of patients with the antiphospholipid syndrome. Blood **104:** 2783–2790.
26. ROTE, N.S., N. KUMAR, S.H. CHANG *et al.* 2002. Monoclonal antibody against annexin V prevents intertrophoblast fusion [abstract]. Lupus **11:** 564.

27. GRIS, J.C., I. QUÉRÉ, M. SANMARCO et al. 2000. Antiphospholipid and antiprotein syndromes in non-thrombotic, non-autoimmune women with unexplained recurrent primary early foetal loss. Thromb. Haemost. **84:** 228–236.
28. KABURAKI, J., M. KUWANA, M. YAMAMOTO et al. 1997. Clinical significance of anti-annexin V antibodies in patients with systemic lupus erythematosus. Am. J. Hematol. **54:** 209–213.
29. LAKOS, G., E. KISS, N. REGECZY et al. 2000. Anti-prothrombin and anti-annexin V antibodies imply risk of thrombosis in patients with systemic autoimmune diseases. J. Rheumatol. **27:** 924–929.
30. ARNOLD, J., Z. HOLMES, W. PICKERING et al. 2001. Anti-beta2-glycoprotein 1 and anti-annexin V antibodies in women with recurrent miscarriage. Br. J. Haematol. **113:** 911–914.
31. OGAWA, H., D. ZHAO, J.S. DLOTT et al. 2000. Elevated anti-annexin V antibody levels in antiphospholipid syndrome and their involvement in antiphospholipid antibody specificities. Am. J. Clin. Pathol. **114:** 619–628.
32. KNUDSEN, U.B., V. HANSEN, S. JUUL et al. 1991. Prognosis of a new pregnancy following previous spontaneous abortions. Eur. J. Obstet. Gynecol. Reprod. Biol. **39:** 31–36.
33. REGAN, L., P.B. BRAUDE & P.L. TREMBATH. 1989. Influence of past reproductive performance on risk of spontaneous abortion. Br. Med. J. **299:** 541–545.
34. BULLETTI, C., C. FLAMIGNI & E. GIACOMUCCI. 1996. Reproductive failure due to spontaneous abortion and recurrent abortion. Hum. Reprod. Update **2:** 118–135.
35. AILUS, K., M. TULPPALA, T. PALOSUO et al. 1996. Antibodies to beta 2 glycoprotein I and prothrombin in habitual abortion. Fertil. Steril. **66:** 937–941.
36. FORASTIERO, R.R., M.E. MARTINUZZO, G.S. CERRATO et al. 1997. Relationship of anti-beta2-glycoprotein I and anti-prothrombin antibodies to thrombosis and pregnancy loss in patients with anti-phospholipid antibodies. Thromb. Haemost. **78:** 967–968.
37. HOLLOWELL, J.G., N.W. STAEHLING, W.H. HANNON et al. 2002. Serum thyrotropin, thyroxine, and thyroid antibodies in the United States population (1988 to 1994): NHANES III. J. Clin. Endocrinol. Metab. **87:** 489–499.
38. RAND, J.H. & X. WU. 2004. Antibody-mediated interference with annexins in the antiphospholipid syndrome. Thromb. Res. **114:** 383–389.

Multiplexed Immunoassay for Detection of Rheumatoid Factors by FIDIS™ Technology

I. ABREU,[a] P. LAROCHE,[b] A. BASTOS,[a] V. ISSERT,[b] M. CRUZ,[c] P. NERO,[c] J. E. FONSECA,[c] J. BRANCO,[c] AND J. A. MACHADO CAETANO[a]

[a]Faculty of Medical Sciences, Department of Immunology, New University of Lisbon, Lisbon, Portugal

[b]Biomedical Diagnostics, Marne-La-Vallée, France

[c]Department of Rheumatology, Egas Moniz Hospital, Lisbon, Portugal

ABSTRACT: Our objective was to (i) compare FIDIS Rheuma, a new multiplexed immunoassay designed for simultaneous detection of IgM class rheumatoid factors (RF) directed against Fc determinants of IgG from humans and animals, with agglutination and ELISA (conventional methods) and (ii) evaluate the clinical sensitivity and specificity of biological markers for rheumatoid arthritis (RA). To do this, FIDIS technology was employed using the Luminex system. It consists of distinct color-coded microsphere sets, a flow cytometer, and digital signal processing hardware and software. Agglutination and ELISA tests were performed with commercial kits. The study included 134 samples from RA patients and 105 from healthy blood donors. For human specificity, we compared FIDIS with latex agglutination and ELISA. Relative sensitivities were 98.9% and 88.5% and specificities were 90.2% and 94.6%, respectively. For animal specificity, we compared FIDIS with Waaler-Rose and ELISA. The results were 84.9% and 71.9% for the sensitivities and 97.5% and 98.4% for the specificities, respectively. Detection of IgG anti-CCP by ELISA and IgG antikeratin by immunofluorescence was also determined in order to compare their clinical sensitivity and specificity with IgM-RF, according to the method used. The results were: IgG anti-CCP 72.3%, 97.2%; IgG antikeratin 36.6%, 100%; latex agglutination 66.4%, 97.2%; Waaler-Rose 55.9%, 96.3%; FIDIS human 73.9%, 92.1%; FIDIS animal 49.2%, 97.2%; ELISA human 93.2%, 95.5%; and ELISA animal 74.6%, 91.3%. The results showed the efficiency of FIDIS with analytical performance equivalent to the conventional methods, but having the advantage of giving quantitative results (IU/mL).

KEYWORDS: rheumatoid factor; rheumatoid arthritis; anti–cyclic citrullinated peptide antibodies; diagnostic tests; autoantibodies

INTRODUCTION

Rheumatoid arthritis (RA) is a chronic inflammatory autoimmune disease characterized by joint destruction, which leads to functional decline and disability as

Address for correspondence: I. Abreu, Faculty of Medical Sciences, Department of Immunology, New University of Lisbon, Lisbon, Portugal. Voice: +351-21-880-30-45; fax: +351-21-885-34-80. iabreu.imuno@fcm.unl.pt

Ann. N.Y. Acad. Sci. 1050: 357–363 (2005). © 2005 New York Academy of Sciences. doi: 10.1196/annals.1313.038

well as increased mortality.[1–4] Together with the clinical features of the disease, serological abnormalities such as the presence of rheumatoid factors (RF) are usually useful in the diagnosis of RA.

RF are detected in the majority of patients with established disease and constitutes one of the American College Rheumatology (ACR) classification criteria.[5]

IgM-RF is the main isotype identified by clinically diagnostic assays for RF detection. Conventional methods for the measurement of IgM-RF have depended upon the agglutination of particles (e.g., latex, bentonite, charcoal, or erythrocytes) coated with human or animal (usually rabbit) IgG. Latex particle agglutination and Waaler-Rose methods are the most commonly used.[6,7] ELISA has also been utilized for the detection of different isotypes of RF.

Besides the RF, another group of autoantibodies was detected in serum of patients with RA: the antikeratin antibodies (AKA) and, more recently, the anti–cyclic citrullinated peptide (anti-CCP) antibodies, a newer diagnostic marker for AR.[8,9]

The aim of this study was to compare FIDIS™ Rheuma, a new multiplexed immunoassay designed for the simultaneous quantitative determination of IgM class RF directed against Fc determinants of IgG from humans and animals, with conventional methods, and to evaluate the clinical sensitivity and specificity of different serological markers for RA.

MATERIALS AND METHODS

Patients

A total of 239 serum samples were studied: 134 patients with RA diagnosed according to the revised criteria formulated by the ACR[5] and 105 healthy blood donors.

FIDIS™ Rheuma Assay System

FIDIS™ technology uses the Luminex 100™ system (Luminex Corporation, Austin, TX), which consists of distinct uniform-size (5.5 µm) color-coded microspheres (potentially 100 different sets) and a benchtop flow cytometer interfaced with a computer containing digital signal processing hardware and software.[10,11] Each set of microspheres is classified on the basis of its orange and red unique fluorescence intensity, which allows the identification of which analyte is analyzed. At the same time, a green laser excites the external reporter fluorescence to quantify the specific reaction related to each analyte.

Reagents

Each antigen (Fc fragment from human or rabbit IgG) was conjugated by a covalent bond to an individual set of microspheres through its surface functional carboxyl groups. The two antigen-coupled microsphere sets are then mixed to constitute the final microsphere reagent. The detection of IgM-RF that have bound the target antigens was revealed by using anti-human IgM conjugated to phycoerythrin (PE). A dilution buffer was used to dilute unknown samples and the prediluted conjugate. Finally, a calibration system allowed quantification of each antigenic specificity after validation of quality control. Results were expressed in international units per mL (IU/mL) according to the first British Standard for Rheumatoid Arthritis (64/2). Cut-off values were determined by the manufacturer by using 142 samples (64 from blood donors and 78 selected for their potential biological interferences: cryoglobulinemia, hypergammaglobulinemia, IgG and IgM monoclonal immunoglobulins, complement, immune complexes) tested with the above procedure. Positive reactions were defined as a fluorescence signal greater than the 99.5th percentile distribution of the samples population for each antigenic antibody specificity. A value of 30 IU/mL was attributed to the signal corresponding to the cutoff value, calculated on the 142 samples and according to the standard 64/2.

Assay Procedure

Twenty µL of microsphere reagent was mixed with 100 µL of calibrator sample, prediluted controls, and samples (1/200) in a filter membrane microtiter plate. After 30 min of incubation at room temperature (RT), microspheres were washed for 30 s by filtration, suspended in 200 µL of a solution of anti-human IgM-PE, and incubated again for 30 min at RT. The reactions were then directly analyzed by the flow cytometer: at least 100 microspheres set in 10 to 20 s according to the number of sets. During this time, the system first categorized each microsphere set according to its orange and red fluorescent color; it then determines the average green fluorescence from PE conjugate, providing a quantitative determination of each autoantibody specificity. Test reports can be automatically generated through the FIDIS™ database management software.

Determination of Antibodies

Rheumatoid Factors (RF)

For IgM-RF detection, agglutination tests using particles sensitized with human IgG (Rhumalatex from Fumouze, France) and rabbit IgG (Polyartitre from Fumouze, France) were performed. Commercial ELISA assays were also used to detect IgM-RF anti-human IgG (Euroimmun, Germany) and anti-rabbit IgG (QuantaLite, Inova Diagnostics, San Diego, CA). Both the agglutination and ELISA assays were performed according to the manufacturer's instructions. On the evaluation of IgM-RF anti-rabbit IgG by ELISA, serum samples with a value of >12 IU/mL were considered positive. The cutoff suggested by the manufacturer is >7 IU/mL. The ELISA assays were performed in duplicate.

Antikeratin Antibodies (AKA)

IgG AKA were determined using indirect immunofluorescence (IIF). As substrate, rat esophagus sections were employed (Biosystems, Spain). Serum samples were diluted 1:10.

Anti-CCP Antibodies

Anti-CCP2 antibodies were detected by a commercial ELISA containing synthetic peptides (Inova Diagnostics, San Diego, CA). The ELISA was performed according to the manufacturer's instructions. Serum samples with a test result of >25 U/mL

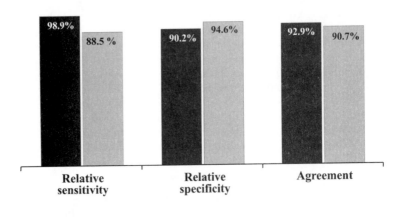

FIGURE 1. Relative sensitivities, specificities, and agreement, comparing the FIDIS Rheuma human vs. latex agglutination and ELISA human IgG.

were considered positive and further designated as the "standard" cutoff. All the assays were performed in duplicate.

RESULTS

Comparing the FIDIS™ Rheuma technology for the detection of IgM-RF anti-human IgG with the latex particle agglutination test (RA test), we found the relative sensitivity and relative specificity to be 98.8% and 90.2%, respectively. When compared to the ELISA, the relative sensitivity and relative specificity were 88.5% and 94.6%, respectively. The agreement was 92.9% for FIDIS Rheuma vs. latex agglutination particles, and 90.7% for FIDIS Rheuma vs. ELISA (FIG. 1).

Concerning the IgM-RF anti-animal IgG, the results from the relative sensitivity, relative specificity, and agreement, obtained by comparing the FIDIS Rheuma with the Waaler-Rose, were 84.9%, 97.5%, and 92.4%, respectively. For the comparison between FIDIS Rheuma and ELISA, the results found were 71.9%, 98.4%, and 81.2%, respectively (FIG. 2). The clinical sensitivity and specificity of the three biological markers for the RA [i.e., RF (evaluated for the three methods in comparison), AKA, and anti-CCP] are shown in TABLE 1.

DISCUSSION

The diagnosis of RA relies mainly on clinical manifestations and serological markers. RF are still the most widely used serological test as an aid for the diagnosis of RA. Most routine laboratory tests in current use are the hemagglutination and the

TABLE 1. Clinical sensitivity and specificity of three biological markers of RA (RF, AKA, and anti-CCP antibodies)

	Sensitivity	Specificity
Rheumatoid factor		
FIDIS Rheuma human	73.9%	92.1%
FIDIS Rheuma animal	49.2%	97.2%
RA test	66.4%	97.2%
Waaler-Rose	55.9%	96.3%
ELISA human IgG	93.2%	95.5%
ELISA animal IgG	74.6%	91.3%
CCP-ELISA	72.3%	97.2%
Keratin-IIF	36.6%	100%

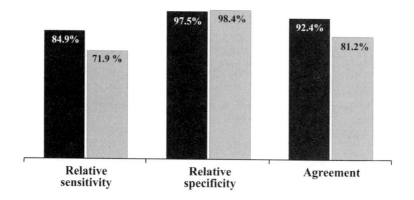

■ FIDIS RHEUMA ANIMAL VS WAALER ROSE
▨ FIDIS RHEUMA ANIMAL VS ELISA ANIMAL IgG

FIGURE 2. Relative sensitivities, specificities, and agreement, comparing the FIDIS Rheuma animal vs. Waaler-Rose and ELISA animal IgG.

latex agglutination, which detected mainly IgM-RF.[12,13] In these techniques, end points are not objectively determined because an observer decides when agglutination is present and this judgment will vary among observers. The ELISA is a more objective method for determining the levels of different RF isotypes. IgM-RF concentration can be expressed in IU/mL on the basis of the World Health Organization reference RF serum.

The performance of FIDIS Rheuma human compared with the latex test and the ELISA anti-human IgG was quite good: relative sensitivity (latex 98.9%; ELISA 88.5%), relative specificity (latex 90.2%; ELISA 94.6%), and agreement (latex 92.9%; ELISA 90.7%). For the IgM-RF anti-animal IgG, the performance was also

good comparing FIDIS with Waaler-Rose, but less good for the comparison to the
ELISA: relative sensitivity (Waaler-Rose 84.9%; ELISA 71.9%), relative specificity
(Waaler-Rose 97.5%; ELISA 98.4%), and agreement (Waaler-Rose 92.4%; ELISA
81.2%). Our results show that methods detecting RF anti-human IgG are more sensitive, but less specific, than the assays using rabbit IgG as antigen, as has previously
been described by other authors.[14–17]

The importance of different RA-associated antibodies as diagnostic markers for
RA has been extensively analyzed. We evaluated the clinical sensitivity and specificity
of RF, AKA, and anti-CCP. Our results for AKA sensitivity (36.6%) and specificity
(100%) are in agreement with reports from other authors.[18–20] All the serological
markers tested showed high clinical specificity. For the IgM-RF anti-human IgG, the
difference of sensitivity between FIDIS Rheuma (73.9%) and ELISA (93.2%) can
be due to the higher sensitivity of ELISA; from 15 samples that were FIDIS negative
and ELISA positive, 14 were also negative by the latex test.

In this study, the clinical sensitivity and specificity of anti-CCP2 were 72.3% and
97.2%, respectively, which are values within the range described by others.[21–23] The
anti-CCP autoantibody system has received a great deal of study recently, and the
superiority of anti-CCP2 to RF in the diagnosis of RA has been reported.[24,25] Although there is an important overlap between the presence of RF and anti-CCP antibodies in the serum of RA patients, evidence has suggested that RF and anti-CCP
antibodies are two separate autoantibody systems.[26] Data from De Rycke et al.[26]
indicate that the RF and anti-CCP antibodies may provide different and, eventually,
complementary biological information on the disease process in RA. The anti-CCP
could act as a disease specific marker for RA, whereas IgM-RF titers could be
related to disease activity.

In RA, most IgM-RF have specificity for human and rabbit IgG.[27] The presence
of both RF specificities at the same time helps in the RA diagnosis. The IgM-RF is
related to the disease activity, having recently reported a decrease in IgM-RF titers
during infliximab treatment.[26,27] Thus, the FIDIS technology seems to be very useful
for IgM-RF detection. Our results have shown the efficiency of FIDIS Rheuma
human/animal with analytical performances equivalent to the conventional methods.
On the other hand, it has the advantage of identifying and quantifying (IU/mL), at
the same run, both RF specificities, thereby saving time.

REFERENCES

1. FUCHS, H.A. & J.S. SERGENT. 1997. Rheumatoid arthritis: the clinical picture. In Arthritis
   and Allied Conditions: A Text Book of Rheumatology, pp. 1041–1070. Williams &
   Wilkins. Baltimore.
2. CALLAHAN, L.F. et al. 1996. Formal education and five-year mortality in rheumatoid
   arthritis: mediation by helplessness scale score. Arthritis Care Res. 9: 463–472.
3. KVALVIK, A.G. et al. 2000. Mortality in a cohort of Norwegian patients with rheumatoid
   arthritis followed from 1977 to 1992. Scand. J. Rheumatol. 29: 29–37.
4. GABRIEL, S.E. et al. 1999. Mortality in rheumatoid arthritis: have we made an impact
   in four decades? J. Rheumatol. 26: 2529–2533.
5. ARNET, F.C. et al. 1988. The American Rheumatism Association 1987 revised criteria
   for classification of rheumatoid arthritis. Arthritis Rheum. 31: 315–324.
6. ROSE, H.M. et al. 1948. Differential agglutination of normal and sensitized sheep
   erythrocytes by sera of patients with rheumatoid arthritis. Proc. Soc. Exp. Biol. Med.
   68: 1–11.

7. WAALER, E. 1940. On the occurrence of a factor in human serum activating the specific agglutination of sheep blood corpuscles. Acta Pathol. Scand. **17:** 172–178.
8. SCHELLEKENS, G.A. *et al.* 2000. The diagnostic properties of rheumatoid arthritis antibodies recognizing a cyclic citrullinated peptide. Arthritis Rheum. **43:** 155–163.
9. BIZZARO, N. *et al.* 2001. Diagnostic accuracy of the anti-citrulline antibody assay for rheumatoid arthritis. Clin. Chem. **47:** 1089–1093.
10. FULTON, R.J. *et al.* 1997. Advanced multiplexed analysis with the FlowMetrix™ system. Clin. Chem. **43:** 1749–1756.
11. SPAIN, M. & R.L. MCDADE. 2000. A workstation approach to bioassays. IVD Technology (July/August 2000).
12. EGELAND. T. & M. MUNTHE. 1983. The role of the laboratory in rheumatology: rheumatoid factors. Clin. Rheum. Dis. **9:** 135–160.
13. AILUS, K. *et al.* 1991. Measuring rheumatoid factor in nonrheumatoid subjects: immuno-turbidimetric assay, latex slide test, and enzyme linked immunosorbent assay compared. Clin. Chem. **37:** 1766–1769.
14. GOODMAN, L.A. *et al.* 1987. Analysis of combined rheumatoid factor determinations by the rheumatoid arthritis latex and sheep cell agglutination tests and the American Rheumatism Association criteria for rheumatoid arthritis. J. Rheumatol. **14**(2): 234–239.
15. KLEEVELAND, G. *et al.* 1988. Quantitation of rheumatoid factors (RF) of IgM, isotypes IgA and IgG by a simple and sensitive ELISA: discrimination between false and true IG-RF. Scand. J. Rheumatol. Suppl. **75:** 15–24.
16. JONES, M.G. *et al.* 1990. Specificity of rheumatoid factors in relation to the disease state in rheumatoid arthritis. Ann. Rheum. Dis. **49:** 757–762.
17. WOLFE, F. *et al.* 1991. The latex test revisited. Arthritis Rheum. **34**(8): 951–960.
18. VINCENT, C. *et al.* 1989. High diagnostic value in rheumatoid arthritis of antibodies to stratum corneum of rat oesophagus epithelium, so-called "anti-keratin antibodies". Ann. Rheum. Dis. **48:** 712–722.
19. KURKI, P. *et al.* 1992. Immunopathology of rheumatoid arthritis: antikeratin antibodies precede the clinical disease. Arthritis Rheum. **35:** 914–917.
20. AHO, K. *et al.* 1994. Marker antibodies for rheumatoid arthritis: diagnostic and pathogenic implications. Semin. Arthritis Rheum. **31:** 315–324.
21. HAYASHI, N. & S. KUMAGAI. 2003. New diagnostic tests for rheumatoid arthritis. Rinsho Byori **51**(10): 1030–1035.
22. GIRELLI, F. *et al.* 2004. Is anti–cyclic citrullinated peptide a useful laboratory test for diagnosis of rheumatoid arthritis? Allerg. Immunol. (Paris) **36**(4): 127–130.
23. KUMAGAI, S. *et al.* 2004. Topics of immunological tests for rheumatoid arthritis. Rinsho Byori **52**(10): 836–843.
24. SUZUKI, K. *et al.* 2003. High diagnostic performance of ELISA detection of antibodies to citrullinated antigens in rheumatoid arthritis. Scand. J. Rheumatol. **32:** 197–204.
25. DE RYCKE, L. *et al.* 2004. Rheumatoid factor and anti-citrullinated protein antibodies in rheumatoid arthritis: diagnostic value, associations with radiological progression rate, and extra-articular manifestations. Ann. Rheum. Dis. **63:** 1587–1593.
26. DE RYCKE, L. *et al.* 2005. Rheumatoid factor, but not anti–cyclic citrullinated peptide antibodies, is modulated by infliximab treatment in rheumatoid arthritis. Ann. Rheum. Dis. **64:** 299–302.
27. GRIPENBERG, M. *et al.* 1979. A simple enzyme immunoassay for the demonstration of rheumatoid factor. J. Immunol. Methods **31:** 109–118.

Antinuclear Antibodies in Domestic Animals

LAUREL J. GERSHWIN

Department of Pathology, Microbiology, and Immunology, School of Veterinary Medicine, University of California, Davis, California, USA

ABSTRACT: Antinuclear antibodies in domestic animal species have been commonly detected for many years, with the greatest frequency occurring in dogs as well as horses and cats. Most commonly, the assay used in diagnostic laboratories is indirect immunofluorescence on HEP-2 cells, similar to that used in human medicine, but with the exception that species-specific antiglobulin reagents are used instead of antihuman immunoglobulin. To a lesser extent, the *Crithidia luciliae* test for antibodies to double-stranded DNA has been used. Several research groups have used other assays.

KEYWORDS: antinuclear antibodies; dogs; systemic lupus erythematosus

ANTINUCLEAR ANTIBODIES IN THE DOG

Systemic Lupus Erythematosus

A positive antinuclear antibody (ANA) is one criterion for diagnosis of systemic lupus erythematosus (SLE). Thus, it is not surprising that dogs diagnosed with this disease have a high incidence of positive ANA, with a 97–100% rate compared with normal dogs. (From 16% to 20% of normal dogs will have a positive ANA, generally of low titer.)

The specificity of ANA in dogs differs from that seen in humans with SLE in that most dogs with SLE have ANA against histones and/or ribonucleoproteins more often than dsDNA.

Characteristics of the disease in dogs are like the disease in humans, with polyclonal gammopathy and lymphadenopathy generally serving as hallmark observations. One or more of the following will also be present: characteristic skin lesions, polyarthritis, glomerulonephritis, Coombs-positive anemia, and thrombocytopenia. FIGURES 1A and 1B show skin lesions typical of SLE.

Clinical signs associated with SLE in dogs include fever and symmetrical non-erosive polyarthritis (90%), renal failure (65%), skin disease (60%), lymphadenopathy and/or splenomegaly (50%), leukopenia (20%), hemolytic anemia (13%), and thrombocytopenia (4%). Other less common clinical signs include myositis, pericarditis (8%), and neurologic manifestations (1.6%) (summarized in ref. 1).

Address for correspondence: Laurel J. Gershwin, D.V.M., Ph.D., Department of Pathology, Microbiology, and Immunology, 2019 Haring Hall, School of Veterinary Medicine, University of California, Davis, CA 95616. Voice: 530-752-6643; fax: 530-752-3349.
ljgershwin@ucdavis.edu

Ann. N.Y. Acad. Sci. 1050: 364–370 (2005). © 2005 New York Academy of Sciences.
doi: 10.1196/annals.1313.039

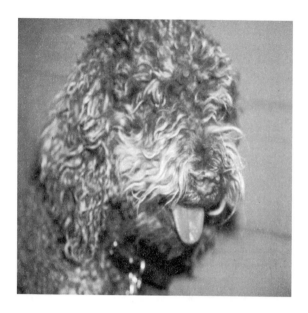

FIGURE 1A. Dog with SLE: ulcerative lesions on nasal planum.

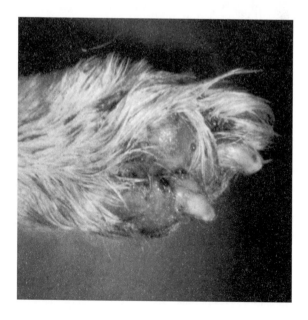

FIGURE 1B. Footpad lesions on the dog shown in FIGURE 1A.

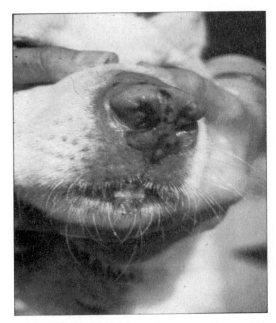

FIGURE 2A. Ulcerative skin lesions in a canine with SLE.

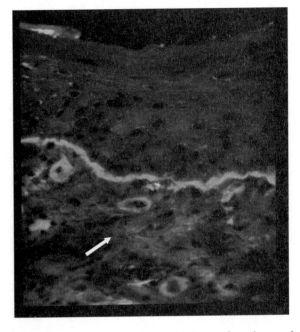

FIGURE 2B. Direct immunofluorescence on skin biopsy from the muzzle of the dog in FIGURE 2A. Characteristic "lupus band" is observed at the dermal-epidermal junction (*arrow*).

Skin lesions associated with SLE in dogs can be biopsied and stained with fluorescein-conjugated anti-canine IgG or anti-C3. These biopsies will commonly show the typical immune complex deposition at the basal lamina and sometimes also complex deposition in small blood vessels in the dermis. In addition, an abundance of mononuclear cells with cytoplasmic fluorescence can sometimes be seen in the dermis. FIGURES 2A and 2B show a typical lesion and immunofluorescence staining of the biopsy.

The polyarthritis seen in SLE is nonerosive, but joint taps reveal high levels of neutrophils in joint fluid. Tapping of the carpus and tarsus of all four legs usually reveals similar inflammatory exudates, in the absence of sepsis. The involvement of multiple joints is typical, often causing the disease to be associated with a "shifting leg lameness".

Although renal failure is not present in all cases of SLE, this may be a result of the stage of disease when diagnosis occurs. A urinalysis will show protein in the urine of cases with kidney involvement. Subsequent biopsy of the kidney followed by direct immunofluorescence for detection of immune complex deposition will show deposition that is irregular in glomeruli. A typical kidney biopsy from a canine SLE case is shown in FIGURE 3.

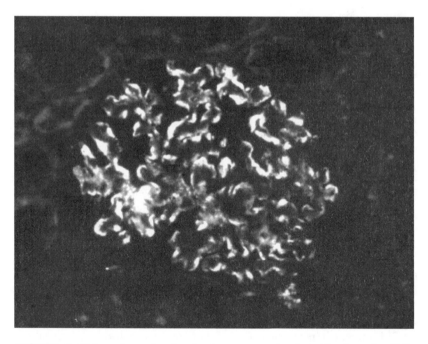

FIGURE 3. Kidney glomerulus showing immune complex deposition in canine SLE.

Other Clinical Syndromes with Positive ANA

There is one report in the literature in which from 30% to 35% of Gordon setter dogs with lupoid onychodystrophy or black hair follicular dysplasia had positive ANA tests.[2]

Infection with certain bacterial and protozoan organisms has been associated with positive ANA tests. Specifically, *Bartonella vinsonii*, *Ehrlichia canis*, and *Leishmania infantum* have been associated with positive ANA in dogs. In a recent retrospective study of patient records with these infections and concurrent ANA test results, it was found that 75% of the *B. vinsonii* reactors, 16.7% of the *E. canis* reactors, and none of the *R. rickettsii* reactors had concurrent positive ANA tests. It was concluded that dogs reactive to more than one of these pathogens had a greater chance of being ANA-positive.[3] Two earlier studies had failed to show a link between positive *E. canis* serology and positive ANA test.[4,5]

There is a report in the literature in which approximately 10% of sera from beagles with autoimmune thyroiditis have positive ANA in addition to antithyroid antibodies.[6]

Drug Treatment: Phentoin, Griseofulvin, and Antibiotics

There have been reports of the development of positive ANA tests in canines treated with a variety of pharmaceuticals, including phentoin, griseofulvin, and several antimicrobials. However, there is a lack of documented publications to substantiate these observations.

Staining Patterns and Specificities for Canine Antinuclear Antibodies

Less is known about disease associations with ANA pattern in dogs than in humans. In general, the homogeneous or rim pattern is more commonly associated with SLE than nonspecific or other diseases, whereas the speckled pattern is more often associated with other autoimmune disease.

In an effort to examine whether particular ANA staining patterns correspond with particular nuclear antigen specificities, a study was performed by Hansson and Karlsson-Parra.[7] It was found that precipitating antibodies, identified by Ouchterlony double immunodiffusion with nuclear antigen, were associated with ANA with speckled pattern. One of the subgroups identified by immunodiffusion showed reactivity with ribonucleoprotein, and none of the immunodiffusion-positive sera reacted with chromosomal antigens.[7]

Do Dogs Living with Human Patients with SLE Have a Greater Chance of Developing Canine SLE?

This question was posed in a recent study by Chiou *et al.*,[8] who studied 59 pet dogs owned by 37 SLE patients and 187 pet dogs owned by non-SLE patients.[7] Approximately 19% of the dogs owned by SLE patients were ANA-positive compared with approximately 5% of dogs owned by non-SLE patients. Of these, 5% of the SLE patient–owned pets were diagnosed with SLE, compared with none (0%) of the non-SLE-owner dog population. These data were compared with the general population of hospital outpatients who had an incidence of approximately 5% ANA positive and slightly less than 1% diagnosed with SLE. This extremely interesting study suggests that there may be some environmental triggers common to the environment of the SLE patients and their pets.

ANTINUCLEAR ANTIBODIES IN THE HORSE

The association with positive ANA and SLE is also seen in the equine species. In horses diagnosed with SLE, the most common presentation is a generalized skin condition with Coombs-positive anemia and positive ANA. Other relevant body systems that may be affected include joints (synovitis), kidneys (glomerulonephritis), and generalized lymphadenopathy.

ANTINUCLEAR ANTIBODIES IN THE CAT

Systemic lupus erythematosus occurs in the cat, but is rare. Coombs-positive anemia is a common presentation. Other clinical manifestations include fever, skin lesions, thrombocytopenia, polyarthritis, and renal failure (glomerulonephritis). In the cat, the manifestation of joint involvement may be sufficiently subtle in that it is only recognized by joint fluid aspiration. Positive ANA is present.

In hyperthyroidism, which is relatively frequent in cats, treatment with propylthiouracil is common. Development of positive ANA after this therapy has been reported. The propylthiouracil treatment appears to induce a lupus-like disease, which is accompanied by antibodies to native DNA. The presence of lymphadenopathy and a Coombs-positive anemia are hallmarks.[9]

SUMMARY

There are four points to be made in summary:

(1) The ANA test is used in the diagnosis of SLE in dogs, horses, and cats.
(2) Positive ANA in the absence of SLE is common in these species.
(3) There are similarities and differences in antigen specificity of ANAs in canine sera when compared with human sera.
(4) More work needs to be done to better characterize the importance of ANA in animals.

REFERENCES

1. TIZARD, I.R. 2004. Veterinary Immunology: An Introduction. Seventh edition. Saunders/ Elsevier. Philadelphia/New York.
2. OVREBO BOHNHORST, J., I. HANSSEN & T. MOEN. 2001. Antinuclear antibodies (ANA) in Gordon setters with symmetrical lupoid onychodystrophy and black hair follicular dysplasia. Acta Vet. Scand. **42:** 323–329.
3. SMITH, B.E., M.B. TOMPKINS & E.B. BREITSCHWERDT. 2004. Antinuclear antibodies can be detected in dog sera reactive to *Bartonella vinsonii* subsp. *berkhoffii*, *Ehrlichia canis*, or *Leishmania infantum* antigens. J. Vet. Intern. Med. **18:** 47–51.

4. KELLY, P.J., S.D. CARTER, P.A. BOBADE, *et al.* 1994. Absence of antinuclear antibodies in dogs infected with *Ehrlichia canis.* Vet. Rec. **134:** 382.
5. HARRUS, S., M.J. DAY, T. WANER & H. BARK. 2001. Presence of immune-complexes, and absence of antinuclear antibodies, in sera of dogs naturally and experimentally infected with *Ehrlichia canis.* Vet. Microbiol. **83:** 343–349.
6. VAJNER, L. 1997. Lymphocytic thyroiditis in beagle dogs in a breeding colony: findings of serum autoantibodies. Vet. Med. **42:** 333–338.
7. HANSSON, H. & A. KARLSSON-PARRA. 1999. Canine antinuclear antibodies: comparison of immunofluorescence staining patterns and precipitin reactivity. Acta Vet. Scand. **40:** 205–212.
8. CHIOU, S.H., J.L. LAN, S.L. LIN, *et al.* 2004. Pet dogs owned by lupus patients are at a higher risk of developing lupus. Lupus **13:** 442–449.
9. AUCOIN, D.P., R.L. RUBIN, M.E. PETERSON, *et al.* 1988. Dose-dependent induction of anti-native DNA antibodies in cats by propylthiouracil. Arthritis Rheum. **31:** 688–692.

The Interaction of Pemphigus Autoimmunoglobulins with Epidermal Cells

Activation of the Fas Apoptotic Pathway and the Use of Caspase Activity for Pathogenicity Tests of Pemphigus Patients

MARINA FRUŠIĆ-ZLOTKIN,[a] ROCHEL PERGAMENTZ,[a] BENO MICHEL,[b] MICHAEL DAVID,[c] DANIEL MIMOUNI,[c] FRANÇOIS BRÉGÉGÈRE,[a] AND YORAM MILNER[a]

[a]Myers Skin Biology and Biochemistry Laboratory, Life Sciences Institute, Hebrew University of Jerusalem, 91904 Jerusalem, Israel

[b]Michel Skin Care Incorporated, Beachwood, Ohio 44122, USA

[c]Department of Dermatology, Rabin Medical Center, 49100 Petach-Tikva, Israel

ABSTRACT: Pemphigus is a fatal autoimmune disease in which autoimmunoglobulins PV-IgG (binding to desmoglein 3) and PF-IgG (binding to desmoglein 1) in pemphigus vulgaris and pemphigus foliaceus, respectively, cause intraepidermal blisters, cell–cell separation (acantholysis), and cell death. The mechanism of acantholytic lesion formation has not yet been elucidated. Recently, we have reported that an apoptotic mechanism might be operative in PV-IgG–induced acantholysis: (1) in patients' lesional and some perilesional skin portions, the FasR pathway is activated as its components were enriched; (2) in cultured keratinocytes, PV-IgG upregulates effectors of the FasR pathway (including the mitochondrial loop), as found by immunodetermination (cytochemistry, Western blot of pathway effectors) and determination of caspases 1, 3, and 8 activity/activation; (3) in organ cultures of skin incubated with PV-IgG, activated caspase 8 was found also in perilesional cells and coaggregated with bound PV-IgG; (4) caspase 8 activation in DISCs precedes caspase 3 activation in keratinocytes in cultures upon incubation with PV-IgG. Because caspase activation was shown to accompany lesion formation in cell and organ cultures incubated with PV-IgG, we used caspase activity to monitor the pathogenicity of PV-IgG in relation to PV-IgG binding to epithelia. A rough correlation was found between sera titers, determined by IIF and by immunoblot binding to desmoglein 3, and activation of caspase 3.

KEYWORDS: apoptosis; acantholysis; pemphigus IgG; autoimmunity

Address for correspondence: Prof. Yoram Milner, Life Sciences Institute, Campus Edmond Safra, Hebrew University of Jerusalem, 91904 Jerusalem, Israel. Voice: +972-2-658-5051; fax: +972-2-658-5429.

milner@vms.huji.ac.il

Ann. N.Y. Acad. Sci. 1050: 371–379 (2005). © 2005 New York Academy of Sciences.
doi: 10.1196/annals.1313.040

INTRODUCTION

Pemphigus vulgaris (PV) is an autoimmune blistering disease of the skin characterized by detachment of epidermal keratinocytes and formation of acantholytic intraepidermal blisters.[1] Direct immunofluorescence tests reveal deposition of epidermal intercellular IgG autoantibodies.[2] These PV-IgG are directed against adherent molecules of the desmosomes, desmoglein 3 (Dsg3) and/or desmoglein 1 (Dsg1, the pemphigus foliaceus antigen), of the cadherin superfamily. When mucosal blisters appear, circulating autoimmune IgG are against Dsg3; when both anti-Dsg1 and 3 are present, formation of a mucocutaneous blister ensues.[2,3]

Up to now, the exact molecular mechanism leading to epidermal acantholysis and blister formation is still unclear. A simple hypothesis was that acantholysis is triggered by the mere binding of PV-IgG to adhesive sites of Dsg3 and/or Dsg1, resulting in impairment of its function (steric hindrance),[3,4] followed by epidermal cell separation. It has been also hypothesized that PV-IgG binding to the Dsg3-plakoglobin complex results in releasing of a plasminogen activator (PA) that, in turn, causes serum plasminogen activation and then separation of epidermal cells, that is, acantholysis.[5] However, studies demonstrating induction of acantholysis and blister formation in knockout mice depleted of PA by passive transfer of PV-IgG[6] ruled out this mechanism. A further hypothesis suggests a role for intracellular signaling response, which involves the activation of phospholipase C pathway after the binding of PV-IgG to Dsg1 and 3.[7,8] Recently, Sanchez-Carpintero et al. have shown that inhibitors of tyrosine kinases and phospholipase C prevented PV-IgG–induced acantholysis, lending further support to the signaling theory of acantholysis.[9]

We have reported that Fas apoptotic pathway might be operative in the acantholytic process.[1] We were able to demonstrate that PV lesions in patients' skin contain apoptotic keratinocytes and effectors activated apparently before observing cell–cell detachment. Using keratinocyte cultures and skin organ cultures, we have shown that PV-IgG–induced acantholysis was associated with cellular accumulation of significant proapoptotic markers: FasR, FasL, Bax, and P53 proteins. Also, enrichment in caspase 8 in the membranal death complex (DISC, death inducing signaling complex) and activation of caspases 3 and 1 have been shown.[1] It was concluded that PV-IgG–induced acantholysis might proceed through death signaling pathway. In other words, apoptosis could be the cause of acantholysis and not a secondary phenomenon.

In this study, we aimed to kinetically determine the activity of caspase 3 in the process of acantholysis and to assess its time of activation by PV-IgG. We show here that caspase 8 and probably caspase 3 are induced by incubation with PV-IgG in a keratinocyte cell line culture before major cell–cell separation. Caspase 3 activity thus could be used as an indicator for PV-IgG pathogenicity evaluation.

RESULTS

Apoptotic Mechanism Controls Acantholysis

First, we inspected regular histological sections of lesional patients' skin, stained by hematoxylin and eosin (FIGS. 1a and 1b). Numerous apoptotic cells and bodies are obvious in the blister fluid (seen as degraded cells and nuclei with condensed chromatin). We have shown previously[1] that these cells and some in the roof of the acantholytic lesion contain elevated levels of apoptotic effectors such as FasR and FasL, FADD, Bax, and caspases 8, 1, and 3. The most striking evidence for the induction of the apoptotic pathway by PV-IgG in epidermal cells is seen in FIGURES 1c and 1d. One can see that, in perilesional epidermal cells of skin in organ culture incubated for 32 h with PV-IgG, the PV-IgG binding sites (Dsg3) are saturated with IgG on the cellular plasma membrane (labeled with FITC-conjugated secondary anti-

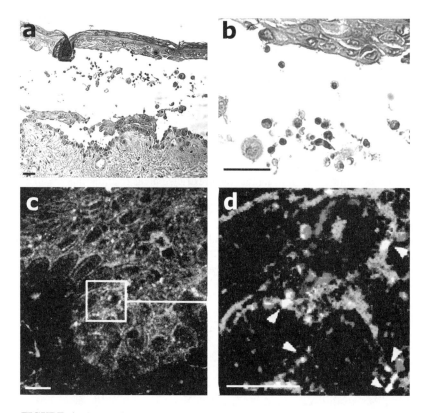

FIGURE 1. Apoptotic markers appearance in PV patients' skin cells and apoptotic DISC formation in organ culture induced by PV-IgG. (**a, b**) Paraffin-embedded skin sections (5–6 µm) of PV lesional epidermis stained by eosin and hematoxylin. Acantholytic cells display apoptotic features (condensed chromatin, fragmented nuclei, apoptotic bodies) in lesional skin of pemphigus vulgaris patients. (**c, d**) Double immunofluorescent staining of 4% PFA–fixed, paraffin-embedded sections (5–6 µm) of skin from organ culture treated with 5 mg/mL PV-IgG for 32 h. Membranal recruitment of an early apoptotic DISC member: caspase 8 (labeled by TRITC-conjugated secondary antibody) is localized on the inner aspect of the cell membrane, and PV-IgG (labeled by FITC-conjugated anti-human antibody) is bound to the outer side of cell membrane. The *arrowheads* in part "d" point to their coaggregation on plasma membrane in suprabasal cell layers (superposition of green FITC and red TRITC labels appears yellow). At that time point, no acantholysis was observed. Control cultures, incubated with N-IgG, showed diffuse weak staining in both labels (not shown). Bars: (a, b) 50 µm; (c, d) 20 µm.

bodies). In parallel, the caspase 8 of the death complexes is aggregated on the inner aspect of cell membrane (DISC formation; labeled with TRITC-conjugated secondary antibodies) and elevated quantitatively (control sections showing weak and diffuse staining are not shown). Part of this aggregation is coincident: Dsg3 and caspase 8 appear in same clusters, indicating the coaggregation of Dsg3 and caspase 8 (seen as yellow fluorescence, white arrowheads).

Caspase 3 Activation by PV-IgG in Keratinocyte Cultures

If indeed the apoptotic mechanism is activated by the incubation with PV-IgG, one must observe an increase in the activity of the "executioner" caspase 3 in skin. When keratinocytes and skin organ cultures were incubated with normal (N-IgG), PV-IgG, or rabbit anti-Dsg3 extracellular portion antibodies (donated by Dr. Prabhakar, University of Texas Medical Branch, Galveston, TX) (FIG. 2), one could readily observe the formation of acantholytic lesions in PV-treated cultures (FIGS. 2b and 2c, in cell culture; FIGS. 2e and 2f, in organ culture; *black asterisks*). In parallel, the appearance of caspase 3 (activity determined in cell lysates) is also represented. Some three- to fourfold increase of caspase 3 was noted in cell cultures incubated with PV-IgG. The lower degree of caspase 3 activation in the organ culture possibly reflects the limited amount of cells in the organ culture relative to the confluent keratinocyte cultures and the fact that only restricted areas of epidermis are afflicted by the acantholytic lesion.

Because caspases are activated in the cells upon PV-IgG binding to cell membrane, we could follow the advance of the acantholytic process by determination of caspases activity. Indeed, a timewise follow-up on caspases activation (activity) upon PV-IgG addition to keratinocyte cell line HaCaT cultures showed a sequential mode of caspase activation. Initially, caspase 8 is being activated at 7–12 h upon PV-

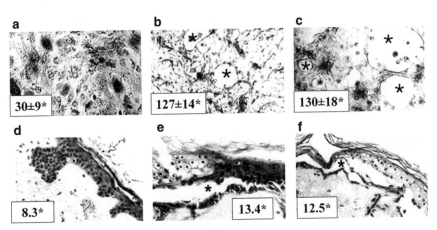

FIGURE 2. Lesion formation in PV-IgG–treated cell and organ cultures (*) is coupled to elevated caspase 3 activity. Normal human keratinocytes, passage 2 (**a, b, c**) and skin organ cultures (**d, e, f**) were incubated for 52 h with N-IgG (**a, d**), PV-IgG (**b, e**), and rabbit anti-desmoglein 3 antibody (**c, f**). Their respective caspase 3 activity (*) determined in cell lysates is shown in each micrograph.

TABLE 1. Correlation of PV sera immunoreactivity and caspase 3 activation by PV-IgG

PV-IgG	Serum Dsg3 immunoreactivity[a]	Serum IIF titer[b]	Caspase 3 activity (% of control)
Di0503	+++	1:640	440
Pr1104	++++	1:640	327
Do0304	+++	1:320	402
Ta0504	+++	1:320	378
La1103	++	1:160	198
Gr1104	+	1:160	185
Oh0400	++	1:80	220
Ha0504	+	1:40	107
Gu1104	+	1:20	98
Ba1104	−	neg.	104

NOTE: Confluent HaCaT cultures were incubated with 7.5 mg/mL PV-IgG; control cultures were incubated with 7.5 mg/mL N-IgG for 24 h in 96-well plates. Other assay conditions were as described in FIGURE 3.

[a]Immunoreactivity with the 130 kDa in Western blot with epidermal membrane extracts (arbitrary densitometric units).

[b]Indirect immunofluorescence titer on monkey esophagus.

IgG addition (FIG. 3a). Caspase 3, on the other hand, shows a delayed activation at 24 h (FIG. 3b) as one would expect as a real-time event in FasR pathway activation in the cells and conditions used.

It seems that the true time of executioner caspase accumulation is close to the onset of cell apoptosis and death as indicated by the follow-up after the number of cells present in the cell culture plate determined by methylene blue assay. As can be seen (FIG. 3c), the final cell death/acantholysis started at 24 h, concurrent with the major caspase 3 activation.

Caspase 3 Determination Can Be Used for Pathogenicity Tests of PV-IgG

The induction of keratinocyte apoptosis by PV-IgG and the participation of caspases in the processes were further investigated by checking the correlation between PV sera titer (determined by IIF), Dsg3 Western blot reactivity, and the enzyme activity level. Because the determination of caspase 3 activity (and as a matter of fact almost all caspases) is easily performed and caspase 3 is the most prevalent final executioner caspase, we decided that this enzyme would serve the purpose well. As can be seen in TABLE 1, there is a rough correlation between sera titers (and Dsg3 in immunoblots) and caspase 3 activity in the group of 1:160 titer sera versus those in the group of 1:320 – 1:640, the latter ones displaying twice the level of caspase activity. The sera with 1:40 – 1:60 titers were not active in caspase 3 mobilization after 24-h incubation, which coincided with their inability to cause acantholysis (not shown here). We have now obtained a group of sera of 1:640/1:1280 titer, which conformed to this correlation being even more active (data not shown).

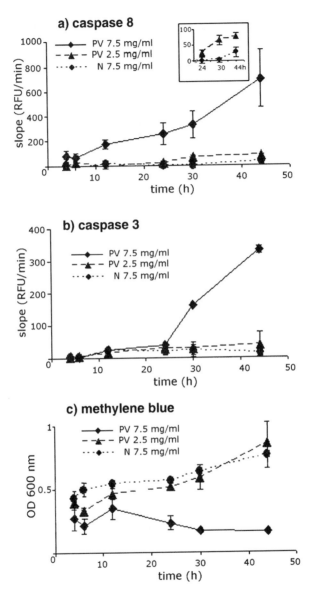

FIGURE 3. Time course of caspase 3 and 8 activation by PV-IgG in HaCaT cells. Eighty percent confluent HaCaT cell cultures were incubated with 2.5 or 7.5 mg/mL PV-IgG (IIF titer 1:320) or 7.5 mg/mL pooled human IgG (N-IgG) for the periods indicated above. The incubation was in 96-well dishes in DMEM medium devoid of FCS. Caspase 8 **(a)** and caspase 3 **(b)** activities were evaluated directly in the culture wells by adding 2.5 μM Z-IETD-AFC or Ac-DEVD-AMC, respectively; 0.02% Triton X-100; and 10 mM DTT (final concentrations). Enzymatic rates were normalized to the number of cells. **(c)** The methylene blue results show a loss of cells after 24-h incubation with PV-IgG (7.5 mg/mL). The insert in part "a" shows the delayed and low activation of caspase 8 by 2.5 mg/mL PV-IgG.

DISCUSSION

The data provided in this study strongly support the notion presented previously that apoptosis induction leads to acantholysis rather than the reverse. Thus, the appearance of preapoptotic cells, enriched in caspase 8 deposition in the so-called DISCs, death complexes, of perilesional cells, is indeed a first-degree indication obtained in skin organ cultures. Furthermore, as can be seen from FIGURE 3a, the caspase 8 activation could be shown in cultures incubated with PV-IgG already at 5 to 10 h. At this time point, no cell–cell detachment, cell separation, or lesion formation was observed microscopically.

These findings focus again on the question of the triggering mechanism of the acantholytic process, whether in tissue, organ, or cell culture. The induction of acantholysis by both PF-IgG and exfoliative toxin of *Staphylococcus aureus* (which has trypsin-like proteolytical activity and specifically hydrolyzes Dsg1 within hours after injection into neonatal mice)[10] perhaps shows the effect of pemphigus-IgG binding to desmoglein as well as the need for desmoglein alteration (enzymatic or conformational change) to initiate a lesional process (apoptosis?) in epidermal cells. The feasibility of this "conformational change mechanism" was evident also from the induction of phosphorylation of Dsg3 upon PV-IgG binding[11] and the abrogated phosphorylation of Dsg3 by methylprednisolone, which prevented skin lesions.[12] Thus, the conformational change in desmoglein and the onset of signaling cascade induced by PV-IgG binding lead to cell–cell separation and eventually apoptosis. However, our data shown in FIGURE 1 suggest that rather a reverse sequence takes place, namely, that apoptosis precedes cell–cell separation.

Comparing the levels of caspase 3 activity with the titer of PV-IgG antibodies in the sera of patients (determined by IIF) and Dsg3 immunoreactivity (determined by Western blot) shows a correlation between caspase 3 activity, titer of antibodies, and Dsg3 immunoreactivity. It appears that pathogenicity of PV-IgG can be determined by the assessment of caspase 3 activity in keratinocyte or cell line cultures in an easy-to-do *in vitro* "bioassay" in 96-well plates.

The pathogenicity of PV-IgG antibodies of a particular patient is an indication of the severity of the disease and might be a predictive marker for the prognosis of the patient. There are *in vitro* and *in vivo* assays by which PV-IgG pathogenicity can be tested: (1) induction of acantholysis in keratinocytes and organ skin cultures incubated with PV-IgG isolated from the tested patient serum,[13,14] and (2) passive transfer to nude or neonatal mice model in which PV-IgG is injected intradermally to induce skin blisters.[15] The outcome in these assays is evaluated microscopically or clinically, which gives a qualitative measurement rather than quantitative results. These are elaborated methods that require specialized laboratories.

PV-IgG pathogenicity can quantitatively be measured by detection of anti-Dsg3 immunoreactivity by different methods. The oldest one is the IIF test. Although the titer of antibodies in the sera of patients is in many instances proportional to the severity of the disease,[16] there are too many exceptions found in the measurement of titer to be regarded as an absolutely reliable index for the severity of the disease,[17] and it could not always be used as a guide for therapeutic judgment.[18] The ELISA technique, which was developed for specific detection of anti-Dsg3 and 1, appears to be a sensitive and highly specific assay mainly for the diagnosis of pemphigus vulgaris and pemphigus foliaceus.[19] There are only a few publications that show a high correlation of titer with the acantholytic activity of the disease.[19,20]

Immunoprecipitation of recombinant Dsg3 and Western blot analysis of pemphigus antigen extracted from the epidermis are also used for the determination of PV-IgG immunoreactivity/presence. However, both tests are expensive and prolonged and provide semiquantitative values.

In view of the above, it appears that testing caspase 3 activity in a cell culture incubated with PV-IgG in ELISA plates may serve as an easy and convenient assay for assessing patients' PV-IgG pathogenicity. Together with Dsg ELISA and IIF assays, the caspase 3 activity test may be a useful tool in the hands of the clinicians for the management of pemphigus patients. Additional studies are under way to further establish this correlation. Further work is needed also to establish the potential use of caspase inhibitors in the treatment of pemphigus.

ACKNOWLEDGMENTS

This work was partially supported by Israel-US BSF Grant No. 1998190 and by the David and Inez Myers Fund of Cleveland, OH, USA.

REFERENCES

1. WANG, X.F. et al. 2004. Possible apoptotic mechanism in epidermal cell acantholysis induced by pemphigus vulgaris autoimmunoglobulins. Apoptosis 9: 131–143.
2. UDEY, M.C. & J.R. STANLEY. 1999. Pemphigus—diseases of antidesmosomal autoimmunity. JAMA 282: 572–576.
3. STANLEY, J.R. 1997. Update: structure and function of pemphigus vulgaris antigen. J. Dermatol. 24: 741–743.
4. PAYNE, A.S. et al. 2004. Desmosomes and disease: pemphigus and bullous impetigo. Curr. Opin. Cell Biol. 16: 536–543.
5. LO MUZIO, L. et al. 2002. Strict correlation between uPAR and plakoglobin expression in pemphigus vulgaris. J. Cutan. Pathol. 29: 540–548.
6. MAHONEY, M.G., Z.H. WANG & J.R. STANLEY. 1999. Pemphigus vulgaris and pemphigus foliaceus antibodies are pathogenic in plasminogen activator knockout mice. J. Invest. Dermatol. 113: 22–25.
7. ESAKI, C. et al. 1995. Pharmacologic evidence for involvement of phospholipase C in pemphigus IgG–induced inositol 1,4,5-trisphosphate generation, intracellular calcium increase, and plasminogen activator secretion in DJM-1 cells, a squamous cell carcinoma line. J. Invest. Dermatol. 105: 329–333.
8. MILNER, Y. et al. 1999. Pemphigus—an autoimmune disease of the skin: cell-cell separation versus membranal signaling and apoptosis in acantholysis. In The Decade of Autoimmunity, pp. 197–207. Elsevier Science. Amsterdam/New York.
9. SANCHEZ-CARPINTERO, I. et al. 2004. In vivo blockade of pemphigus vulgaris acantholysis by inhibition of intracellular signal transduction cascades. Br. J. Dermatol. 151: 565–570.
10. AMAGAI, M. et al. 2000. Toxin in bullous impetigo and staphylococcal scalded-skin syndrome targets desmoglein 1. Nat. Med. 6: 1275–1277.
11. AOYAMA, Y., M.K. OWADA & Y.A. KITAJIMA. 1999. A pathogenic autoantibody, pemphigus vulgaris–IgG, induces phosphorylation of desmoglein 3, and its dissociation from plakoglobin in cultured keratinocytes. Eur. J. Immunol. 29: 2233–2240.

12. NGUYEN, V.T. *et al.* 2004. Pemphigus vulgaris IgG and methylprednisolone exhibit reciprocal effects on keratinocytes. J. Biol. Chem. **279:** 2135–2146.
13. DIAZ, L.A. & C.L. MARCELO. 1978. Pemphigoid and pemphigus antigens in cultured epidermal cells. Br. J. Dermatol. **98:** 631–637.
14. SCHILTZ, J.R .& B. MICHEL. 1976. Production of epidermal acantholysis in normal human skin *in vitro* by the IgG fraction from pemphigus serum. J. Invest. Dermatol. **67:** 254–260.
15. ANHALT, G.J. *et al.* 1982. Induction of pemphigus in neonatal mice by passive transfer of IgG from patients with the disease. N. Engl. J. Med. **306:** 1189–1196.
16. WEISSMAN, V. *et al.* 1978. The correlation between the antibody titers in sera of patients with pemphigus vulgaris and their clinical state. J. Invest. Dermatol. **71:** 107–109.
17. CRESWELL, S.N. *et al.* 1981. Correlation of circulating intercellular antibody titres in pemphigus with disease activity. Clin. Exp. Dermatol. **6:** 477–483.
18. FITZPATRICK, R.E. & V.D. NEWCOMER. 1980. The correlation of disease activity and antibody titers in pemphigus. Arch. Dermatol. **116:** 285–290.
19. ISHII, K. *et al.* 1997. Characterization of autoantibodies in pemphigus using antigen-specific enzyme-linked immunosorbent assays with baculovirus-expressed recombinant desmogleins. J. Immunol. **159:** 2010–2017.
20. D'AGOSTO, G. *et al.* 2004. Evaluation of recombinant antigen-based assays for diagnosis of bullous autoimmune diseases. Clin. Diagn. Lab. Immunol. **11:** 762–765.

Evaluation of the BioPlex™ 2200 ANA Screen

Analysis of 510 Healthy Subjects: Incidence of Natural/Predictive Autoantibodies

O. SHOVMAN,[a] B. GILBURD,[a] O. BARZILAI,[a] E. SHINAR,[b] B. LARIDA,[c]
G. ZANDMAN-GODDARD,[a] S. R. BINDER,[c] AND Y. SHOENFELD[a,d]

[a]Center for Autoimmune Diseases, Department of Medicine "B",
Chaim Sheba Medical Center, Tel-Hashomer, Israel

[b]National Blood Bank, Ramat Gan, Israel

[c]Bio-Rad Laboratories, Hercules, California 94547, USA

[d]Sackler Faculty of Medicine, Incumbent of the Laura Schwarz-Kip Chair for Research of
Autoimmune Diseases, Tel-Aviv University, Tel-Aviv, Israel

ABSTRACT: The BioPlex™ 2200 ANA Screen is a fully automated system that
determines levels for 13 different autoimmune antibodies of established clinical
significance. The objective of this study was to determine the specificity of the
BioPlex™ 2200 ANA Screen assay and to analyze the antibody profile samples
collected from healthy subjects against comparative ELISA and IIF screening
methods. A total of 510 specimens were randomly selected from a cohort of
apparently healthy blood bank donors. Samples were distributed to five age
brackets. All samples were tested using Bio-Rad's ANA Screen kit. Specificity
was compared to IIF and ELISA results. Most of the samples were found
negative in all ANA screening systems (84.5% by IIF, 92.5% by BioPlex™ 2200
ANA Screen kit, and 94.5% by ELISA). The frequency of positive results was
highest (15.5%) using IIF, in comparison to almost similar results (5.5% vs.
7.5%) achieved by ANA ELISA and BioPlex™ 2200 ANA Screen kits. The positive rate of autoantibodies was significantly reduced when analyzed by different
combinations of ANA screen assays (from 2.35% using IIF + BioPlex ANA
Screen tests to 0.98% by using all three tests). Using the BioPlex™ 2200 ANA
Screen system, we were able to identify samples with high levels of individual
antibodies: anti-dsDNA at 20–63 IU/mL, antichromatin at 4–8 AI, anti-
SmRNP at 2–6 AI, and anti-RNPA at 2–4.5 AI. Importantly, from 7 IIF and
ELISA positive sera, 5 of these were also BioPlex 2200 positive, suggesting that
the BioPlex is seeing the samples that are of the greatest interest, using the
established techniques. The specificity of the BioPlex 2200 ANA Screen analysis
of 13 different analytes (dsDNA, centromere B, chromatin, Jo1, ribosomal P,
RNP 68, RNP A, Scl-70, Sm, SmPNP, SS-A52, SS-A60, SS-B) is comparable
($P < 0.252$) to the ELISA ANA screening test. Like the ELISA, the BioPlex 2200
has a lower ($P < 0.001$) positive rate than IIF for the autoantibody screening.

KEYWORDS: ANA; autoantibodies; autoimmunity; predictive value; healthy;
multiplexed assay

Address for correspondence: Yehuda Shoenfeld, M.D., FRCP, Head, Department of Medicine
"B" and Center for Autoimmune Diseases, Chaim Sheba Medical Center, Tel-Hashomer 52621,
Israel. Voice: +972-3-5302652; fax: +972-3-5352855.
shoenfel@post.tau.ac.il

Ann. N.Y. Acad. Sci. 1050: 380–388 (2005). © 2005 New York Academy of Sciences.
doi: 10.1196/annals.1313.120

INTRODUCTION

Measurement of autoantibodies provides supporting evidence in the diagnosis and monitoring of systemic rheumatic diseases. The presence of autoantibodies in the sera of healthy subjects in low–medium titers is reported frequently.[1] The role and predictive value of this incidental finding of autoantibodies is uncertain.

In the last several years, a different constellation has been raised, namely, that the presence of autoantibodies in healthy populations might be a marker of future autoimmune disease.[2,3] Initially, this notion has been supported by data showing increased concentration of anti-DNA antibodies before the clinical onset of SLE[4] and autoantibodies against IgM rheumatoid factor[5] or anti–cyclic citrullinated peptide (anti-CCP)[5,6] prior to the clinical onset of rheumatoid arthritis. Pregnancy-triggered autoimmune conditions such as postpartum rheumatoid arthritis[7] and thyroid autoimmune disease[8] have been predicted by the existence of respective autoantibodies: rheumatoid factor and antithyroid-peroxidase antibodies (anti-TPO) detected in previously healthy pregnant women. Therefore, an identification of specific antibodies might allow the proper selection of patients with preclinical natural history, risk stratification of potential autoimmune diseases, follow-up of specific populations, and possibly preventive trials in the future. Hence, high-throughput technology in which hundreds of autoantibodies can be analyzed simultaneously is necessary.

The multiplexed assay plays an important role in laboratory work. Considerable data confirm the advantage of the multiplexed technology and its applications in diverse fields of medicine, including cancer research, cytokines, gene expression, and genetic and infectious diseases.[9–14] An application of multiplexed technology in the field of autoimmunity suggests that this assay may be suitable as a sensitive screening method for detection of numerous autoantibodies in patients with autoimmune diseases.[15–18] It has been demonstrated that multiplexed technology offers a useful tool for the detection of ANA and extractable nuclear antigens in autoimmune diseases.[15,16] Furthermore, an assessment of the multiplexed system in patients with Sjögren's syndrome[17] and SLE[18] confirmed its specificity, sensitivity, and reproducibility for measuring autoantibodies.

The BioPlex 2200 multiplexed system was developed for high-throughput analysis of 13 autoimmune analytes simultaneously in a single tube. The current evaluation of the BioPlex 2200 system for assessment of Epstein-Barr immunologic status[19] or IgM *Toxoplasma gondii* antibodies[20] proposed its potential for the diagnosis and surveillance of infectious diseases.

The objective of this study was to determine the specificity of the BioPlex 2200 ANA Screen assay in the analysis of an antibody profile in 510 samples collected from healthy subjects against comparative enzyme immunoassay (ELISA) and indirect immunofluorescence (IIF) screening methods.

METHODS

A total of 510 specimens were randomly selected from a cohort of apparently healthy blood bank donors. Samples were distributed to five age brackets, as shown in TABLE 1. All samples were tested using the BioPlex™ 2200 system (BioPlex) (Bio-Rad Laboratories, Hercules, CA). Specificity was compared to IIF (Kallestad

TABLE 1. Characterization of healthy subjects

Age (years)	Male (no.)	Female (no.)	Total
20–30	24	101	125
30–40	25	98	123
40–50	25	95	120
50–60	25	99	124
60–70	5	13	18
Total	104	406	510

TABLE 2. Frequency of autoantibodies in healthy subjects evaluated by different ANA screening methods

Method	Positive rate
IIF	15.5% (79)
ELISA	5.5% (28)
BioPlex ANA Screen	7.5% (38)

HEp-2 cell line substrate, Bio-Rad Laboratories, Redmond, WA) and ELISA (Autoimmune EIA ANA Screening Test, Bio-Rad Laboratories, Hercules, CA) results determined at the Chaim Sheba Medical Center.

The BioPlex™ 2200 system employs multiplexed bead technology to simultaneously perform measurements of 13 autoantibodies in a single tube as previously described.[21] The overall specificity of the BioPlex 2200 ANA Screen kit was calculated by considering each of the 13 analytes as a separate test performed on each sample (e.g., 510 samples × 13 autoantibodies = 6630 results). Fisher's exact test was used for comparison of frequency of positive autoantibody rate.

RESULTS

Five hundred ten samples from healthy subjects were evaluated for presence of autoantibodies by three different assays (IIF, ELISA, and BioPlex 2200 ANA Screen kit). The majority of the samples were found negative in all ANA screening systems (84.5% by IIF, 92.5% by BioPlex 2200 ANA Screen kit, and 94.5% by ELISA). The frequency of positive results (TABLE 2) was highest (15.5%) using IIF, in comparison to almost similar results (5.5% vs. 7.5%) obtained by using ANA ELISA and BioPlex 2200 ANA Screen kits. It is remarkable that the positivity rate of the BioPlex is similar to the ELISA ANA kit, given that it is based on 13 times as many determinations. The positive rate of autoantibodies (TABLE 3) was significantly reduced after analysis with different combinations of ANA screening assays (from 2.35% using IIF + BioPlex ANA Screen tests to 0.98% by using all three tests). Importantly, from 7 IIF and ELISA positive sera, 5 of these were also BioPlex positive, suggesting that the BioPlex is seeing the samples that are of the greatest interest, using the established techniques. Low positive rates of all 13 autoantibodies were found in the

TABLE 3. Frequency of elevated autoantibody titers determined by different combinations of ANA screening methods

Methodology	Positive rate
IIF + BioPlex ANA Screen	2.35% (12)
ELISA + BioPlex ANA Screen	1.96% (10)
IFA + ELISA	1.37% (7)
IIF + ELISA + BioPlex ANA Screen	0.98% (5)

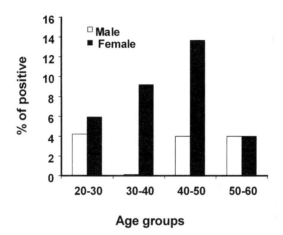

FIGURE 1. The prevalence of positive rate of autoantibodies in different age groups as evaluated by the BioPlex 2200 ANA Screen kit.

BioPlex 2200 ANA Screen kit. For 9 of 13 analytes, the positivity rate was <1.0%. These 9 include all the analytes that are associated with scleroderma and myositis (centromere, Scl-70, Jo-1) as well as 2 markers that are most specific for SLE (ribosomal P and Sm). This confirms that a positive finding by BioPlex for these analytes is likely to have a very high positive likelihood ratio (TABLE 4). The 40 positive results (0.6%) obtained with the BioPlex are out of a total of 6630 (510 × 13) determinations, indicating that the specificity by analyte is >99.4%. The significantly higher positive rate (FIG. 1) of autoantibodies was detected in females by the BioPlex ANA Screen test (30–40 and 40–50 year-groups). Using the BioPlex 2200 ANA Screen kit, we were able to identify samples with high levels of individual antibodies: anti-DNA, 20–63 IU/mL (FIG. 2A); antichromatin, 4–8 AI (FIG. 2B); anti-SmRNP, 2–6 AI (FIG. 2C); and anti-RNP A, 2–4.5 AI (FIG. 2D).

DISCUSSION

The capability of multiplexed technology to analyze several parameters simultaneously might permit large-scale prospective studies of healthy individuals.

TABLE 4. Frequency of the elevated titers of individual antibodies in healthy subjects

BioPlex ANA Screen individual analyte	Positive rate
dsDNA	1.0% (5)
Centromere B	0.2% (1)
Chromatin	1.4% (7)
Jo1	0.0% (0)
Ribosomal P	0.2% (1)
RNP 68	0.2% (1)
RNP A	1.8% (9)
Scl-70	0.2% (1)
Sm	0.2% (1)
SmRNP	1.2% (6)
SS-A52	0.2% (1)
SS-A60	0.6% (3)
SS-B	0.8% (4)
Overall (6630)	0.6% (40)

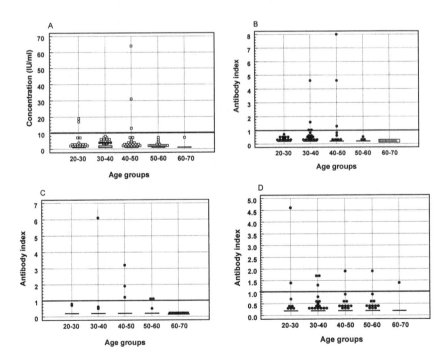

FIGURE 2. Elevated level of individual antibodies determined by the BioPlex 2200 Screen kit: **(A)** anti-dsDNA; **(B)** antichromatin; **(C)** anti-SmRNP; and **(D)** anti-RNP A.

In the present study, we evaluated a new method using a panel of multiplexed flow cytometer–based immunoassays combined with computer-assisted pattern recognition. A number of important lessons are clear from these observations: BioPlex 2200 ANA Screen analysis of 510 sera from well-distributed healthy blood donors for 13 different analytes (dsDNA, centromere B, chromatin, Jo1, ribosomal P, RNP 68, RNP A, Scl-70, Sm, SmPNP, SS-A52, SS-A60, SS-B autoantibodies) yielded low "false-positive" results of less than 2% (e.g., anti-dsDNA, 1%; antichromatin, 1.6%; anti-RNP A, 1.8%; others, <0.2%). These observations were comparable to auto-antibody screening obtained by ELISA and IIF. We found that the positive rate of autoantibodies was significantly reduced after analysis with different combinations of ANA screening assays (from 2.35% using IIF + BioPlex ANA Screen tests to 0.98% by using all three tests).

The prevalence of the positive rate of autoantibodies evaluated by the BioPlex 2200 ANA Screen kit was in correlation with the reported prevalence of different autoantibodies in healthy subjects.[1]

Therefore, our results allowed us to conclude that the BioPlex ANA Screen test is suitable as a sensitive screening test to confirm or to exclude the presence of large numbers of autoantibodies simultaneously. Based on these observations, several questions should be raised: What is the significance of positive results in the screening of a healthy patient and could these findings be of a predictive value? Do the 5, 10, or 12 "false-positive" results obtained by 2 or 3 methods or the high levels of antibodies (anti-DNA, chromatin, SmRNP, or RNP A) detected in sera of healthy patients predict development of an overt disease (e.g., SLE or other autoimmune diseases), or is the existence of these antibodies epiphenomenal and thus lacking in diagnostic importance? Will the findings of sequential antibody formation in asymptomatic persons improve future clinical outcomes and, if so, how?

Recently, the presence of specific serum antibodies was shown to precede the clinical onset of a variety of autoimmune diseases by many years. Hence, the existence of autoantibodies may be considered to be a marker for future development of these diseases in presently healthy individuals. The concept of a crescendo auto-immunity culminating in clinical illness was proposed by Arbuckle *et al.*,[4] who reported about progressive accumulation of specific autoantibodies, especially anti-DNA, prior to the onset of SLE. Nielen *et al.* found antibodies against IgM rheumatoid factor and anti-CCP in serum samples of patients with rheumatoid arthritis taken at a median of 4–5 years before disease onset.[5] The negative predictive value of these tests was 75% and the positive predictive value was 100%. Several pregnancy-related conditions have been studied, such as postpartum rheumatoid arthritis,[7] thyroid autoimmune disease,[8] and type 1 diabetes after gestational diabetes.[22] It has been demonstrated that future autoimmune disease can be predicted with respective auto-antibody assay at delivery. In our recent study, we proved that anti-*Saccharomyces cerevisiae* (ASCA) and antineutrophil cytoplasmic antibodies (ANCA) may predict the development of inflammatory bowel disease (IBD) years before the disease is clinically diagnosed and may even forecast the clinical course.[23] Furthermore, it was suggested that an immunological screening strategy and treatment follow-up can aid in the prevention of disease development or delay disease progression. For instance, detection of the highly specific diagnostic anti-pyruvate-dehydrogenase (PDH)[24] autoantibodies may precede primary biliary cirrhosis. An early initiation of a relatively benign therapy of ursodeoxycholic acid may delay the development of the fatal autoimmune disease.[25] Several large-scale trials are under way in which individuals with two or more diabetes-associated antibodies are receiving immuno-modulating therapy, such as nasal insulin in the Type 1 Diabetes Prediction and Prevention Project in Finland.[26]

Thus, on the one hand, an identification of patients that are prone to develop auto-immune disease may be important for follow-up, early diagnosis, and promising prevention by utilization of immune-modulating therapy. On the other hand, most patients who were tested positive for different autoantibodies never developed a disease. A positive result might have several meanings: It might be a clinical false-positive result, the patient may harbor an autoimmune condition at the time of test-ing, or it might predict a future disease. Perhaps, testing and follow-up of specific populations such as pregnant women or those with organ-specific autoimmune disease cannot be extrapolated to the general population, which is at lower risk of disease.[2] Additionally, autoimmune diseases may be characterized by dissimilar pat-tern of autoantibodies—for instance, more than 100 different autoantibodies found in SLE patients.[27] In general, the question related to the clinical importance of the presence of antibodies in asymptomatic subjects may only be resolved by additional prospective studies, with the follow-up of autoantibody titers as well as clinical symptoms in evaluated individuals. In this way, an application of BioPlex 2200 ANA Screen multiplexed technology is a useful tool for high-throughput screening of healthy populations.

CONCLUSIONS

The specificity of BioPlex 2200 ANA Screen analysis of 13 different analytes (dsDNA, centromere B, chromatin, Jo1, ribosomal P, RNP 68, RNP A, Scl-70, Sm, SmPNP, SS-A52, SS-A60, SS-B) is comparable ($P < 0.252$) to the ELISA ANA screening test. Like the ELISA, the BioPlex 2200 has a lower ($P < 0.001$) positive rate than IIF for the autoantibody screening.

For 9 of 13 analytes, the positivity rate was <1.0%. These 9 include all the ana-lytes that are associated with scleroderma and myositis (centromere, Scl-70, Jo-1) as well as 2 markers that are most specific for SLE (ribosomal P and Sm). This con-firms that a positive finding by BioPlex for these analytes is likely to have a very high positive likelihood ratio.

ACKNOWLEDGMENTS

O. Shovman and B. Gilburd contributed equally to this work.

REFERENCES

1. ABU-SHAKRA, M. & Y. SHOENFELD. 1993. Introduction to natural autoantibodies. *In* Natural Autoantibodies, pp. 15–33. CRC Press. Boca Raton, Florida.
2. SCOFIELD, R.H. 2004. Autoantibodies as predictors of disease. Lancet **363:** 1544–1546.
3. SHOENFELD, Y. & A. TINCANI. 2005. Autoantibodies—the smoke and the fire. Auto-immunity **38:** 1–2.

4. ARBUCKLE, M.R., M.T. MCCLAIN, M.V. RUBERTONE *et al.* 2003. Development of autoantibodies before the clinical onset of systemic lupus erythematosus. N. Engl. J. Med. **349:** 1526–1533.
5. NIELEN, M.M., D. VAN SCHAARDENBURG, H.W. REESINK *et al.* 2004. Specific autoantibodies precede the symptoms of rheumatoid arthritis: a study of serial measurements in blood donors. Arthritis Rheum. **50:** 380–386.
6. RANTAPAA-DAHLQVIST, S., B.A. DE JONG, E. BERGLIN *et al.* 2003. Antibodies against cyclic citrullinated peptide and IgA rheumatoid factor predict the development of rheumatoid arthritis. Arthritis Rheum. **48:** 2741–2749.
7. IIJIMA, T., H. TADA, Y. HIDAKA *et al.* 1998. Prediction of postpartum onset of rheumatoid arthritis. Ann. Rheum. Dis. **57:** 460–463.
8. KITA, M., D.G. GOULIS & A. AVRAMIDES. 2002. Post-partum thyroiditis in a Mediterranean population: a prospective study of a large cohort of thyroid antibody positive women at the time of delivery. J. Endocrinol. Invest. **25:** 513–519.
9. DUNBAR, S.A., C.A. VANDER ZEE, K.G. OLIVER *et al.* 2003. Quantitative, multiplexed detection of bacterial pathogens: DNA and protein applications of the Luminex LabMAP system. J. Microbiol. Methods **53:** 245–252.
10. YE, F., M.S. LI, J.D. TAYLOR *et al.* 2001. Fluorescent microsphere–based readout technology for multiplexed human single nucleotide polymorphism analysis and bacterial identification. Hum. Mutat. **17:** 305–316.
11. PICKERING, J.W., T.B. MARTINS, M.C. SCHRODER & H.R. HILL. 2002. Comparison of a multiplex flow cytometric assay with enzyme-linked immunosorbent assay for quantitation of antibodies to tetanus, diphtheria, and Haemophilus influenzae type b. Clin. Diagn. Lab. Immunol. **9:** 872–876.
12. DE JAGER, W., H. TE VELTHUIS, B.J. PRAKKEN *et al.* 2003. Simultaneous detection of 15 human cytokines in a single sample of stimulated peripheral blood mononuclear cells. Clin. Diagn. Lab. Immunol. **10:** 133–139.
13. PRETL, K., K.A. CHESTERTON, J.T. SHOLANDER *et al.* 2003. Accurate, rapid characterization of HLA-specific antibodies using Luminex technology. Hum. Immunol. **64:** s108.
14. SEIDEMAN, J. & D. PERITT. 2002. A novel monoclonal antibody screening method using the Luminex-100 microsphere system. J. Immunol. Methods **267:** 165–171.
15. ROUQUETTE, A.M., C. DESGRUELLES & P. LAROCHE. 2003. Evaluation of the new multiplexed immunoassay, FIDIS, for simultaneous quantitative determination of antinuclear antibodies and comparison with conventional methods. Am. J. Clin. Pathol. **120:** 676–681.
16. SHOVMAN, O., B. GILBURD, G. ZANDMAN-GODDARD *et al.* 2005. Multiplexed AtheNa Multi-Lyte immunoassay for ANA screening in autoimune diseases. Autoimmunity **38:** 105–109.
17. GILBURD, B., M. ABU-SHAKRA, Y. SHOENFELD *et al.* 2004. Autoantibodies profile in the sera of patients with Sjögren's syndrome: the ANA evaluation—a homogeneous, multiplexed system. Clin. Dev. Immunol. **11:** 53–56.
18. MARTINS, T.B., R. BURLINGAME, C.A. VON MUHLEN *et al.* 2004. Evaluation of multiplexed fluorescent microsphere immunoassay for detection of autoantibodies to nuclear antigens. Clin. Diagn. Lab. Immunol. **11:** 1054–1059.
19. KLUTTS, J.S., R.S. LIAO, W.M. DUNNE, JR. & A.M. GRONOWSKI. 2004. Evaluation of a multiplexed bead assay for assessment of Epstein-Barr virus immunologic status. J. Clin. Microbiol. **42:** 4996–5000.
20. KAUL, R., P. CHEN & S.R. BINDER. 2004. Detection of immunoglobulin M antibodies specific for *Toxoplasma gondii* with increased selectivity for recently acquired infections. J. Clin. Microbiol. **42:** 5705–5709.
21. BINDER, S.R., M.C. GENOVESE, J.T. MERRILL *et al.* 2005. Automated multiplex analysis of 13 autoantibodies with computer-assisted interpretation. Lupus. Submitted.
22. FERBER, K.M., E. KELLER, E.D. ALBERT & A.G. ZIEGLER. 1999. Predictive value of human leukocyte antigen class II typing for the development of islet autoantibodies and insulin-dependent diabetes postpartum in women with gestational diabetes. J. Clin. Endocrinol. Metab. **84:** 2342–2348.
23. ISRAELI, E., I. GROTTO, B. GILBURD *et al.* 2005. Anti–*Saccharomyces cerevisiae* and antineutrophil cytoplasmic antibodies as predictors of inflammatory bowel disease. GUT. In press.

24. ZURGIL, N., R. BAKIMER, M. KAPLAN et al. 1991. Anti–pyruvate dehydrogenase auto-
    antibodies in primary biliary cirrhosis. J. Clin. Immunol. **11:** 239–245.
25. POUPON, R.E., K.D. LINDOR, A. PARES et al. 2003. Combined analysis of the effect of
    treatment with ursodeoxycholic acid on histologic progression in primary biliary
    cirrhosis. J. Hepatol. **39:** 12–16.
26. KUPILA, A., P. MUONA, T. SIMELL et al. 2001. Feasibility of genetic and immunological
    prediction of type I diabetes in a population-based birth cohort. Diabetologia **44:**
    290–297.
27. SHERER, Y., A. GORSTEIN, M.J. FRITZLER & Y. SHOENFELD. 2004. Autoantibody explosion
    in systemic lupus erythematosus: more than 100 different antibodies found in SLE
    patients. Semin. Arthritis Rheum. **34:** 501–537.

Autoimmunity and Coxsackievirus Infection in Primary Sjögren's Syndrome

ANTIGONI TRIANTAFYLLOPOULOU[a,b] AND
HARALAMPOS M. MOUTSOPOULOS[a]

[a]Department of Pathophysiology, National University of Athens Medical School, Athens, Greece

[b]Department of Medicine, Montefiore Medical Center, Albert Einstein College of Medicine, Bronx, New York, USA

ABSTRACT: Exocrine gland epithelial cells are the target of autoimmune pathology in primary Sjögren's syndrome (pSS). Their activated phenotype has incited the notion that they are infected by a virus. We recently presented evidence that coxsackieviruses may persistently infect the salivary glands of pSS patients. We hypothesize that coxsackieviruses may play a permissive role for the perpetuation and possibly the induction of autoimmune disease in pSS.

KEYWORDS: Sjögren's syndrome; autoimmunity; coxsackieviruses; epithelial cell activation

INTRODUCTION

Primary Sjögren's syndrome (pSS) is characterized by epithelial cell destruction and periepithelial lymphocytic infiltrates in multiple organ targets, of which most prominent are the salivary and lacrimal glands. The disease is thought to be auto-immune partly because autoantibodies are consistently detected in the serum and the salivary glands, and mostly because the antigenic triggers of chronic inflammation and epithelial cell destruction are largely unknown.

The majority of the mononuclear infiltrating cells are CD4+ cytotoxic T cells that express perforin and granzyme B.[1] There are limited studies in humans to suggest that these T cells are autoreactive. Analysis of the T cell clonotype by PCR–single strand conformation polymorphism and sequencing in a study of 4 SS patients inter-estingly showed that some of the T cells are expanding clonally and recognize shared epitopes,[2] one of which was identified as part of the self-antigen Ro (SSA).[3] The rest of those epitopes were not identified.

B cells are polyclonally activated, and produce immunoglobulins in the serum and in situ in the salivary glands, including autoantibodies against the self-antigens Ro (SSA) and La (SSB). As the disease becomes chronic and the antigenic triggers

Address for correspondence: Prof. H. M. Moutsopoulos, Department of Pathophysiology, National University of Athens Medical School, M. Asias 75, Goudi, Athens 11527, Greece. Voice: +30-210-7462513; fax: +30-210-7462664.
hmoutsop@med.uoa.gr

Ann. N.Y. Acad. Sci. 1050: 389–396 (2005). © 2005 New York Academy of Sciences.
doi: 10.1196/annals.1313.090

persist, B cells undergo oligoclonal expansion, organize with T cells and dendritic cells, and form ectopic lymphoid follicles.[1,4,5] Immunohistochemistry studies that used biotinylated Ro and La autoantigens to detect autoreactive B cells showed that only a small minority of B cells were positive.[5] Thus, the antigens that drive the B cell expansion, as in the case of T cells, have yet to be characterized.

EPITHELIAL CELL ACTIVATION IN PRIMARY SJÖGREN'S SYNDROME

While the inflammatory infiltrates expand, epithelial cells are destroyed, largely by undergoing apoptosis. Acinar epithelial cells that are terminally differentiated are affected the most, while ductal epithelial cells may survive until more advanced stages of the disease process.

It has long intrigued the researchers of the syndrome that the pSS epithelial cells, while being the target of the destructive inflammatory response, display markers of activation. In situ hybridization and immunohistochemistry studies revealed that epithelial cells in pSS expresss proinflammatory cytokines IL-1, IL-6, and TNF-α;[1] chemokines, such as BCA-1 and ELC;[6] and costimulatory B7.2 molecules.[1] The latter were constitutively expressed in salivary gland epithelial cell lines and were functional in vitro.[7]

Furthermore, salivary gland epithelial cells in pSS inappropriately express phenotypic markers of antigen-presenting cells. MHC class II molecules are known to be expressed by professional antigen-presenting cells such as dendritic cells, macrophages, and B cells. However, epithelial cells in pSS express MHC II,[1] in agreement with other studies in organ-specific autoimmune diseases, such as Graves' disease, Hashimoto's thyroiditis, and autoimmune diabetes.[8-10] It is unclear whether MHC II induction in nonprofessional antigen-presenting cells is driven intrinsically by the activated epithelial cells themselves, extrinsically by an autoimmune reaction, or even by an unknown infectious agent. Interestingly, in the case of Helicobacter pylori infection, MHC class II molecules are induced on the surface of gastric epithelial cells by the invading Helicobacter and bind the Helicobacter enzyme urease, thereby inducing gastric epithelial cell death through apoptosis.[11,12]

VIRUSES AND INFECTIOUS EPITHELITIS

The presence of a virus has long been postulated as the intrinsic factor that activates the epithelial cells in pSS.[1] Viral infections may cause apoptosis of the infected host cells, but also induction of cytokines and chemokines.[13]

HCV, HIV, and HTLV-1[14-16] have been associated with infectious sialadenitis, but none of those agents was shown to produce the full spectrum of systemic clinical manifestations along with the circulating autoantibodies that characterize pSS. Further, it has been clear that the majority of patients with pSS have no evidence of concomitant HIV or HTLV-1 infection.[17] Despite the above limitations, HCV-associated Sjögren's-like syndrome may be indistinguishable by pSS when looking only at the salivary gland immunopathology and thus deserves some attention in this context.

HCV RNA and core antigen were detected by in situ hybridization and immunohistochemistry, respectively, in the salivary gland epithelial cells from HCV patients.[18] The lymphocytic infiltrates in chronic HCV sialadenitis are CD4 T cell predominant as in pSS, but they tend to score significantly lower than pSS in the degree of inflammation.[19] It is noteworthy that lymphoid follicle–like structures are detected in the liver of chronically HCV-infected patients, but have not been reported in the salivary glands.[20] The B cells in those lesions are clonally restricted,[20] much like the B cells in the salivary glands of chronic pSS.[4] Thus, a possible conclusion is that HCV infection primarily affects the liver and secondarily the salivary glands, while liver involvement, if any, in pSS will manifest as pericholangial[1] and not intrahepatic inflammation.

COXSACKIEVIRUSES AND PRIMARY SJÖGREN'S SYNDROME

We recently presented evidence that coxsackievirus infection is associated with pSS.[21] Differential display experiments revealed a 94-bp fragment of coxsackievirus B4 (CVB4) protease P2A that was differentially expressed in a pSS salivary gland sample, but not in the control sample. In a preliminary group of 8 pSS, 9 secondary SS (sSS), and 8 control subjects, use of RT-PCR for the coxsackieviral conserved noncoding region and sequencing confirmed the presence of coxsackieviral sequences in 7 pSS patients, while sSS and control salivary gland biopsies tested negative for coxsackieviruses (FIG. 1A). Sequencing revealed a 97–99% similarity with the non-coding region of CVB4 in 4 samples and with coxsackievirus A13 (CVA13) in 3 samples. CVB4 is known to be associated with autoimmune diabetes.[22,23] CVA13 has no established human disease association, although it has diabetogenic properties in mice.[24] It is of note that simultaneously collected samples of PBMCs were negative for coxsackieviruses by RT-PCR, making an acute infection in pSS patients less likely (D. Liakos *et al.*, manuscript in progress).

Immunohistochemistry in salivary gland biopsies for the common enteroviral VP1 capsid protein antigen was performed using a monoclonal antibody (DAKO, clone 5D8/1). This antibody recognizes an epitope in the N-terminal of capsid protein VP1, which is conserved in the enterovirus genus. Its specificity and sensitivity for the detection of enteroviruses in epithelial cell culture and tissue samples have been the object of prior reports,[25–30] including immunohistochemistry studies for the detection of CVB3 in formalin-fixed myocardial biopsies from patients with dilated cardiomyopathy and Western blot experiments on CVB3-infected epithelial cell cultures.

In our study, positive staining with the anti-VP1 antibody was observed in 11 out of 12 pSS samples, 1 out of 8 sSS samples, and 0 out of 16 controls. In positive biopsies, both the infiltrating lymphocytes and the ductal epithelial cells stained positive, while the majority of acinar epithelial cells were negative (FIGS. 1C–1F).[21]

Does Persistent Coxsackievirus Infection Play a Role in pSS Immunopathology?

In contrast to the traditional belief that coxsackieviruses are only mediators of acute infectious syndromes, multiple studies have shown that they are able to establish persistent noncytolytic infections *in vitro*,[13,31–34] which may result in auto-immunity induction *in vivo*.[22,23,35,36]

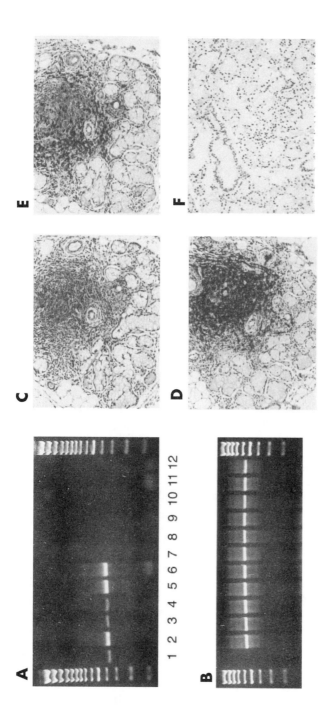

FIGURE 1. Detection of enteroviruses in salivary gland biopsies from pSS and control patients. (**A**) Representative example of RT-PCR of the 5′ noncoding region of enteroviral RNA. All primary pSS samples were positive (lanes 2–6), while disease controls were negative (lanes 7–12). Lane 1 shows amplification of CVB4 as a positive control. (**B**) RT-PCR for the b-actin housekeeping gene was performed in all samples to verify the integrity and equal loading of RNA. (**C**) Representative immunohistochemistry of a pSS salivary gland biopsy, with the anti-VP1 antibody staining positive both ductal epithelial cells and infiltrating mononuclear cells. (**D**) Serial section in the same experiment with anti-CD20 antibody showing that anti-VP1 positive cells have the same spatial distribution as B lymphocytes. (**E**) Serial section of the same biopsy showing anti-CD3 staining for T lymphocytes. (**F**) Immunohistochemistry with anti-VP1 antibody in a control salivary gland biopsy. (Original magnification: ×40.)

In genetically predisposed, but not spontaneously diabetic mice that express a restricted diabetogenic TCR specific to an islet antigen and have subclinical insulitis, infection with CVB4 induced diabetes.[37] Horwitz et al.[38] showed that activation of autoreactive T cells by CVB4 was the result of a bystander effect that required virus-induced islet cell damage and could not be reproduced by nonspecific release of cytokines in situ.

In the case of autoimmune dilated cardiomyopathy, persistent CVB3 infection of cardiac myocytes in mice was found to induce autoreactive antibodies and T lymphocytic infiltrates in the myocardium.[39–41] In this case, besides immune-mediated pathology, myocardial damage through direct viral cytotoxicity may also play a role: transgenic mice expressing coxsackieviral cDNA specifically in cardiomyocytes developed excitation-contraction coupling abnormalities.[42] Further, the enteroviral protease 2A was shown to cleave human dystrophin in vitro and in vivo.[43]

We hypothesize that in pSS, after an initial phase of acute viremia, coxsackieviruses localize in the secondary lymphoid organs and chronically persist in B cells and follicular dendritic cells, similar to the kinetics of CVB3 in chronic cardiomyopathy.[44] Using B lymphocytes as carriers,[45] coxsackieviruses may be transferred to susceptible epithelial cells, in genetically predisposed individuals, where they may establish a noncytolytic persistent infection. The induction of autoimmunity may be related to coxsackievirus interactions with host-cell proteins since cleavage of La protein by enteroviruses has been shown to result in translocation of La from the nucleus to the cytoplasm.[46] The latter event is thought to be vital for the recognition of La as an autoantigen.[1] Epitope spreading may result in further self-antigen recognition by the immune system.[47]

In line with this hypothesis, persistent infection of epithelial cells by coxsackieviruses is a possible trigger of B cell polyclonal activation. As shown by Hunziker et al.,[48] persistent noncytopathic LCMV infection of pancreatic islet cells resulted in polyclonal hypergammaglobulinemia and production of autoantibodies. Furthermore, expansion of CD4+ cytotoxic T cells may result due to the persistent state of inflammation induced by a chronic viral infection, as shown in the cases of HIV-1, EBV, and CMV.[49] Finally, the tropism of coxsackieviruses for B lymphocytes and follicular dendritic cells[44] may play a pivotal role in their successful evasion of the antiviral immune response and may chronically stimulate the formation of lymphoid follicles, thus perpetuating the autoimmune pathology in the site of autoantigen induction.

CONCLUSIONS

Primary Sjögren's syndrome is an interesting model of organ-specific autoimmune disease that is accompanied by epithelial cell destruction and activation, polyclonal B cell and CD4+ cytotoxic T cell expansion, organization of B lymphocytes and dendritic cells into lymphoid follicles, polyclonal hypergammaglobulinemia, and circulating autoantibodies. We presented data showing that persistent coxsackievirus infection is associated with the syndrome and provided a hypothetic mechanism for the induction of autoimmunity in pSS by persistent coxsackieviruses. It will be worthwhile to test this hypothesis experimentally in animals since it may allow us to dissect autoimmunity generated by viruses and antiviral immunopathology mediated by the persistence of an invading microorganism.

ACKNOWLEDGMENTS

We thank Dr. Nikos Tapinos for critical review of the manuscript and helpful discussions.

REFERENCES

1. TAPINOS, N.I., M. POLIHRONIS, A.G. TZIOUFAS et al. 1999. Sjögren's syndrome: auto-immune epithelitis. Adv. Exp. Med. Biol. **455:** 127–134.
2. MATSUMOTO, I., K. TSUBOTA, Y. SATAKE et al. 1996. Common T cell receptor clonotype in lacrimal glands and labial salivary glands from patients with Sjögren's syndrome. J. Clin. Invest. **97**(8): 1969–1977.
3. SUMIDA, T., T. NAMEKAWA, T. MAEDA et al. 1996. New T-cell epitope of Ro/SSA 52 kDa protein in labial salivary glands from patients with Sjögren's syndrome. Lancet **348:** 1667.
4. STOTT, D., F. HIEPE, M. HUMMEL et al. 1998. Antigen-driven clonal proliferation of B cells within the target tissue of an autoimmune disease. J. Clin. Invest. **102**(5): 938–946.
5. SALOMONSSON, S., M.V. JONSSON, K. SKARSTEIN et al. 2003. Cellular basis of ectopic germinal center formation and autoantibody production in the target organ of patients with Sjögren's syndrome. Arthritis Rheum. **48**(11): 3187–3201.
6. XANTHOU, G., M. POLIHRONIS, A.G. TZIOUFAS et al. 2001. "Lymphoid" chemokine messenger RNA expression by epithelial cells in the chronic inflammatory lesion of the salivary glands of Sjögren's syndrome patients. Arthritis Rheum. **44**(2): 408–418.
7. KAPSOGEORGOU, E., H.M. MOUTSOPOULOS & M.N. MANOUSSAKIS. 2001. Functional expression of a costimulatory B7.2 (CD86) protein on human salivary gland epithelial cells that interacts with the CD28 receptor, but has reduced binding to CTLA4. J. Immunol. **166:** 3107–3113.
8. PUJOL-BORRELL, R., I. TODD, M. LONDEI et al. 1986. Inappropriate major histocompat-ibility complex class II expression by thyroid follicular cells in thyroid autoimmune disease and by pancreatic β cells in type I diabetes. Mol. Biol. Med. **3:** 159.
9. HANAFUSA, T., R. PUJOL-BORRELL, L. CHIOVATO et al. 1983. Aberrant expression of HLA-DR antigen on thyrocytes in Graves' disease: relevance for autoimmunity. Lancet **2:** 1111.
10. MARKMANN, J., D. LO, A. NAJI et al. 1988. Antigen presenting function of class II MHC expressing pancreatic beta cells. Nature **336:** 476.
11. FAN, X., S.E. CROWE, S. BEHAR et al. 1998. The effect of class II major histocompat-ibility complex expression on adherence of Helicobacter pylori and induction of apoptosis in gastric epithelial cells: a mechanism for T helper cell type 1–mediated damage. J. Exp. Med. **187**(10): 1659–1669.
12. FAN, X., H. GUNASENA, Z. CHENG et al. 2000. Helicobacter pylori urease binds to class II MHC on gastric epithelial cells and induces their apoptosis. J. Immunol. **165**(4): 1918–1924.
13. ZANONE, M., E. FAVARO, P. CONALDI et al. 2003. Persistent infection of human micro-vascular endothelial cells by coxsackie B viruses induces increased expression of adhesion molecules. J. Immunol. **171:** 438–446.
14. HADDAD, J., P. DENY, C. GUNZ-GOTHEIL et al. 1992. Lymphocytic sialadenitis of Sjögren's syndrome associated with chronic hepatitis C virus liver disease. Lancet **339:** 321–323.
15. OHYAMA, Y., S. NAKAMURA, H. HARA et al. 1998. Accumulation of human T lympho-tropic virus type 1–infected T cells in the salivary glands of patients with human T lymphotropic virus type 1–associated Sjögren's syndrome. Arthritis Rheum. **41**(11): 1972–1978.
16. TALAL, N., M.J. DAUPHINEE, H. DANG et al. 1990. Detection of serum antibodies to retroviral proteins in patients with primary Sjögren's syndrome. Arthritis Rheum. **33:** 774–781.

17. KORDOSSIS, T., S. PAIKOS, K. ARONI et al. 1998. Prevalence of Sjögren's-like syndrome in a cohort of HIV-1 positive patients: descriptive pathology and immunopathology. Br. J. Rheumatol. **37:** 691–695.

18. ARRIETA, J., E. RODRIGUEZ-INIGO, N. ORTIZ-MOVILLA et al. 2001. In situ detection of hepatitis C virus RNA in salivary glands. Am. J. Pathol. **158:** 259–264.

19. SCOTT, C.A., C. AVELLINI, L. DESINAN et al. 1997. Chronic lymphocytic sialoadenitis in HCV-related chronic liver disease: comparison with Sjögren's syndrome. Histopathology **30:** 41–48.

20. RACANELLI, V., D. SANSONNO, C. PICOLLI et al. 2001. Molecular characterization of B clonal expansions in the liver of chronically hepatitis C virus–infected patients. J. Immunol. **167:** 21–29.

21. TRIANTAFYLLOPOULOU, A., N. TAPINOS & H.M. MOUTSOPOULOS. 2004. Evidence for coxsackievirus infection in primary Sjögren's syndrome. Arthritis Rheum. **50**(9): 2897–2902.

22. YOON, J.W., M. AUSTIN, T. ONODERA & A.L. NOTKINS. 1979. Virus-induced diabetes mellitus: isolation of a virus from the pancreas of a child with diabetic ketoacidosis. N. Engl. J. Med. **300:** 1173–1179.

23. JAECKEL, E., M. MANNS & M. VON HERRATH. 2002. Viruses and diabetes. Ann. N.Y. Acad. Sci. **958:** 7–25.

24. BOCHAROV, E.F., I.P. SHORIN, I.A. SOLODOVNIKOVA et al. 1988. Diabetogenic properties of coxsackie A13 and coxsackie B4 viruses in experimental infection in mice. Vopr. Virusol. **33**(4): 469–474.

25. ZHANG, H., Y. LI, D.R. MCCLEAN et al. 2004. Detection of enterovirus capsid protein VP1 in myocardium from cases of myocarditis or dilated cardiomyopathy by immunohistochemistry: further evidence of enterovirus persistence in myocytes. Med. Microbiol. Immunol. (Berl.) **193**(2/3): 109–114.

26. BOURLET, T., J. GHARBI, S. OMAR et al. 1998. Comparison of a rapid culture method combining an immunoperoxidase test and a group specific anti-VP1 monoclonal antibody with conventional virus isolation techniques for routine detection of enteroviruses in stools. J. Med. Virol. **54:** 204–209.

27. ZHANG, H., Y. LI, T. PENG et al. 2000. Localization of enteroviral antigen in myocardium and other tissues from patients with heart muscle disease by an improved immunohistochemical technique. J. Histochem. Cytochem. **48:** 579–584.

28. SAMUELSON, A., M. FORSGREN & M. SALLBEREG. 1995. Characterization of the recognition site and diagnostic potential of an enterovirus group–reactive monoclonal antibody. Clin. Diagn. Lab. Immunol. **2:** 385–386.

29. TRABELSI, A., F. GRATTARD, M. NEJMEDDINE et al. 1995. Evaluation of an enterovirus group–specific anti-VP1 monoclonal antibody, 5D8/1, in comparison with neutralization and PCR for rapid identification of enterovirus in cell culture. J. Clin. Microbiol. **33:** 2454–2457.

30. YOUSEF, G.E., I.N. BROWN & J.F. MOWBRAY. 1987. Derivation and biochemical characterization of an enterovirus group–specific monoclonal antibody. Intervirology **28:** 163–170.

31. FRISK, G., A.M. LINDBERG & H. DIDERHOLM. 1999. Persistence of coxsackievirus B4 infection in rhabdomyosarcoma cells for 30 months. Arch. Virol. **144:** 2239–2245.

32. BRILOT, F., W. CHEHADEH, C. CHARLET-RENARD et al. 2002. Persistent infection of human thymic epithelial cells by coxsackievirus B4. J. Virol. **76**(10): 5260–5265.

33. HARRATH, R., T. BOURLET, O. DELEZAY et al. 2005. Coxsackievirus B3 replication and persistence in intestinal cells from mice infected orally and in the human CaCo-2 cell line. Submitted.

34. CHEHADEH, W., J. KERR-CONTE, F. PATTOU et al. 2000. Persistent infection of human pancreatic islets by coxsackievirus B is associated with alpha interferon synthesis in cells. J. Virol. **74**(21): 10153–10164.

35. LESLIE, K., R. BLAY, C. HAISH et al. 1989. Clinical and experimental aspects of viral myocarditis. Clin. Microbiol. Rev. **2**(2): 191–203.

36. ANDREOLETTI, L., P. WATTRE, C. DECOENE et al. 1995. Detection of enterovirus-specific RNA sequences in explanted myocardium biopsy specimens from patients with dilated or ischemic cardiomyopathy. Clin. Infect. Dis. **21:** 1315–1317.

37. HORWITZ, M., L. BRADLEY, J. HARBERTSON *et al.* 1998. Diabetes induced by coxsackievirus: initiation by bystander damage and not molecular mimickry. Nat. Med. **4**(7): 781–785.
38. HORWITZ, M., A. ILIC, C. FINE *et al.* 2002. Presented antigen from damaged pancreatic cells activates autoreactive T cells in virus-mediated autoimmune diabetes. J. Clin. Invest. **109**: 79–87.
39. NEUMANN, D.A., N.R. ROSE, A.A. ANSARI *et al.* 1994. Induction of multiple heart autoantibodies in mice with coxsackievirus B3– and cardiac myosin–induced autoimmune myocarditis. J. Immunol. **152**: 343–350.
40. WOLFGRAM, L.J., K.W. BEISEL & N.R. ROSE. 1985. Heart-specific autoantibodies following murine coxsackievirus B3 myocarditis. J. Exp. Med. **161**(5): 1112–1121.
41. HUBER, S.A. & P.A. LODGE. 1984. Coxsackievirus B-3 myocarditis in BALB/c mice: evidence for autoimmunity to myocyte antigens. Am. J. Pathol. **116**(1): 21–29.
42. WESSELY, R., K. KLINGEL, L.F. SANTANA *et al.* 1998. Transgenic expression of replication-restricted enteroviral genomes in heart muscle induces defective excitation-contraction coupling and dilated cardiomyopathy. J. Clin. Invest. **102**: 1444–1453.
43. BADORFF, C., N. BERKELY, S. MEHROTRA *et al.* 2000. Enteroviral protease 2A directly cleaves dystrophin and is inhibited by a dystrophin-based substrate analogue. J. Biol. Chem. **275**(15): 11191–11197.
44. ANDERSON, D.R., J.E. WILSON, C.M. CARTHY *et al.* 1996. Direct interactions of coxsackievirus B3 with immune cells in the splenic compartment of mice susceptible or resistant to myocarditis. J. Virol. **70**(7): 4632–4645.
45. KLINGEL, K., S. STEPHAN, M. SEUTER *et al.* 1996. Pathogenesis of murine enterovirus myocarditis: virus dissemination and immune cell targets. J. Virol. **70**(12): 8888–8895.
46. SHIROKI, K., T. ISOYAMA, S. KUGE *et al.* 1999. Intracellular redistribution of truncated La protein produced by poliovirus 3C pro-mediated cleavage. J. Virol. **73**(3): 2193–2200.
47. TOPFER, F., T. GORDON & J. MCCLUSKEY. 1995. Intra- and intermolecular spreading of autoimmunity involving the nuclear self-antigens La (SS-B) and Ro (SS-A). Proc. Natl. Acad. Sci. USA **92**: 875–879.
48. HUNZIKER, L., M. RECHER, A. MACPHERSON *et al.* 2003. Hypergammaglobulinemia and autoantibody induction mechanisms in viral infections. Nat. Immunol. **4**(4): 343–349.
49. APPAY, V., J. ZAUNDERS, L. PAPAGNO *et al.* 2002. Characterization of CD4+ CTLs *ex vivo.* J. Immunol. **168**: 5954–5958.

Human and Nonhuman Primate Lentiviral Infection and Autoimmunity

NATTAWAT ONLAMOON,[a] KOVIT PATTANAPANYASAT,[a] AND
AFTAB A. ANSARI[b]

[a]Faculty of Medicine, Siriraj Hospital, Mahidol University, Bangkok, Thailand

[b]Department of Pathology and Laboratory Medicine, Emory University
School of Medicine, Atlanta, Georgia 30322, USA

ABSTRACT: The goal of this communication is to summarize the following—the
types of autoimmune responses that have been characterized in human HIV-1
infection; the potential mechanisms that were initially thought to be the basis
for such autoimmune responses; the prevalence and incidence of conventional
autoimmune diseases with HIV-1 infection; the spectrum of autoimmune disorders following the institution of HAART and its associated mechanisms; the
role of such autoimmunity in SIV-infected nonhuman primates; and the molecular basis for autoimmune responses, such as the role of exosomes in lentiviral
disease.

KEYWORDS: HIV-1; SIV; human; nonhuman; primates; autoimmune; infection;
lentivirus

INTRODUCTION

The consequences of lentiviral infections, such as HIV-1 in humans and SIV in
Asian rhesus or pig-tailed macaques, are remarkably similar.[1] Both of these lentiviruses cause an AIDS-like disease exemplified by depletion of CD4[+] T cells, a
gradual loss of memory T cell response, a state of immunodeficiency, increased susceptibility to opportunistic infections, diarrhea, weight loss, and ultimately death.
Ever since the discovery of the etiology of AIDS, there have been several studies that
have documented the occurrence of autoantibodies against a number of self-
antigens,[2–5] the presence of cytotoxic T cells[6–8] with specificity for autologous non-
infected CD4[+] T cells (believed to contribute to CD4[+] T cell loss), and the association of HIV-1 infection with a number of autoimmune diseases, such as rheumatoid
arthritis, SLE, etc.[9] Induction of such immune responses in the setting of immunodeficiency was considered somewhat of a paradox because such patients have been
noted to gradually lose antigen-specific memory T cell responses and demonstrate
reduced responses to primary immunization with conventional vaccines that correlated with CD4 counts and viral loads. These associations of HIV-1 infection with

Address for correspondence: Aftab A. Ansari, Department of Pathology and Laboratory Medicine,
Emory University School of Medicine, Atlanta, GA 30322.
pathaaa@emory.edu

Ann. N.Y. Acad. Sci. 1050: 397–409 (2005). © 2005 New York Academy of Sciences.
doi: 10.1196/annals.1313.091

autoimmune diseases, often with contradictory interpretations, were considered complex because of a variety of findings; an example is listed here to provide one explanation for the loss of interest in defining relationships between HIV infection and autoimmune disease. Thus, it was noted that patients with rheumatoid arthritis (RA) demonstrate activated CD4$^+$ T cell and macrophage/dendritic lineage cells in the synovium during acute disease flare-ups. These are the precise lineages that are the target of HIV infection and, as such, they become an excellent target for HIV infection with several consequences. First of all, they would serve to increase viral loads and, second, the local inflammatory responses against HIV would be additive to the autoimmune-mediated inflammatory response, making the disease worse. Antiviral therapy for such patients has in select cases shown to lead to not only a decrease in viral load, but also to lead to remission from their autoimmune rheumatoid disease. However, the introduction of highly active antiretroviral therapy (HAART) has in these cases of RA exacerbated the rheumatoid disease.[10] Interest in the role of autoimmunity in the pathogenesis of HIV- and SIV-induced disease in human and nonhuman primates thus waned, until recently, not only because of the discovery of such complexities in clinical presentations, but also because of the more urgent need to define antiviral chemotherapies and to develop effective vaccines.

Two issues have brought back a renewed interest in the role of autoimmunity in HIV disease. Thus, first a relatively longer follow-up study of patients placed on HAART led to the discovery that such therapy leads to a disease termed "immune reconstitution syndrome", which has clinical features typical of autoimmune diseases.[11] This syndrome has also been termed "immune restoration disease" and "immune restoration inflammatory syndrome" (IRIS), all of which are basically the same clinical disease reflecting different scales of disorders of the immune system. Second, an increased understanding of the molecular basis by which lentiviruses are packaged has led to the discovery of a role for "exosomes",[12] which could potentially play an ever-increasing role not only in the pathogenesis of HIV, but in the induction of autoimmune disease. These two issues are discussed below in some detail. Thus, the goal of this communication is to summarize the following: our knowledge of the types of autoimmune responses that have been characterized in human HIV-1 infection; the potential mechanisms that were initially thought to be the basis for such autoimmune responses; the prevalence and incidence of conventional autoimmune disease with HIV-1 infection; the spectrum of autoimmune disorders following the institution of HAART and its associated mechanisms; the role of such autoimmunity in SIV-infected nonhuman primates; and, last, our current understanding of the molecular basis for autoimmune responses, such as the role of exosomes in lentiviral disease.

TARGETS OF AUTOIMMUNE RESPONSES

Basically, autoantibodies that have been identified in the sera of HIV-1-infected patients can be divided into three distinct but overlapping groups of autoantigens. These include autoantibodies against cell surface molecules such as CD4, MHC class I and II, TCR, and Fas, to name a few;[13–17] organ-specific autoantibodies such as antiplatelet antibodies, anti–cardiac myosin antibodies, anti–smooth muscle–specific antibodies, and anti–erythroid cell–specific antibodies;[18–20] and, lastly, nonorgan-specific antibodies such as antinuclear antibodies, antihistone antibodies, anti–double-stranded DNA antibodies,[21–24] and antiphospholipid antibodies.[25] Each of these categories of antibodies has been characterized to contribute to the pathogenesis of human HIV-1 infection. Thus, autoantibodies against cell surface molecules have been reasoned to lead to depletion of CD4[+] T cells[26] by either complement-mediated activation or antibody-dependent cellular cytotoxicity–mediated effector mechanisms.[27,28] Autoantibodies against platelets and cardiac tissue myosin have been thought to contribute to thrombocytopenic purpura and myocarditis. Other autoantibodies have been thought to contribute to systemic autoimmune disease. Some of the issues that remain unresolved in reviewing the results of all these studies is whether the extent and severity of autoimmune disease is worse if the autoimmune disease precedes HIV infection and whether the autoimmune disease that is seen in HIV-infected patients is due to an existing predilection to develop autoimmune disease and was not induced by HIV infection, and thus was a comorbid condition. These issues are difficult to address objectively because most autoimmune diseases are manifest at later stages of life than cohorts that acquire HIV infection, and the number of cases that can be studied to address such issues at any given single clinical center appear limited.

POTENTIAL MECHANISMS IMPLICATED IN THE AUTOIMMUNITY OF HIV-1-INFECTED PATIENTS

To a large extent, the mechanisms which investigators outlined as the basis for the occurrence of autoimmune disease in HIV-infected patients were no different than those discussed for standard autoimmune diseases. Thus, one of the major hypotheses put forward was that of a role for molecular mimicry in the induction of autoimmune antibodies in the plasma of HIV-1-infected patients. Hence, similarity between a number of HIV proteins and self-molecules was identified.[28,29] This included the finding of the reactivity of anti-gp41 antibody against human MHC molecules.[28] Detailed structural and sequence analysis of the HIV-1 gp-41/gp120 led to the concept of a high degree of homology between self-molecules and HIV-1.[30,31] These findings were followed by the reports of the occurrence of anti-idiotypic antibodies against gp-120 and the role such anti-idiotypic antibodies may play in the induction of autoimmune responses secondary to binding of such antibodies to the CD4 molecule. Thus, the view that was put forward was that "molecular complementarity" exists between the binding sequence of HIV-1 gp120 and the CD4 molecule and that anti-idiotypic antibodies against gp120 would have the potential of binding to the CD4 molecule and lead either directly or indirectly to the elimination of the CD4[+] T cells and/or dysregulate the induction of immune responses, contributing to the generation of autoimmune disease.[32] A third mechanism that received considerable attention concerned the potential ability of select HIV-1-encoded proteins to serve as "superantigens". The HIV-1-encoded proteins included gp120[33] and HIV-1 "nef".[34] While the mechanisms by which HIV gp120 serves as a superantigen have been defined primarily in terms of the ability of the gp120 molecule to bind selectively to the VH3 Ig gene-encoding family and to B cells that express VH3 Ig,[35] the ability of the HIV-1-encoded "nef" gene has been somewhat controversial.[36] Some studies have also documented polyclonal B cell activation as a consequence of HIV-1 infection and have reasoned this activity to lead to hypergammaglobulinemia, which has been well characterized in HIV-1-infected individuals.[37] More recently, a role for regulatory T cells (Tregs) has been implicated in HIV-1-infected patients. This issue is important because a major role of a dysregulation of this cell subset has been implicated in a variety of autoimmune diseases;[38] such cells are known to maintain tolerance to self-antigens and control autoimmunity. Thus, it has been shown in one study that removal of CD4[+] CD25hi–expressing cells from the PBMCs of HIV-1-infected patients resulted in enhanced HIV- and CMV-specific immune response.[39] In addition, in a separate study, it was shown that the presence of a significant frequency of such Tregs was beneficial to HIV-1-infected patients because they suppressed and thus regulated T cell activation, proliferation, and cytokine synthesis, and their presence was correlated with decreased viral load.[40] Thus, while such cells may suppress virus-specific immune responses, they also suppress cell activation, thereby leading to less viral replication and lower viral loads. The precise role of such Tregs in regulating autoimmunity in HIV-1-infected individuals can only be hypothesized at this point because detailed studies of this subset in HIV-infected individuals with autoimmune disease—in particular, in the era of HAART—remain to be performed.

HIV INFECTION AND THE INCIDENCE OF AUTOIMMUNE DISEASE

As stated above, a plethora of autoantibodies has been catalogued from the sera from HIV-1 infected patients. These include antibodies against cardiolipin, DNA, small nucleoriboproteins (snRNPs), thyroglobulin, thyroid peroxidase, myosin, erythropoietin, to name a few.[41] Similarly, a number of autoimmune diseases have been documented in HIV-1-infected patients. These include systemic lupus erythematosus (SLE), rheumatoid arthritis (RA), vasculitis, PBC, antiphospholipids syndrome, polymyositis, Graves' disease, ITP, etc.[41] Early on, it was reasoned that loss of immunocompetence in HIV-infected individuals would make them more susceptible to opportunistic infections that could, in turn, lead to either the induction or exacerbation of an underlying autoimmune disease due to the likelihood of molecular mimicry. While most of the above data are derived from either single case reports and a limited number of prevalence studies, for example, the studies that document the prevalence of cryoglobulinemia and serological markers of autoimmune disease in 97 HIV-1-infected patients[42] and the study of autoimmune hemolytic anemia associated with HIV-1 infection,[43] there have been limited studies in the past on the true incidence of autoimmune diseases in HIV-1-infected patients. The reasons for this are not clear, but are likely due to the difficulty in the proper diagnosis of autoimmune disease in HIV-1-infected patients, or that autoimmune diseases and HIV target different populations, or that the immunological disorders are skewed and polarized such that they result in excluding each other. The prevalence/incidence is therefore too low and would require extensive and costly epidemiologic studies. Clearly, the epidemiological data appear to support this latter view. Thus, based on the available data and mathematical calculations performed in 1993, if there were 500,000 SLE patients and 220,000 AIDS patients in the United States, there would at least be 400 concurrent cases of HIV and SLE.[44] This is clearly not the case because only 6 cases were reported in the period that this study was performed. Other reports similarly confirmed the low occurrence of SLE in HIV-infected patients[45] and that chemotherapy in fact led to reactivation of SLE in the few patients who were co-infected.[46] However, as stated above, now that we have had sufficient time to follow HIV-1-infected patients following the advent of HAART and have noticed the emergence of autoimmune disease in these patients,[47] it is becoming increasingly clear that the reconstitution of the immune system in such patients is not optimal and has given rise to the introduction of a new lexicon in medicine termed "immune reconstitution disease".

IMMUNE RESTORATION DISEASE (IRD) OR IMMUNE RESTORATION INFLAMMATORY SYNDROME (IRIS)

The fact that HAART-based therapy led to a marked decrease in the incidence of opportunistic infections (O.I.'s) and the resolution of O.I.'s in HIV-1-infected patients following HAART provided strong evidence that such chemotherapeutic strategies were effective in restoring immune responses in such patients.[48] This view was further supported by the findings of increased CMV-specific cellular responses in HIV-1-infected patients co-infected with CMV accompanied by the lowering of CMV viremia.[49] However, soon thereafter, a number of reports emerged on a series of "atypical" infections in patients following placement on HAART-based therapies that were considered inflammatory disorders in response to O.I.'s and thought to be initially due to partial and incomplete immune reconstitution.[50] Since then, there has been a growing acceptance that a distinct clinical syndrome exists which appears to accompany patients that are placed on HAART who respond to such therapy by lowering of viral loads and regaining immune competence. The response of such patients to the pathogen in question is of pathogenic consequence and in select cases leads to death and can be viewed as an uncontrolled immune response against the pathogen. The syndrome has been given different names by different investigators, and until the pathogenic mechanisms are fully defined this problem will likely continue. It is also clear that learning the mechanisms by which such an overzealous immune response is initiated may lead to refined methodologies for the therapy and management of such patients. French *et al.*[51] have divided the clinical immune restoration disease syndromes into three different types. One type includes syndromes with an infectious etiology and thus it is termed infectious IRD; a second type includes those with a granulomatous inflammation of the lungs and is termed sarcoid IRD; and the last category includes syndromes in which a new autoimmune disease occurs and/or an existing autoimmune disease is exacerbated, shortly after HAART-based therapies; it has been termed autoimmune IRD. Under infectious IRD, a description of mycobacterial infections is included, such as *Mycobacterium avium* complex, *Mycobacterium tuberculosis*, and *M. leprae*,[52] cryptococcal infections, pneumocystis, hepatitis B and C infections, CMV, varicella zoster, herpes simplex, JC viral infections, and a few others (reviewed in French *et al.*[51]). Under sarcoid IRD, the disease is distinct from typical HIV-associated sarcoidosis because it involves $CD4^+$ T cells instead of $CD8^+$ T cells and could be secondary to treatment with IL-2 as an adjunct therapy. The most common diseases included among the autoimmune IRD are SLE, polymyositis, and RA, followed by Guillain-Barré and Graves' disease. Of interest has been the finding of reactivity against the CD4 molecule in HIV-1-infected patients on HAART.[53] These patients have been a subject of a T cell vaccination protocol with the rationale that incomplete CD4[+] T cell recovery in these patients was secondary to immune response against the CD4 molecule and that immunizing them with glutaraldehyde-treated enriched populations of their own anti-CD4 reactive cells (auto–anti-idiotypic therapy protocol) would be beneficial. Also of interest was the finding that such immunizations led to a decrease in anti-CD4 immunity in 5 of 7 patients with no effect on viral load.[53] These are novel approaches that require additional studies to precisely assess the usefulness of such an approach. In general, it appears that infectious disease etiology–based IRDs occur relatively early following the institution of HAART, whereas non-infectious disease–based etiologies of IRD occur relatively late post-institution of HAART, although this may be an overgeneralization. It is also clear that therapeutic management of such patients is going to be rather complex. Thus, it will depend on the reason for the occurrence of the IRD, of which there may be many. Secondarily, it could be due to incomplete immune reconstitution (holes in the immunological repertoire), contribution of genetic traits, selective loss of synthesis and/or response of a select number of cytokines such as Th1 versus Th2, a role for dysfunctional regulatory T cells, abnormal synthesis and/or response to growth factors, or a combination of these. Thus, additional studies are required to gain a better understanding of the mechanisms of these diseases before therapeutic strategies can be devised.

ROLE OF AUTOIMMUNITY IN SIV-INFECTED NONHUMAN PRIMATES

To date, there have been very few studies performed on characterizing the prevalence of autoimmune disease in SIV-infected nonhuman primates. There are several reasons. First, the focus on the use of SIV-infected nonhuman primates has been to utilize them to study candidate vaccines and antiretroviral drugs; this is appropriate because of the clinical need and importance of such studies. Second, the viral isolates that are being utilized are those that cause rapid disease so that answers to the efficacy of antiretroviral drugs and vaccines can be acquired in a timely fashion. Thus, the time course of experimental SIV infection and disease is relatively rapid compared with HIV-infected humans. It is unlikely that the disease pathogenesis secondary to autoimmune disease would be readily apparent in such a short time frame. In this context, it is important to note that whereas pathology directly related to auto-immune disease has been rarely reported, there clearly have been reports of the occurrence of autoimmune antibodies in SIV-infected nonhuman primates. These reports include the finding of autoimmune antibodies against histone H2B only in the sera of SIV-infected rhesus macaques, but not uninfected macaques.[54] Of importance was the finding that such antibodies were not found in the sera of SIV-infected sooty mangabeys. This issue is discussed below. Other autoimmune manifestations that have been reported include the finding of autoimmune hemolytic anemia in SIV-infected rhesus macaques, which was determined to be multifactorial.[55,56] There have also been reports of increased prevalence of cardiac disease in SIV-infected rhesus macaques.[57] However, it is not clear whether this disease is secondary to autoimmune responses against cardiac tissue, due to myocyte loss secondary to innocent bystander effects or due to increased susceptibility to cardiotropic viruses that initiate the disease, which leads to myocarditis and later to cardiomyopathy.

An issue that has not been recognized widely in the HIV/AIDS research community is the complete lack of any signs of autoimmune disease in select African species of nonhuman primates including the species studied by our lab for the last two decades. Thus, sooty mangabey monkeys bred in captivity at the Yerkes Primate Center of Emory University are naturally infected with SIV, but to date have never shown any signs of SIV-associated clinical disease or of any autoimmune disease.[58,59] This is not due to viral loads, route of infection, or lack of SIV-specific humoral immune response. Thus, some mangabeys have had viral loads of >1 million viral copies/mL of plasma for years and have yet to show any signs of clinical disease. Clearly, such viral loads lead to disease and death of Asian macaques infected with SIV. Groups of SIV-seronegative mangabeys have been experimentally infected intravenously with SIVmac239, but again, while they do get infected and develop viral and cellular viral loads and anti-SIV–specific antibody responses similar to SIVmac239-infected rhesus macaques, they have not shown any signs of clinical disease to date. Thus, there is a paradox within this species. If the SIV-specific immune response is protective of disease, then why do they continue to have high viral loads? If they have high viral loads, then why do they not develop disease? In the context of this review, why do these animals not develop any clinical signs of autoimmune disease if chronic infection is reasoned to be required to lead to autoimmune disease in HIV-1-infected humans? Thus, these issues need to be addressed. It is important to point out in this regard that our laboratory has screened sera from SIV-infected rhesus macaques and sooty mangabeys. Only the sera from SIV-infected rhesus macaques appear to contain antibodies either against the cell line in which the virus is prepared (if a cell line is used for the preparation of the viral stock) or against rhesus PBMCs if day 3 PHA blasts from rhesus macaques are used to grow the viral stocks. The potential of such antibodies to induce pathology *in vivo* has not been defined, and therefore the significance of such antibodies is not clear at present. Preliminary studies appear to suggest that such antibodies are primarily directed at MHC class I and II molecules and against costimulatory molecules such as CD80 and CD86. Such antibodies may contribute to immune suppression characteristic of such SIV-infected rhesus macaques.

MOLECULAR BASIS FOR THE AUTOIMMUNE RESPONSE: THE EXOSOME HYPOTHESIS

It is becoming increasingly clear that host proteins are in fact a significant component of lentiviruses as they emerge from infected cells. In addition, these virus particles either bud from the cell surface or exit from the cell in the form of multi-vesicular bodies (MVB) depending on the cell lineage in which they replicate (see FIG. 1). Thus, while these virus particles normally bud from the cell surface of both CD4[+] T cells and macrophages, they form MVB when they are packaged within the macrophage lineage of cells.[12] These MVB have been termed "exosomes" and are reasoned to be the "Trojan horses" for the infectious cycle in HIV infection.[60] Exosomes like microparticles have also been shown to carry with them chemokine receptor molecules such as CXCR4, which are critical for entry of X4 tropic viruses into the appropriate target cells.[61] Thus, coculture of such CXCR4 containing microparticles has been shown to transfer such chemokine receptors to cell lineages

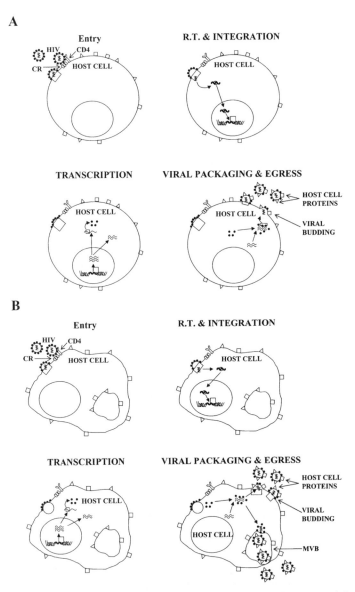

FIGURE 1. Steps in the infection, replication, and production of HIV-1 particles in (**A**) CD4+ T cells and (**B**) macrophages. The viral life cycle basically has four steps: entry; reverse transcription (RT) and integration into the host cell genome; viral transcription; and finally viral assembly and egress from the host cell. The figures are meant to signify differences in the assembly of the virus within CD4+ T cells and macrophages. Thus, as seen in the figure, virus predominantly exits from the CD4+ T cells via budding, but incorporates within it a number of host cell membrane proteins. In the case of macrophages, the virus can not only exit via budding, but also can form multivesicular bodies (MVB), which have also been termed "exosomes". In this case, the virus also incorporates a variety of host cell proteins. Such host cell proteins carrying exosomes are hypothesized to play a role in the induction of immune responses against self-proteins.

that do not otherwise express such chemokine receptors and, importantly, such receptors are then decorated on the otherwise infection-resistant cell in a form that makes these cells now susceptible to HIV-1 infection. What is relevant for this review is that when such viruses replicate and emerge from these lineages they incorporate and carry with them a variety of host proteins. Of great interest is that the type of host proteins incorporated includes those that are involved in normal immune responses such as MHC class I/class II molecules, costimulatory molecules, etc., as well as molecules that are part of "lipid rafts" and constituents of the "immunological synapse". These packaged virions are by themselves capable of inducing novel immune responses because the host cell MHC molecules that are part of the virions bear peptides that are likely also to be part of host cellular proteins, and in the presence of costimulatory molecules they maintain the potential to induce immune responses. There have been a few studies that have used exosomes as immunogens and have successfully utilized them as therapeutic vehicles for cancer.[62,63] They have been found to be highly potent, inducing immune responses in the pg range.[64] It has been suggested that this increased efficiency is due to the molecular nature of the assembly of the MHC and costimulatory molecules encompassing the virions. Also of great interest is that there are marked differences in the type of host proteins that get incorporated into such virions depending on the cell lineage in which they replicate. These findings have prompted a re-examination of the quality and specificity of the host immune response against lentiviruses by those involved in defining the role of host proteins in the immune response against lentiviruses. Our laboratory has become involved in the comparative analysis of the nature of the host proteins that get incorporated in virions emerging from CD4[+] T cells and macrophage lineages both from SIV-infected disease-resistant sooty mangabeys that do not demonstrate any autoimmune responses and from SIV-infected disease-susceptible rhesus macaques that do develop autoimmune responses. The rationale is that the findings from such a study will help define the potential reasons for the difference in the ability to induce autoimmune responses and, more importantly, the distinct clinical outcome in these two species. Also, germane to this review, it may provide us with some clues as to the mechanisms of induction of autoantibodies in SIV-infected macaques, but not SIV-infected mangabeys. Preliminary data from such electrospray mass spectrometric analysis (extracts analyzed by ESI-MS, positive mode) already have shown differences in the types of proteins that are incorporated in SIV replicating within cells from macaques and mangabeys. Thus, whereas virions from CD4[+] T cells from rhesus macaques appear to contain predominantly host cell cytoskeleton proteins, they also contain CD80 and a number of additional costimulatory molecules. SIV preparations from mangabeys on the other hand also contain cytoskeleton proteins; however, these are different from those from macaques and, in addition, contain proteins that are unique from proteins found in SIV preparations of macaque CD4[+] T cells, but that have still to be identified.

CONCLUSIONS

The importance of a role for autoimmunity in the pathogenesis of lentiviral infection has had an undulating history. While autoimmune antibodies were recognized to exist in the sera of patients with HIV-1 infection and in SIV-infected nonhuman primates, their importance in contributing to the pathogenesis of lentiviral infection and vice versa was not clearly defined. There were also reports that HIV-1 infection induced immunosuppression that in fact led to remission of a number of autoimmune diseases. While limited formal prevalence and/or incidence studies on the occurrence of autoimmune diseases in HIV-1-infected patients were conducted, it was generally considered that such occurrences were rare, most likely because the two diseases occurred in different population groups. More recently, however, two issues have once again rekindled the interest for the role of autoimmune disease in lentiviral infections. This includes the finding of the phenomenon of "immune restoration disease" and the more detailed understanding of the molecular mechanisms by which lentiviruses are assembled, packaged, and exit from the cells in which they replicate; this gives rise to the concept that these virions, especially in the form of exosomes, may play an important role in the immune response not only against the viral proteins, but also against self-proteins that become incorporated within the virions. Findings on these two issues contribute to our current concept of HIV pathogenesis.

ACKNOWLEDGMENTS

This work was supported by a grant from the National Institutes of Health (No. NIH-AI-27057).

N. Onlamoon is on leave from Mahidol University.

REFERENCES

1. McClure, H.M., D.C. Anderson, P.N. Fultz, et al. 1989. Spectrum of disease in macaque monkeys chronically infected with SIV/SMM. Vet. Immunol. Immunopathol. **21:** 13–24.
2. Kloster, B.E., R.H. Tomar & T.J. Spira. 1984. Lymphocytotoxic antibodies in the acquired immune deficiency syndrome (AIDS). Clin. Immunol. Immunopathol. **30:** 330–335.
3. Dorsett, B., W. Cronin, V. Chuma, et al. 1985. Anti-lymphocyte antibodies in patients with the acquired immune deficiency syndrome. Am. J. Med. **78:** 621–626.
4. Kiprov, D.D., R.E. Anderson, P.R. Morand, et al. 1985. Antilymphocyte antibodies and seropositivity for retroviruses in groups at high risk for AIDS. N. Engl. J. Med. **312:** 1517.
5. Tomar, R.H., P.A. John, A.K. Hennig, et al. 1985. Cellular targets of antilymphocyte antibodies in AIDS and LAS. Clin. Immunol. Immunopathol. **37:** 37–47.
6. Israel-Biet, D., A. Venet, K. Beldjord, et al. 1990. Autoreactive cytotoxicity in HIV-infected individuals. Clin. Exp. Immunol. **81:** 18–24.
7. Zarling, J.M., J.A. Ledbetter, J. Sias, et al. 1990. HIV-infected humans, but not chimpanzees, have circulating cytotoxic T lymphocytes that lyse uninfected CD4+ cells. J. Immunol. **144:** 2992–2998.
8. Grant, M.D., F.M. Smail & K.L. Rosenthal. 1994. Cytotoxic T-lymphocytes that kill autologous CD4+ lymphocytes are associated with CD4+ lymphocyte depletion in HIV-1 infection. J. Acquir. Immune Defic. Syndr. **7:** 571–579.
9. Morrow, W.J., D.A. Isenberg, R.E. Sobol, et al. 1991. AIDS virus infection and autoimmunity: a perspective of the clinical, immunological, and molecular origins of the autoallergic pathologies associated with HIV disease. Clin. Immunol. Immunopathol. **58:** 163–180.

10. WEGRZYN, J., J.M. LIVROZET, J.L. TOURAINE, *et al.* 2002. Rheumatoid arthritis after 9 years of human immunodeficiency virus infection: possible contribution of tritherapy. J. Rheumatol. **29:** 2232–2234.
11. STOLL, M. & R.E. SCHMIDT. 2004. Adverse events of desirable gain in immunocompetence: the immune restoration inflammatory syndromes. Autoimmun. Rev. **3:** 243–249.
12. NGUYEN, D.G., A. BOOTH, S.J. GOULD, *et al.* 2003. Evidence that HIV budding in primary macrophages occurs through the exosome release pathway. J. Biol. Chem. **278:** 52347–52354.
13. CHAMS, V., T. JOUAULT, E. FENOUILLET, *et al.* 1988. Detection of anti-CD4 autoantibodies in the sera of HIV-infected patients using recombinant soluble CD4 molecules. AIDS **2:** 353–361.
14. GOLDING, H., F.A. ROBEY, F.T. GATES III, *et al.* 1988. Identification of homologous regions in human immunodeficiency virus I gp41 and human MHC class II beta 1 domain. I. Monoclonal antibodies against the gp41-derived peptide and patients' sera react with native HLA class II antigens, suggesting a role for autoimmunity in the pathogenesis of acquired immune deficiency syndrome. J. Exp. Med. **167:** 914–923.
15. LOPALCO, L., C. DE SANTIS, R. MENEVERI, *et al.* 1993. Human immunodeficiency virus type 1 gp120 C5 region mimics the HLA class I alpha 1 peptide-binding domain. Eur. J. Immunol. **23:** 2016–2021.
16. LAKE, D.F., S.F. SCHLUTER, E. WANG, *et al.* 1994. Autoantibodies to the alpha/beta T-cell receptors in human immunodeficiency virus infection: dysregulation and mimicry. Proc. Natl. Acad. Sci. USA **91:** 10849–10853.
17. STRICKER, K., E. KNIPPING, T. BOHLER, *et al.* 1998. Anti-CD95 (APO-1/Fas) autoantibodies and T cell depletion in human immunodeficiency virus type 1 (HIV-1)–infected children. Cell Death Differ. **5:** 222–230.
18. VAN DER LELIE, J., J.M. LANGE, J.J. VOS, *et al.* 1987. Autoimmunity against blood cells in human immunodeficiency-virus (HIV) infection. Br. J. Haematol. **67:** 109–114.
19. CURRIE, P.F., J.H. GOLDMAN, A.L. CAFORIO, *et al.* 1998. Cardiac autoimmunity in HIV related heart muscle disease. Heart **79:** 599–604.
20. SIPSAS, N.V., S.I. KOKORI, J.P. IOANNIDIS, *et al.* 1999. Circulating autoantibodies to erythropoietin are associated with human immunodeficiency virus type 1–related anemia. J. Infect. Dis. **180:** 2044–2047.
21. CASSANI, F., L. BAFFONI, E. RAISE, *et al.* 1991. Serum non-organ specific autoantibodies in human immunodeficiency virus 1 infection. J. Clin. Pathol. **44:** 64–68.
22. ARGOV, S., A. SCHATTNER, R. BURSTEIN, *et al.* 1991. Autoantibodies in male homosexuals and HIV infection. Immunol. Lett. **30:** 31–35.
23. MULLER, S., P. RICHALET, A. LAURENT-CRAWFORD, *et al.* 1992. Autoantibodies typical of non-organ-specific autoimmune diseases in HIV-seropositive patients. AIDS **6:** 933–942.
24. KYRIAKIS, K., A. TOSCA, J. KATSANTONIS, *et al.* 1992. Detection of autoimmunity parameters in the acquired immunodeficiency syndrome (AIDS). Int. J. Dermatol. **31:** 113–116.
25. HASSOUN, A., Z. AL-KADHIMI & J. CERVIA. 2004. HIV infection and antiphospholipid antibody: literature review and link to the antiphospholipid syndrome. AIDS Patient Care STDS **18:** 333–340.
26. DALGLEISH, A.G. 1995. Autoimmune mechanisms of depletion of CD4 cells in HIV infection. Br. J. Haematol. **91:** 525–534.
27. DANIEL, V., C. SUSAL, R. WEIMER, *et al.* 1995. Sequential occurrence of IgM, IgM/IgG, and gp120-IgM/IgG complement complexes on CD4+ lymphocytes in relation to CD4+ blood lymphocyte depletion in HIV+ hemophilia patients: results of a 10-year study. Immunol. Lett. **47:** 97–102.
28. BLACKBURN, R., M. CLERICI, D. MANN, *et al.* 1991. Common sequence in HIV 1 GP41 and HLA class II beta chains can generate crossreactive autoantibodies with immuno-suppressive potential early in the course of HIV 1 infection. Adv. Exp. Med. Biol. **303:** 63–69.
29. SILVESTRIS, F., R.C. WILLIAMS, JR. & F. DAMMACCO. 1995. Autoreactivity in HIV-1 infection: the role of molecular mimicry. Clin. Immunol. Immunopathol. **75:** 197–205.

30. POWELL, P.D., J.C. DEMARTINI, P. AZARI, *et al.* 2000. Evolutionary stable strategy: a test for theories of retroviral pathology which are based upon the concept of molecular mimicry. J. Theor. Biol. **202:** 213–229.

31. MAKSIUTOV, A.Z., A.G. BACHINSKII & S.I. BAZHAN. 2002. Searching for local similarities between HIV-1 and human proteins: application to vaccines. Mol. Biol. (Mosk.) **36:** 447–459.

32. SUSAL, C., G.W. HOFFMAN, V. DANIEL, *et al.* 1993. Complementarities and network interactions in AIDS. J. Autoimmun. **6:** 601–610.

33. TOWNSLEY-FUCHS, J., M.S. NESHAT, D.H. MARGOLIN, *et al.* 1997. HIV-1 gp120: a novel viral B cell superantigen. Int. Rev. Immunol. **14:** 325–338.

34. TANABE, T., B.A. TORRES, P.S. SUBRAMANIAM, *et al.* 1997. V beta activation by HIV Nef protein: detection by a simple amplification procedure. Biochem. Biophys. Res. Commun. **230:** 509–513.

35. NESHAT, M.N., L. GOODGLICK, K. LIM, *et al.* 2000. Mapping the B cell superantigen binding site for HIV-1 gp120 on a V(H)3 Ig. Int. Immunol. **12:** 305–312.

36. LAPATSCHEK, M.S., S. DURR, G. SUTTER, *et al.* 2001. Functional evaluation of HIV/SIV Nef as superantigen. Virology **282:** 329–337.

37. LANE, H.C., H. MASUR, L.C. EDGAR, *et al.* 1983. Abnormalities of B-cell activation and immunoregulation in patients with the acquired immunodeficiency syndrome. N. Engl. J. Med. **309:** 453–458.

38. BAECHER-ALLAN, C. & D.A. HAFLER. 2004. Suppressor T cells in human diseases. J. Exp. Med. **200:** 273–276.

39. AANDAHL, E.M., J. MICHAELSSON, W.J. MORETTO, *et al.* 2004. Human CD4+ CD25+ regulatory T cells control T-cell responses to human immunodeficiency virus and cytomegalovirus antigens. J. Virol. **78:** 2454–2459.

40. KINTER, A.L., M. HENNESSEY, A. BELL, *et al.* 2004. CD25(+)CD4(+) regulatory T cells from the peripheral blood of asymptomatic HIV-infected individuals regulate CD4(+) and CD8(+) HIV-specific T cell immune responses *in vitro* and are associated with favorable clinical markers of disease status. J. Exp. Med. **200:** 331–343.

41. ZANDMAN-GODDARD, G. & Y. SHOENFELD. 2002. HIV and autoimmunity. Autoimmun. Rev. **1:** 329–337.

42. BONNET, F., J.J. PINEAU, J.L. TAUPIN, *et al.* 2003. Prevalence of cryoglobulinemia and serological markers of autoimmunity in human immunodeficiency virus infected individuals: a cross-sectional study of 97 patients. J. Rheumatol. **30:** 2005–2010.

43. SAIF, M.W. 2001. HIV-associated autoimmune hemolytic anemia: an update. AIDS Patient Care STDS **15:** 217–224.

44. BARTHEL, H.R. & D.J. WALLACE. 1993. False-positive human immunodeficiency virus testing in patients with lupus erythematosus. Semin. Arthritis Rheum. **23:** 1–7.

45. PALACIOS, R. & J. SANTOS. 2004. Human immunodeficiency virus infection and systemic lupus erythematosus. Int. J. STD AIDS **15:** 277–278.

46. PALACIOS, R., J. SANTOS, P. VALDIVIELSO, *et al.* 2002. Human immunodeficiency virus infection and systemic lupus erythematosus: an unusual case and a review of the literature. Lupus **11:** 60–63.

47. DIRI, E., P.E. LIPSKY & R.E. BERGGREN. 2000. Emergence of systemic lupus erythematosus after initiation of highly active antiretroviral therapy for human immunodeficiency virus infection. J. Rheumatol. **27:** 2711–2714.

48. JACOBSON, M.A. & M. FRENCH. 1998. Altered natural history of AIDS-related opportunistic infections in the era of potent combination antiretroviral therapy. AIDS **12**(suppl. A): S157–S163.

49. WEINBERG, A., D.A. WOHL, S.M. WHINNEY, *et al.* 2003. Cytomegalovirus-specific IFN-gamma production is associated with protection against cytomegalovirus reactivation in HIV-infected patients on highly active antiretroviral therapy. AIDS **17:** 2445–2450.

50. STONE, S.F., P. PRICE & M.A. FRENCH. 2004. Immune restoration disease: a consequence of dysregulated immune responses after HAART. Curr. HIV Res. **2:** 235–242.

51. FRENCH, M.A., P. PRICE & S.F. STONE. 2004. Immune restoration disease after antiretroviral therapy. AIDS **18:** 1615–1627.

52. COUPPIE, P., S. ABEL, H. VOINCHET, *et al.* 2004. Immune reconstitution inflammatory syndrome associated with HIV and leprosy. Arch. Dermatol. **140:** 997–1000.

53. ABULAFIA-LAPID, R., Z. BENTWICH, Y. KEREN-ZUR, *et al.* 2004. T-cell vaccination against anti-CD4 autoimmunity in HIV-1 infected patients. J. Clin. Virol. **31**(suppl. 1): S48–S54.
54. FULTZ, P.N., R.B. STRICKER, H.M. MCCLURE, *et al.* 1990. Humoral response to SIV/SMM infection in macaque and mangabey monkeys. J. Acquir. Immune Defic. Syndr. **3**: 319–329.
55. HILLYER, C.D., A.R. BRODIE, A.A. ANSARI, *et al.* 1991. Severe autoimmune hemolytic anemia in SIVsmm9-infected *Macaca mulatta*. J. Med. Primatol. **20**: 156–158.
56. HILLYER, C.D., S.A. KLUMPP, J.M. HALL, *et al.* 1993. Multifactorial etiology of anemia in SIV-infected rhesus macaques: decreased BFU-E formation, serologic evidence of autoimmune hemolysis, and an exuberant erythropoietin response. J. Med. Primatol. **22**: 253–256.
57. SHANNON, R.P., M.A. SIMON, M.A. MATHIER, *et al.* 2000. Dilated cardiomyopathy associated with simian AIDS in nonhuman primates. Circulation **101**: 185–193.
58. ANSARI, A.A., N. ONLAMOON, P. BOSTIK, *et al.* 2003. Lessons learnt from studies of the immune characterization of naturally SIV infected sooty mangabeys. Front. Biosci. **8**: s1030–s1050.
59. ANSARI, A.A. 2004. Autoimmunity, anergy, lentiviral immunity and disease. Autoimmun. Rev. **3**: 530–540.
60. GOULD, S.J., A.M. BOOTH & J.E. HILDRETH. 2003. The Trojan exosome hypothesis. Proc. Natl. Acad. Sci. USA **100**: 10592–10597.
61. ROZMYSLOWICZ, T., M. MAJKA, J. KIJOWSKI, *et al.* 2003. Platelet and megakaryocyte-derived microparticles transfer CXCR4 receptor to cancer cells and make them susceptible to infection by X4-HIV. AIDS **17**: 33–42.
62. CHO, J.A., D.J. YEO, H.Y. SON, *et al.* 2004. Exosomes: a new delivery system for tumor antigens in cancer immunotherapy. Int. J. Cancer. In press.
63. CHAPUT, N., N.E. SCHARTZ, F. ANDRE, *et al.* 2004. Exosomes as potent cell-free peptide-based vaccine. II. Exosomes in CpG adjuvants prime naïve Tc1 lymphocytes leading to tumor rejection. J. Immunol. **172**: 2137–2146.
64. ALINE, F., D. BOUT, S. AMIGORENA, *et al.* 2004. *Toxoplasma gondii* antigen-pulsed–dendritic cell–derived exosomes induce a protective immune response against *T. gondii* infection. Infect. Immun. **72**: 4127–4137.

Autoimmune Nature of Influenza Atherogenicity

VICTOR S. GUREVICH,[a] VLADIMIR M. PLESKOV,[b] AND
MARGARITA V. LEVAYA[a]

[a]Center of Atherosclerosis and Lipid Disorders, Department of Cardiology,
Mechnicov's State Medical Academy, Saint Petersburg, Russia

[b]Laboratory of Pathomorphology, The Gripp Research Institute, Saint Petersburg, Russia

ABSTRACT: It has been observed during influenza epidemics and in a number
of population and clinical trials that this prevalent viral infection was associated
with increased death rates from cardiovascular diseases. The clinical and
experimental data that may explain accelerated coronary atherosclerosis in
influenza infection with implications involving autoimmune mechanisms are
analyzed in this article. Both cellular and humoral autoimmune modes could
be proposed to participate in the onset or progression of atheromatous lesions
due to influenza infection.

KEYWORDS: atherosclerosis; influenza; autoantibodies to oxidized LDL;
molecular mimicry; autoimmunity

INTRODUCTION

Influenza is the most common viral infection. As observed during influenza epidemics as well as shown in a number of population and clinical studies, it is associated with increased death rates from cardiovascular diseases.[1–3] On the other hand, it is generally accepted now that viral injury to the vessel wall is often the important component of atherogenesis.[4,5] In this article, we consider our own and literary clinical and experimental data from the point of view that atherogenicity of influenza infection is based on autoimmune mechanisms.

THE ROLE OF AUTOIMMUNE REACTIONS IN ATHEROGENESIS

The idea that circulating LDL must undergo some kind of structural modification before it becomes completely atherogenic was put forward by Brown and Goldstein in 1983.[6] Subsequently, so-called "scavenger receptors" were discovered and identified.[7,8] The concept of LDL oxidation was supported by many lines of evidence[9] and later it was shown that autoantibodies are generated against oxidized LDL and

Address for correspondence: Prof. Victor S. Gurevich, M.D., Ph.D., Center of Atherosclerosis and
Lipid Disorders, Chair of Cardiology, Mechnicov's State Medical Academy, 194291 pr. Kultury 4,
CMSD-122, Saint Petersburg, Russia. Voice: +7-812-559-9759; fax: +7-812-227-1201.
gur@cards.lanck.net

Ann. N.Y. Acad. Sci. 1050: 410–416 (2005). © 2005 New York Academy of Sciences.
doi: 10.1196/annals.1313.092

that the titers are correlated with the extent of atherosclerosis.[10] Now, it is well known that atherosclerotic lesions are filled with immune cells (macrophages and T cells) that can orchestrate inflammatory responses and initiate plaque destabilization.[11–13] Experimental and clinical studies have identified several other candidate lipid antigens and autoantibodies suggested to play important roles in atherogenesis. Antibodies against oxidized LDL, cardiolipin, heat-shock proteins, β_2-glycoprotein I, and lupus anticoagulant are thought to be the main antibodies associated with the enhanced risk of atherosclerosis and cardiovascular disease.[14–16]

EVIDENCE FOR ASSOCIATION OF INFLUENZA AND CORONARY HEART DISEASE

There is at present good evidence about an association between influenza and coronary events. More than two decades ago, Vullers *et al.*[3] described a striking temporal relationship between the onset of major coronary attack and influenza infection in patients aged from 53 to 75 years with chronic heart disease leading to a severe and even to a fatal course.

Ten years later, a retrospective analysis was made of 387 case reports of patients with coronary heart disease (CHD) admitted to the infectious department with the diagnosis of influenza.[5] In all the patients, the diagnosis was verified serologically with the aid of the hemagglutination inhibition test. Exacerbation of CHD was seen in the period of early convalescence in 60% of cases (days 5–13 of the disease). As compared to parainfluenza, influenza provoked the deterioration of CHD significantly more often.

Recently and worthy of note, analysis of a population study based on data from the United States showed an association between the age distribution of mortality due to an influenza pandemic in 1918–19 in the 10- to 49-year age bracket and the distribution of CHD mortality from 1920 to 1985 in survivors from the corresponding birth cohorts.[17,18]

According to data of Keatinge (2002), approximately half of excess winter deaths are due to coronary thrombosis, and the peak of winter mortality is about two days after the peak of a cold spell.[19] Among the main reasons of such a coincidence, the author considers hemoconcentration during cold exposure rather than respiratory infection. However, we know from other studies that the latter may also be one of the causes of atherothrombosis.[20,21]

On the opinion of Madjid *et al.*,[22] the relationship between influenza and CHD meets the main following criteria: strength of association, consistency, temporal sequence, coherence, biologic plausibility, and experimental evidence. Multivariate conditional logistic regression analysis revealed that the presence of heart disease is an independent prognostic factor for influenza-associated hospitalization and death in a general practice–based case-control study.[23] Some authors consider influenza even as a trigger for acute myocardial infarction.[24] In our own single-blind randomized study, IgG antibodies to influenza type A virus have been determined by enzyme-linked immunosorbent assay in 56 and 51 patients with and without clinical, laboratory, and instrumental signs of atherosclerosis progression, respectively. It has been shown that mean anti-IgG titers to influenza A virus are significantly higher in the group with documented progression of atherosclerosis in comparison with the con-

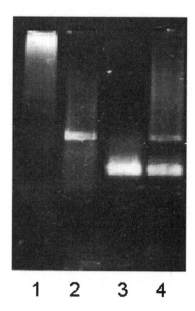

FIGURE 1. Detection of influenza genes in atherosclerotic plaques by RT-PCR.[25] RNA amplification products were detected by ethidium bromide staining of 3% agarose gel and visualized by ultraviolet transillumination. Lane 1: negative control; lane 2: influenza A (H1N1); lane 3: influenza A (H3N2); lane 4: positive control.

trol group. Also, we detected influenza A viral genomes in the vessel wall samples with histologically confirmed atherosclerotic injuries obtained during coronary bypass operation from ascendant aorta by reverse transcriptase–polymerase chain reaction (RT-PCR) with the use of primers for hemagglutinin of H1N1, H3N2 type A influenza viruses[25] (FIG. 1).

In addition, we found in the literature a description of one noncoronary cardiac death evidently associated with influenza. A previously healthy 27-year-old patient developed an acute cardiac failure at 1 week after onset of influenza-like respiratory infection, and died on her fourth day in hospital. Intravital differential diagnosis included myocardial infarction because of ECG changes and massive elevation of myocardial enzymes. However, the autopsy revealed severe myocarditis and intact coronary arteries. Influenza A virus was isolated from the myocardial tissue. At microscopic examination, the myocardium was heavily infiltrated with lymphocytes and an immunological mechanism of myocardial damage was suggested.[26]

INFLUENZA AND ATHEROGENIC IMMUNE AND AUTOIMMUNE REACTIONS

Both cellular and humoral autoimmune mechanisms could be proposed to partic-ipate in the onset or progression of atheromatous lesions due to influenza infection. In order to analyze mechanisms governing tolerance and autoimmunity to self-

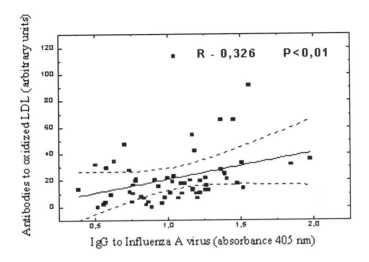

FIGURE 2. Correlation between antibody levels to oxidized LDL and to influenza virus type A in patients with progressing atherosclerosis.[31]

antigens, Caton *et al.*[27] have generated lineages of transgenic mice that express the influenza virus hemagglutinin (HA) as a neo-self-antigen. This study has revealed that specific subsets of HA-specific T and B cells are negatively selected from the primary repertoires of HA transgenic mice. However, substantial populations of HA-specific T and B cells evade negative selection and can be activated by virus immunization. Understanding the capacity of these autoreactive lymphocytes to differentiate and participate in antigen-specific immune responses will provide important insights into mechanisms by which autoimmunity might be induced by influenza viruses bearing structural similarities with self-antigens.[28] It has been also shown in the experimental studies that influenza infection in mice can lead to a marked increase in arterial macrophage trafficking[29] as well as to monocyte activation that may be associated with atherosclerosis and plaque rupture in the group with progressing atherosclerosis in comparison with the control group.[30] In our clinical study, the positive correlation between antibodies to influenza A virus and antibodies to oxidized LDL titers has been demonstrated in patients with laboratory and clinically documented progression of atherosclerosis[31] (FIG. 2). Autoimmune cross-reaction between the influenza viral HA and the apolipoprotein B was considered by Azambuja[18] as a linkage between influenza and atherogenic hypercholesterolemia.

Despite HDL (unlike LDL) not becoming antigenic, this lipoprotein can intensively influence atherogenic autoimmune reactivity because normal HDL contains at least four enzymes as well as apolipoproteins that can prevent the formation of the LDL-derived oxidized phospholipids or inactivate them *in vivo* after they are formed.[32] It has been recently shown that HDL can lose its protective potential due to influenza infection. Therefore, it is proposed that LDL-derived oxidized phospholipids and HDL may be part of a system of nonspecific innate immunity.[33] Obviously, any disbalance in this system may activate the opportunity of autoimmune reactions and increase the susceptibility to atherosclerosis.

VACCINATION AGAINST INFLUENZA AND PROGRESSING ATHEROSCLEROSIS

Naghavi et al.[34] were among the first who hypothesized that influenza vaccination might reduce the incidence of myocardial infarction in patients with established coronary atherosclerosis. A case-control study was performed by these authors on 218 CHD patients during the influenza season in 1997–98. Patients who experienced new myocardial infarction or unstable angina were included in the case group, and those who did not experience acute coronary syndrome were assigned to the control group. Adjusted for a history of influenza vaccination in previous years, multivariate logistic regression revealed the risk of myocardial infarction to be positively associated with current hypertension, hypercholesterolemia, and smoking, and negatively associated with influenza vaccination. Recently, the analysis of the first prospective clinical trial on influenza vaccination in acute coronary syndromes (FLUVACS) was published. This trial has provided evidence that influenza vaccination together with standard therapy may be useful during the winter season to reduce the risk of death and major cardiac events in patients with acute myocardial infarction. Information available in the FLUVACS database was analyzed to evaluate the efficacy of flu vaccination in different subgroups. Vaccination against influenza was effective in reducing the incidence of the composite end point (death, nonfatal myocardial reinfarction, or recurrent angina prompting urgent revascularization) at 6 months after inclusion. The regression model showed a greater benefit of vaccination in patients with no ST-segment elevation, those older than 65 years, nonsmokers, and patients with a high risk of thrombosis.[35] However, the data of Jackson et al.[36] demonstrated no association between influenza vaccination and risk of recurrent coronary events. In addition, Ritter et al.[37] described a case of myocardial infarction after influenza vaccination. Thus, in the context of this article, a connection between influenza vaccination and autoimmune reactions is worthy of attention. The association between influenza vaccination and autoimmune reactions has been reported a number of times.[38] These data even allowed Plotkin et al.[39] to put forward the idea that influenza vaccine can act as the trigger to the development of rhabdomyolysis on a background of combined statin/fibrate therapy. However, in another study, it was shown that influenza vaccine does not produce myopathy in patients taking statins.[40]

POSSIBLE MECHANISMS OF ATHEROGENIC INFLUENZA AUTOIMMUNITY

It may be concluded from the data reviewed here that the following main potential autoimmune mechanisms exist whereby influenza plays a role in the development and progression of atherosclerotic vascular injury: (1) in some cases, the effect may simply be that of enhancing the lipid peroxidation as a result of inflammatory response of the body to viral infection and subsequent production of autoantibodies to modified LDL as well as to other autoantigens (e.g., the heat-shock protein family);

(2) the effect may also result from direct vessel wall colonization that may initiate local cell autoimmune reaction by activation of antigen-presenting cells; (3) in addition, we suggest that the molecular mimicry when a structural similarity between influenza viral antigens and some self-antigens occurs may be the stimulus to atherogenic auto-immune reaction leading to the initiation, progression, or destabilization of athero-sclerotic plaques. Future studies are expected to elucidate further the relationship between influenza infection, autoimmune machinery, and atherogenic vascular injury.

ACKNOWLEDGMENTS

We thank John M. Sands for his careful review of the manuscript.

REFERENCES

1. TILLETT, H.E., J.W. SMITH & C.D. GOOCH. 1983. Excess deaths attributable to influenza in England and Wales: age at death and certified cause. Int. J. Epidemiol. **12:** 344–352.
2. BONDARENKO, S.S. & F.A. TUMANOV. 1993. The effect of influenza and para-influenza on the course of ischemic heart disease. Ter. Arkh. **64:** 81–83.
3. VULLERS, R., B. BULTMANN, H. FISCHER *et al.* 1980. Influenza A virus infection, a precip-itating factor for the major heart attack. Muench. Med. Wochenschr. **122:** 1415–1417.
4. FABRICANT, C.G., J. FABRICANT, M.M. LITRENTA *et al.* 1978. Virus-induced atherosclerosis. J. Exp. Med. **148:** 335–340.
5. JARA, L.J., G. MEDINA, O. VERA-LASTRA *et al.* 2003. Atherosclerosis and antiphospholipid syndrome. Clin. Rev. Allergy Immunol. **25:** 79–88.
6. BROWN, M.S. & J.L. GOLDSTEIN. 1983. Lipoprotein metabolism in the macrophage: implications for cholesterol deposition in atherosclerosis. Annu. Rev. Biochem. **52:** 223–261.
7. KODAMA, T., P. REDDY, C. KISHIMOTO *et al.* 1988. Purification and characterization of a bovine acetyl low density lipoprotein receptor. Proc. Natl. Acad. Sci. USA **85:** 9238–9242.
8. KRIEGER, M. & J. HERZ. 1994. Structures and functions of multiligand lipoprotein receptors: macrophage scavenger receptors and LDL receptor–related protein (LRP). Annu. Rev. Biochem. **63:** 601–637.
9. STEINBERG, D. & J.L. WITZTUM. 1990. Lipoproteins and atherogenesis: current concepts. JAMA **264:** 3047–3052.
10. SALONEN, J.T., S. YLA-HERTTUALA, R. YAMAMOTO *et al.* 1992. Autoantibody against oxidized LDL and progression of carotid atherosclerosis. Lancet **339:** 883–887.
11. NICOLETTI, A., S. KAVERI, G. CALIGIURY *et al.* 1998. Immunoglobulin treatment reduces atherosclerosis in apo E knockout mice. J. Clin. Invest. **102:** 910–918.
12. VAN DER WAL, A.C., P. DAS, D.B. VAN DE BERG *et al.* 1989. Atherosclerotic lesions in humans: *in situ* immunophenotypic analysis suggesting an immune mediated response. Lab. Invest. **61:** 166–170.
13. ZHOU, X., A. NICOLETTI, R. ELHAGE *et al.* 2000. Transfer of CD4$^+$ T cells aggravates atherosclerosis in immunodeficient apoprotein E knockout mice. Circulation **102:** 2919–2922.
14. GEORGE, J. & Y.S. SHOENFELD. 1995. Atherosclerosis as autoimmune disease. Harefuah **129:** 257–259.
15. TSUTSUMI, A., E. MATSUURA, K. ICHIKAWA *et al.* 1996. Antibodies to β_2-glycoprotein I and clinical manifestations in patients with systemic lupus erythematosus. Arthritis Rheum. **39:** 1466–1474.
16. FROSTEGARD, J. 2002. Autoimmunity, oxidized LDL, and cardiovascular disease. Autoimmun. Rev. **4:** 233–237.
17. AZAMBUJA, M.I. & B.B. DUNCAN. 2002. Similarities in mortality patterns from influenza in the first half of the 20th century and the rise and fall of ischemic heart disease in

the United States: a new hypothesis concerning the coronary heart disease epidemic. Cad. Saude Pub. **18:** 557–577.

18. AZAMBUJA, M.I. 2004. Spanish flu and early 20th-century expansion of a coronary heart disease–prone subpopulation. Tex. Heart Inst. J. **31:** 14–21.

19. KEATINGE, W.R. 2002. Winter mortality and its causes. Int. J. Circumpolar. Health **61:** 292–299.

20. HAIDER, A.W., M.G. LARSON, C.J. O'DONNELL et al. 1999. The association of chronic cough with the risk of myocardial infarction: the Framingham Heart Study. Am. J. Med. **106:** 279–284.

21. HUGHES, S. 2003. Novel cardiovascular risk factors. J. Cardiovasc. Nurs. **18:** 131–138.

22. MADJID, M., I. ABOSHADY, I. AWAN et al. 2004. Influenza and cardiovascular disease: is there a causal relationship? Tex. Heart Inst. J. **31:** 4–13

23. HAK, E., T.J. VERHEIJ, G.A. VAN ESSEN et al. 2001. Prognostic factors for influenza-associated hospitalization and death during an epidemic. Epidemiol. Infect. **126:** 261–268.

24. DVORAKOVA, A. & R. POLEDNE. 2004. Influenza—a trigger for acute myocardial infarction. Atherosclerosis **172:** 391–392.

25. GUREVICH, V.S., V.M. PLESKOV, M.V. LEVAYA et al. 2002. Influenza virus infection in progressing atherosclerosis. Kardiologia **42:** 21–24.

26. ENGBLOM, E., T.O. EKFORS, O.H. MEURMAN et al. 1983. Fatal influenza A myocarditis with isolation of virus from the myocardium. Acta Med. Scand. **213:** 75–78.

27. CATON, A., D.M. CERASOLI & F.F. SHIH. 1998. Immune recognition of influenza hemagglutinin as a viral and a neo-self-antigen. Immunol. Res. **17:** 23–32.

28. REED, A.J., M.P. RILEY & A.J. CATON. 2000. Virus-induced maturation and activation of autoreactive memory B cells. J. Exp. Med. **192:** 1763–1774.

29. VAN LENTEN, B.J., A.C. WAGNER, G.M. ANANTHARAMAIAH et al. 2002. Influenza infection promotes macrophage traffic into arteries of mice that is prevented by D-4F, an apolipoprotein A-I mimetic peptide. Circulation **106:** 1127 –1132.

30. BOUWMAN, J.J., F.L. VISSEREN, M.C. BOSCH et al. 2002. Procoagulant and inflammatory response of virus-infected monocytes. Eur. J. Clin. Invest. **32:** 759–766.

31. GUREVICH, V., V. PLESKOV & S. URAZGILDEEVA. 2004. The role of immune response to influenza virus in progression of atherosclerosis [abstract]. Clin. Exp. Rheumatol. **22:** 13.

32. KLIMOV, A.N., V.S. GUREVICH, A.A. NIKIFOROVA et al. 1993. Antioxidative activity of high density lipoproteins in vivo. Atherosclerosis **100:** 13–18.

33. NAVAB, M., J.A. BERLINER, G. SUBBANAGOUNDER et al. 2001. HDL and the inflammatory response induced by LDL-derived oxidized phospholipids. Arter. Thromb. Vascul. Biol. **21:** 481–488.

34. NAGHAVI, M., Z. BARLAS & S. SIADATY. 2000. Association of influenza vaccination and reduced risk of recurrent myocardial infarction. Circulation **102:** 3039–3045.

35. GURFINKEL, E. & R.L. DE LA FUENTE. 2004. Two-year follow-up of the FLU Vaccination Acute Coronary Syndromes (FLUVACS) registry. Tex. Heart Inst. J. **31:** 28–32.

36. JACKSON, L.A., O. YU & S.R. HECKBERT. 2002. Influenza vaccination is not associated with a reduction in the risk of recurrent coronary events. Am. J. Epidemiol. **156:** 634–640.

37. RITTER, O., A. BONZ, J. STROTMANN et al. 2003. Myocardial infarction after influenza vaccination. Z. Kardiol. **92:** 962–965.

38. GEIER, M.R., D.A. GEIER & A.C. ZAHALSKY. 2003. Influenza vaccination and Guillain Barré syndrome small star, filled. Clin. Immunol. **107:** 116–121.

39. PLOTKIN, E., J. BERNHEIM, S. BEN-CHETRIT et al. 2000. Influenza vaccine—a possible trigger of rhabdomyolysis induced acute renal failure due to the combined use of cerivastatin and bezafibrate. Nephrol. Dial. Transplant. **15:** 740–741.

40. CHAZAN, B., R. WEISS & H. TABENKIN. 2002. Influenza vaccine does not produce myopathy in patients taking statins. J. Fam. Pract. **51:** 986–988.

Bovine Spongiform Encephalopathy, Multiple Sclerosis, and Creutzfeldt-Jakob Disease Are Probably Autoimmune Diseases Evoked by *Acinetobacter* Bacteria

ALAN EBRINGER, TAHA RASHID, AND CLYDE WILSON

Division of Health and Life Sciences, King's College, University of London, London, United Kingdom

ABSTRACT: Bovine spongiform encephalopathy (BSE) belongs to a group of conditions named together as transmissible spongiform encephalopathies (TSE). They are fatal neurodegenerative diseases that include "scrapie" in sheep, Creutzfeldt-Jakob disease (CJD) and kuru in humans, and chronic wasting disease in deers. BSE-affected animals suffer from "hindquarters" paralysis, which is also one of the main features of "experimental allergic encephalomyelitis" (EAE). EAE is considered an animal model of multiple sclerosis (MS) and lower limb ataxia is often observed in MS patients. The presence of clinical and histopathological similarities in these diseases suggests a common pathology. Specific brain peptides, which produce EAE, were shown to have "molecular mimicry" with the soil and skin saprophytic microbe, *Acinetobacter*. BSE-affected animals and patients suffering from MS have been found to have elevated levels of antibodies to both *Acinetobacter* and *Pseudomonas* bacteria, as well as autoantibodies to both white and gray matter brain components. The hypothesis is proposed that *Acinetobacter/Pseudomonas* bacteria may have evoked both BSE and MS through the mechanism of "molecular mimicry" and autoimmunity in a similar way to *Streptococcus* microbes producing rheumatic fever and Sydenham's chorea. The possibility that CJD patients may show similar features remains to be determined.

KEYWORDS: bovine spongiform encephalopathy; Creutzfeldt-Jakob disease; multiple sclerosis; autoimmunity; *Acinetobacter*

INTRODUCTION

Bovine spongiform encephalopathy (BSE) is a chronic fatal neurological disease that appeared in British cattle in the 1980s following the introduction of a modified "meat and bonemeal" (MBM) produced from abattoir materials containing brain, spinal cord, pancreas, thymus, and intestines with their contents.[1] The abattoir material was called "green offal" due to its high content of chlorophyll-containing

Address for correspondence: Alan Ebringer, Infection and Immunity Group, Division of Health and Life Sciences, King's College London, 150 Stamford Street, London SE1 9NN, United Kingdom. Voice: +020-7848-4302; fax: +020-7848-4500.
alan.ebringer@kcl.ac.uk

Ann. N.Y. Acad. Sci. 1050: 417–428 (2005). © 2005 New York Academy of Sciences.
doi: 10.1196/annals.1313.093

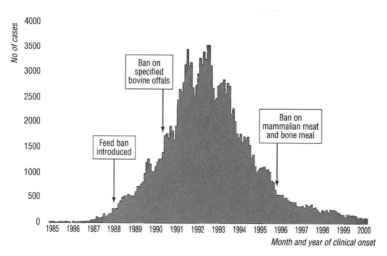

FIGURE 1. Chronology of the bovine spongiform encephalopathy (BSE) epidemic in the United Kingdom. (Adapted with permission from Brown, P. 2001. BMJ **322:** 841–844.)

grass found in the intestinal contents. Following homogenization and heat treatment, the MBM was given to cattle as a food additive in an attempt to increase the protein content of cattle feed.

By 1988, some 60,000 cows had been identified as suffering from BSE and the "Ministry of Agriculture, Fisheries, and Food" (MAFF) scientists suggested that "brains" in the "green offal" could have been contaminated by "prions" from sheep having had "scrapie" and thereby probably caused the disease in British cattle.[2]

A statutory ban on the use of this MBM was introduced in 1988, and the incidence of BSE reached its peak in the year 1992, but from then on the disease progressively decreased, although not to zero levels (Fig. 1). The drop in new cases of BSE was progressive until 2001, when there were more cases in the rest of the "European Union" than in the United Kingdom.

However, in 1996, a new disease was described in humans living in Great Britain that resembled sporadic Creutzfeldt-Jakob disease (s-CJD); however, instead of affecting elderly patients, it seemed to be found predominantly in young people below the age of 40 years.[3] The possibility was raised that it could have been caused by the consumption of BSE-affected beef since it appeared from epidemiological studies that at least 1 million BSE-affected cattle had been slaughtered in abattoirs and entered the human food chain. Furthermore, Americans were banned from donating blood if they had been on holidays in Europe. The BSE problem continues to dominate public concern about food safety throughout the world.

SCRAPIE AS A MODEL OF "TSE"

The origin of BSE is unknown, but it has been suggested that it could have been caused by viruses,[4] the use of organophosphate pesticides,[5] or the consumption of offal from scrapie-affected sheep, which could have been inadvertently included during the preparation of MBM feedstuffs.[6] Such offal material may have contained denatured "scrapie prions", also known as PrP[sc], which could have caused the disease.

Scrapie is a chronic neurological disease of sheep and goats characterized by generalized ataxia, which is endemic in parts of Europe and the United States. The animals appear to be unsteady, tremble especially when excited, and often rub themselves against posts and trees—hence the name of "scrapie".[7] Scrapie was first described in England in 1732, while a similar disease known as "la Tremblante" was known in France way back in the 1690s during the reign of Louis XIV.

The most characteristic findings at postmortem is the presence of intraneuronal vacuoles. The spongy appearance of the neuropil is due to vacuolation of the neuronal processes. Studies in the 1960s had shown that "experimental scrapie" could be produced in goats injected with brain tissues from apparently normal goats.[8] The authors pointed out that similarities existed between the agents of scrapie and those of EAE. Since EAE is considered as an animal model of multiple sclerosis (MS), a disease recognized to be an autoimmune disease, such an observation in this ovine condition raises the question of whether scrapie may also be an autoimmune disease.

In the 1980s, Gajdusek's group from Washington had demonstrated that scrapie animals[9] and patients with kuru and CJD possessed autoantibodies to gray matter neurofilaments.[10] The origin of these brain autoantibodies was unclear since no environmental agent causing scrapie has so far been isolated, despite an intensive search for pathogenic viruses.

EXPERIMENTAL ALLERGIC ENCEPHALOPATHY: AN ANIMAL MODEL OF MULTIPLE SCLEROSIS

Experimental allergic encephalomyelitis (EAE) is considered as an animal model of MS.[11] This experimental model was discovered almost by accident 125 years ago by Pasteur and his colleagues in Paris.[12] Pasteur was trying to immunize patients who had been bitten by rabid dogs and wolves. In an endeavor to produce antirabies immunity in the patients bitten by rabid dogs, he had available the brains of only 2 rabid animals: a rabid dog and a rabid wolf. In an endeavor to increase the quantity of rabies material, he injected the brains of the 2 rabid animals into some 60 rabbits. He then used the rabbit brain homogenates to immunize patients who had been bitten by rabid dogs or wolves. Some patients developed, as expected, antirabies immunity, but a small number of subjects developed a neurological disease, which was characterized by ataxia and in some cases led to a fatal outcome. An extensive literature is present in the scientific journals describing these serious complications and, by the 1940s, the "World Health Organization" (WHO) in Geneva had between 200 and 300 cases of patients who had died from a disease known as "postrabies vaccination allergic encephalomyelitis".

The cause for this unexpected and lethal response was not explained till the 1930s, when it was shown that injection of foreign brain homogenates will evoke an immune response in the immunized animal by the production of antibrain autoantibodies, which will damage the brain tissues of the host.[13]

In the 1950s, it became apparent that this was a general observation in immunology. Immunization with any organ homogenate would produce an autoimmune disease in the target organ. The classical work of Rose and Witebsky from Buffalo demonstrated that peripheral injection of homogenates of thyroid tissue produced an experimental disease in animals that was similar to the human autoimmune disease, Hashimoto's thyroiditis.[14]

It was only after the work of Medawar on allogeneic skin transplants that this phenomenon was recognized as an example of the homograft response by which the recipient recognizes foreign "transplantation antigens" and mounts a powerful rejection immune response against the transplant.[15]

Injection of brain homogenates from animals with BSE or scrapie led to a neurological disease and this was described as transmission of the disease. However, the question arises whether this is not an example of "allergic encephalomyelitis", the disease that Pasteur had observed 100 years ago, after immunization with brain homogenates.

THE LINK BETWEEN SPONGIFORM CHANGES IN "EAE", BOVINE MYELIN, AND *ACINETOBACTER*

In "acute EAE", observed 1 to 3 weeks following immunization with brain homogenates, there is perivascular infiltration with inflammatory cells leading eventually to the formation of fibrotic plaques resembling those observed in MS patients. This is one of the main reasons why EAE is considered to be an animal model of MS.

However, in "chronic EAE", observed 3 to 6 months following immunization, characteristic "spongiform changes" have been described, at least in rabbits[16] and then in guinea pigs,[17] by Raine's group from New York.

One of the main components in the central nervous system responsible for the production of EAE is a basic protein present in the white matter of the brain. In 1970, Eylar's group from San Diego identified a highly active peptide from bovine myelin that, when injected in microgram quantities into guinea pigs, would produce hindlegs paralysis, tremors, weight loss, and eventually death.[18] These features of hindquarters paralysis, tremors, weight loss, and death are also features described in cattle affected by BSE. Furthermore, the biological activity of this peptide was retained when it was heated to 100°C for 1 hour or treated with 8 M urea, and these are properties also described for prions. Clearly, this suggests that bacterial protein antigens will be present in the modified MBM preparations and evoke immune responses following food consumption. The observation that the maximal response is obtained with the IgA isotype in BSE cattle is consistent with a gut-mediated trigger factor.[19]

The hypothesis was proposed that there may be in the environment a microbe having proteins resembling brain tissues, similar to the situation of *Streptococcus* in rheumatic fever and Sydenham's chorea.[20] Computer analysis of proteins in Swiss-Prot database, using the Eylar sequence as a probe, revealed that the microbe *Acinetobacter* that is present in soil or on the skin had such a sequence in the molecule 4-carboxy-mucono-lactone decarboxylase.[6] Subsequently, a similar sequence was found in γ-carboxy-mucono-lactone decarboxylase of *Pseudomonas*.[21] Both groups of microbes *Acinetobacter* and *Pseudomonas* belong to the same family of gram-negative bacteria and share many antigens.

The discovery that a common environmental microbe *Acinetobacter* had a sequence showing molecular mimicry with bovine brain antigens suggested a possible mechanism as to how cattle could have developed BSE. Offal material from abattoirs used in the preparation of the MBM feedstuffs given to cattle could have become inadvertently contaminated by *Acinetobacter*. Although heat treatment was still applied, albeit at a lower temperature, to the preparation of the MBM, the demonstration by Eylar and coworkers that the myelin peptides were highly resistant to heat denaturation meant that these bacterial fragments retained their biological activity in being able to induce EAE. The presence of such biologically active fragments in MBM meant that the cows would not only make antibodies against them, but (because of molecular mimicry or similarity between brain tissues and *Acinetobacter*) any antibodies produced, especially of the IgG isotype, which can cross the "blood-brain barrier", would also attack the brain and cause a neurological disease.

ANTIBODIES TO *ACINETOBACTER* AND AUTOANTIBODIES TO BRAIN ANTIGENS IN "BSE"

The demonstration that *Acinetobacter*, a common environmental microbe, had antigens cross-reacting with mammalian brain tissues raised the question of whether BSE animals had been exposed to it or to fragments of the bacterium. An approach was made to the MAFF in the United Kingdom with the suggestion that an alternative explanation was possible for the onset of BSE in British cows.

Approval was given for a small pilot study. Antibodies to *Acinetobacter calcoaceticus* were found to be significantly elevated in the 29 BSE-affected animals when compared to the 18 BSE-negative animals ($p < 0.001$), 30 organically raised cows aged less than 30 months ($p < 0.001$), and 28 organically raised cows aged more than 30 months ($p < 0.001$), but no such elevations were found against 2 control bacteria—*E. coli* and *Agrobacterium*. Organically raised cows had never been fed with the modified MBM material. High levels of autoantibodies were also found against bovine neurofilaments, which are components of the gray matter, and against bovine myelin, which are components of the white matter of the brain.[22] The highest relative increased levels of antibodies were found in the IgA isotype and this suggested that they had been produced by the gut immune system, following exposure of *Acinetobacter* antigens present in the MBM feeds to the gut mucosa and not as a result of brain damage by prions.

In a second study,[19] antibody responses were measured against 7 different bacteria—*Klebsiella, Proteus, Serratia, Escherichia, Bacillus, Pseudomonas,* and *Acinetobacter*—in 128 BSE-positive animals, 63 BSE-negative animals, and 64 healthy controls. Significantly elevated levels of antibodies to *Acinetobacter* were found in the BSE-affected animals when compared to BSE-negative animals ($p < 0.001$) and healthy controls ($p < 0.001$). Antibodies to *Pseudomonas* were also elevated, although these titers were not as high as those found against *Acinetobacter* bacteria. *Pseudomonas* species belong to the same family as *Acinetobacter* bacteria and this could explain this response. The important specificity observation is that BSE-affected animals did not have antibody elevations against 6 bacteria: 5 from this study—*Klebsiella, Proteus, Serratia, E. coli,* and *Bacillus*; and 1 *Agrobacterium* from a previous study.[22] Furthermore, an amino acid homology (RPVDQ) has been identified between the *Acinetobacter* enzyme, vinyl transferase (positions 121–125), and the bovine prion molecule (positions 175–179). Elevated levels of antibodies to these peptides were found in 189 BSE-positive cows when compared to 127 BSE-negative cattle ($p < 0.001$) or 87 healthy control animals ($p < 0.001$).[23] These studies show that specific antibodies to *Acinetobacter* and maybe *Pseudomonas* bacteria as well as autoantibodies to brain antigens are present in BSE-affected animals. It is clear that BSE-affected cattle have been exposed to *Acinetobacter* antigens, probably present in the MBM supplements fed to the cows. The use of MBM supplements was legally banned in 1988 and no residual MBM material has been available for further analysis.

The demonstration of specific antibodies to a microbe bearing antigens cross-reacting with brain tissues, as well as the presence of autoantibodies to brain components, in a disease showing clinical features resembling those found in EAE and MS, would tend to suggest that BSE could at least be considered as an autoimmune disease that has been evoked by *Acinetobacter* bacteria (FIG. 2).

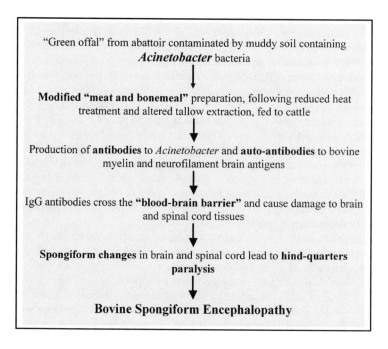

FIGURE 2. Schematic sequential steps in the pathogenesis of bovine spongiform encephalopathy (BSE).

IMPLICATIONS OF *ACINETOBACTER* ANTIBODIES
IN "BSE" TO HUMAN DISEASES

The discovery that brain antigens have sequences, which resemble molecules found in *Acinetobacter* and *Pseudomonas* bacteria, has opened a new way of looking at neurological diseases in humans and animals. Many clinical studies attest to the observation that lower limb ataxia is one of the features of MS in humans, and hind-quarters paralysis occurs in both EAE- and BSE-affected animals.

In a pilot study carried out on sera obtained from 53 MS patients, 2 patients with s-CJD, 10 patients with viral encephalitis, 20 patients with cerebrovascular accidents (CVA), and 25 healthy blood donors, elevated levels of antibodies to *Acinetobacter* were found in the MS and s-CJD patients, but not in those with viral encephalitis or strokes, when compared to blood donors.[24]

A more detailed study measured antibody responses to 5 different strains of *Acinetobacter*, *Pseudomonas*, *E. coli*, myelin basic protein, and neurofilaments in 26 MS patients, 20 patients with CVA, 10 patients with viral encephalitis, and 25 healthy controls. In MS patients, elevated levels of antibodies against all 5 strains of *Acinetobacter*, as well as antibodies to *Pseudomonas*, were observed (but no elevations against *E. coli*) when compared to blood donors. Furthermore, specific elevations of autoantibodies to white matter myelin basic protein and gray matter neurofilaments were found in the MS patients, but not in those with strokes or encephalitis.[25] In a more recent study, antibody levels against mimicking peptide sequences from *Acinetobacter* ($p < 0.001$), *Pseudomonas* ($p < 0.001$), myelin basic protein (MBP) ($p < 0.001$), and myelin oligodendrocyte glycoprotein (MOG) ($p < 0.001$) were found to be elevated in sera of patients with MS when compared to those patients with CVA or to healthy controls. Antisera raised in mice against *Acinetobacter* mimicking peptides were found to be significantly inhibited by peptides from the MBP or *Pseudomonas* microbe. Moreover, MOG peptides were found to inhibit antibodies against the mimicking sequences present in *Acinetobacter*, but no inhibition was observed when human papilloma virus peptides were used as controls.[26]

It would thus appear that, in patients with MS and in cattle affected by BSE, elevated levels of antibodies to *Acinetobacter* and autoantibodies to brain components can be demonstrated. These results taken together with the clinical similarities have led to the working hypothesis that BSE and MS are related diseases, associated with exposure to bacteria possessing antigens cross-reacting with brain tissues (FIG. 2).

In humans, *Acinetobacter* species usually produce respiratory tract infections, especially in patients lying in intensive care units. Over 50% of MS patients in England suffer from sinusitis[27] and similar results have been published from Scotland.[28] Furthermore, investigations of American patients with sinusitis by antral tap and endoscopically directed nasal cultures show predominantly *Acinetobacter* and *Pseudomonas* bacteria.[29] If these results can be confirmed, then this opens up entirely new therapeutic possibilities. The use of anti-*Acinetobacter* therapy such as antibiotics, drainage of sinuses, immunosuppressive drugs, and other measures could be evaluated in the earliest stages of MS, before irreversible neurological changes had occurred in such patients. Rheumatic fever and Sydenham's chorea have disappeared in the Western world by the early use of antibiotics, and it is possible that a similar approach might work in patients affected by MS or CJD.

A POSSIBLE LINK BETWEEN "MS" AND "SPORADIC-CJD"

Both MS and s-CJD have been reported to show some similarities in the pheno-typic features, such as the occurrence of signs of cognitive and intellectual deficits, signs of brain-stem and cerebellar involvements, and features of Parkinson's disease as well as dementia and ataxia.[30] Furthermore, the disease in some patients with severe MS was found to have a downhill course with resultant death in early stages of the disease,[31] similar to the rapidly progressive and fatal outcome in CJD.

The involvement of the myelin sheath, which is a characteristic feature in MS, has also been observed in the nervous tissues of panencephalopathic CJD.[32] Involvement of the white matter has been reported to occur in cases with CJD,[33] while the gray matter is involved in patients with MS.[34] Inflammatory cells and molecules appear to accumulate at the pathological sites of patients with MS[35] as well as in patients with CJD.[36,37] Although the appearance of oligoclonal bands is characteristic for MS,[38] the observation of other markers such as 14-3-3 protein molecules in the CSF of patients with CJD[39] and MS[40] appears to be a shared feature.

Furthermore, patients with MS[26] and s-CJD[24] were found to have significantly elevated levels of antibodies to *Acinetobacter* bacteria as well as autoantibodies to brain antigens such as MBP and neurofilaments when compared to corresponding healthy controls.

THE PROBLEM WITH VARIANT-"CJD"

A new disease, variant-CJD, has been described and over 100 patients have so far died from this condition.[3] It has been suggested that consumption of meat from BSE-affected animals may have caused the disease. However, nutritional studies carried out by the "National CJD Surveillance Unit" in Edinburgh and published in their yearly reports have failed to show higher meat consumptions in v-CJD patients compared to controls.[41] Furthermore, some v-CJD patients had been vegetarians for a number of years.

In a review of the v-CJD problem, G. Venters, an epidemiologist who had investigated the *E. coli 0157* epidemic in Lanarkshire, has cast some doubt on the link between BSE and v-CJD.[42] The scientific issue relating to the v-CJD problem is the following question: To what neurological group did the 100 v-CJD patients who died from the disease belong? Is v-CJD a separate, autonomous disease, "sui generis" so to speak, or does it belong to a larger group? Since some patients with s-CJD[24] and MS[26] have elevated levels of antibodies to *Acinetobacter*, a working hypothesis is proposed that v-CJD patients may also have antibodies to *Acinetobacter* bacteria. If they do have such antibodies, then the conclusion follows that v-CJD as well as s-CJD and MS are somehow associated with exposure to *Acinetobacter* bacteria.

Approximately 700 persons per year die in England and Wales from MS, which is about 2 persons per day (Department of Health Statistics, U.K.—1995: 685; 1996: 712; 1997: 703; 1998: 801; 1999: 758; 2000: 696). Some 7% of MS patients die before the age of 40 years, which is approximately 1 person per week. Since the majority of v-CJD patients were below the age of 40 years, could they have belonged to the group of MS patients who died before the age of 40 years? Professor Scholz from Munich has pointed out that the distribution of v-CJD in the United Kingdom

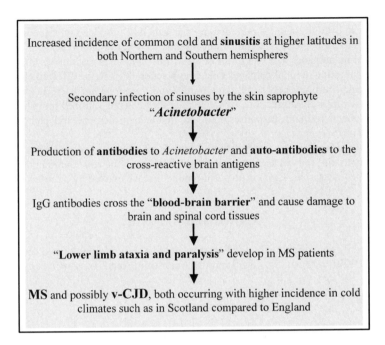

FIGURE 3. Schematic pathogenetic sequences in the development of multiple sclerosis (MS) and possibly Creutzfeldt-Jakob disease (CJD) triggered by *Acinetobacter* infection in cold climates.

shows the highest incidence in Scotland,[43] which does not tally with the distribution of BSE-affected cattle that occurred predominantly in the south of England.[44] However, the distribution of v-CJD does fit quite well the distribution of MS in the United Kingdom. It is well known that there is more MS in Scotland than in England and there is more MS in Minnesota than in Texas. The north-south distribution appears to hold for the Northern hemisphere and the reverse is found in the Southern hemisphere. MS is seven times more common in Tasmania and Southern New Zealand[45] than in tropical Queensland, in populations coming predominantly from Anglo-Celtic stock. Whether this latitudinal effect could be linked to greater prevalence of upper respiratory infections and chronic sinusitis during winter months by *Acinetobacter/Pseudomonas* bacteria awaits further studies (FIG. 3). If such a link can be demonstrated in other populations, then this opens up a novel way of treating MS and CJD patients in the early stages of their disease.

CONCLUSIONS AND FUTURE PERSPECTIVES

Various studies suggest the possibility of a similar triggering factor and pathogenetic mechanism in BSE, CJD, and MS via *Acinetobacter* infection, molecular mimicry, and autoimmunity.

The proposed pathogenetic mechanism is that susceptible patients when exposed to repetitive or high load of *Acinetobacter* bacteria will produce increased levels of antibodies to the bacterial antigenic molecules as well as autoantibodies to the cross-reacting brain antigens. The end result of these immunological reactions is inflammation, degeneration, axonal damages, and even vacuolations in the affected areas.

Molecular mimicry between *Acinetobacter* and *Pseudomonas* bacteria and brain antigens suggests that infections by these microbes causing chronic sinusitis could have produced immune responses that led to the neurological and pathological features of MS.

The demonstration of a link between *Acinetobacter* bacteria and BSE has opened a new way to the study of MS. A similar approach should be considered in the study of sporadic and variant-CJD, as an autoimmune disease evoked by an infection.

ACKNOWLEDGMENTS

This work was supported by the Department of the Environment, Food, and Rural Affairs (DEFRA) (No. CSA 4302) and the American Friends of King's College.

REFERENCES

1. WELLS, G.A., T. SCOTT, T. JOHNSON et al. 1987. A novel progressive spongiform encephalopathy in cattle. Vet. Rec. **121:** 419–420.
2. PRUSINER, S.B. 1982. Novel proteinaceous infectious particles cause scrapie. Science **216:** 136–143.
3. WILL, R.G., J.W. IRONSIDE, M. ZEIDLER et al. 1996. A new variant of Creutzfeldt-Jakob disease in the UK. Lancet **347:** 921–925.
4. DICKINSON, A.G. & V.M. MEIKLE. 1971. Host genotype and agent effects in scrapie incubation: change in allelic interaction with different strains of agent. Mol. Gen. Genet. **112:** 73–79.
5. PURDEY, M. 1994. Are organo-phosphates involved in the causation of bovine spongiform encephalopathy (BSE)? Hypothesis based upon literature review and limited trials on BSE cattle. J. Nutr. Med. **4:** 43–82.
6. EBRINGER, A., J. PIRT, C. WILSON et al. 1997. Bovine spongiform encephalopathy: is it an autoimmune disease due to bacteria showing molecular mimicry with brain antigens? Environ. Health Perspect. **105:** 1172–1174.
7. PATTISON, I.H. 1988. Fifty years with scrapie: a personal reminiscence. Vet. Rec. **123:** 661–666.
8. PATTISON, I.H. & G.C. MILLSON. 1962. Distribution of the scrapie agent in the tissues of experimentally inoculated goats. J. Comp. Pathol. **72:** 233–244.
9. AOKI, T., C.J. GIBBS, J. SOTELO et al. 1982. Heterogeneic autoantibody against neurofilament protein in the sera of animals with experimental kuru, Creutzfeldt-Jakob disease, and natural scrapie infection. Infect. Immun. **38:** 316–324.
10. SOTELLO, J., C.J. GIBBS & D.C. GAJDUSEK. 1980. Autoantibodies against axonal neurofilaments in patients with kuru and Creutzfeldt-Jakob disease. Science **210:** 190–193.
11. REINDL, M., C. LININGTON, U. BREHM et al. 1999. Antibodies against the myelin oligodendrocyte glycoprotein and the myelin basic protein in multiple sclerosis and other neurological diseases: a comparative study. Brain **122:** 2047–2056.
12. PEARCE, J.M. 2002. Louis Pasteur and rabies: a brief note. J. Neurol. Neurosurg. Psychiatry **73:** 82.
13. WESTONHURST, E. 1932. The effects of the injection of normal brain emulsion into rabbit with specific reference to the aetiology of the paralytic accidents of the antirabic treatment. J. Hyg. **32:** 33–44.

14. ROSE, N.R. & E. WITEBSKY. 1956. Studies on organ specificity. V. Changes in the thyroid glands of rabbits following active immunization with rabbit thyroid extracts. J. Immunol. **76:** 417–427.
15. MEDAWAR, P.B. 1958. The homograft reaction. Proc. R. Soc. (Lond.) **149:** 145–166.
16. PRINEAS, J., C.S. RAINE & H. WISNIEWSKI. 1969. An ultrastructural study of experimental demyelination and remyelination. 3. Chronic experimental allergic encephalomyelitis in the nervous system. Lab. Invest. **21:** 472–483.
17. RAINE, C.S., D.H. SNYDER, M.P. VALSAMIS *et al.* 1974. Chronic experimental allergic encephalomyelitis in inbred guinea pigs: an ultrastructural study. Lab. Invest. **31:** 369–380.
18. EYLAR, E.H., J. CACCAM, J.J. JACKSON *et al.* 1970. Experimental allergic encephalomyelitis: synthesis of disease-inducing site of the basic protein. Science **168:** 1220–1223.
19. WILSON, C., L.E. HUGHES, T. RASHID *et al.* 2003. Antibodies to *Acinetobacter* bacteria and bovine brain peptides, measured in bovine spongiform encephalopathy (BSE) in an attempt to develop an ante-mortem test. J. Clin. Lab. Immunol. **52:** 23–40.
20. EBRINGER, A., J. PIRT, C. WILSON *et al.* 1998. Bovine spongiform encephalopathy: comparison between the "prion" hypothesis and the autoimmune theory. J. Nutr. Environ. Med. **8:** 265–276.
21. EBRINGER, A., L. HUGHES, T. RASHID *et al.* 2005. *Acinetobacter* immune responses in multiple sclerosis—etiopathogenetic role and its possible use as a diagnostic marker. Arch. Neurol. **62:** 33–36.
22. TIWANA, H., C. WILSON, J. PIRT *et al.* 1999. Autoantibodies to brain components and antibodies to *Acinetobacter calcoaceticus* are present in bovine spongiform encephalopathy. Infect. Immun. **67:** 6591–6595.
23. WILSON, C., L. HUGHES, T. RASHID *et al.* 2004. Antibodies to prion and *Acinetobacter* peptide sequences in bovine spongiform encephalopathy. Vet. Immunol. Immunopathol. **98:** 1–7.
24. EBRINGER, A., T. RASHID, C. WILSON *et al.* 2004. Multiple sclerosis, sporadic Creutzfeldt-Jakob disease, and bovine spongiform encephalopathy: are they autoimmune diseases evoked by *Acinetobacter* microbes showing molecular mimicry to brain antigens. J. Nutr. Environ. Med. **14**(4): 293–302.
25. HUGHES, L.E., S. BONELL, R.S. NATT *et al.* 2001. Antibody responses to *Acinetobacter* spp. and *Pseudomonas aeruginosa* in multiple sclerosis: prospects for diagnosis using the myelin-*Acinetobacter*-neurofilament antibody index. Clin. Diag. Lab. Immunol. **8:** 1181–1188.
26. HUGHES, L.E., P.A. SMITH, S. BONELL *et al.* 2003. Cross-reactivity between related sequences found in *Acinetobacter* sp., *Pseudomonas aeruginosa*, myelin basic protein, and myelin oligodendrocyte glycoprotein in multiple sclerosis. J. Neuroimmunol. **144:** 105–115.
27. GAY, D., G. DICK & G. UPTON. 1986. Multiple sclerosis associated with sinusitis: case-controlled study in general practice. Lancet **i:** 815–819.
28. CALLAGHAN, T.S. 1986. Multiple sclerosis and sinusitis. Lancet **ii:** 160–161.
29. CASIANO, R.R., S. COHN, E. VILLASUSO *et al.* 2001. Comparison of antral tap with endoscopically directed nasal culture. Laryngoscope **111:** 1333–1337.
30. EBRINGER, A., T. RASHID, C. WILSON *et al.* 2005. A possible link between multiple sclerosis and Creutzfeldt-Jakob disease based on clinical, genetic, pathological, and immunological evidence involving *Acinetobacter* bacteria. Med. Hypotheses **64:** 487–494.
31. BARNETT, M.H. & J.W. PRINEAS. 2004. Relapsing and remitting multiple sclerosis: pathology of the newly forming lesion. Ann. Neurol. **55:** 458–468.
32. LIBERSKI, P.P. & D.C. GAJDUSEK. 1997. Myelinated axon undergoes complete demyelination in the panencephalopathic, but it is merely subjected to the Wallerian degeneration in the polioencephalopathic type of transmissible spongiform encephalopathies. Pol. J. Pathol. **48:** 163–171.
33. MACCHI, G., A.L. ABBAMONDI, G. DI TRAPANI *et al.* 1984. On the white matter lesions of the Creutzfeldt-Jakob disease: can a new subentity be recognized in man? J. Neurol. Sci. **63:** 197–206.

34. DAVIES, G.R., L. RAMIO-TORRENTA, A. HADJIPROCOPIS *et al.* 2004. Evidence for grey matter MTR abnormality in minimally disabled patients with early relapsing-remitting multiple sclerosis. J. Neurol. Neurosurg. Psychiatry **75**: 998–1002.
35. PRINEAS, J.W., W.I. MCDONALD & R.J.M. FRANKLIN. 2002. Demyelinating diseases. *In* Greenfield's Neuropathology, pp. 471–541. Arnold. London.
36. VAN EVERBROECK, B., E. DEWULF, P. PALS *et al.* 2002. The role of cytokines, astrocytes, microglia, and apoptosis in Creutzfeldt-Jakob disease. Neurobiol. Aging **23**: 59–64.
37. LEWICKI, H., A. TISHON, D. HOMANN *et al.* 2003. T cells infiltrate the brain in murine and human transmissible spongiform encephalopathies. J. Virol. **77**: 3799–3808.
38. CORREALE, J. & M.M.B. MOLINAS. 2002. Oligoclonal bands and antibody responses in multiple sclerosis. J. Neurol. **249**: 375–389.
39. GREEN, A.J. 2002. Cerebrospinal fluid brain-derived proteins in the diagnosis of Alzheimer's disease and Creutzfeldt-Jakob disease. Neuropathol. Appl. Neurobiol. **28**: 427–440.
40. BARTOSIK-PSUJEK, H. & J.J. ARCHELOS. 2004. Tau protein and 14-3-3 are elevated in the cerebrospinal fluid of patients with multiple sclerosis and correlate with intrathecal synthesis of IgG. J. Neurol. **251**: 414–420.
41. UK CREUTZFELDT-JAKOB DISEASE SURVEILLANCE UNIT. 1999. Eighth Annual Report [www.cjd.ed.ac.uk].
42. VENTERS, G.A. 2001. New variant Creutzfeldt-Jakob disease: the epidemic that never was. Br. Med. J. **323**: 858–861.
43. EBRINGER, A., T. RASHID & C. WILSON. 2004. Bovine spongiform encephalopathy as an autoimmune disease evoked by *Acinetobacter*: implications for multiple sclerosis and Creutzfeldt-Jakob disease. *In* Infection and Autoimmunity, pp. 383–394. Elsevier. Amsterdam/New York.
44. ANDERSON, R.M., C.A. DONNELLY, N.M. FERGUSON *et al.* 1996. Transmission dynamics and epidemiology of BSE in British cattle. Nature **382**: 779–788.
45. MILLER, D.H., S.R. HAMMOND, J.G. MCLEOD *et al.* 1990. Multiple sclerosis in Australia and New Zealand: are the determinants genetic or environmental? J. Neurol. Neurosurg. Psychiatry **53**: 903–905.

Index of Contributors